URGENT CARE MEDICINE

URGENT CARE MEDICINE

ROBERT P. OLYMPIA, MD
Professor
Department of Emergency Medicine and Pediatrics
Penn State College of Medicine/Penn State Hershey
Medical Center
Hershey, Pennsylvania

RORY O'NEILL, DO, MBA
Medical Director of Quality
Department of Urgent and Express Care
UPMC of Central PA
Harrisburg, Pennsylvania

MATTHEW L. SILVIS, MD
Professor
Departments of Family and Community Medicine &
Orthopedics and Rehabilitation
Penn State Health
Hershey, Pennsylvania

ELSEVIER

Elsevier
1600 John F. Kennedy Blvd.
Ste 1800
Philadelphia, PA 19103-2899

URGENT CARE MEDICINE SECRETS, SECOND EDITION   ISBN: 978-0-443-10752-8

Notice

Practitioners and researchers must always rely on their own experience and knowledge in evaluating and using any information, methods, compounds, or experiments described herein. Because of rapid advances in the medical sciences, in particular, independent verification of diagnoses and drug dosages should be made. To the fullest extent of the law, no responsibility is assumed by Elsevier, authors, editors, or contributors for any injury and/or damage to persons or property as a matter of product liability, negligence or otherwise, or from any use or operation of any methods, products, instructions, or ideas contained in the material herein.

Previous edition copyrighted 2018.

Senior Content Strategist: Marybeth Thiel
Senior Content Development Specialist: Jinia Dasgupta
Senior Project Manager: Beula Christopher
Design Direction: Renee Duenow

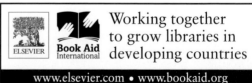

Printed in India

Last digit is the print number: 9 8 7 6 5 4 3 2 1

To my wife, Jodi, my Little Love and "Mo Chuisle" (my blood, my pulse), for supporting me with unconditional love and for allowing me to pursue my professional and personal dreams. Any success in my life is because of you, and your belief in me has allowed me to overcome any obstacle in life. "Love is putting someone else's needs before yours." —Olaf, Frozen; "Because when I look at you, I can feel it. And I look at you and I'm home." —Dory, Finding Nemo

To my children, Abigail and Madelyn. I am so lucky and blessed to be your daddy. You inspire me every day to be the best person I can be. My world is complete because you are part of my life. I am so proud of the young women you have become, but never forget, you will always be my babies. "You are my greatest adventure." —Mr. Incredible, The Incredibles; "Don't just fly, soar." —Dumbo

To my parents (Manuel and Delia), my grandparents (Manuel, Avelina, Teofilo, Gliceria), Coco, my sisters (Patricia, Catherine, Nicole, Lauren), my brothers (Rob, Mark, Matthew, Andy), Grant, Isabel, Gracie, Sienna, Drew, Moriah, Quinn, and Theo, Bob and Nancy Brady, and extended family from all over the world. Thank you for your unwavering love and support, and for being amazing role models. I hope I have made you all proud. "Ohana means family. Family means nobody gets left behind." —Lilo, Lilo & Stitch

To my mentors, Drs. Magdy Attia, Steven Selbst, Waseem Hafeez, and Jeff Avner. Thank you for believing in me. "All it takes is faith and trust." —Peter Pan

To every student, resident, and fellow that I have trained and mentored through the years. You challenge me every day to be the best teacher, researcher, and physician I can be. "Venture outside your comfort zone. The rewards are worth it." —Rapunzel, Tangled

To all of the emergency department staff that I have worked with over my 25-year career at the DuPont Hospital for Children, Christiana Care Hospital, Children's Hospital at Montefiore, Newark Beth Israel Medical Center, and Penn State Hershey Medical Center. I am the physician I am today because of the compassion, dedication, hard work, and selflessness that I have learned from each and every one of you. We make an amazing team. "The flower that blooms in adversity is the most rare and beautiful of all." —The Emperor, Mulan

"All our dreams can come true, if we have the courage to pursue them." "It's kind of fun to do the impossible." —Walt Disney.

—Robert P. Olympia

To Carina, Padraig, and Finn, who make my life truly special. To my parents, Craig and Christine, who raised a man of dedication and drive. And to those who are finding their way through the maze of medicine, I hope this reference guides your journey.

—Rory O'Neill

To my parents, who instilled in me a passion for lifelong learning, and to my wife (Christine) and children (Nicholas, Benjamin, and Emory), who fill my life with love.

—Matthew L. Silvis

CONTRIBUTORS

Spencer Adoff, MD, FACEP
Director of Operations
Department of Emergency
Georgia Emergency Associates;
Assistant Medical Director
St. Joseph's/Candler Health System;
Assistant Clinical Professor
Medical College of Georgia;
Medical Director
ExperCARE Urgent Care
Savannah, Georgia

Tabassum F. Ali, MD
Ophthalmologist
Department of Ophthalmology
Delaware Ophthalmology Consultants
Wilmington, Delaware

J. Elizabeth Allen, DO, FACEP
Assistant Professor of Emergency Medicine
Department of Emergency Medicine
Penn State Hershey Medical Center
Mechanicsburg, Pennsylvania

Siraj Amanullah, MD, MPH
Associate Professor
Department of Emergency Medicine, Pediatrics, and
    Health Services, Policy and Practice
Alpert Medical School of Brown University, Brown School
    of Public Health, Hasbro Children's Hospital/Rhode
    Island Hospital
Providence, Rhode Island

Jennifer F. Anders, MD
Assistant Professor
Division of Pediatric Emergency Medicine
Johns Hopkins Children's Center
Baltimore, Maryland

Roselyn A. Appenteng, MD
Clinical Fellow
Division of Pediatric Emergency Medicine
Johns Hopkins University
Baltimore, Maryland

Nadine Aprahamian, MD, FAAP
Assistant Professor
Harvard Medical School;
Urgent Care/Hospitalist
Department of Emergency Medicine
Boston Children's Hospital
Boston, Massachusetts;
Director of Pediatrics – Inpatient
Department of Pediatrics,
Site Director of BU Medical Students
Winchester Hospital
Winchester, Massachusetts

Joseph Ash, MD
Resident Physician
Department of Emergency Medicine
Penn State Hershey Medical Center
Hershey, Pennsylvania

Jeffrey R. Avner, MD, FAAP
Chair
Department of Pediatrics
Maimonides Children's Hospital
Brooklyn, New York

Michael C. Bachman, MD, MBA
Chief Operating Officer
PM Pediatric Care
Lake Success, New York

Richard G. Bachur, MD
Chief
Division of Emergency Medicine
Boston Children's Hospital;
Professor
Harvard Medical School
Boston, Massachusetts

Ellen Maria Benitah Bulbarelli, MD
Medical Doctor Researcher
Department of Family Medicine/Sports
    Medicine
Mayo Clinic;
Medical Doctor Resident
Department of Family Medicine
Einstein Medical Center Philadelphia
Philadelphia, Pennsylvania

Justine Bensur, DO, MSMedEd
Fellow, Family Medicine Surgical Obstetrics
Department of Family Medicine
Ellis Medicine
Schenectady, New York

Harsh Bhakta, DO
Emergency Medicine Specialist
Department of Emergency
Baylor Scott and White
McKinney, Texas

Toral Bhakta, DO
Chair
Department of Emergency Medicine
Baylor Scott and White All Saints Medical Center
Fort Worth, Texas;
Assistant Professor
Department of Emergency Medicine
TCU Burnett School of Medicine
Dallas, Texas

Jodi Brady-Olympia, MD
Assistant Professor of Pediatrics
Department of Pediatrics
Penn State College of Medicine
Hershey, Pennsylvania

Kathryn S. Brigham, MD
Instructor
Department of Pediatrics
Harvard Medical School;
Assistant Pediatrician
Department of Pediatrics, Division of Adolescent and
    Young Adult Medicine
Massachusetts General Hospital
Boston, Massachusetts

Travis K. Bryan, DO
Primary Care Sports Medicine Fellow
University of North Carolina
Chapel Hill, North Carolina

Jeffrey I. Campbell, MD, MPH
Attending Physician
Pediatric Infectious Diseases
Boston Medical Center
Boston, Massachusetts

Morgan Chambers, MD, MEd
PGY-3, Chief Resident
Family and Community Medicine
Penn State Hershey Medical Center
Hershey, Pennsylvania

Cindy D. Chang, MD
Clinical Fellow
Department of Emergency Medicine
Cincinnati Children's Hospital Medical Center;
Clinical Instructor
Department of Emergency Medicine
University of Cincinnati
Cincinnati, Ohio

Bradley Chappell, DO, MHA, FACOEP, FACEP
Vice Chair of Clinical Operations
Department of Emergency Medicine
Harbor-UCLA Medical Center
Torrance, California;
Associate Professor of Emergency Medicine
David Geffen School of Medicine
UCLA
Westwood, California

Joel M. Clingenpeel, MD, MPH, MS.MEdL
Fellowship Director
Department of Pediatric Emergency Medicine;
Associate Professor
Department of Pediatrics
Eastern Virginia Medical School
Norfolk, Virginia

Jeff Cloyd, MD
Assistant Professor
Department of Emergency Medicine
University of Tennessee Medical Center
Knoxville, Tennessee

Douglas Comeau, DO, CAQSM, FAAFP, FAMSSM
Director
University Health Services and Primary Care Sports
    Medicine
Boston College
Chestnut Hill, Massachusetts;
Clinical Associate Professor
Department of Family Medicine
Boston University Chobanian and Avedisian School of
    Medicine
Boston, Massachusetts

Deanna L. Corey, MD, CAQSM
Physician
Department of Health Services
Tufts University
Medford, Massachusetts;
Physician
Department of Urgent Care
Emerson Hospital
Littleton, Massachusetts

Monica Corsetti, MD
Emergency Medicine Physician
Department of Emergency Medicine
Penn State Health
Camp Hill, Pennsylvania

Teresa Coyle, DO
Sports Medicine Fellow
Department of Sports Medicine
UPMC
Harrisburg, Pennsylvania

Mina M. Cunningham, MD
Assistant Professor of Family Medicine
Department of Family Medicine
St. Louis University
O'Fallon, Illinois

Marvin Dang, DO
Primary Care Sports Medicine Physician, Clinical
    Assistant Professor
Department of Orthopedics
NYU Langone Health
New York, New York

Joshua Davis, MD
Emergency Medicine Physician
Department of Emergency Medicine
Vituity;
Clinical Instructor
University of Kansas School of Medicine
Wichita, Kansas

Jessica Deitrick, DO
Physician
Department of Emergency
Penn State Hershey Medical Center
Hershey, Pennsylvania

Nicolas Delacruz, MD
Fellow
Department of Emergency Medicine
NYU Langone Health/Bellevue Hospital
New York, New York

Kaynan Doctor, MD, MBBS, BSc
Attending Physician
Pediatric Emergency Medicine
Division of Emergency Medicine
Nemours Children's Hospital, Delaware
Wilmington, Delaware;
Assistant Professor
Department of Pediatrics
The Sidney Kimmel Medical College at Thomas Jefferson
    University
Philadelphia, Pennsylvania

Jennifer Dunnick, MD, MPH
Assistant Professor of Pediatrics
Division of Pediatric Emergency Medicine
UPMC Children's Hospital of Pittsburgh
Pittsburgh, Pennsylvania

Michele J. Fagan, MD
Attending Physician
Department of Pediatric Emergency
Maimonides Medical Center
Brooklyn, New York

Daniel M. Fein, MD
Associate Professor
Department of Pediatrics
Albert Einstein College of Medicine;
Interim Division Chief
Division of Pediatric Emergency Medicine
Children's Hospital at Montefiore
Bronx, New York

Jennifer N. Fishe, MD
Associate Professor
Department of Emergency Medicine
University of Florida College of Medicine – Jacksonville
Jacksonville, Florida

Sylvia E. Garcia, MD
Assistant Professor
Department of Pediatric Emergency Medicine
Icahn School of Medicine at Mount Sinai
New York, New York

Michelle Georgia, DO
Fellow
Department of Pediatric Emergency Medicine
Children's Hospital of the King's Daughters
Norfolk, Virginia

Scott Goldstein, DO, FACEP, FAEMS, EMT-PHP
Director
Division of EMS/Disaster Medicine
Department of Emergency Medicine
Jefferson Einstein Hospital;
Clinical Associate Professor
Department of Emergency Medicine
Sidney Kimmel College of Medicine
Philadelphia, Pennsylvania

Brian A. Gottwalt, DO
Resident
Department of Family Medicine
Wake Forest University
Winston-Salem, North Carolina

Laurie Seidel Halmo, MD, FAAP
Assistant Professor
Department of Pediatrics
University of Colorado School of Medicine
Aurora, Colorado

Selena Hariharan, MD, MHSA
Professor of Pediatrics
Department of Pediatrics
University of Cincinnati College of Medicine;
Professor of Pediatrics
Department of Emergency Medicine
Cincinnati Children's Hospital Medical Center
Cincinnati, Ohio

Shenel A. Heisler, DO
Pediatrics Resident
Department of Pediatrics
Children's Hospital at Montefiore
Bronx, New York

Kristin Herbert, DO, MPH
Attending Physician
Department of Pediatric Emergency Medicine
Children's Hospital of the King's Daughters;
Assistant Professor
Department of Pediatrics, Division of Emergency
    Medicine
Eastern Virginia Medical School
Norfolk, Virginia

Bruce E. Herman, MD
Professor and Vice-Chair of Education
Department of Pediatrics
University of Utah School of Medicine
Salt Lake City, Utah

Sixtine Valdelièvre Herold, MD, MS
Physician
Department of Emergency Medicine
Boston Children's Hospital
Boston, Massachusetts;
Associate Director of Pediatric Emergency
    Medicine
Department of Emergency Medicine
South Shore Hospital
South Weymouth, Massachusetts

Toni Clare Hogencamp, MD
Senior Physician
PM Pediatric Urgent Care
PM Pediatric Care
Dedham, Massachusetts

Bret C. Jacobs, DO, MA
Family Medicine and Primary Care Sports Medicine
    Physician
Department of Family Medicine
One Medical;
Clinical Assistant Professor
Family Medicine and Community Health
Icahn School of Medicine at Mount Sinai
New York, New York

Leah Kaye, MD, FAAP
Assistant Professor
Department of Pediatrics, Division of Academic General
 Pediatrics
Penn State Health Children's Hospital, Penn State College
 of Medicine
Hershey, Pennsylvania

Jessica J. Kirby, DO, FACEP
Chair
Department of Emergency Medicine
John Peter Smith Health Network;
Associate Clinical Professor
Department of Emergency Medicine
Texas Christian University
Fort Worth, Texas

Ryan P. Kirby, MD, FAAEM, FACEP
Chief of Academics (Emeritus)
Department of Emergency Medicine
John Peter Smith Health Network
Fort Worth, Texas

Jessica Knapp, CAQSM
Department of Sports Medicine
MAHEC Asheville
Asheville, North Carolina

Atsuko Koyama, MD, MPH
Clinical Assistant Professor
Department of Child Health
University of Arizona, College of Medicine–Phoenix
Phoenix, Arizona

Karen Y. Kwan, BS, MD
Assistant Professor of Pediatrics
Children's Hospital Los Angeles;
Division of Emergency and Transport Medicine
Keck School of Medicine
Los Angeles, California

Mark E. Lavallee, MD, CSCS, FACSM, FAMSSM
Chairman
Sports Medicine Society
USA Weightlifting
Colorado Springs, Colorado;
Member
Executive Medical Committee
International Weightlifting Federation
Lausanne, Switzerland;
Clinical Assistant Professor
Department of Family Medicine
Drexel University College of Medicine
Philadelphia, Pennsylvania;
Faculty
UPMC Pinnacle Sports Medicine Fellowship
UPMC Pinnacle
Harrisburg, Pennsylvania

Alexander Lee, MD
Resident Physician
Department of Emergency Medicine
Penn State Health Milton S. Hershey
Medical Center
Hershey, Pennsylvania

Laura J. Lintner, DO
Assistant Professor
Department of Family and Community Medicine
Wake Forest University School of Medicine
Winston-Salem, North Carolina

Sean Lisse, MD
Assistant Professor
Department of Radiology and Biomedical Imaging
Yale School of Medicine
New Haven, Connecticut

Andrew Lutzkanin, MD, FAAFP
Associate Professor
Department of Family and Community Medicine
Penn State College of Medicine
Hershey, Pennsylvania

Michelle N. Marin, MD
Pediatric Emergency Medicine Physician
Department of Emergency Medicine
HCA Palms West Hospital
Loxahatchee, Florida

Saamia Masoom, MD
Fellow
Division of Pediatric Emergency Medicine
Baylor College of Medicine/Texas Children's Hospital
Houston, Texas

Michael Mesisca, DO, MBA, MS, CCHP-P
Department Chair
Department of Emergency Medicine
Riverside University Health System;
Chief Medical Officer
Correctional Health Services
Riverside University Health System
Moreno Valley, California

Sarah Dennis Meskill, MD, MS
Assistant Professor
Department of Pediatrics, Division of Pediatric Emergency
 Medicine
Texas Children's Hospital/Baylor College of Medicine
Houston, Texas

Jonathan L. Mezrich, MD, JD, MBA, LLM
Associate Professor
Department of Radiology and Biomedical Imaging
Yale School of Medicine
New Haven, Connecticut

Christopher M. Miles, MD
Associate Program Director
Primary Care Sports Medicine Fellowship;
Associate Professor
Department of Family and Community Medicine
Wake Forest University School of Medicine
Winston-Salem, North Carolina

Emily M. Miller, MD
Health Sciences Assistant Clinical Professor
Departments of Family Medicine and
 Orthopaedics
University of California, Los Angeles
Los Angeles, California

Nathan J. Morrison, DO, M.Eng
Physician
Department of Emergency Medicine
Penn State Hershey Medical Center
Hershey, Pennsylvania

Ariella Nadler, MD
Pediatric Emergency Medicine Provider
Department of Pediatric Emergency Medicine
Advocate Medical Group
New York, New York

Heli Naik, DO, CAQSM
Assistant Director of Family Medicine
Department of Family Medicine and Sports Medicine
RWJBH Somerset Family Medicine Residency
Somerville, New Jersey

Chadd E. Nesbit, MD, PhD, FACEP, FAEMS
System EMS Director/EMS Fellowship Program Director
Department of Emergency Medicine
Allegheny Health Network
Pittsburgh, Pennsylvania

Thuy L. Ngo, DO, MEd
Assistant Professor
Department of Pediatrics
Johns Hopkins University School of Medicine
St. Petersburg, Florida

Rory O'Neill, DO, MBA
Medical Director of Quality
Department of Urgent and Express Care
UPMC of Central PA
Harrisburg, Pennsylvania

Lauren P. Oberle, MD
Assistant Professor
Department of Family Medicine
Denver Health
Denver, Colorado;
Assistant Professor
Department of Family Medicine
University of Colorado School of Medicine
Aurora, Colorado

Robert P. Olympia, MD
Professor
Department of Emergency Medicine and Pediatrics
Penn State College of Medicine/Penn State Hershey
    Medical Center
Hershey, Pennsylvania

Cayce Onks, DO, MS, ATC
Associate Professor
Department of Family Medicine and Orthopedics
Penn State Health
Palmyra, Pennsylvania;
Program Director
Primary Care Sports Medicine Fellowship
Hershey, Pennsylvania

John A. Park, MD
Attending Physician
Department of Pediatric Emergency Medicine
Westchester Medical Center
Valhalla, New York

Jay Pershad, MD, MMM, CPE
Professor
Department of Emergency Medicine, Pediatrics
George Washington University
Washington, District of Columbia

Christopher Pitotti, MD, FACEP
Attending Physician
Department of Medical Toxicology
Washington Poison Center
Seattle, Washington

Christopher M. Pruitt, MD
Professor
Department of Pediatrics, Division of Emergency Medicine
Medical University of South Carolina;
Medical Director
Department of Emergency Services
Shawn Jenkins Children's Hospital
Charleston, South Carolina

George G.A. Pujalte, MD, FACSM, FAMSSM, FAAFP
Associate Professor
Department of Family Medicine;
Assistant Professor
Department of Orthopedics and Sports Medicine
Mayo Clinic College of Medicine and Science
Jacksonville, Florida

Joni E. Rabiner, MD
Associate Professor
Department of Emergency Medicine, Division of Pediatric
    Emergency Medicine
Columbia University Irving Medical Center
New York, New York

Lilia Reyes, MD, FAAP
Assistant Professor of Pediatrics and Emergency
    Medicine
Penn State Hershey Medical Center
Penn State College of Medicine
Hershey, Pennsylvania

Ruby F. Rivera, MD
Assistant Professor
Department of Pediatrics
Children's Hospital at Montefiore
Bronx, New York

Munaza Batool Rizvi, MD
Assistant Professor
Department of Pediatric Emergency Medicine
Columbia University Irving Medical Center, Vagelos
    College of Physicians and Surgeons
New York, New York

Emily Rose, MD
Associate Professor of Clinical Emergency Medicine
    (Educational Scholar)
Department of Emergency Medicine
LA County + USC Medical Center;
Director for Pre-Health Undergraduate Studies
Department of Medical Education
Keck School of Medicine of the University of Southern
    California
Los Angeles, California

Jerri A. Rose, MD
Associate Professor
Department of Pediatric Emergency Medicine
UH-Rainbow Babies and Children's Hospital/Case Western
    Reserve University School of Medicine
Cleveland, Ohio

Rachel Rothstein, MD, MPH
Resident
Department of Pediatrics
Children's Hospital of Philadelphia
Philadelphia, Pennsylvania

David A. Sanchez, MSPAS, PA-C
Lead Physician Assistant
Department of Urgent Care
UPMC
Mechanicsburg, Pennsylvania

Jennifer E. Sanders, MD
Associate Professor
Departments of Emergency Medicine, Pediatrics and
    Medical Education
Icahn School of Medicine at Mount Sinai
New York, New York

Sandra K. Schumacher, MD, MPH, CTropMed
Department of Emergency Medicine
Boston Children's Hospital;
Assistant Professor
Harvard University
Boston, Massachusetts

Kara K. Seaton, MD, FAAP
Fellowship Director
Department of Pediatric Emergency Medicine
Children's Minnesota;
Adjunct Assistant Professor
Department of Pediatrics
University of Minnesota
Minneapolis, Minnesota

Peter H. Seidenberg, MD, MA, FAAFP, FACSM, RMSK
Professor and Chair
Department of Family Medicine
Louisiana State University of Health Sciences School of
    Medicine
Shreveport, Louisiana

Jacob Silverman, MD
Resident Physician
Department of Emergency Medicine
Penn State College of Medicine
Hershey, Pennsylvania

Matthew L. Silvis, MD
Professor
Departments of Family and Community Medicine and
    Orthopedics and Rehabilitation
Penn State Health
Hershey, Pennsylvania

Tori Beth L. Snoad, MD
Resident Physician
Department of Emergency
Penn State Health Hershey
Hummelstown, Pennsylvania

Kaitlyn R. Swimmer, MD
Resident Physician
Department of Pediatrics
Penn State Hershey Medical Center
Hershey, Pennsylvania

Jeremy Swisher, MD
Resident Physician
Department of Family and Community Medicine
Wake Forest University School of Medicine
Winston-Salem, North Carolina

Jillian E. Sylvester, MD, CAQSM, FAAFP
Clinical Assistant Professor
Department of Orthopedics
University of North Carolina
Chapel Hill, North Carolina

Ellen Szydlowski, MD
Associate Professor
Department of Pediatrics, Division of Emergency
    Medicine
Children's Hospital of Philadelphia
Philadelphia, Pennsylvania

Ee Tein Tay, MD
Assistant Professor
Department of Emergency Medicine and Pediatrics
NYU School of Medicine;
Clinical Site Chief
Emergency Medicine and Pediatrics
Health+Hospitals/Bellevue
New York, New York

Heath C. Thornton, MD
Associate Professor
Departments of Family and Community Medicine and
    Orthopedic Surgery
Wake Forest University School of Medicine
Winston-Salem, North Carolina

Jesse Tran, DO
Emergency Physician
Department of Emergency
Via Christi Wichita
Wichita, Kansas

Thomas Trojian, MD, MMB, CAQSM, FACSM, FAMSSM, RMSK
Clinical Director
Student Health Service
Temple University
Philadelphia, Pennsylvania

Peggy Tseng, MD
Attending Physician
Department of Emergency Medicine
LAC USC
Los Angeles, California

Sahel Uddin, DO
Resident Physician
Department of Family and Community Medicine
Penn State Hershey Medical Center
Hershey, Pennsylvania

Bryan Upham, MD, MSCE
Associate Professor
Department of Pediatrics
Eastern Virginia Medical School;
Attending Physician
Department of Pediatrics, Division of Pediatric
Emergency Medicine
Children's Hospital of the King's Daughters
Norfolk, Virginia

Charles W. Webb, DO, FAMSSM, FAAFP, CAQSM
Director
Sports Medicine Fellowship;
Associate Professor
Division of Sports Medicine, Department of Family
Medicine
LSU Health Science Center Shreveport
Shreveport, Louisiana

Robert D. Wilkinson, DO
Medical Director
Department of Pediatric Emergency Medicine
The Children's Medical Center at Summerlin
Hospital
Las Vegas, Nevada

R. Blake Windsor, MD
Associate Professor
Department of Pediatrics
University of South Carolina School of Medicine-Greenville;
Medical Director, Pediatric Pain and Headache Medicine
Department of Pediatrics
Prisma Health
Greenville, South Carolina

PREFACE

During the pandemic, we as a society and profession encountered struggles and hardships that come once in a lifetime, if not rarer. We battled and persevered like characters from our favorite comic books and came out stronger on the other side. Through it all, we cared for the ill and injured in our communities, risking our own lives for the benefit of others. Urgent care medicine continued to be an important part of health care throughout the pandemic, increasing the number of centers while advancing medicine through research and technology.

We wanted our second edition of *Urgent Care Medicine Secrets* to reflect these advancements in the field while focusing on what made our first edition successful: the simplicity of the question-and-answer format, targeting health care providers from different levels of experience and different specialty backgrounds while providing a wealth of knowledge based on the current evidence found in the emergency medicine, sports medicine, and urgent care medicine literature.

Once again, I am blessed to embark on this journey with two colleagues I admire and respect tremendously. Rory O'Neill is a board-certified emergency medicine physician, working both clinically and administratively in the arenas of emergency medicine and urgent care medicine. Matthew Silvis is board-certified in both family medicine and primary care sports medicine, balancing his professional career with clinical medicine, education, administration, and research. We searched far and wide for contributors who have demonstrated scholarship in their careers and are experts in their fields. Our contributors represent varied backgrounds, covering general pediatrics, emergency medicine, pediatric emergency medicine, family medicine, urgent care medicine, sports medicine, and anesthesiology.

Based on your feedback from our first edition, we added several topics, such as the history of urgent care medicine, adult head and neck trauma, adult chest and abdominal trauma, toxicology, general concepts in diagnostic imaging, and obstetrical complaints. The second edition is divided into six sections. The first section includes general concepts in urgent care medicine (the history of urgent care medicine, the business of urgent care medicine, office emergency and disaster preparedness, and the recognition and stabilization of adult and pediatric emergencies). The second and third sections focus on chief complaints, divided into adult and pediatrics. The fourth section focuses on primary care sports medicine, covering common injuries and sports-related infections and illnesses. The fifth section focuses on minor trauma and procedures, including wound assessment/burns/animal bites, laceration repair, orthopedic fracture reduction and splinting, incision and drainage, foreign body removal, dental procedures, and utilization of analgesia and sedation. The last section focuses on miscellaneous topics that may be of interest to the urgent care medicine health care provider, including mental health urgencies, toxicology, travel medicine, general concepts in diagnostic imaging, utilization of diagnostic ultrasound, and obstetrical complaints.

Thank you to those who have utilized *Urgent Care Medicine Secrets* in your educational advancements and clinical practice. We hope that the second edition will be a valuable tool for those working in the urgent care medicine setting and optimize care delivered to each and every patient who presents to an urgent care center.

Robert P. Olympia, MD
May 26, 2023

CONTENTS

V PROCEDURES

VI MISCELLANEOUS

TOP 100 SECRETS

Robert P. Olympia, Rory O'Neill, Matthew L. Silvis

TOP 100 SECRETS FOR URGENT CARE MEDICINE SECRETS

1. While most patients present to urgent care centers (UCC) with non-life-and-limb-threatening conditions, approximately 2–4% of patients are transferred from UCCs to the emergency department (ED) due to a need for a higher level of care (Chapter 1).
2. Two mnemonics developed by Rothstein et al. to help educate the community on chief complaints appropriate for urgent care centers and EDs are "URGENT CARES" and "STOP AT AN ED STAT" (Chapter 1).
3. A recently published bibliometric study found that between 2000 and 2020, there were 144 published studies pertaining to UCM in 94 peer-reviewed journals. The rate of publication increased over the past decade, and the majority of studies were retrospective; 48.6% of studies were considered clinical, and the most common topics were urgent care utilization (specifically effectiveness and disease-based), diagnostic testing (specifically HIV and STD), and antibiotic stewardship (Chapter 1).
4. The success of an urgent care business is dependent on providing top-notch customer service. Locations must be convenient, clean service must be fast and efficient, staff must be attentive and empathetic, and the level of care must be excellent (Chapter 2).
5. Urgent care centers must be able to rapidly recognize, assess, stabilize, and transfer patients presenting to their center with medical and traumatic emergencies beyond the capability of the center (Chapter 3).
6. In an adult patient presenting with chest pain, quickly ruling out STEMI and occlusive myocardial infarction on a 12-lead ECG must be a priority (Chapter 4).
7. While the differential diagnosis for syncope or altered mental status in an adult is broad, there is no "standard workup" for either chief complaint. A thorough focused history and physical exam are crucial to making the diagnosis (Chapter 4).
8. In children with altered mental status, the "AEIOU TIPS" mnemonic may be helpful in formulating a differential diagnosis (Chapter 5).
9. In children who sustain a simple febrile seizure, the only diagnostic testing that should be performed is testing to determine the source of the fever, if needed. Neuroimaging and EEG are not indicated (Chapter 5).
10. Headaches in adults can be treated with oxygen (Chapter 6).
11. Continuous nonpositional dizziness can be a posterior stroke (Chapter 6).
12. Visual acuity should be part of every eye exam (Chapter 7).
13. Of tympanic membrane perforations in adults, 80–90% will heal spontaneously in 4–6 weeks (Chapter 8).
14. Acute rhinitis in adults is most commonly allergic (Chapter 8).
15. Canker sores are treated with topical anesthetics and cleansing rinses (Chapter 9).
16. Viral upper respiratory infections and bronchitis are the most common overall causes of cough and shortness of breath (Chapter 10).
17. Any female of childbearing age should have a pregnancy test performed (Chapter 11).
18. Ultrasound is the preferred initial advanced imaging for suspected ureterolithiasis (Chapter 12).
19. The absence of hematuria does not preclude the presence of urolithiasis (Chapter 12).
20. The most common cause of vaginal discharge or malodor is bacterial vaginosis (Chapter 13).
21. In general, simple cutaneous abscesses require incision and drainage for treatment, but not all abscesses require antibiotics. Utilization of the loop drainage technique may improve cosmetic outcomes and prevent subsequent intervention. Adjuncts such as ultrasound can help identify a drainable pocket of fluid (Chapter 14).
22. Antiviral treatment should be initiated within 72 hours of rash onset to be most effective in cases of herpes zoster (Chapter 14).
23. Globe rupture is an ophthalmologic emergency (Chapter 15).
24. "Occult" rib fractures are unlikely to be clinically significant if there are no signs of pneumothorax, hemothorax, or contusion seen on x-ray (Chapter 16).
25. With musculoskeletal complaints that involve the upper and lower extremities, always conduct a proper neurovascular examination, and consider compartment syndrome (the six Ps—pain out of proportion, pallor, paresthesias, pulselessness, paralysis, and poikilothermia, and remember that all six are not necessary to make the diagnosis) (Chapter 17).
26. X-rays are the initial diagnostic test of choice for musculoskeletal injuries. MRI may be considered if conservative therapy does not improve symptoms after 3–5 days (Chapter 17).
27. Erythema migrans if identified is an indicator for antibiotic treatment without laboratory confirmation (Chapter 18).
28. No one has ever contracted rabies from a dog, cat, or ferret who was able to be observed for 10 days (Chapter 18).

29. Fever itself is not dangerous to an otherwise healthy child, and the specific temperature value (as opposed to its presence or absence) is generally not important (Chapter 19).

30. The height of pediatric fever has limited use in determining management; other clinical features, especially the child's clinical appearance, are better predictors (Chapter 19).

31. Most acute headaches in the pediatric patient are due to viral infections (mostly upper respiratory infections). With a normal neurologic exam, pediatric headaches rarely warrant emergent imaging (Chapter 20).

32. Apply proparacaine or tetracaine drops to a fluorescein strip when staining a painful eye to avoid excessive discomfort from the drops and to successfully visualize ocular surface abrasions under a Wood's lamp (Chapter 21).

33. Pediatric preseptal cellulitis can be treated with outpatient oral antibiotics. If there are concerns for orbital cellulitis, urgent referral to the emergency department is warranted for imaging and intravenous antibiotics (Chapter 21).

34. The treatment of choice for otitis media, bacterial sinusitis, and GABHS pharyngitis in children is amoxicillin (Chapter 22).

35. Rheumatic fever does not occur in children less than 3 years of age, and therefore young children in this age group should not be tested or treated for GABHS pharyngitis (Chapter 22).

36. Ultrasound is the diagnostic test of choice for pediatric neck masses. If you are concerned for a deep mass you cannot palpate, or the child presents with difficulty breathing, difficulty swallowing, or significant limitation of range of motion, transfer for computed tomography (Chapter 23).

37. Chest x-rays are not indicated in pediatric patients with suspected pneumonia unless they are exhibiting severe distress, persistent hypoxia, outpatient treatment failure, or any other indication that the patient would need hospital admission for therapy (Chapter 24).

38. In the routine treatment of bronchiolitis, there is no role for beta-agonists, systemic steroids, inhaled steroids, nebulized hypertonic saline, or nebulized epinephrine (Chapter 24).

39. Pediatric chest pain associated with exertion warrants careful evaluation for a cardiopulmonary etiology (Chapter 25).

40. Constipation is one of the most common causes of childhood abdominal pain and is a diagnosis of exclusion (Chapter 26).

41. Consider referred abdominal pain from extraabdominal sources, such as pneumonia, Streptococcal pharyngitis, DKA if a patient has a history or concurrent symptoms of a URI, sore throat, or viral illness (Chapter 26).

42. Ileocolic intussusception should always be considered in a young child (between 6 and 36 months) with isolated vomiting (Chapter 27).

43. Parental report of oliguria is the least predictive sign of pediatric dehydration (Chapter 27).

44. Urinary tract infections can present with subtlety in young children. Unexplained fever or vomiting in a preverbal or diapered child is ample reason to consider UTI (Chapter 28).

45. Pregnancy should be ruled out regardless of the patient's sexual history or absence of menarche if other signs of puberty are present (Chapter 29).

46. Petechiae below the nipple should raise concerns for serious bacterial infection in infants with fever (Chapter 30).

47. Blood cultures, cutaneous aspirates, and biopsies are not routinely recommended in immunocompetent patients with cellulitis (Chapter 30).

48. The most common cause of atraumatic limp in children is transient synovitis, developmental dysplasia of the hip (DDH) in infants, and Legg-Calvé-Perthes (LCP) in young school-aged children. Slipped capital femoral epiphysis (SCFE) in preteens and teens can cause a limp (Chapter 31).

49. Pediatric head trauma guidelines, such as those published by PECARN, can be helpful to minimize the use of CT scans in children at low risk for significant injury (Chapter 32).

50. Consider cervical spine injuries in children presenting with a concerning mechanism (especially diving or axial loading) who complain of neck pain, have focal neurologic findings, or torticollis (Chapter 32).

51. Consider nonaccidental trauma in children younger than 2 years of age with rib fractures, abdominal pain/bruising, associated serious injury such as long bone fractures or intracranial injury, and no history of significant accidental mechanism of injury (Chapter 33).

52. The pliability of the pediatric skeleton results in unique fracture patterns including "plastic" fractures (torus, greenstick, and bowing) and fractures involving the growth plate, which are described using the Salter-Harris classification (Chapter 34).

53. Brief resolved unexplained events (BRUE), formerly known as apparent life-threatening events (ALTE), unexpected episodes that are frightening to the caregiver, include apnea, color change, marked change in muscle tone, and choking or gagging (Chapter 35).

54. The Buffalo treadmill test helps guide early activity in concussion and the return-to-play protocol is a stepwise return to play that takes 24 hours for each stage (Chapter 36).

55. There is no evidence for a specific medication for concussion treatment (Chapter 36).

56. Sports with the highest rate of acute cervical spine injuries include American football, wrestling, diving, ice hockey, skiing/snowboarding, and gymnastics (Chapter 37).

57. The NEXUS (National Emergency X-Radiography Utilization Study) criteria and the Canadian C-Spine Rule are highly sensitive decision-making tools that provide guidelines for when to immobilize and obtain imaging following acute injury (Chapter 37).

58. Most patients with low back pain do not need imaging (Chapter 38).

59. Encourage patients with low back pain to stay active. Bed rest is NOT helpful for acute low back pain (Chapter 38).
60. Beginning an active eccentric loading rehabilitation program early in the course of Achilles tendonitis has been shown to have long-term benefits (Chapter 39).
61. Localized tenderness to palpation over lateral epicondyle and pain with resisted wrist and third finger extension can help diagnose lateral epicondylitis (Chapter 39).
62. Apophysitis is an overuse injury in skeletally immature athletes that warrants rest and activity modification until pain is no longer present, to prevent further irreversible injury (Chapter 40).
63. In evaluating the patient with acute shoulder pain, the mechanism of injury and age of the patient can help you determine the likely diagnosis (Chapter 41).
64. In any fracture or dislocation, neurovascular status should be thoroughly assessed and, if compromised, the fracture or dislocation should be emergently reduced (Chapter 41).
65. A fall on an outstretched hand can lead to injuries of the hand, wrist, forearm, elbow, arm, and shoulder (Chapter 42).
66. The most common fractures associated with a fall on an outstretched hand include the clavicle, elbow, and scaphoid (Chapter 42).
67. Scaphoid fractures often do not show on initial radiographs (Chapter 43).
68. Mallet fingers often are treated nonoperatively, but jersey fingers need a surgical referral (Chapter 43).
69. If possible, always obtain weight-bearing radiographs of the knee (Chapter 44).
70. If septic arthritis is suspected, arthrocentesis for fluid analysis followed by parental antibiotics and urgent referral for surgical debridement is warranted (Chapter 44).
71. A child with septic arthritis will usually appear more ill than those with transient synovitis. Hip aspiration is the gold standard for diagnosis (Chapter 45).
72. Ankle imaging should only be done when the Ottawa Criteria are met (Chapter 46).
73. Cryotherapy, bracing or taping, and early mobilization are the mainstays of therapy for acute ankle sprains (Chapter 46).
74. In cold exposure injuries, do not allow thawed skin to refreeze, and do not use excess heat, cold, or massage or provide direct heat (Chapter 47).
75. If a patient has a temperature >104°F, persistent vomiting, or altered mental status, alert emergency medical services for immediate transfer (Chapter 47).
76. When distinguishing between viral and bacterial upper respiratory tract infections, it is important to note that bacterial infections are less common, last longer than the usual 7- to 10-day course for a viral infection, and are associated with a history of persistent purulent rhinorrhea and facial pain (Chapter 48).
77. It is important to perform a culture of furuncles' and carbuncles' secretions, and drain lesions, for complete resolution (Chapter 48).
78. Utilization of validated imaging guidelines (i.e., Ottawa Ankle/Knee rules, Pittsburgh Rules for knee trauma, Canadian C-spine Rule) can reduce unnecessary imaging (Chapter 49).
79. Identification of specific fractures around the knee on x-ray can help in diagnosing other ligamentous and meniscal pathology only seen with advanced imaging (Chapter 49).
80. Pain control and anxiolytics are important considerations for treating injured pediatric patients with wounds, burns, animal bites, and envenomations (Chapter 50).
81. It is important to assess the percentage of total body surface area that burns occupy in children, which can be done by various methods including the "rule of nines," the "hand method," and Lund Browder charts (Chapter 50).
82. In young children in whom suture removal may be a challenge, it is reasonable to use absorbable suture material for facial and scalp lacerations (Chapter 51).
83. A benzodiazepine can be used to overcome muscle spasms in mandibular dislocations, greatly facilitating reduction (Chapter 52).
84. Children may not exhibit the classic "4 Ps" (pallor, paresthesias, pulseless, pain with passive stretch) of compartment syndrome. The earliest signs are the "3 As" (increased agitation, anxiety, analgesic requirement) (Chapter 53).
85. A recently published meta-analysis demonstrated that providing systemic antibiotics after incision and drainage more than doubled clinical cure rates. Providers should consider the use of antibiotics while balancing the risks of side effects and adverse events (Chapter 54).
86. Factors that affect the method and urgency of removal of a foreign body include the type of material (e.g., button battery versus food item), location, risk of further injury to surrounding tissue, long-term sequelae, and potential for infection (Chapter 55).
87. Most lacerations of the buccal mucosa, gingiva, and tongue heal well without intervention (Chapter 56).
88. Multimodal treatments should always be used to treat pain without opioids or to reduce the opioid to the minimum required dose (Chapter 57).
89. The WHO analgesic ladder is an effective treatment approach for acute and cancer-related pain (Chapter 57).
90. Normal labs, weight, and EKG do not exclude the diagnosis of an eating disorder (Chapter 58).
91. There are certain circumstances in which confidentiality may be breached, including when disclosure is required by law such as with abuse or homicidal ideation, or when the provider has concern for risk or harm to the adolescent such as suicidal ideation or high-risk behavior (Chapter 58).
92. Screen for acetaminophen and salicylate exposure in all patients in whom self-harm or intentional ingestion is suspected (Chapter 59).

93. Many common toxicologic therapies such as activated charcoal, naloxone, and n-acetylcysteine can and should be started in the urgent care setting prior to transfer to a higher level of care (Chapter 59).

94. It is crucial to inquire about the countries traveled to, time of travel, travel activities, and basic health status to determine what illnesses need to be considered in a returning traveler who is sick (Chapter 60).

95. When reviewing imaging, search patterns are important. For example, when reviewing a chest x-ray, using a systemic approach (e.g., ABCD) is helpful to avoid overlooking subtle findings. Find one you're comfortable with and use it consistently (Chapter 61).

96. Be aware that rings like to fracture/dislocate in more than one place. When a patient has an unstable ankle fracture, obtain imaging of the proximal tibia/fibula, as forces may have translated up the fibular shaft. Similarly, in cases of a wrist/forearm fracture or dislocation, imaging at the elbow is warranted (Chapter 61).

97. On ultrasound, fluid appears hypoechoic or anechoic (black), soft tissues and muscles are gray, and bones and air appear hyperechoic (white) on ultrasound (Chapter 62).

98. POCUS (Point-of-Care Ultrasound) can be used to rule in pathology due to its high specificity for most applications (Chapter 62).

99. Administer Rhogam to Rh-negative women experiencing early pregnancy loss or ectopic pregnancy (Chapter 63).

100. Infections of the urinary tract are more common during pregnancy, with asymptomatic bacteriuria occurring in 2–7% of patients. Left untreated, 30–40% will develop a symptomatic infection (Chapter 63).

URGENT CARE MEDICINE: THE PAST, PRESENT, AND FUTURE

Rory O'Neill, DO, MBA, Robert P. Olympia, MD, Professor

1. **What is urgent care medicine?**
   Urgent care medicine (UCM) incorporates clinical services provided at urgent care centers (UCCs) into a growing specialty consisting of administration, education, research and scholarship, and community service. Urgent care services are defined as (1) a medical examination, diagnosis, and treatment for non-life- or -limb-threatening illnesses and injuries that are within the capability of a UCC that accepts unscheduled, walk-in patients seeking medical attention during all posted hours of operation and is supported by on-site evaluation services, including radiology and laboratory services; and (2) any further medical examination, procedure, and treatment to the extent they are within the capabilities of the staff and facilities available at the UCC.

THE PAST

2. **How did urgent care centers get their start?**
   The first urgent care centers began popping up in the 1970s. These were sometimes known as "walk-in" or "fast care" clinics. Health care leaders as well as physician entrepreneurs looked to fill a void in the medical delivery model. Before, urgent care patients had to either get an appointment with their primary care physician or go to the emergency department. The former was often hard to get and the latter was often unnecessary for the condition needing treatment.

3. **What are factors that contributed to the growth of urgent care centers in the last two decades throughout the United States?**
   Factors contributing to the growth of urgent care centers in the last two decades throughout the United States include shortages of primary care providers, fewer weekend and evening primary care hours, high costs of emergency department visits, wait times at emergency departments, insurance companies realizing cost savings of deferring patients to urgent care, and patient scheduling flexibility.

THE PRESENT

4. **What is the current state of urgent care medicine in the United States?**
   As per the Urgent Care Association (UCA), the leading organization for UCM since 2004, the current state of UCM has been described in the "Urgent Care Industry White Paper: the essential role of the UCC in population health (2019)," and summarized here:
   a) As of June 2019, there are approximately 9279 UCCs in the US.
   b) UCCs have reported a median patient volume of 35 patients per day, increasing during late fall and winter, with an estimated total of 112 million patient visits per year in the US. This represents 23% of all primary care visits and 12.6% of all outpatient physician visits.
   c) Ninty-four percent of UCCs in the US report an average wait time of 30 minutes or less.
   d) The majority of consumers presenting to UCCs are millennials (ages 18–34 years) and younger Gen Xers (ages 35–44 years).
   e) The presence of UCCs in the community has decreased ED visits by 30%.
   f) Forty percent of UCCs in the US are physician-owned and 37% are hospital-owned.
   g) Over the past decade, there has been an increase in the number of pediatric-specific UCCs employing pediatric EM physicians, such as PM pediatrics and UCCs associated with children's hospitals in the US.
   h) The majority of UCCs employ physicians trained in family medicine and emergency medicine as well as other licensed health care professionals, including physician assistants, nurse practitioners, registered nurses, and radiology technicians. Sixty-two percent of UCCs utilize a hybrid model of physicians and advanced practice clinicians.
   i) The majority of UCCs provide the following on-site laboratory testing: complete blood counts, comprehensive metabolic profiles, diabetic testing (Hemoglobin A1c), urine pregnancy, urinalysis, rapid strep and throat cultures, and rapid viral testing. Several UCCs offer Tuberculosis testing, drug screens, and STD testing.
   j) The majority of UCCs provide x-ray imaging, while an increasing number of UCCs offer CT scan, MRI, and ultrasound services.
   k) The majority of UCCs utilize radiology and laboratory technologists.

l) Other services provided by most UCCs include preplacement physicals, urinary drug screening and postinjury testing, annual employment physicals, flu and other vaccine immunizations, and workforce health education on injury/illness prevention.

5. **What emergencies presenting to urgent care centers require transport to local emergency departments?**
While most patients present to the UCC with non-life- and -limb-threatening conditions, approximately 2–4% of patients are transferred from UCCs to the ED due to a need for a higher level of care.

A single-center study found that for *adult referrals* from a UCC to an ED, the most common diagnoses for complex referrals (requiring resources not commonly available at UCCs) were nonspecific abdominal pain requiring a workup for a surgical abdomen, complex lacerations, and complex fractures. The most common diagnoses for critical referrals (requiring intensive care, surgery, or invasive procedure) were acute appendicitis, fractures requiring operative management, and cholecystitis (Siegfried et al., 2019).

A single-center study found that for *pediatric referrals* from a UCC to an ED, the most common diagnoses for essential referrals (requiring resources not commonly available at UCCs) were closed extremity fractures, nonsurgical unspecified abdominal pain, and gastroenteritis (Olympia et al., 2018)

6. **Are there transfers from urgent care centers to emergency departments that are considered nonessential (not requiring resources, such as laboratory investigations, procedures, medications, subspecialty consultations, hospitalization, or resuscitation, available at a higher level of care center)?**
The most common nonessential referrals for *pediatric patients* were gastroenteritis, brain concussion, upper respiratory infection, acute febrile illness, and nonsurgical, unspecified abdominal pain (Olympia et al., 2018). The most common nonessential referrals for *adult patients* were simple lacerations, nonspecific abdominal pain, simple fractures, nonemergent rashes, and corneal ulcer abrasions (Siegfried et al., 2019). The authors suggest that educational strategies for clinicians working at UCCs, utilizing validated risk stratification tools and prediction models, be implemented to decrease nonessential ED referrals.

7. **Why do patients with emergencies requiring a higher level of care present to urgent care centers?**
In addition to the convenience of access provided at UCCs and the growing frustration with EDs and primary care provider offices, there exists confusion as to what are appropriate or inappropriate chief complaints managed in UCCs. A recently published study concluded that there exists much variability on the websites of the top 30 urgent care organizations regarding acuity-appropriate triage of chief complaints to the UCC or ED (Rothstein et al., 2021). Two mnemonics developed by Rothstein et al. to help educate the community are "URGENT CARES" and "STOP AT AN ED STAT" (Table 1.1; infographics provided in the article by Rothstein et al.).

Table 1.1 Two Mnemonics to Triage Patients to Either the Emergency Department or Urgent Care Center Based on Chief Complaint

"URGENT CARES" (PRESENTING PROBLEMS THAT UCCS CAN EVALUATE AND TREAT)	"STOP AT AN ED STAT" (PRESENTING PROBLEMS NEEDING A HIGHER LEVEL OF CARE THAN UCCS CAN PROVIDE)
Urinary/vaginal symptoms	Shock
Rashes	Trouble swallowing
Gastrointestinal complaints	Overdose
Extremity injury	Pain
Nose bleeds	Altered mental status
Temperature (fever)	Tormented thoughts
Cough and cold symptoms	Abnormal walking
Allergy symptoms	Numbness
Respiratory illness	Environmental emergency
Earaches	Difficulty breathing
Skin Infections	Seizures or syncope
	Trauma
	Anaphylaxis
	Tachycardia or tachypnea

Excludes: Any complaints above combined with confusion, poor blood flow to extremities, dehydration, difficulty breathing or swallowing, unbearable pain (especially headache, neck pain, chest pain, and abdominal pain), serious weakness, numbness, lightheadedness, dizziness or changes in vision or speech, uncontrollable bleeding, trauma with significant deformities.

Table 1.2 Most Common Topics of Research Conducted in Urgent Care Medicine Published 2000–2020

RESEARCH TOPIC	SUBTOPIC
Utilization (n = 34)	Effectiveness (n = 9) Disease-based (n = 7) Alternative care (n = 6) Access to care (n = 5) Patient flow (n = 5) Patient preference (n = 2)
Testing (n = 20)	HIV (n = 7) Sexually transmitted infections (n = 6) Group A strep (n = 2) Influenza (n = 2) Radiology (n = 1) Respiratory illness(n = 1) Blood pressure (n = 1)
Antibiotic stewardship (n = 17)	
Treatment (n = 12)	Medication (n = 8) Intervention (n = 2) Contraception (n = 1) Mental health (n = 1)
Specific disease incidence (n = 9)	Acute coronary syndrome (n = 1) Asthma (n = 1) Bacteremia (n = 1) Congestive heart failure (n = 1) Escherichia coli (n = 1) Influenza/RSV (n = 1) Mental health (n = 1) Ocular (n = 1) Oncology (n = 1)
Patient satisfaction (n = 7)	
UCC referrals (n = 7)	

8. **Has research been conducted in the field of urgent care medicine?**
   A recently published bibliometric study (McNickle et al., 2021) found that between 2000 and 2020, there were 144 published studies pertaining to UCM in 94 peer-reviewed journals, and the rate of publications increased over the past decade. The majority of studies were retrospective (55.5%), followed by study-specific (24.3%), prospective (15.3%), and quality improvement (4.9%). Publications were categorized as clinical (48.6%) and nonclinical (51.4%). Adults were the most frequently identified study population (33.3%), followed by pediatrics (18%) and both adults and pediatrics (16.7%). The top publishing journals were *Pediatric Emergency Care* (n = 9), *Annals of Emergency Medicine* (n = 8), *JAMA Pediatrics* (n = 4), *Journal of Emergency Medicine* (n = 4), and *Pediatrics* (n = 4).

9. **What are the most common topics of research conducted in urgent care medicine?**
   See Table 1.2.

10. **Are there urgent care societies? Are they involved in credentialing?**
    The Urgent Care Association (UCA) is the "largest, most notable trade and professional association in urgent care." They engage in many aspects of urgent care advocacy, education, and research. They also oversee an extensive accreditation process, certifying urgent care centers. The American Academy of Urgent Care Medicine (AAUCM) is "the leading society for physicians, physician assistants, and nurse practitioners practicing urgent care medicine." Their stated goals include increasing training standards, bettering patient care, and providing its members with tools to succeed in urgent care practice.

11. **Are there urgent care CME, conferences, or other educational offerings?**
    Yes. While there are many urgent care educational opportunities, the Urgent Care Boot Camp, Urgent Care RAP Podcast, and Urgent Care LLSA through HIPPO are widely popular. The most well-known in-person conference is the Urgent Care Association (UCA) annual conference, which is typically in the spring.

THE FUTURE

12. **What is the ET3 model, and how may this affect urgent care centers in the future?**
On January 1, 2021, a 5-year pilot plan was instituted called the Emergency Triage, Treat, and Transport (ET3) program model. This voluntary payment model provides flexibility to EMS to address emergency health care needs of Medicare Fee-for-Service beneficiaries following a 911 call. The program allows partnered EMS providers the ability to transport patients to an alternative site for care, including UCCs, primary care offices, or community mental health centers, based on the presenting chief complaint. The ET3 model hopes to decrease overcrowding and resource utilization in EDs, provide person-centered care by giving the patient control of their health care through the availability of options, encourage appropriate utilization of services, and increase the efficiency of the EMS system to focus on high-acuity cases. Implementation of this model will affect how UCCs are operated and staffed; more to come.

13. **Is there a role for telemedicine in urgent care medicine?**
According to the Urgent Care Association, as of 2019, 8% of UCCs offer telemedicine options, although this service likely has increased due to the COVID-19 pandemic. While "tele-urgent care" increases access to effective, convenient, high-quality urgent care and protects patients from current and emerging infectious diseases, identified obstacles to optimizing this method of health care include greater investments in technology infrastructure (high-speed broadband and hardware, IT expertise, clinicians developing proficiencies in utilizing this technology), clinicians adapting communication and examination techniques from in-person care to "tele-urgent care" encounters, and mismatched expectation leading to added tension (especially regarding prescriptions and diagnostic testing) (Laub et al., 2020).

KEY POINTS

1. While most patients present to the UCC with non-life- and -limb-threatening conditions, approximately 2–4% of patients are transferred from UCCs to the ED due to a need for a higher level of care.
2. Two mnemonics developed by Rothstein et al. to help educate the community are "URGENT CARES" and "STOP AT AN ED STAT."
3. A recently published bibliometric study found that between 2000 and 2020, there were 144 published studies pertaining to UCM in 94 peer-reviewed journals, the rate of publication increased over the past decade, the majority of studies were retrospective, 48.6% of studies were considered clinical, and the most common topics were urgent care utilization (specifically effectiveness and disease-based), diagnostic testing (specifically HIV and STD), and antibiotic stewardship.

BIBLIOGRAPHY

About UCA. www.ucaoa.org/About-UCA. Accessed September 28, 2022
Laub N, Agarwal AK, Shi C, et al. Delivering urgent care using telemedicine: insights from experienced clinicians at academic medical centers. *J Gen Intern Med.* 2020;37(4):407–413.
McKeeley S. Urgent Care Centers: An Overview. *Am J Clin Med.* 2012;9(2):80–81.
McNickle LA, Chiang KC, McNulty EM, et al. Publishing trends in the field of urgent care medicine from 2000–2020: a bibliometric analysis. *Am J Emerg Med.* 2021;46:233–237.
Olympia RP, Wilkinson R, Dunnick J, et al. Pediatric Referrals to the Emergency Department from Urgent Care Centers. *Pediatr Emerg Care.* 2018;34(12):872–877.
Resnick. Urgent Care: the evolution of a revolution. *Isr J Health Policy Res.* 2013;2:39.
Rothstein R, Zhen K, Kim RY, et al. Acuity-appropriate triage of chief complaints found on urgent care center organization websites. *Am J Emerg Med.* 2021;43:276–280.
Siegfried IB, Jacobs J, Olympia RP. Adult referrals to an emergency department from urgent care centers. *Am J Emerg Med.* 2019 Oct;37(10):1949–1954.
Welcome to the AAUCM. www.aaucm.org. Accessed September 28, 2022.
Urgent Care Association (2019). Urgent Care Industry White Paper: The essential role of the urgent care center in population health. https://www.ucaoa.org/LinkClick.aspx?fileticket=Q4TP7cypW94%3D&portalid=80. Accessed September 9, 2022.

THE BUSINESS OF URGENT CARE

Michael C. Bachman, MD, MBA

CHAPTER 2

1. **What are the key components of a business plan?**
    When developing a business plan for a new urgent care (UC) business, it is important to include the following components: concept (description of the project, the problem you are solving, benefits to customers, and why it will succeed), market assessment (industry overview, target market, competition, potential market size, and expected penetration), strategy, operations, marketing activities, corporate structure, financial data, and risks involved.

2. **What expenses should be considered prior to opening a new UC center?**
    Cost of the build-out, furniture, fixtures, equipment, opening supplies, software and training, attorney fees, deposits, architect and filing fees.

3. **What expenses should be considered after the opening of a new UC center?**
    It is very important to calculate the expected ramp-up losses. These should include personnel expenses (salary, payroll taxes, benefits, malpractice coverage), rent and related costs, marketing expenses, supplies, billing and collections, miscellaneous fees, and accounts receivable.

4. **Is urgent care a variable- or fixed-cost business?**
    Urgent care is primarily a fixed-cost business. The only true variable cost is supplies. Personnel are semifixed because, as volume grows, new staff need to be added incrementally. Because urgent care is a fixed-cost business, profitability is volume driven. Once fixed costs are covered, a very high percentage of additional revenue will increase profits. It is important for an urgent care business to determine its initial breakeven volume and then recalculate as staffing increases.

5. **What are the different sources of capital to fund an urgent care business?**
    Sources of capital include friends and family, bank loans, finance companies, landlord contributions, equipment leasing, angel investors, venture capital, and private equity. For a newer company, the best sources of funding are investment by the founders, bank loans, and landlord contributions. As the company grows to a multiple-site practice, the other funding sources may become better options.

6. **You figure out how much cash you need until you expect to break even and are able to secure the funds from friends and family. Should you be ready to take the leap?**
    No, you need to anticipate issues that may arise and increase your costs. Examples include permit or construction delays that result in a delayed opening even while paying rent, unanticipated capital or operating expenses, a slower ramp-up than predicted, and delays in reimbursement from insurance companies. It is essential to have contingency funds to cover these unexpected expenses, as much as 50% more than your calculated needs.

7. **What demographic data are essential to determine the ideal site for a new UC center?**
    Important demographics to consider are the total population within your catchment area, population trends (i.e., is the local population growing?), average age of the population, income levels, and population density (i.e., people per square mile). It is important to determine your catchment area: that is, where patients will come from, driving distance, and ease of travel to get to your site. Local behaviors are important to consider, such as if the local population drives, relies on public transportation, or walks to destinations. Sources of demographic data include real estate brokers, commercial real estate web listings, and the US Census Bureau.

8. **After deciding on the location of your new UC center, what specific site characteristics should you evaluate?**
    Key characteristics include accessibility, visibility from major roads, adequate parking, and the size and shape of available space. The condition of the building should be considered to determine if there will be exterior work needed and if there are adequate utilities. Based on your business model, you need to determine if your business should be placed in a freestanding building, retail shopping center, or medical office building. If you choose a retail center, consider your cotenants and the customer activity in the center. Local zoning and use laws should be reviewed to determine if your use is permitted in the space, if any variances will be required, and what types of building signage are allowed.

9. **What are the important leasing considerations for a new UC site?**
    It is important to consider the desired term of the lease. If investing in the space build-out, you want to benefit from that investment as long as possible, but you don't want to be locked in for too long if things don't work out. Termination rights for the lease need to be determined as well as a guarantee to reimburse the landlord for their investment in the deal. Rent will also include a proportionate share of real estate tax and common area maintenance and often increases over time by a predetermined percentage. Rent start should be delayed until after

building and sign permits are issued and ideally until after build-out and outfitting are complete and the business is ready to open. Construction allowances from the landlord should also be negotiated and can be delivered in the form of cash or free rent and may be rolled into the base rent.

10. **What is EBITDA?**
EBITDA stands for earnings before interest, taxes, depreciation, and amortization. It serves as a common measure of a company's profitability before deductions that are considered superfluous to the business decision-making process.

11. **Are profits all that matter?**
Profits = Revenue – Expenses. Revenue is the amount of money earned, but it is not necessarily the money collected. It is important to understand that being profitable does not mean the business is guaranteed to succeed. Cash is extremely important to help cover capital expenditures, accounts payable, loan repayments, etc. Profits may not be realized until accounts receivable are realized and expenses are covered.

12. **What are the important business metrics to be followed?**
   - Visit patterns: determine monthly growth, hourly volumes, seasonal patterns, and zip code analysis
   - Revenue: average revenue per visit, average time to collect
   - Expenses: personnel costs per visit, supply cost per visit
   - Marketing: advertising effectiveness

13. **Describe the different ways of contracting reimbursement with payers**
UC businesses can contract with payers as fee for service or at a case rate. With fee for service, each service provided is paid for separately. A case rate provides a flat amount per visit, covering a group of procedures and services. While fee for service may generate higher reimbursements, case rates provide ease of coding and billing and lower risk of audits. In certain markets, UC businesses may not participate with insurance companies and may offer various self-pay rates.

14. **What are the legal considerations for an urgent care business?**
Legal considerations include malpractice and liability coverage, licensing requirements, the corporate practice of medicine, and local laws regarding medication dispensing and e-prescribing. It is very important to understand the state and local laws where your UC center is located. Many states have "no surprise billing laws" that require patients to be notified if the UC center is part of a hospital and will charge an additional facility fee if out of network, and of any extra fees that may be charged for certain procedures or diagnostic tests.

15. **Does your UC business need a compliance program?**
Any UC center that gets reimbursements from Medicare or Medicaid must have a compliance program. They should have a Code of Conduct that provides rules for all employees to follow, to comply with fraud and abuse laws and other legal mandates. The compliance program should provide ongoing employee education on fraud and abuse laws, as they may change over time.

16. **What are the important methods for marketing your UC business?**
Marketing methods include branding the UC business with an identifiable logo, signage, print advertising, direct mail, web and social media, grassroots and community outreach, and public relations. Increasing numbers of customers seek health care providers online, so it is important to have a modern and easy-to-navigate website that is an extension of the brand. Equally important is for the website to have a mobile-friendly format. The website should be developed with search engine optimization in mind. The social media landscape is rapidly growing and becoming a low-cost effective marketing tool for UC businesses.

17. **What are drivers of customer satisfaction in urgent care?**
It is essential to understand what urgent care customers' values include: convenient and clean locations, speed of service, attention and empathy of staff, and excellent care. The design and appearance of the physical space impact the customers' first impressions, and the site layout must be conducive to efficient treatment and facilitate effective communication between staff and patients. All staff should understand the mission of the company and the values and priorities of the company. Staffing with the right people who receive the right training will help ensure excellent service. Staff should be happy and motivated and always willing to go above and beyond customer expectations.

KEY POINTS

1. Develop a thorough business plan, consider both upfront expenses and ongoing expenses that will occur after opening, and make sure to have contingency funds to cover unexpected expenses that may arise.
2. Choose your location wisely, considering local demographics, travel habits, ease of access, and characteristics of the specific site.
3. Your UC business must practice in accordance with state and federal laws including meeting all the licensure, insurance, compliance, billing, and credentialing requirements.
4. The success of an urgent care business is dependent on providing top-notch customer service. Locations must be convenient, clean service must be fast and efficient, staff must be attentive and empathetic, and the level of care must be excellent.

CHAPTER 3

OFFICE EMERGENCY AND DISASTER PREPAREDNESS

Robert P. Olympia, MD, Chadd E. Nesbit, MD, PhD, FACEP, FAEMS

TOP SECRETS

1. Urgent care centers must be able to rapidly recognize, assess, stabilize, and transfer patients presenting to their center with medical and traumatic emergencies beyond the capability of the center.
2. Communication among staff, local EMS, and the receiving hospital is important when dealing with an office emergency and arranging patient transfer.

1. **A 4-year-old boy presents to your urgent care center after falling from monkey bars 1 hour prior. He sustained a blunt head injury, but there was no loss of consciousness. While in your waiting area, he proceeds to have a generalized tonic-clonic seizure, has multiple episodes of vomiting, turns blue, and stops breathing. You detect no peripheral pulses. How often do serious emergencies occur in urgent care centers?**
   Although not meant to replace emergency departments, urgent care centers may need to provide the acute assessment and management of moderately to severely ill or injured infants and children. While studies examining the etiology of pediatric emergencies, including those considered life-threatening, that present to urgent care centers have not been published, retrospective studies have found that the rate of emergencies in primary care practices providing care to children ranges from less than 1 per office per year to more than 30 per office per year, with the most common reported emergencies being respiratory distress, severe dehydration, seizures, severe trauma, abdominal pain, syncope, and behavioral/psychiatric disorders. A published study of urgent care centers in the US showed that 71% of respondents reported that their center has contacted 911 or community EMS to transport a critically ill or injured child to a definitive care facility. A more recent publication found a transport rate of <1% for pediatric patients to a hospital by EMS from pediatric ambulatory settings. These transports were generally for respiratory issues, seizures, and psychiatric complaints.

2. **Do emergencies occur more or less frequently in the adult urgent care setting?**
   Emergencies in the adult population are frequently encountered in outpatient offices and in the urgent care setting. A Canadian study from the Ottawa area recorded more than 3000 calls for "life-threatening" emergencies to family practice offices over the 3-year period of the study. In addition, an Australian study found that 95% of family practice offices had seen an emergency in the preceding 12 months. Although these studies were conducted in the primary care office setting, they may help give us an estimate of the frequency of emergencies in the urgent care center setting. The Urgent Care Association of America notes that 4% of patients are either "directed or transferred from an urgent care center to an emergency department."

3. **What types of adult emergencies are seen in the urgent care setting?**
   Almost any kind of emergency could conceivably present to an urgent care center. The patient who presents with "indigestion" may experience a cardiac arrest, as his complaint is really a myocardial infarction. The patient who presents with a headache or weakness may be having a stroke. Allergic reactions may rapidly progress to airway obstruction. One must also consider that patients may be brought into the urgent care center from traumatic events such as motor vehicle collisions that occur in close proximity to the center. A Canadian study found that general illness, cardiovascular, respiratory, neurological, and endocrine problems were the five most common reasons for adult life-threatening emergencies to occur in the outpatient office setting.

4. **What kind of equipment should be readily available in the urgent care setting in the event of a life-threatening emergency?**
   The urgent care center must be prepared to act in emergency situations involving both adult and pediatric populations. Therefore, it is important to have equipment that is appropriate for all age ranges from neonate to adult populations. Table 3.1 lists emergency equipment that should be maintained in the urgent care setting. In some emergency situations, airway management is necessary. Often this can be achieved by the use of airway adjuncts and effective bag valve mask ventilation. If the center is staffed by physicians who are certified in endotracheal intubation, having the equipment needed for placing an endotracheal tube is a consideration.

5. **What emergency medications should an urgent care center stock for use in an office emergency?**
   Tables 3.2 and 3.3 list recommended medications that should be readily available in the event of an adult or pediatric emergency. The Joint Commission recommends that, whenever possible, emergency medications are available in unit-dose, age-specific, ready-to-administer forms.

Table 3.1 Suggested Office Equipment for Adult and Pediatric Emergencies

SUGGESTED EQUIPMENT FOR ADULT AND PEDIATRIC URGENT CARE OFFICE EMERGENCIES

Automatic External Defibrillator (AED) or a Cardiac Monitor with Defibrillator
Bag valve mask ventilators in multiple sizes with masks for infants through adults
Blood pressure cuffs (various sizes)
Color-coded resuscitation tape (pediatrics)
Gloves, masks, and eye protection
Glucometer
IV access equipment (IV catheters, butterfly needles)
IV tubing
Nasopharyngeal airway set
Nebulizer sets
Oropharyngeal airway set
Oxygen delivery devices (nasal cannula, simple mask, nonrebreather masks) in appropriate sizes
Oxygen tank(s) for portable use
Portable suction device with catheter
Pulse oximeter (adult and pediatric sizes)

Additional Equipment to Consider

Cervical collars and backboards
Endotracheal tubes (various sizes)
Laryngoscope with curved and straight blades (various sizes)
Magill forceps

Table 3.2 Suggested Medications for Adult Emergencies

Drugs and Fluids

Acetaminophen
Albuterol (MDI or nebulized)
Aspirin (chewable 81 mg)
Ceftriaxone (IM or IV)
Corticosteroids (IV and PO)
Dextrose (25% and 50% for IV use)
Diazepam, IV (Valium)
Diphenhydramine (IV and PO) Benadryl
Epinephrine (EpiPen)
Epinephrine (Cardiac 1:10,000)
Naloxone
Nitroglycerin (spray or sublingual tablets)
Saline (IV fluid)

Other Medications to Consider

Atropine
Flumazenil (Romazicon)
Glucagon
Lidocaine
Narcotics such as morphine

6. **What kind of training should the office staff have to deal with emergencies?**
   The Urgent Care Association of America notes that approximately 80% of urgent care centers employ a combination of physicians, physician assistants, and nurse practitioners. The remaining 20% are staffed by physicians only. They recommend that all providers and staff in urgent care centers be trained to provide basic life support in emergency situations until EMS arrives. Furthermore, the most senior clinical provider in the office on a given day should additionally be trained in Advanced Cardiac Life Support (ACLS) and Pediatric Advanced Life Support (PALS). Additional certification for the stabilization of trauma victims, such as the Advanced Trauma Life Support (ATLS) course, may be helpful. If possible, Advanced Practice Clinicians, nurses, and technicians ideally should be certified in lifesaving courses as well. Maintenance of certification is imperative, as the standards for these courses are frequently updated to reflect the latest basic science findings and may change significantly from one version to the next.

Table 3.3 Essential (E) and Suggested (S) Emergency Medications as per the American Academy of Pediatrics

DRUGS/FLUIDS	RECOMMENDATION
Oxygen source	E
Nebulized/inhaled β-agonist	E
Epinephrine (1:1000)	E
Activated charcoal	S
IV/IM ceftriaxone	S
IV lorazepam	S
Rectal diazepam	S
IV methylprednisolone	S
IV dextrose	S
Epinephrine (1:10,000)	S
Atropine	S
Naloxone	S
Normal saline	S
IM midazolam	S

7. **Your office manager would like to develop a quality improvement initiative, developing written emergency plans for adult and pediatric emergencies and performing monthly mock codes. What should this initiative be based on?**
As outlined above, there are a number of emergencies that may occur in the urgent care setting, and your office staff must be prepared to handle medical and traumatic emergencies that may present or occur at your facility. Simulation of emergencies has been shown to improve performance in the office and outpatient settings. Simulations should take place on a regular basis, but ideally should not be announced to staff so as to be more realistic. Following these simulations or mock codes, quality improvement strategies should be discussed and changes implemented to ensure patient safety and to improve morbidity and mortality outcomes.

8. **An adult patient presents to your center with expressive aphasia. Their spouse tells the secretary that this started as they were shopping in a nearby store. Does your staff have assigned roles in emergency situations?**
Having the office staff assigned to particular tasks may help reduce confusion during an emergency in the urgent care setting. A staff member should be assigned to alert the physician of the problem. Alternatively, the office may have a panic button to summon personnel to a predesignated location in the event of an emergency. The physician or senior clinician should be the team leader, assisted by Advanced Practice Clinicians depending on the office staff model. Nurses should be assigned to gather equipment, prepare medications, and document during the emergency. A secretary should be assigned to call 911 and lead EMS to the room where the patient is located. Records of any procedures or medications given should be sent with the patient to the ED.

9. **Your staff has just resuscitated a patient from a cardiac arrest after he had a heart attack. How are patients transported from the center to an appropriate hospital?**
It is important to understand the capabilities of the EMS agency that provides service to the locale where the urgent care is located. If the center is in an urban area, it is likely that it is covered by an Advanced Life Support (ALS) service staffed by paramedics who are ACLS and PALS trained and have a relatively short response time. More remote locations may only be served by an ambulance staffed by EMTs providing Basic Life Support services. ALS, if available, may be available only with a delayed response time. Staff may need to be prepared to take care of the patient for a longer period of time prior to EMS arrival. Staff should also be familiar with the capabilities of local hospitals regarding specialty designations such as trauma, pediatric trauma, stroke, or cardiac catheterization centers to ensure that patients are transferred to an appropriate facility. Local EMS is generally very aware of these designations. In some critical time-sensitive situations, air medical transport may be indicated depending on the distance to definitive specialty care such as a trauma or stroke center. Again, this is likely best done in conjunction with local EMS agencies.

Table 3.4 Common Presenting Signs and Symptoms of Class A Biological Agents

AGENT	INFLUENZA-LIKE ILLNESS	RAPIDLY PROGRESSIVE PNEUMONIA	BLOODY DIARRHEA	FEVER, RASH, MENINGITIS	HEPATITIS
Anthrax	50–90%	10–20%		10–50%	
Botulism (see note)	Not seen	Not seen	Not seen	Not seen	Not seen
VHF	>90%	10–50%	50–100%	Highly variable	Variable
Pneumonic Plague	10–50%	100%		<10%	Not seen
Smallpox	50–90%	<10%	10–50%	>90%	
Pneumonic tularemia	25–50%	100%			

VHF, Viral hemorrhagic fever (Ebola, Marburg).
Botulism classically presents with the triad of bulbar nerve palsy and descending paralysis, lack of fever, and a clear sensorium. The signs listed above are typically not seen with botulism.

10. Your patient is on the stretcher and ready to be transported. What information should staff send to the ED along with the patient?
    A recent paper revealed that ED physicians want to know the reasons that a patient is being referred from the urgent care center to the emergency department. They would also like to receive a copy of the urgent care center chart. A phone call from the center and having contact information for the center that the patient was being sent from were additional pieces of information that receiving ED physicians would like to have.

11. Besides medical emergencies, are there other emergencies that the urgent care office should anticipate and prepare for?
    The Joint Commission has standards for urgent care centers for disaster preparedness. This is an "all hazards" type approach to disasters, which may be internal (loss of power, water, infrastructure failure) or external (storms, flooding, or snow), causing disruptions in service. A survey of centers published in 2016 shows that only 27% of centers had a disaster plan involving their centers and the surrounding community. Less than 25% of centers took part in local disaster drills. Less than half of the centers had a disaster plan that they practiced more than once a year. Suggested areas for improvement included developing and practicing disaster plans, familiarization with community disaster plans and shelters, providing surveillance for chemical and biological acts of terrorism, and assisting the community with disaster planning.

12. I've heard about syndromic surveillance. What is this and why is it important? Do urgent care centers do this?
    Syndromic surveillance is defined by the World Health Organization as "the continuous, systematic collection, analysis and interpretation of health-related data needed for the planning, implementation, and evaluation of public health practice." It is an early warning system for public health events such as the spread of disease. It may also serve as a means of detection of biological or chemical attacks. The Public Health Information Network of the CDC is one such program that collects real-time data from a variety of acute and urgent care settings. A 2016 paper found that 17% of urgent care centers that returned the survey participated in some type of syndromic surveillance.

13. Are there signs that might be suspicious for a covert biological or chemical attack?
    Covert biological and chemical attacks are very difficult to detect. The presentation of large numbers of patients to a facility with similar complaints may be suggestive of such an attack. Large numbers of patients presenting with fevers, cough, and myalgias may be nothing unusual in mid-January, but if this is happening in August, it may be something that needs to be investigated. Maintaining a high degree of suspicion is your best defense against this kind of activity. Participation in a syndromic surveillance network helps strengthen the safety net for detection of these events. Table 3.4 lists common presenting signs and symptoms for the CDC Class A Biological Weapons.

14. What type of equipment should an urgent care center have readily available for a public health event like the recent COVID-19 pandemic?
    As we have learned since the onset of the COVID-19 pandemic in early 2020, health care facilities overall in the US were not adequately prepared for an epidemic of this scale. Urgent care centers in particular faced challenges obtaining PPE and N-95 masks. Many centers experienced significant lability in volume as well as difficulty navigating the frequent changes in guidance from the CDC, state, and local public health agencies.

Having a supply of PPE, especially N-95 or equivalent masks or elastomeric respirators with appropriate filters, is critical for staff safety and preservation of the health care workforce that is needed to care for the increased volumes that hospitals and urgent care centers have seen since the fall of 2020. Having a plan for increasing throughput is also recommended. As with any surge or disaster plan, tabletop exercises and drills will result in more efficient implementation of the plan when it is actually needed. Urgent care centers should also work with local public health, EMS, and disaster management agencies to ensure that they are included in all disaster preparedness and planning.

KEY POINTS

1. Urgent care centers must be able to rapidly recognize, assess, stabilize, and transfer patients presenting to their center with medical and traumatic emergencies beyond the capability of the center.
2. Communication among staff, local EMS, and the receiving hospital is important when dealing with an office emergency and arranging patient transfer.
3. Consistent oversight, planning, and quality improvement/management are crucial in emergency and disaster preparedness.

BIBLIOGRAPHY

Committee on Pediatric Emergency Medicine. Pediatric care recommendations for freestanding urgent care facilities. *Pediatrics.* 2014;133(5):950–953.

Dunnick J, Olympia RP, Wilkinson R, Brady J. Low compliance of urgent care centers in the United States with recommendations for office-based disaster preparedness. *Pediatr Emerg Care.* 2016;32(5):298–302.

Gardener R, Choo EK, Gravenstein S, Baier RR. Why is this patient begin sent here? Communication from urgent care to the emergency department. *J Emerg Med.* 2016;50:416–421.

LaVelle BA, McLaughlin JJ. Simulation-Based Education Improves Patient Safety in Ambulatory Care. In: Henriksen K, Battles JB, Keyes MA et al., eds. *Advances in Patient Safety: New Directions and Alternative Approaches (Vol. 3: Performance and Tools).* Rockville (MD): Agency for Healthcare Research and Quality (US); 2008. Available from http://www.ncbi.nlm.nih.gov/books/NBK43667/.

Liddy C, Dreise H, Gaboury I. Frequency of in-office emergencies in primary care. *Can Fam Physician.* 2009;55:1004–1005.e1-e4.

Monachino A, Caraher C, Ginsberg J, Bailey C, White E. Medical Emergencies in the Primary Care Setting: An Evidence Based Practice Approach Using Simulation to Improve Readiness. *J Pediatr Nurs.* 2019;49:72–78. doi:10.1016/j.pedn.2019.09.017. Epub 2019 Oct 25. PMID: 31670140.

Sturge D. Pandemic Impact on Urgent Care and 4 Strategies to Protect Revenue. Accessed 8/27/2022 at https://www.hmpgloballearningnetwork.com/site/ihe/commentary/pandemic-impact-urgent-care-and-4-strategies-protect-revenue-moving-forward.

Saidinejad M, Paul A, Gausche-Hill M, Woolridge D, Heins A, Scott WR, Friesen P, Rayburn D, Conners G, Petrack E, Horeczko T, Stoner M, Edgerton E, Joseph M. Consensus Statement on Urgent Care Centers and Retail Clinics in Acute Care of Children. *Pediatr Emerg Care.* 2019;35(2):138–142. doi:10.1097/PEC.0000000000001656. PMID: 30422946.

Scaramuzzo LA, Wong Y, Voitle KL, Gordils-Perez J. Cardiopulmonary arrest in the outpatient setting: Enhancing patient safety through rapid response algorithms and simulation teaching. *Clin J Onc Nursing.* 2014;18:61–64.

Shamji H, Baier RR, Gravenstein S, Gardner RL. Improving the quality of care and communication during patient transitions: best practices for urgent care centers. *Jt Comm J Qual Patient Safety.* 2014;40:319–324.

Toback S. Medical emergency preparedness in office practice. *Am Fam Physician.* 2007;75:1679–1684.

Wilkinson R, Olympia RP, Dunnick J, Brady J. Pediatric care provided at urgent care centers in the United States: compliance with recommendations for emergency preparedness. *Pediatr Emerg Care.* 2016;32(2):77–81.

Yuknis ML, Weinstein E, Maxey H, Price L, Vaughn SX, Arkins T, Benneyworth BD. Frequency of Pediatric Emergencies in Ambulatory Practices. *Pediatrics.* 2018;142(2):e20173082. doi:10.1542/peds.2017-3082. PMID: 30030368.

CHAPTER 4

ADULT EMERGENCIES PRESENTING TO URGENT CARE CENTERS

Joshua Davis, MD, Jesse Tran, DO

CASE

A 29-year-old man with history of asthma is brought to the urgent care center for trouble breathing that started a couple of hours ago. He did not have his inhaler with him while he was out, and he got worse on his way home, so he stopped at your urgent care center. On arrival, he is found to be in moderate distress. Heart rate is 110 bpm; respiratory rate is 30 bpm; BP is 122/88 mmHg; SpO_2 is 80% in room air; and temperature is 37.2 degrees Centigrade. His heart is in regular rhythm and tachycardic. His respiratory exam shows tachypnea with shallow breathing, retractions, decreased breath sounds, and expiratory wheezing bilaterally. You need to decide what your next course of action is.

GENERAL APPROACH

1. **What is the focus of care for adults presenting to urgent care with life-threatening emergencies?**
   The priorities of the treatment of emergencies in urgent care centers include early recognition; stabilization within the resources provided; and rapid, safe disposition. Most true medical emergencies cannot be handled definitively with the resources provided in most urgent care centers. Thus, early recognition of these cases is key so the patient can receive definitive care in a timely manner.

2. **How do you recognize a medical emergency?**
   Keys to early recognition include identification of "red flag" signs or symptoms such as abnormal vital signs, maintaining a broad differential, and knowledge of common emergencies and what resources are available in your urgent care center. Other high-risk presentations include chest pain, neurologic symptoms, and those at extremes of age. Protocols for high-risk situations can help in the early recognition of subtle emergencies that may be outside the scope of urgent care center resources.

3. **What are the priorities of stabilization in medical emergencies?**
   The keys to medical stabilization are the basics of life support and resuscitation. This includes "C-A-B" (Circulation, Airway, and Breathing). What type of resuscitation can be provided will be based on available resources. Patients with low blood pressure may need IV access and fluids, if available. Epinephrine can be used, also, if available. Any obstruction to the airway should be removed and the patient may need to have respiratory support including supplemental oxygen or mask ventilation. Be mindful that mask ventilation can support respirations—even in an awake patient—until other noninvasive support, such as continuous or bilevel positive airway pressure, or intubation is available.
   "DEFG" is an often-missed corollary in emergency situations, which stands for "Don't ever forget the glucose." Blood glucose is a key component in many medical emergencies.
   In an emergency, it is important to engage all resources and staff available. This includes early activation of the emergency medical services (EMS) system. Teamwork and high-fidelity, closed-loop communication are important components of high-quality resuscitation care.

4. **How do you appropriately disposition a patient to a higher level of care?**
   All patients with medical emergencies should be transported by ambulance to the nearest emergency department (ED) with capabilities to handle the patient. Sending a patient to the ED via private vehicle is always a risky decision. In this case, any patient deterioration en route could result in harm to the patient, delay in care, and liability to the sending clinician. The EMS team can help determine an appropriate hospital based on the patient's needs. Having preexisting relationships with local hospitals can help streamline care for time-sensitive conditions like STEMI and stroke.
   Any relevant diagnostic tests and a list of treatments administered (medication administration record; MAR) should be sent with the patient. A verbal handoff report should always be given to the receiving hospital for any patient sent to the ED, ideally before the patient leaves the urgent care center. However, stabilization and transport should not be delayed in time-sensitive cases in order to give a verbal handoff. This verbal report can help streamline care and ensure the patient ends up at a hospital that has the resources to adequately care for the patient.

Clinicians should be familiar with local laws and the specifics of their facility. Most urgent care centers (as opposed to EDs) are not covered under the EMTALA (Emergency Medical Treatment and Labor Act) law. Thus, direct communication and obtaining an accepting physician are not required in order to transport the patient. However, while direct communication may not be a legal requirement, it is an expected standard for patient safety.

5. **How do you prepare for medical emergencies in urgent care?**
Clinicians need to be familiar with the resources available at their urgent care center. This includes knowing the location and organization of emergency supplies. Routine practice, even with simulation or mental practice and visualization, is an important method to improve the quality of emergency medical care. This is especially important for high-risk, low-volume situations and procedures like resuscitation. Teamwork can be improved in these situations when the team practices together.

CHEST PAIN

6. **What is the approach to the patient with chest pain?**
Any patient who appears acutely ill and complains of chest pain needs to be taken seriously. The basic approach to resuscitation above should be followed, including the C-A-B approach. A 12-lead electrocardiogram (ECG) should be obtained in any adult patient with chest pain, particularly those who are ill, have abnormal vital signs, have a history of coronary disease, or are elderly. A chest radiograph (x-ray) is routinely indicated as well.

7. **What are the potentially life-threatening causes of chest pain?**
Pulmonary embolism (PE), myocardial infarction (MI), pneumothorax, hemothorax, aortic dissection, esophageal rupture, pneumonia, and cardiac tamponade can cause life-threatening chest pain.

8. **What are the criteria for ST-segment elevation myocardial infarction on ECG?**
An ST-segment elevation myocardial infarction (STEMI) is identified by ST-segment elevation in two or more contiguous leads (Fig. 4.1). Threshold values vary based on age and gender, but in general, if the elevation is >1 mm in two leads on the ECG, there is a high index of suspicion for STEMI.
   It is important to note that recent literature has identified many ECG findings of occlusive myocardial infarction that are not STEMI but still provide mortality and morbidity, and these will benefit from immediate reperfusion (catheterization) (Figs. 4.2 and 4.3). The ECG machine is imperfect in identifying STEMI and even more unreliable in identifying these findings of occlusive myocardial infarction that are not STEMI. The urgent care clinician must continuously hone his or her ECG interpretation skills. Reliance on the ECG machine reading will lead to many misdiagnoses.

9. **What actions should be taken for a patient with chest pain and an occlusive myocardial infarction or STEMI on ECG?**
Arrange transportation to the nearest hospital with a cardiac catheterization laboratory (Cath lab), where percutaneous coronary intervention (PCI, stenting) can be performed. Call ahead to the hospital to alert them of the incoming patient. Provide a full dose of aspirin (162–325 mg). Place the patient on a cardiac monitor for rapid transport.

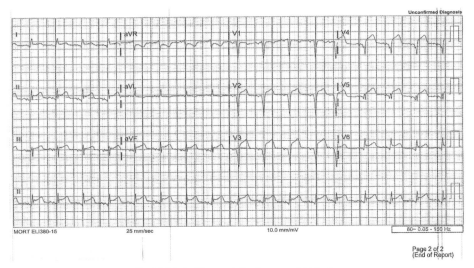

Fig. 4.1 Anterior ST-segment elevation myocardial infarction.

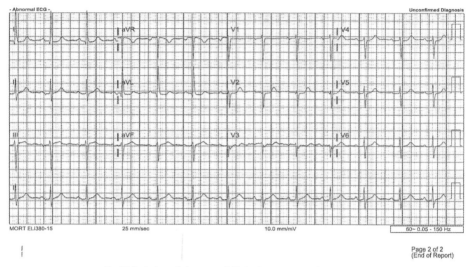

Fig. 4.2 Posterior occlusive myocardial infarction (not meeting STEMI criteria).

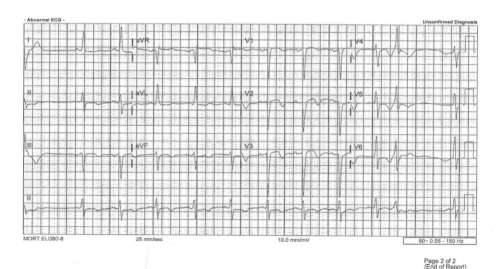

Fig. 4.3 Wellen's T waves–diagnostic of anterior occlusive myocardial infarction (not meeting STEMI criteria).

There are several traditional components of ACS care that are controversial. Analgesia can be given if needed. This may include nitroglycerin if no contraindications, or opioid pain medication. Some evidence suggests morphine may inhibit antiplatelet agents and may not be the ideal agent, though evidence for this is weak. Analgesia and nitroglycerin do not improve outcomes, though. There is evidence that supplemental oxygen provides no benefit unless the patient is hypoxemic. It also may increase infarct size.

10. **Which patients with chest pain of possible cardiac origin and a nondiagnostic ECG need to be transported to the hospital?**
There are several scores designed to risk-stratify patients with possible acute coronary syndrome. A standardized approach is recommended by experts and national guidelines. The most commonly used score in emergency medicine is the HEART score, but other scores include the GRACE, EDACS, and TIMI scores. Each has its pros and cons.

The HEART score is an acronym that stands for History, ECG, Age, Risk Factors, and Troponin (Table 4.1). Patients with a HEART score of 3 or less and reliable follow-up can safely be referred for prompt outpatient care.

Table 4.1 History, ECG, Age, Risk Factors, and Troponin (HEART) for Risk Stratification of Acute Coronary Syndrome in Patients With Chest Pain

CRITERIA	Score (Points)		
	0	1	2
History[1]	Not suspicious or slightly suspicious	Moderately suspicious	Highly suspicious
ECG	Normal	Non-specific repolarization disturbance[2]	Significant ST deviation not related to left ventricular hypertrophy, left bundle branch block, or digoxin
Age	<45 years old	45–64 years old	>64 years old
Risk factors[3]	No known risk factors	1–2 risk factors	3 or more risk factors
Troponin[4]	Within normal limits	1–2x normal limit	>2x normal limit

[1]High-risk historical features include retrosternal pain, pressure, radiation to jaw/left shoulder/arms, duration 5–15 min, initiated by exercise/cold/emotion, perspiration, nausea/vomiting, reaction on nitrates within mins, patient recognizes symptoms. Low-risk features include well-localized, sharp, nonexertional, no diaphoresis, no nausea or vomiting, and reproducible with palpation.
[2]Left bundle branch block, typical changes suggesting left ventricular hypertrophy, repolarization disorders suggesting digoxin, unchanged known repolarization disorders.
[3]Hypertension, dyslipidemia, diabetes, obesity (BMI >30 kg/m^2), smoking, parent or sibling with CVD before age 65.
[4]Updated versions of the HEART score use three times the normal limit.
Patients with a HEART score of 3 or less have <1–2% chance of major adverse cardiac events in 30 days.
Source: Six AJ, Backus BE, Kelder JC. Chest pain in the emergency room: value of the HEART score. *Neth Heart J.* 2008;16(6):191–196. doi:10.1007/BF03086144.

All other patients with chest pain of possible cardiac origin should be evaluated in an ED with prolonged cardiac monitoring capabilities.

A troponin may not be available in the urgent care setting. Thus, historical features may need to be used to stratify patients of risk for ACS. A systematic review shows features such as radiation to either or both arms, vomiting, diaphoresis, and chest pain similar to prior MI may suggest patients who are at high risk for acute coronary syndrome. Any patient over 65 years old, those with known coronary disease, and smokers are high-risk patients. Response to nitroglycerin has often historically been used to predict if ACS is the cause of chest pain. However, data show this is not accurate, and the American Heart Association Guidelines clearly state, "Relief with nitroglycerin is not necessarily diagnostic of myocardial ischemia and should not be used as a diagnostic criterion."

Cardiac arrest and sudden cardiac death can be the rare outcome of acute coronary syndrome. There is often not a second chance to recover from this. Thus, any patient with uncertainty regarding chest pain and acute coronary syndrome should be sent (via ambulance) to the ED for expert consultation and prolonged monitoring.

11. **What is an approach to the evaluation of pulmonary embolism (PE) in the urgent care setting?**
A patient with PE may present with pleuritic chest pain, tachycardia, unilateral leg swelling, and hypoxemia, but there is no single history or exam finding that is sensitive or specific to PE. Risk factors for pulmonary embolism include recent prolonged (>4 hours) travel, immobility, travel, estrogen use, pregnancy, smoking, cancer, obesity, and hypercoagulability. In the ED, the Pulmonary Embolism Rule-out Criteria (PERC rule) has been validated in order to identify patients who are at very low risk for PE and do not need further testing as the risks of testing outweigh the benefits (Box 4.1). PE can be potentially life-threatening, and any patient with concern for PE should be evaluated in the ED.

Box 4.1 Pulmonary Embolism Rule-Out Criteria (PERC)

- Age ≥50
- HR ≥100
- O$_2$ sat on room air <95%
- Prior history of venous thromboembolism
- Trauma or surgery within 4 weeks
- Hemoptysis

- Exogenous estrogen
- Unilateral leg swelling

If no criteria are present and the pretest probability is <15%, the patient is low-risk for PE and does not require any further testing.

STROKE

12. **What is a stroke or cerebrovascular accident (CVA)?**
A stroke is defined as brain cell death due to a blockage or rupture of a blood vessel that supplies that area of the brain. There are two types of strokes. Ischemic stroke, which is caused by a clot obstructing the flow of blood to the brain, causes about 80% of strokes. Hemorrhagic stroke comprises the other 20% and is due to the rupture of a blood vessel leading to blood leakage in the brain and thus preventing blood flow to that area.

13. **What is a transient ischemic attack (TIA)?**
TIA is often colloquially referred to as "mini-stroke" by patients. The current definition of TIA is a transient episode of neurologic dysfunction caused by focal brain, spinal cord, or retinal ischemia, without acute infarction. Patients with TIA have a very high risk of recurrent stroke; up to 15 % in 90 days, with the vast majority of these occurring in the first 3–7 days.

14. **What are the most important pieces of history to ask regarding a patient with suspected stroke?**
In addition to gathering the history of recent events and symptoms the patient is experiencing, the exact time that the patient was last noted to be feeling at baseline (last known well) is a crucial piece of information that affects treatment. It is very important to differentiate symptom onset from last known well. This is because within up to 4.5 hours last known normal, treatment with thrombolytics, while controversial, may have improved outcomes for patients diagnosed with ischemic stroke and is still considered standard care in most centers. There is also convincing evidence that patients with large vessel occlusions also benefit from mechanical thrombectomy within 24 hours of symptoms.

15. **What are the signs and symptoms concerning for a stroke or TIA?**
Unilateral weakness or sensory deficits, facial droop, or speech problems are the most common symptoms of stroke (Table 4.2). The National Institute of Health Stroke Scale (NIHSS) is commonly used to identify stroke-like symptoms (Table 4.3). This is generally focused on anterior circulation strokes. An NIHSS greater than 6 is often considered concerning for a large vessel occlusion. Other signs and symptoms of stroke or TIA include vision changes, vertigo, nausea, vomiting, ataxia, and altered mental status.

16. **What are common stroke "mimics"?**
Hypoglycemia, seizure, syncope, intracranial mass, complex migraine, psychiatric disorder, metabolic disorder, peripheral vertigo, sepsis, encephalopathy, transient global amnesia, drugs, alcohol, and dementia.

17. **What are the priorities in the management of a patient with suspected stroke or TIA in urgent care?**
Rule out hypoglycemia by checking a glucose level. After initial stabilization, patients with acute (i.e., less than 24-hour onset), potentially disabling neurologic symptoms should be transported emergently via ambulance to a stroke-capable center to determine if any interventions may benefit the patient. Stroke is a time-sensitive diagnosis, particularly if there are disabling symptoms. Time should not be spent evaluating alternative causes of stroke or mimics (other than hypoglycemia) if acute stroke is a concern and the patient is eligible for acute stroke interventions.

An advanced and rational approach to acute neurologic symptoms would include an assessment of eligibility from thrombolysis or mechanical thrombectomy and stratification of whether stroke is a leading differential diagnosis. Patients with subjective, nondisabling symptoms, or those who are not eligible for acute interventions, could potentially have some workup or treatment initiated in the urgent care setting if a stroke is not highly suspected. This will depend on the resources available at a given urgent care center, the comfort level of the clinician, and shared decision making with the patient. It is always best to err on the side of caution and rapidly transport a patient via ambulance to the ED if there is any question or concern.

Table 4.2 B-FAST Signs and Symptoms Concerning for Stroke or TIA

B	Balance problems
F	Face drooping
A	Arm weakness
S	Speech difficulty
T	Time to call 911/arrange rapid transport to the emergency department

Table 4.3 National Institutes of Health Stroke Scale

CRITERIA	Score (Points)				
	0	**1**	**2**	**3**	**4**
Level of consciousness	Alert	Arouses to minor stimulation	Requires repeated stimulation to arouse; movements to pain	Posturing or unresponsive	
Orientation (ask month and age)	Answers both right	1 question right	0 questions right or unable to answer		
Command following ("blink eyes" and "squeeze hand")	Performs both tasks	Performs 1 task	Performs 0 tasks		
Gaze	Normal	Partial gaze palsy can be overcome	Partial gaze palsy cannot be overcome		
Visual fields	Normal	Partial hemianopia	Complete hemianopia	Bilaterally blind	
Facial palsy	Normal	Minor paralysis	Partial paralysis	Complete or bilateral paralysis	
Left arm strength (drift)	No drift	Drifts but does not hit bed	Drifts to bed or some effort against gravity	No effort against gravity	No effort
Right arm strength (drift)	No drift	Drifts but does not hit bed	Drifts to bed or some effort against gravity	No effort against gravity	No effort
Left leg strength (drift)	No drift	Drifts but does not hit bed	Drifts to bed or some effort against gravity	No effort against gravity	No effort
Right leg strength (drift)	No drift	Drifts but does not hit bed	Drifts to bed or some effort against gravity	No effort against gravity	No effort
Limb ataxia	No ataxia	Ataxia in 1 limb	Ataxia in both limbs		
Sensation	No sensation loss	Mild sensation loss	Complete sensation loss or unresponsive		
Aphasia	Normal	Mild/moderate aphasia	Severe aphasia	Mute or unresponsive	
Dysarthria	Normal	Mild/moderate dysarthria	Severe dysarthria or mute		
Extinction/ inattention	Normal	Extinction to bilateral stimuli	Profound hemi-attention or extinction to >1 modality		

Scores range from 0 (no deficits) to 42 (severe deficit).
Scores 6 or greater are concerning for large or moderate to severe stroke.
Adapted from National Institute of Neurological Disorders and Stroke rt-PA Stroke Study Group. Tissue plasminogen activator for acute ischemic stroke. *N Engl J Med.* 1995;333(24):1581–1587. doi:10.1056/NEJM199512143332401.

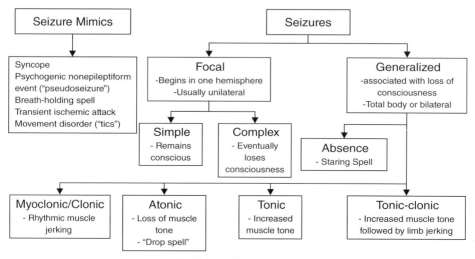

Fig. 4.4 Seizure types and mimics.

SEIZURE

18. **What are the commonly encountered seizure types, and what do these look like to an observer?**
    Not all seizures look the same, and urgent care providers should be able to identify the common seizure patterns and mimics described in Fig. 4.4.

19. **What are the common causes of seizures?**
    While many of these seizure types can look similar, it is important to recognize that not all seizures are caused by epilepsy. Seizures can be caused by electrolyte disturbances (namely hypoglycemia or hyponatremia), infection, stroke, brain masses, substance use or toxins, or alcohol or benzodiazepine withdrawal.

20. **How can you help a patient who is actively seizing in urgent care?**
    First, utilize the C-A-B approach to resuscitation. Make sure the patient's airway is clear. Apply supplemental oxygen. Unless the patient is at risk of imminent trauma (e.g., falling out of a bed), restraining or moving them while seizing can cause harm. Check blood glucose when safe and able and treat with dextrose if patient is hypoglycemic. Once the patient is in a safe position, administer an appropriate dose of whatever benzodiazepine is available at the urgent care center. In an actively seizing patient, this can be done via rectal, intravenous, intranasal, or intramuscular routes. Midazolam is the most rapidly acting benzodiazepine, if available.

ALTERED MENTAL STATUS

21. **What is an approach to assessing mental status in a patient "altered from baseline"?**
    The most important part of an altered mental status workup is a focused history and physical exam, along with a blood glucose level. Find a family member, friend, or health care worker who knows the patient well and has seen them recently. Get an idea of the patient's prior functional baseline, what exactly is different, and when it started. Be aware that patients and family will often use terms like "disoriented" and "lethargic" in ways that are not consistent with their traditional medical definitions. Thus, specific questioning is needed. Further, it is also common that a visiting family member may not know the patient's baseline.
    The physical exam should be thorough with a focus on mental status and an appropriate neurologic exam. Orientation, gait, strength, sensation, cranial nerves, reflexes, coordination, and speech are key components of an acute mental status examination.

22. **What is the appropriate disposition for a patient with altered mental status?**
    The differential for altered mental status is exceedingly long and will likely be unable to be completely evaluated in the urgent care setting. Thus, most patients with altered mental status should be evaluated in an ED.

Table 4.4 Differentiating Syncope vs. Seizure

SYNCOPE	SEIZURE
No aura	Aura
Post-loss of consciousness jerks	Pre-loss of consciousness jerks
Asynchronous jerks	Synchronous jerks
Tongue bite at the tip or no tongue biting	Tongue bite lateral
Flaccid	Stiff
Quick recovery	Postictal (confused period)
	Transient elevation in lactic acid, anion gap, creatinine phosphokinase, and prolactin
	Urinary incontinence

SYNCOPE

23. **What is syncope?**
Syncope is defined as sudden, brief loss of consciousness due to transient global cerebral hypoperfusion with spontaneous complete recovery that is not attributed to another cause (i.e., seizure or stroke).

24. **How does one differentiate between syncope and seizure?**
A syncopal episode can sometimes be confused with a seizure. Fortunately, some features of the episode can help differentiate the two (Table 4.4).

25. **What is an appropriate approach to the patient with syncope presenting to the urgent care center?**
There is no "standard" workup for a patient presenting with syncope. Most guidelines recommend a thorough history, physical examination, and ECG. Female patients of childbearing age should have a pregnancy test performed. If an etiology for syncope is identified, the patient should be managed according to the causal condition. Some patients may need laboratory testing or prolonged cardiac monitoring. Rarely, patients may need neuroimaging or other advanced testing. Most patients can be managed in the outpatient setting.

26. **How does one best risk stratify a patient who presents with syncope?**
Cardiac causes of syncope, namely ventricular dysrhythmias, are among the most feared and risky causes of syncope. This will be present in a minority of patients. Multiple risk stratification tools for patients with syncope have been developed; however, none have been proven to perform better than clinical judgment. Overall, admission to the hospital has not been shown to benefit patients with syncope. Nevertheless, there are some features that are considered high-risk or low-risk for cardiogenic syncope. Elderly patients and those with heart disease (coronary disease or heart failure), anemia, family history of early cardiac death, and unheralded syncope are high-risk patients. Young patients and those with clear orthostatic or vasovagal syncope are considered lower-risk.
   Abnormal ECG findings should prompt further investigation (Table 4.5). Some findings on ECG that are not considered high-risk include first-degree AV nodal block, rare premature ventricular contractions, or sinus arrhythmia. The ECG machine is quite reliable in reading intervals, but it will often miss or misdiagnose other subtle high-risk findings.

27. **What is the disposition of a patient presenting with syncope?**
The disposition for the patient should consider the clinical gestalt, perceived risk, cost, potential adverse events, available resources in urgent care, access to outpatient care, and patient preference. As noted above, most patients do not benefit from inpatient hospitalization, but further testing in the ED may be helpful. Any patient with concerning ECG findings should be evaluated in the ED.

RESPIRATORY DISTRESS

28. **What are the top priorities in the approach to a patient presenting in respiratory distress?**
Place the patient in a position of comfort. Perform head tilt/chin lift and/or jaw thrust to ensure an open airway. Remove any obvious material obstructing the airway but avoid blind finger sweep. Apply oxygen as necessary. A bag-valve mask can be used to support respirations and ventilation, even in an awake patient, until other more advanced forms of respiratory support are available. Treat the underlying cause with the resources available. Respiratory distress should almost always be treated in the ED. Very rarely, patients with reversible causes of respiratory distress can be stabilized and discharged home. This is outside the scope of most urgent care centers.

Table 4.5 Low- and High-Risk Features of Syncope

LOW-RISK FEATURES	HIGH-RISK FEATURES
Age <40 years	Age > 40 years
Characteristics of syncope: • Only while standing • Standing from supine/sitting • Nausea/vomiting before syncope • Feeling warm before syncope • Triggered by stress/pain • Triggered by cough/defecation/micturition	• During exertion • In supine position • New onset chest discomfort • Palpitations or no symptoms before syncope • Associated with shortness of breath
Past history: • Prolonged history of recurrent syncope similar to current episode	• Family history of sudden death • Congestive heart failure • Aortic stenosis • Left ventricular outflow tract disease • Dilated cardiomyopathy • Hypertrophic cardiomyopathy • Arrhythmogenic right ventricular cardiomyopathy • Ejection fraction <35% • Ventricular arrhythmias • Coronary artery disease • Congenital heart disease • Previous myocardial infarction • Pulmonary hypertension • Previous ICD implantation
	Vital signs and laboratory findings: • Anemia (hemoglobin <9 g/dL) • Systolic blood pressure <90 mm Hg • Sinus bradycardia (<40 bpm)
	ECG features: • New bundle branch block • Brugada pattern • Ischemic changes • New non-sinus rhythm • Prolonged QTc (>450 ms) • Prolonged QRS (>120 ms) • U waves • Peaked T waves • >10% ventricular ectopy

29. **What potentially life-threatening diagnoses must be considered for a patient in respiratory distress presenting to an urgent care center and their associated interventions?**

    Asthma, COPD (chronic obstructive pulmonary disease), heart failure, pneumonia, pneumothorax, pulmonary embolism, and anaphylaxis. Clinicians would be wise to remember nonpulmonary causes of respiratory distress, like acidosis. Checking blood glucose may be helpful in identifying DKA as a cause of respiratory distress.

30. **How does one diagnose and treat someone with severe asthma or COPD?**

    Obstructive lung diseases like asthma and COPD often present with tachypnea and wheezing. Sometimes decreased air entry or hypoxemia may be present. Patients will most often already have a diagnosis of these diseases and have home treatments. Chest x-ray, if available, will be normal or show hyperinflation. After stabilization, the treatment for asthma and COPD includes bronchodilators (albuterol, ipratropium) and rapid steroid administration. While the bioavailability of steroids is equal for oral and parenteral routes, patients in severe distress should ideally be given parenteral medications in order to prevent worsening of their respiratory status or aspiration. Advanced therapies for asthma and COPD that may be available in some urgent care centers include epinephrine and rapid administration of IV magnesium (2 grams over 20 minutes). Noninvasive ventilation (CPAP and BiPAP) has been shown to reduce the need for intubation and improve the time to improvement in patients with severe asthma and COPD.

31. **What is the diagnostic and treatment approach to the patient with acute heart failure/ pulmonary edema?**

    Patients with acute heart failure typically present with rales, jugular venous distention, orthopnea, and bilateral lower extremity edema. They may present with hypertension or hypoxemia. They often, but not always, have a known diagnosis of congestive heart failure. Chest x-ray, if available, will show enlarged heart and pulmonary vascular congestion or pulmonary edema and sometimes pleural effusions. These patients often will not tolerate lying flat and it may worsen their respiratory status. Reducing afterload can help patients in distress from heart failure. Hypertensive patients with heart failure benefit from afterload reduction with nitroglycerin. Diuretics, if available, may be administered, but are not a priority in patients in distress. Respirations may need to be supported. As above, this can be done via bag-valve mask until other more advanced forms of respiratory support are available. Noninvasive ventilation (CPAP and BiPAP) has been shown to reduce the need for intubation and improve outcomes in patients with acute heart failure.

32. **What is the diagnostic and therapeutic approach to pneumothorax in the urgent care center?**

    Patients with pneumothorax will have absent breath sounds on one side and tachypnea. Tall male patients and those with COPD are at risk of spontaneous pneumothorax, and trauma is another common cause of pneumothorax. Severe pneumothorax may cause "tension physiology." In this case, the patient will be in severe distress, may have jugular venous distention, may have tracheal deviation, and often will be hypotensive. Patients with simple pneumothorax can often be initially treated with high-flow oxygen (regardless of oxygen saturation levels). Patients with tension physiology need immediate decompression. An experienced clinician can perform needle decompression to stabilize a patient in this situation. All patients with pneumothorax should be transported to the ED. At a minimum, they will need prolonged observation. Some patients will need a chest tube to reinflate the lungs.

ANAPHYLAXIS

33. **What is anaphylaxis?**

    Anaphylaxis is a serious allergic reaction that is rapid in onset and potentially life-threatening. It is a multisystem disorder that involves symptoms from cutaneous, respiratory, cardiovascular, gastrointestinal, and central nervous systems.

34. **What are the most common causes of anaphylaxis?**

    Food (e.g., nuts, fish, shellfish, dairy, eggs), medications (e.g., penicillins), and insect stings and bites (e.g., bees, vespids, stinging ants) are the most common causes of anaphylaxis.

35. **What are the diagnostic criteria for anaphylaxis?**

    Diagnostic criteria are listed in Table 4.6. It is important to memorize these criteria. Patients can have atypical presentations (i.e., vomiting and rash) and still meet the criteria for anaphylaxis. Early identification and treatment of all patients with anaphylaxis is key to improving outcomes and preventing deterioration.

36. **What are the main treatment priorities for a patient in anaphylaxis?**

    Timely administration of epinephrine is the treatment for anaphylaxis. Epinephrine is administered at a dose of 0.01 mg/kg of 1:1000 solution (up to 0.5 mg for adults) into the intramuscular space of midanterolateral thigh or deltoid and repeated every 5–15 minutes as needed. If available, crystalloid fluids (5–10 mL/kg) should be given via large bore IV. Respiratory distress should be addressed as discussed above. Any other medications should not delay the administration of epinephrine.

Table 4.6 Diagnostic Criteria for Anaphylaxis	
Acute onset symptoms with involvement of the skin, mucosal tissue, or both AND at least one of these:	• Respiratory compromise (e.g., dyspnea, bronchospasm, stridor, hypoxemia) • Hypotension or symptoms of end-organ dysfunction (e.g., hypotonia, syncope)
Rapid onset of 2 or more symptoms after exposure to a likely allergen for that patient:	• Cutaneous or mucosal involvement (e.g., urticaria, angioedema, pruritus) • Respiratory compromise (e.g., dyspnea, bronchospasm, stridor, hypoxemia) • Hypotension or symptoms of end-organ dysfunction (e.g., hypotonia, syncope) • Persistent gastrointestinal symptoms (e.g., abdominal pain, vomiting)
Hypotension after exposure to known allergen for that patient	

Second-line medications such as albuterol should be given to a patient in bronchospasm. An antihistamine with the addition of an H2 blocker can be given for cutaneous symptoms. Diphenhydramine is often used, though guidelines suggest second- or third-generation antihistamines (loratadine, cetirizine, desloratadine, fexofenadine, levocetirizine) are preferred. Corticosteroids may prevent rebound or recurrence of symptoms and can be given as needed. Again, none of these medications should delay timely administration of epinephrine. A common pitfall in the treatment of anaphylaxis is to give an antihistamine and a corticosteroid and delay or avoid epinephrine administration. This should never be done in patients meeting the criteria for anaphylaxis.

37. **How does the disposition differ between patients with anaphylaxis compared to those with a less severe allergic reaction?**
Patients with anaphylaxis should be transferred as soon as possible to the nearest ED with critical care capability. Patients with mild allergic reactions without meeting the criteria for anaphylaxis (i.e., rash alone), with stable or improving symptoms, can be discharged with close follow-up with their primary care doctor. They should always be discharged with strict return precautions and a prescription for a self-injectable dose of epinephrine. They should be taught how to use the device and demonstrate how to do so before discharge. They should also be advised to avoid exposure to their suspected allergen.

SEPSIS

38. **What is the definition of sepsis?**
Sepsis is a syndrome of dysregulated host response to infection leading to life-threatening organ dysfunction. Sepsis can be life-threatening in its most severe forms.

39. **What are the clinical criteria for the diagnosis of sepsis?**
Sepsis is a clinical diagnosis. There is no single tool or test that will diagnose sepsis.

Historically, screening for sepsis was positive when a patient had two or more systemic inflammatory response syndrome (SIRS) criteria (Table 4.7) with suspected or documented infection. However, many experts have suggested this may be overly sensitive and may lead to overtesting and treatment. Thus, another tool has more recently been proposed—the quick Sequential Organ-Failure Assessment (qSOFA)—which can be used to identify adult patients with suspected infection who are likely to have poor outcomes (Table 4.7). This may be preferred in the urgent care setting as no diagnostic tests are needed for this tool. Which tool to use to screen for sepsis remains a controversial topic. Regardless, early recognition and treatment of sepsis can improve outcomes. True sepsis, i.e., with organ dysfunction, will not be able to be treated in the urgent care setting, and patients will need transfer via ambulance to the nearest ED.

40. **What are the main management priorities in the urgent care setting when caring for a patient with suspected sepsis?**
The urgent care clinician can help patient care by establishing IV access, if able, and initiating IV fluid resuscitation. Timely administration of appropriate parenteral antibiotics can be initiated, if available, though obtaining cultures prior to this is preferred. Transportation to the nearest ED is crucial.

CASE CONCLUSION

You place your patient, a 29-year-old with a moderately severe asthma exacerbation, on supplemental oxygen. You administer continuous nebulized albuterol through a face mask. You activate the EMS system. You administer intramuscular dexamethasone. You contact the physician at the nearest local ED and give a verbal handoff report. EMS staff arrive and transport the patient to the ED, where he receives ongoing care and is eventually discharged from the hospital much improved.

Table 4.7 Comparing Sepsis Screening Criteria in Patients With Known or Suspected Infection	
SYSTEMIC INFLAMMATORY RESPONSE SYNDROME (SIRS) (2 OR MORE OF THE FOLLOWING)	**QUICK SEQUENTIAL ORGAN FAILURE ASSESSMENT (QSOFA) (2 OR MORE OF THE FOLLOWING)**
Temperature >38°C or <36°C	Altered mental status
Heart rate >90/min	Systolic blood pressure ≤100 mm Hg
Respiratory rate >20/min or $PaCO_2$ <32 mm Hg	Respiratory rate ≥22/min
White blood cell count >12,000/mm³ or <4000/mm³ or >10% immature bands	

KEY POINTS

1. In any patient presenting with chest pain, quickly ruling out STEMI and occlusive myocardial infarction on a 12-lead ECG must be a priority.
2. A patient with a suspected stroke or TIA with the last known normal within 24 hours should be transported to the closest stroke-capable center as soon as possible for consideration of thrombolytic therapy or thrombectomy.
3. Checking a fingerstick glucose early can rule out hypoglycemia as a treatable cause of any patient presenting with stroke-like symptoms, seizure, and altered mental status.
4. While the differential diagnosis for syncope or altered mental status is broad, there is no "standard workup" for either chief concern. A thorough focused history and physical exam are crucial to making the diagnosis.
5. Benzodiazepines are the first-line treatment for the seizing patient.
6. Rapid recognition of sepsis and early antibiotic administration are key to improving outcomes.
7. The mainstay of treatment for anaphylaxis is 0.5 mg intramuscular epinephrine for adults, repeated every 5–15 minutes as needed.

Acknowledgments

The authors would like to thank Drs. Jeffrey Rixe, MD and Alexander Sheng, MD for their contributions to this chapter in the previous edition.

BIBLIOGRAPHY

American College of Emergency Physicians Clinical Policies Committee; Clinical Policies Subcommittee on Seizures; Clinical policy: Critical issues in the evaluation and management of adult patients presenting to the emergency department with seizures. *Ann Emerg Med.* 2004;43(5):605–625. doi:10.1016/S019606440400068X.

American College of Emergency Physicians Clinical Policies Subcommittee (Writing Committee) on Use of Intravenous tPA for Ischemic Stroke, Brown MD, Burton JH, Nazarian DJ, Promes SB. Clinical Policy: Use of Intravenous Tissue Plasminogen Activator for the Management of Acute Ischemic Stroke in the Emergency Department. *Ann Emerg Med.* 2015;66(3):322–333.e31. doi:10.1016/j.annemergmed.2015.06.031. Erratum in: *Ann Emerg Med.* 2017;70(5):758.

American Heart Association. *Basic Life Support (BLS) Provider Manual*; 2016.

Aslanger EK, Yıldırımtürk Ö, Şimşek B, Bozbeyoğlu E, Şimşek MA, Yücel Karabay C, Smith SW, Değertekin M. Diagnostic accuracy of electrocardiogram for acute coronary occlusion resulting in myocardial infarction (DIFOCCULT Study). *Int J Cardiol Heart Vasc.* 2020;30:100603. doi:10.1016/j.ijcha.2020.100603.

Backus BE, Six AJ, Kelder JC, et al. A prospective validation of the HEART score for chest pain patients at the emergency department. *Int J Cardiol.* 2013;168(3):2153–2158. doi:10.1016/j.ijcard.2013.01.255. Epub 2013 Mar 7.

Costantino G, Sun BC, Barbic F, et al. Syncope clinical management in the emergency department: a consensus from the first international workshop on syncope risk stratification in the emergency department. *Eur Heart J.* 2015(i):ehv378.

Dodd A, Hughes A, Sargant N, Whyte AF, Soar J, Turner PJ. Evidence update for the treatment of anaphylaxis. *Resuscitation.* 2021;163:86–96. doi:10.1016/j.resuscitation.2021.04.010. Epub ahead of print.

Evans L, Rhodes A, Alhazzani W, et al. Surviving sepsis campaign: international guidelines for management of sepsis and septic shock 2021. *Intensive Care Med.* 2021;47(11):1181–1247. doi:10.1007/s00134-021-06506-y. Epub 2021 Oct 2.

Fanaroff AC, Rymer JA, Goldstein SA, Simel DL, Newby LK. Does this patient with chest pain have acute coronary syndrome? The rational clinical examination systematic review. *JAMA.* 2015;314(18):1955–1965.

Han JH, Wilber ST. Altered mental status in older patients in the emergency department. *Clin Geriatr Med.* 2013;29(1):101–136.

Kline JA, Mitchell AM, Kabrhel C, Richman PB, Courtney DM. Clinical criteria to prevent unnecessary diagnostic testing in emergency department patients with suspected pulmonary embolism. *J Thromb Haemost.* 2004;2(8):1247–1255.

Koita J, Riggio S, Jagoda A. The mental status examination in emergency practice. *Emerg Med Clin North Am.* 2010;28(3):439–451.

Mendelson SJ, Prabhakaran S. Diagnosis and Management of Transient Ischemic Attack and Acute Ischemic Stroke: A Review. *J Am Med Assoc.* 2021;325(11):1088–1098. doi:10.1001/jama.2020.26867.

Shaker MS, Wallace DV, Golden DBK, et al. Anaphylaxis-a 2020 practice parameter update, systematic review, and Grading of Recommendations, Assessment, Development and Evaluation (GRADE) analysis. *J Allergy Clin Immunol.* 2020;145(4):1082–1123. doi:10.1016/j.jaci.2020.01.017. Epub 2020 Jan 28.

Shen WK, Sheldon RS, Benditt DG, et al. 2017 ACC/AHA/HRS Guideline for the Evaluation and Management of Patients With Syncope: A Report of the American College of Cardiology/American Heart Association Task Force on Clinical Practice Guidelines and the Heart Rhythm Society. *J Am Coll Cardiol.* 2017;70(5):e39–e110. doi:10.1016/j.jacc.2017.03.003. Epub 2017 Mar 9. Erratum in: *J Am Coll Cardiol.* 2017 Oct 17;70(16):2102-2104.

Singer M, Deutschman CS, Seymour CW, et al. The Third International Consensus Definitions for Sepsis and Septic Shock (Sepsis-3). *J Am Med Assoc.* 2016;315(8):801–810. doi:10.1001/jama.2016.0287.

Thiruganasambandamoorthy V, Kwong K, Wells GA, et al. Development of the Canadian Syncope Risk Score to predict serious adverse events after emergency department assessment of syncope. *Can Med Assoc J.* 2016;188(12):E289–E298. doi:10.1503/cmaj.151469. Epub 2016 Jul 4.

CHAPTER 5

PEDIATRIC EMERGENCIES PRESENTING TO URGENT CARE CENTERS

Jennifer Dunnick, MD, MPH, Bruce E. Herman, MD, Jerri A. Rose, MD

TOP SECRETS

Rapid assessment and stabilization of the airway, breathing, and circulation and transfer to an emergency department should be the top priorities for children presenting to urgent care centers with emergent conditions.

ALTERED MENTAL STATUS

1. **The differential diagnosis for altered mental status is quite broad. How can the etiologies be quickly recalled?**
   There's a mnemonic for that! The "tips on vowels," AEIOU TIPS (Fig. 5.1), is a useful tool for remembering the major categories of causes that should be considered in children presenting with altered mental status.

2. **What are the most common causes of altered mental status in children?**
   The potential causes of altered mental status in children are numerous, including both structural brain disorders and systemic diseases. Trauma, infections, intoxications, and metabolic abnormalities are among the most common reasons for children to present with altered mental status.

3. **What are the signs of altered mental status in infants and young children?**
   In children who cannot yet talk, it can be difficult to discern alterations from their usual. Crying, inconsolability, irritability, lethargy, and/or poor feeding are common manifestations for patients in this age group. Remember to use the parents as a resource because they are the experts on their child's baseline mental status.

4. **What tools can be used to quantify a child's mental status?**
   The Glasgow Coma Scale (GCS) and Alert, Voice, Pain, Unresponsive (AVPU) scale (Table 5.1 and Fig. 5.2) are widely used and accepted tools that can be used to quantify and communicate a child's neurologic status. There is a separate GCS for infants, since verbal response is required in the traditional GCS. These scales allow for the standardized evaluation, documentation, and communication of a child's changing neurologic status over time.

5. **What elements of the medical history are particularly critical to obtain for children presenting with altered mental status?**
   Use the AEIOU TIPS mnemonic again to help guide your history taking. What medications are in the home? Have they had recent sick symptoms? Did you see any abnormal movements? Does the child have a known history of a seizure disorder or diabetes? Has the child suffered any trauma, especially head injuries? While these questions can elicit much of the necessary information, always remember that history alone should not rule out trauma as a cause. Head trauma could be unwitnessed or unreported in the case of nonaccidental trauma.

A: Alcohol, Abuse of substances
E: Epilepsy, Encephalopathy, Electrolytes
I: Infection, Intussusception, Ischemia
O: Overdose, Oxygen deficiency
U: Uremia
T: Trauma, Temperature abnormality, Tumor
I: Infection, Increased intracranial pressure, Insulin-related problems
P: Poisoning, Psychiatric conditions, blood Pressure
S: Shock, Stroke, Space-occupying lesions, Shunt problems

Fig. 5.1 AEIOUTIPS mnemonic.

Table 5.1 Glasgow Coma Scale (GCS) for Infants and Children

	SCORE	INFANT	CHILD
Eye opening	4	Spontaneous	Spontaneous
	3	To speech	To speech
	2	To pain	To pain
	1	None	None
Verbal response	5	Coos and babbles	Oriented, appropriate
	4	Irritable, cries	Confused
	3	Cries in response to pain	Inappropriate words
	2	Moans in response to pain	Incomprehensible sounds
	1	None	None
Motor response	6	Spontaneous and purposeful	Obeys commands
	5	Withdraws to touch	Localizes painful stimulus
	4	Withdraws to pain	Withdraw to pain
	3	Abnormal flexion to pain	Flexion in response to pain
	2	Abnormal extension to pain	Extension in response to pain
	1	None	None

A: Alert
V: Response to verbal stimuli
P: Response to painful stimuli
U: Unresponsive

Fig. 5.2 AVPU mnemonic.

6. **What physical exam findings are important when assessing a child with altered mental status?**
   Some findings, like a head laceration or rhythmic jerking, will be immediately apparent to the provider. Most of the pertinent physical exam will be more subtle, though. Size and reactivity of the pupils can help you assess for possible ingestion or increased intracranial pressure. Increased tone and tachycardia may lead you to be concerned about seizure activity. Cool, mottled skin is worrisome for shock or environmental exposure.

7. **What is the initial approach for managing a child with altered mental status?**
   The initial management of any child presenting with altered mental status should begin with rapid assessment and support of the airway, breathing, and circulation. A full set of vitals should be obtained as quickly as possible. Temperature extremes in either direction can lead to an alteration from baseline mentation. Provide 100% oxygen by nonrebreather face mask to all patients until adequate oxygenation is assured. Intravenous (IV) access will likely need to be established, as many of the causes of altered mental status will require IV fluids or medications. A focused history and careful physical examination must be completed and should guide the selection of laboratory and imaging studies. Almost all these patients will require emergent care, so it is essential to anticipate transfer to the closest emergency department and begin arranging for transport early on.

8. **What laboratory study should be obtained in all children with altered mental status?**
   A rapid serum glucose should be performed in all children presenting with altered mental status. Additional laboratory studies may be useful but are dependent upon the patient's history and physical examination findings.

9. **What clinical clues should raise suspicion for toxic ingestion as the cause of altered mental status in a child?**
   Ingestion of a toxic substance should be strongly considered in children presenting with altered mental status, especially without a preceding history of trauma or illness. Ask the caregiver what medications are in the home, remembering that over-the-counter medications like acetaminophen (Tylenol) and diphenhydramine (Benadryl)

Anaphylaxis is highly likely when any one of the following 2 criteria are fulfilled:

(1) Acute onset of an illness (minutes to several hours) with simultaneous involvement of

the skin, mucosal tissue, or both (e.g., generalized hives, itching or flushing, swollen

lips/tongue/uvula) *AND AT LEAST ONE OF THE FOLLOWING*:

- Respiratory compromise (e.g., dyspnea, wheeze/bronchospasm, stridor, hypoxia)

- Decreased blood pressure or associated symptoms of end-organ dysfunction (e.g.,

    syncope, dizziness, hypotonia, incontinence)

- Severe gastrointestinal symptoms (e.g., crampy abdominal pain, repetitive vomiting),

    especially after exposure to non-food allergens

(2) Acute onset of hypotension or bronchospasm or laryngeal involvement after exposure

to a known or highly probably allergen for that patient (minutes to several hours), even

in the absence of typical skin involvement. (Hypotension= low age-specific systolic BP

or a decrease in systolic BP by 30% or more in infants/children)

Fig. 5.3 Clinical criteria for the diagnosis of anaphylaxis.

can be just as dangerous as prescription medications. Your exam can also be helpful in determining the type of ingestion. Pinpoint pupils with slow respiratory and heart rates are signs concerning for opioid intoxication and should make you think about administering naloxone (Narcan).

ANAPHYLAXIS

10. **What is the most common cause of anaphylaxis in children?**
    Food allergens represent the most common triggers of anaphylaxis among children, teens, and young adults. Other triggers may include medications, insect stings, blood products, immunotherapy, and radiocontrast media. In a significant proportion of cases, the cause is unidentified.

11. **What are the signs and symptoms of anaphylaxis?**
    Anaphylaxis is a clinical syndrome that is highly likely when a patient meets any one of two diagnostic criteria summarized in Fig. 5.3.

12. **What features of anaphylaxis are potentially life-threatening?**
    Anaphylaxis has the potential to result in significant morbidity and even death. Upper airway obstruction (due to edema of the tongue, larynx, and other airway structures), cardiovascular collapse, and respiratory compromise due to bronchospasm are potentially life-threatening complications.

13. **What immediate interventions are required for patients with anaphylaxis?**
    Anaphylaxis is a medical emergency requiring immediate assessment and simultaneous aggressive support of the airway, breathing, and circulation. Intramuscular epinephrine is the first-line treatment for anaphylaxis; it should be given as early as possible (in the anterolateral thigh) to all patients presenting with the characteristic signs and symptoms. Any known or suspected trigger(s) should be removed immediately. Patients with circulatory compromise should be placed in the supine position (or in their position of comfort if they have vomiting or respiratory distress).

14. **Can antihistamines and/or corticosteroids be used as an alternative to epinephrine in children with anaphylaxis?**
No. Neither H_1-receptor antihistamines (such as diphenhydramine) nor corticosteroids are first-line agents for treating anaphylaxis due to a lack of evidence supporting their efficacy. While these medications are commonly used and may be beneficial for specific symptoms, they are *not* replacements for epinephrine and should serve only as adjuncts in treating anaphylaxis. Treatment with IM epinephrine should not be withheld or delayed due to the administration of these medications. Unlike epinephrine, antihistamines will not effectively treat life-threatening cardiovascular or respiratory symptoms such as hypotension or bronchospasm. Furthermore, antihistamines and glucocorticoids have not been found to be reliable interventions for preventing subsequent biphasic reactions.

15. **What laboratory studies are required to confirm the diagnosis of anaphylaxis?**
None! Anaphylaxis is a clinical diagnosis, based primarily on a thorough history (including recent exposures) and recognition of the characteristic signs and symptoms. While elevated serum tryptase and histamine levels may support the diagnosis in some patients, these tests are not universally available, not useful in all patients, not performed emergently, and not specific for anaphylaxis. Their role in the diagnosis of anaphylaxis is limited and should never delay treatment.

16. **What are the main benefits and contraindications to epinephrine use in patients with anaphylaxis?**
Epinephrine use has been shown to decrease both hospitalizations and death among patients presenting with anaphylaxis. There is no absolute contraindication to its use in anaphylaxis. Therefore, it should be administered as the first-line agent for all patients with anaphylaxis.

17. **Can repeat epinephrine doses be given to children with anaphylaxis?**
Yes! Intramuscular epinephrine doses may be repeated every 5–15 minutes for persistent or recurrent symptoms. In children with circulatory compromise and/or for those in whom multiple intramuscular doses have been ineffective, careful administration of intravenous epinephrine may be indicated.

18. **How long should children be observed after treatment for anaphylaxis?**
There is no "standard" time period for observing children after treatment for anaphylaxis. Length of observation should be determined for each child based upon factors including severity of illness at presentation, underlying risk factors, and ability of the family to access care. All patients treated for anaphylaxis should be kept under observation until their symptoms have fully resolved. Those with mild to moderate symptoms resolving completely after treatment may be able to be discharged within 1–2 hours after they have become asymptomatic, while those with more severe reactions (e.g., with hypotension) and/or the need for multiple doses of epinephrine should be monitored for a longer duration.

19. **What information should be provided for patients who are discharged after treatment for anaphylaxis?**
All patients with anaphylaxis should receive education about anaphylaxis and the risk for both biphasic reactions and recurrence. Education about trigger avoidance, a prescription and instructions for self-injectable epinephrine, and thresholds for further care should also be provided. All patients treated for anaphylaxis should be referred to an allergist for follow-up evaluation.

RESPIRATORY DISTRESS

ASTHMA

20. **What is the best initial treatment for an acute asthma exacerbation?**
The mainstays of acute asthma exacerbation therapy are inhaled short-acting β_2 agonists, corticosteroids, and oxygen. The severity of the exacerbation, however, will ultimately dictate treatment. Oxygen as needed to maintain $SaO_2 > 90\%$ should be provided to all patients. Ipratropium can be used in conjunction with inhaled bronchodilators for those with moderate or severe exacerbation. Corticosteroids should be given within the first hour for children presenting with an exacerbation.

21. **How should bronchodilators be administered during an acute exacerbation?**
Short-acting β_2 agonists, commonly albuterol, can be given via nebulizer or by metered-dose inhaler (MDI). Several studies show that albuterol by MDI is better tolerated by patients and has equal efficacy to albuterol given by continuous nebulizer. Patients presenting with a moderate to severe exacerbation require continuous or repetitive inhaled bronchodilators in the first hour. If using an MDI, give a dose every 20 minutes.

22. **When and how should steroids be administered?**
Patients with an asthma exacerbation should receive oral corticosteroids, preferably within the first hour of presentation. IV steroids should be reserved for patients with respiratory arrest or failure. Oral steroids have been found to be equally effective as IV steroids in several studies. A one- or two-dose regimen of dexamethasone is preferred to a 3- to 5-day course of prednisone because of improved patient compliance with equal efficacy.

23. In a patient with asthma, when should a chest x-ray be obtained?

Chest x-rays should not be routinely ordered during the evaluation of an asthma exacerbation, as they do not change clinical management. Imaging should be ordered if you are concerned about pneumothorax, concomitant bacterial pneumonia, or foreign body aspiration. As most pediatric asthma exacerbations are incited by a viral illness, fever alone cannot be used to raise concern for bacterial pneumonia. If a child has a fever with focal lung exam findings that do not improve with bronchodilators, then a chest x-ray can be considered.

24. What are the indications for endotracheal intubation and mechanical ventilation during an asthma exacerbation?

Patients presenting with an asthma exacerbation are very difficult to mechanically ventilate. As such, pharmacologic treatment—including treatment with agents such as magnesium sulfate—should be maximized prior to proceeding to intubation. Failure of maximal treatment, inability to oxygenate, worsening hypercarbia, or declining mental status is an indication for intubation or noninvasive positive pressure ventilation.

BRONCHIOLITIS

25. A 7-month-old boy presents with a fever, nasal congestion, persistent cough, tachypnea, intermittent subcostal retractions, and diffusely scattered bilateral wheezes on lung exam. He had rhinorrhea for 2 days before his fever, cough, and increased work of breathing began. What is his most likely diagnosis?

This infant likely has bronchiolitis, the most common lower respiratory tract infection in children under the age of 2 years. Bronchiolitis is the leading cause of infant hospitalizations in high-income countries. Respiratory syncytial virus (RSV) is the most common cause and is responsible for up to 80% of cases, although other common respiratory viruses can also result in bronchiolitis. Children with bronchiolitis typically present with a prodrome of upper respiratory symptoms (i.e., rhinorrhea, congestion) for up to 2 days, followed by progression to symptoms of lower respiratory tract infection, including persistent cough, fever, tachypnea, and increased work of breathing. Infants with bronchiolitis may develop tachypnea, crackles, wheezing, hypoxia, and signs of increased work of breathing (i.e., retractions, nasal flaring, grunting, head bobbing) due to lower respiratory tract inflammation and increased mucous production.

26. How is bronchiolitis diagnosed?

Bronchiolitis is diagnosed clinically, based on history and physical exam. Viral testing, laboratory studies, chest radiography, and other diagnostic tests are not needed for infants presenting with clinical bronchiolitis.

27. What is the primary treatment for bronchiolitis?

Bronchiolitis treatment is largely supportive, as it is a self-limited viral illness. Supportive care measures include superficial nasal suctioning, nasogastric or intravenous fluids for infants who cannot maintain hydration, and supplemental oxygen for oxygen saturations persistently <92%. The peak severity of bronchiolitis typically occurs between days 3–5 of symptoms, and symptom resolution occurs within 2–3 weeks for the majority of infants affected.

28. Should bronchodilators be given to children with bronchiolitis?

Numerous studies have investigated the efficacy of bronchodilators for the treatment of bronchiolitis. Most randomized controlled trials have failed to show a benefit. While beta-agonists may improve symptoms and clinical scores, they do not change the progression of the disease or improve outcomes such as the need for hospitalization or length of stay. Based on extensive review of the available evidence, national and international guidelines for bronchiolitis management do not recommend the use of bronchodilators.

29. Are corticosteroids useful in bronchiolitis?

Numerous clinical studies have demonstrated no benefit from the use of corticosteroids for bronchiolitis. Further, steroids may prolong viral shedding. As such, national and international evidence-based guidelines recommend against administering corticosteroids to children with bronchiolitis.

30. An 11-month-old girl presents with cough and nasal congestion for 2 weeks. Her history and physical examination support the diagnosis of bronchiolitis. She is afebrile and well appearing without respiratory distress. Her parents ask whether antibiotics should be started, due to the persistence of her cough. Will antibiotics be useful for alleviating her symptoms?

The use of antibiotics in children with bronchiolitis is not recommended unless there is clear and documented evidence of a concomitant serious bacterial infection. Avoiding adverse effects of unnecessary antibiotic use is important for patients, families, and society. Antibiotics will not offer a benefit for this patient and should not be prescribed.

CROUP

31. **What is croup and what are the typical symptoms?**
Croup (laryngotracheitis) is a respiratory illness characterized by barky cough, hoarseness, and inspiratory stridor. These symptoms arise from inflammation in the larynx and subglottic airway. Most cases of croup are caused by viruses, with parainfluenza virus being the most common cause. Croup is seen most commonly in children 6 months to 3 years of age. Other viral symptoms, such as nasal congestion, sore throat, and fever, are typically present.

32. **An 18-month-old boy presents with a 2-day history of rhinorrhea, low-grade fever, hoarseness, and frequent barky cough. He is well appearing with no drooling, no stridor at rest, clear lungs, and no increased work of breathing. There is no history of choking or foreign body aspiration. His history and clinical findings support the diagnosis of viral croup. What treatment is recommended for this child?**
Based on findings from multiple clinical studies, administration of glucocorticoids is recommended for children with croup of any severity in both inpatient and outpatient settings. Clinical trials have demonstrated that glucocorticoids reduce croup symptoms at 2 hours and for at least 24 hours, reduce return visits for care, and shorten hospital stays (when required). Dexamethasone is the mainstay of treatment for croup and can be administered orally. For children who cannot tolerate oral medications and/or who have severe respiratory distress, intramuscular administration of dexamethasone is also an option.

33. **When should racemic epinephrine be given to children with croup, and what must occur after its administration?**
Nebulized racemic epinephrine is reserved for patients with moderate to severe croup, including children with biphasic stridor, stridor at rest, retractions, decreased air entry, or hypoxia. Racemic epinephrine is effective within 30 minutes of administration. However, racemic epinephrine does not alter the disease course, so patients must be monitored closely for a "rebound effect" after the medication wears off. The recommended monitoring time is at least 2 hours after treatment.

34. **Why is hypoxia with croup an emergency?**
Since croup is an upper airway obstructive disease, gas exchange at the level of the alveoli is preserved. Therefore, hypoxia is a sign of impending respiratory failure due to severe upper airway obstruction.

35. **Although croup is the most common cause of stridor in febrile children, what other potentially life-threatening causes of stridor should be considered when assessing a child presenting with stridor?**
See Table 5.2.

SEIZURE

36. **What is the definition of status epilepticus?**
Status epilepticus is defined as a continuous seizure lasting greater than 5 minutes without regaining consciousness in that time or three seizures within a 15-minute period. It is a medical emergency and should be anticipated in any patient presenting with an acute seizure.

Table 5.2 Potentially Life-Threatening Causes of Stridor in Children
LIFE-THREATENING CAUSES OF STRIDOR
Causes typically presenting with fever: Severe croup   Epiglottitis/supraglottitis   Tracheitis   Retropharyngeal abscess   Causes typically presenting without fever: Foreign body   Anaphylaxis   Angioedema   Neck trauma   Neoplasm (compressing trachea/airway)   Thermal or caustic injury to the airway

Adapted from Table 75.3 in Chapter 75: Stridor. Hoppa EC, Perry HE. In: *Fleisher & Ludwig's Textbook of Pediatric Emergency Medicine*, 8th edition, Shaw KN, Bachur RG, eds. Wolters Kluwer; 2021:514.

Table 5.3 Usual First-Line Antiepileptic Medications for the Treatment of Status Epilepticus

DRUG	ROUTE	DOSE	MAXIMUM DOSE
Lorazepam	IV, IN	0.05–0.1 mg/kg	4 mg
Midazolam	IV, IM, IN	0.2 mg/kg	10 mg
	Buccal	0.5 mg/kg	
Diazepam	IV	0.2–0.4 mg/kg	10 mg
	PR	0.5–1 mg/kg	

Data from: Chiang VW. Seizures. In: *Textbook of Pediatric Emergency Medicine.* 6th ed. Philadelphia: Lippincott Williams & Wilkins; 2010:564–570; Mikati MA, Hani AJ. Seizures in Childhood. In: *Nelson Textbook of Pediatrics,* 20th ed. Philadelphia: Elsevier; 2016:2823–2857.

37. **What are the first-line medications for treating status epilepticus?**
See Table 5.3.

38. **What testing should be performed for a first-time, unprovoked afebrile seizure?**
Electrolytes, especially glucose, should be obtained in a patient who is actively seizing. If the seizure has already stopped, there is limited utility in emergent metabolic testing. An electroencephalogram (EEG) is recommended and may be helpful to obtain within 24–48 hours after the seizure. A nonurgent MRI is indicated in patients less than 1 year old, those with focal seizures, and those with unexplained abnormalities on neurologic exam including cognitive function. For patients with a known seizure disorder, a brain MRI is indicated if there is a change in their typical seizure pattern.

39. **What are indications for ordering urgent neuroimaging after a first-time seizure?**
Urgent head imaging is indicated in only a small proportion of children with first-time seizure. Neuroimaging is not generally needed after a first-time seizure in patients who have returned to baseline and have a nonfocal neurologic exam, pending EEG results. The following situations warrant rapid imaging:
- Focal findings on neurologic exam
- Persistent decreased level of consciousness and/or alteration in mental status beyond the expected postictal period
- Signs of increased intracranial pressure
- Posttraumatic seizures not consistent with concussive convulsions
- Cases in which abusive head trauma is suspected, especially in infants <1 year of age (abusive head trauma should be strongly suspected in infants <4 months with any bruising, those with head circumference >85th percentile, those with associated symptoms such as vomiting, as well as those with patterned bruising and/or bruises to the torso, ears, neck, frenulum, angle of the jaw, cheeks, eyelids, or subconjunctivae)
   While MRI of the brain is generally the preferred neuroimaging study in the evaluation of seizures, it may not be available or feasible to obtain immediately following a seizure. If a brain MRI cannot be obtained, a head CT should be performed in children meeting the criteria for rapid imaging above.

40. **What is a febrile seizure?**
A febrile seizure is seizure activity in the setting of a temperature of 38°C or greater and in the absence of other causes of seizure. They are very common, occurring in 3–4% of children between the ages of 6 months and 5 years. There is a 30% risk of recurrence for febrile seizures but only a small increase in the risk of developing epilepsy.

41. **How can you differentiate between a simple and complex febrile seizure?**
In order to meet criteria for a simple febrile seizure, the seizure must be less than 15 minutes in duration and the child can have no more than one seizure in a 24-hour period. Simple febrile seizures are characterized by generalized tonic-clonic activity. Focal seizure activity, prolonged seizure, or multiple seizures are consistent with a complex febrile seizure.

42. **A 2-year-old girl is brought to urgent care after having a 2-minute generalized seizure. She has never had a seizure before. Her mom tells you that she is back to baseline now, about 2 hours after the episode. She is febrile but otherwise well appearing and has a normal neurologic exam. What tests should be performed?**
This child has had a simple febrile seizure. Febrile seizures are diagnosed clinically. The only diagnostic testing that should be performed is testing to determine the source of the fever if needed. Neuroimaging and EEG are not indicated.

43. **What is a concussive convulsion?**

Concussive convulsions are generalized tonic-clonic activity occurring within seconds of head impact. They are also called "impact seizures," though there is controversy as to whether they are truly epileptic activity. A concussive convulsion does not increase a patient's risk of epilepsy and does not require treatment. Medical management and evaluation should be focused on the head injury and concussion.

44. **Can other diagnoses mimic a seizure?**

Up to 25% of "first-time seizures" are later determined to have no evidence of an epileptic event. It is critical to obtain a careful history and exam to determine the diagnosis. Each age group can present with different mimics. Common seizure mimics in infancy are benign sleep myoclonus (short episodes of myoclonus only during sleep) and Sandifer syndrome (back arching with stiffness that is secondary to reflux). Breath-holding spells can be misinterpreted as seizures in young children. In adolescents, vasovagal syncope can be associated with rhythmic jerking but the return to baseline is rapid.

45. **What is Todd paralysis?**

Todd paralysis is a transient paresis or paralysis in the postictal period. Symptoms typically resolve within 24 hours after the seizure.

SEPSIS

46. **What is SIRS?**

SIRS stands for systemic inflammatory response syndrome. Two of the following criteria are necessary, one of which must be temperature instability or abnormal leukocyte count:
- Temperature >38.5°C or <36.0°C
- Tachycardia (>2 standard deviations [SD] above the mean for age)
- Tachypnea (>2 SD above the mean for age)
- Abnormal leukocyte count or >10% immature cells (bands)

Remember that SIRS is not specific to infection and can be present in settings such as trauma, burns, leukemia, and other diseases. Many children presenting with fever will meet SIRS criteria.

47. **How do you differentiate between sepsis, severe sepsis, and septic shock?**

Sepsis = SIRS + an infectious source (either presumed or proven)
Severe sepsis = sepsis + cardiovascular dysfunction or respiratory dysfunction or dysfunction in 2 other organ systems
Septic shock = sepsis + cardiovascular compromise

A child with sepsis and any of the following criteria is in septic shock.
- Hypotension
- Altered mental status
- Flash capillary refill or capillary refill >2 seconds
- Bounding or weak peripheral pulses
- Wide pulse pressure
- Urine output <1 mL/kg/hr

48. **What vital sign abnormality can be a sign of early septic shock?**

Unexplained tachycardia. As stroke volume decreases due to capillary leak and third spacing, heart rate increases to maintain cardiac output.

49. **Can blood pressure be reliably used to diagnose early septic shock in a child?**

Unlike in adults, hypotension is a late sign of septic shock in children. Initially, pediatric patients can typically compensate through tachycardia and vasoconstriction. Hypotension indicates uncompensated shock and should be a warning to you that your patient is in a prearrest phase.

50. **You have diagnosed a child with septic shock. What should your initial management include?**

Always start with ABCs. The first hour is critical and a patient in shock requires emergency medical care. After establishing that the patient has an adequate airway and is breathing, apply oxygen via facemask and obtain vascular access. Within the first hour, patients should receive broad-spectrum antibiotics and rapid fluid resuscitation. Give 10–20 mL/kg isotonic fluid boluses intravenously over 5–10 minutes, targeting a total of 40–60 mL/kg in the first hour. Frequent reassessments are essential to monitor for signs of fluid overload, such as hepatomegaly or rales. Obtaining blood cultures prior to starting antibiotics is ideal but should not delay antibiotic administration.

51. **What are the empiric antibiotics that should be used for neonates and children presenting with septic shock?**

See Table 5.4.

Table 5.4 Empiric Antibiotic Therapy for Sepsis

AGE	BACTERIAL ETIOLOGY	ANTIBIOTIC CHOICE
Child	Staphylococcal pneumoniae, Neisseria meningitidis, Haemophilus influenzae type b, Staphylococcus aureus, group A streptococcus (GAS)	Third-generation cephalosporin + vancomycin • Add aminoglycoside if concerned about nosocomial or gram-negative infection • Add clindamycin for toxic shock syndrome
Neonate	Group B streptococcus (GBS), gram-negative enteric organisms, Listeria species, Herpes simplex virus	Ampicillin + third-generation cephalosporin • Add vancomycin for nosocomial infection or late-onset sepsis • Add acyclovir for infants under 28 days

52. **A 20-day-old infant presents with a temperature of 38.0°C rectally. Other than fever, her exam is benign. What is the risk of serious bacterial illness (SBI) in this infant?**
In febrile infants (≤60 days old), approximately 10% will have an SBI. The risk increases in infants <28 days old. Of infants with an SBI, urinary tract infections are the most common, followed by bacteremia and, rarely, meningitis. Herpes simplex virus (HSV) infection must also be considered in infants <28 days old. Well appearance and lack of other symptoms should not be used to rule out SBI or HSV in this age group.

SYNCOPE

53. **What is syncope?**
Syncope is a sudden, transient loss of consciousness and postural muscle tone that reverses without intervention. Its pathophysiologic mechanism involves a temporary decrease in cerebral blood flow or glucose supply, which the brain constantly depends on to function normally. Approximately 15–25% of children and adolescents will experience at least one episode of syncope by early adulthood.

54. **What causes syncope in children?**
The causes of syncope range from completely benign (most cases) to life-threatening. Although cardiac causes for syncope are relatively common in adults, most syncope in pediatric patients is benign and *not* due to cardiac pathology. Autonomic-mediated reflex syncope (also known as vasovagal syncope) accounts for the majority of all pediatric syncope cases. Other causes of syncope can be classified into several broad categories, including situational, cardiac, neurologic, psychogenic, metabolic, toxicologic, and miscellaneous.

55. **Most causes of syncope in children are benign. However, what life-threatening causes must be ruled out?**
In children with syncope, the following life-threatening cases should be excluded:
• Long QT syndrome
• Cardiomyopathy (hypertrophic cardiomyopathy) or critical aortic stenosis
• Wolff-Parkinson-White syndrome
• Coronary artery anomalies
• Complete atrioventricular block
• Seizures
• Intracranial hemorrhage and/or increased intracranial pressure
• Drug ingestion
• Carbon monoxide poisoning

56. **What "red flags" for underlying cardiac pathology should one be aware of when evaluating a pediatric patient with syncope?**
Syncope that occurs suddenly without warning—including episodes without any presyncopal prodrome—should be assumed to be due to cardiac pathology until proven otherwise. Syncope occurring during exercise, while in a supine position, or that is associated with chest pain, dyspnea, cyanosis, or palpitations is also concerning for a cardiac etiology. Family history of sudden death or arrhythmia is also a "red flag." Children with any of these red flags should be evaluated promptly by a pediatric cardiologist.

57. **What evaluation is required in children and adolescents with syncope?**
A careful history, complete physical examination, and electrocardiogram (ECG) will help identify serious underlying causes of syncope in the majority of patients. An ECG is highly useful in identifying cardiac causes of syncope and

should be obtained in all children presenting with syncope and "red flags." Screening laboratory tests and neuro-imaging studies are generally not indicated in pediatric patients presenting with syncope unless there is concern for a specific underlying cause based on history and physical examination.

58. You have completed an ECG on a 13-year-old girl who "passed out" while running at soccer practice. You note that her QTc is 0.600 seconds. She takes no medications but does have a family history of arrhythmias. What should you do next?
Consult cardiology immediately. This patient has several red flags including syncope during exercise, an abnormal ECG, and a positive family history.

KEY POINTS

1. Immediately obtain a glucose level on children presenting with altered mental status or who are actively seizing.
2. Epinephrine is the only medication for anaphylaxis that has been shown to reduce mortality and hospitalizations; all other medication options only treat the symptoms.
3. Always prioritize ABCs (airway, breathing, circulation) when managing critically ill children.

BIBLIOGRAPHY

Bachur RG, Shaw KN, Chamberlain J. *Fleisher & Ludwig's Textbook of Pediatric Emergency Medicine*. 8th ed. Lippincott Williams & Wilkins; 2020.
Berger RP, Fromkin J, Herman B, et al. Validation of the Pittsburgh Infant Brain Injury Score for Abusive Head Trauma. *Pediatrics*. 2016; 138(1):e20153756.
Cardona V, Ansotegui IJ, et al. World allergy organization anaphylaxis guidance 2020. *World Allergy Organ J*. 2020;13:100472.
Dalziel SR, Haskell L, et al. Bronchiolitis. *Lancet*. 2022;400:392–406.
Dubey V, Nau E, Sycip M. Altered Mental Status in Children After Traumatic Brain Injury. *Pediatr Ann*. 2019;48(5):e192–e196.
Dunnick J, Mazzarini A. Altered Mental Status. In: Olympia RP, Lubin JS, eds. *Prehospital Emergency Medicine Secrets*. 2022:132–134.
Fine A, Wirrell EC. Seizures in Children. *Pediatr Rev*. 2020;41(7):321–347.
Gates A, Johnson DW, Klassen TP. Glucocorticoids for croup in children. *JAMA Pediatr*. 2019;173(6):595–596.
Kuppermann N, Dayan PS, Levine DA, et al. A Clinical Prediction Rule to Identify Febrile Infants 60 Days and Younger at Low Risk for Serious Bacterial Infections. *JAMA Pediatr*. 2019;173(4):342–351.
Pardue Jones B, Fleming GM, et al. Pediatric acute asthma exacerbations: Evaluation and management from emergency department to intensive care unit. *J Asthma*. 2016;53(6):607–617.
Pediatric Emergencies: A Practical, Clinical Guide, 1st ed. Rose E, ed. Oxford University Press. 2021.
Pierce MC, Kaczor K, Lorenz DJ, et al. Validation of a Clinical Decision Rule to Predict Abuse in Young Children Based on Bruising Characteristics. *JAMA Netw Open*. 2021;4(4):e215832.
Ralston SL, et al. Clinical practice guideline: the diagnosis, management, and prevention of bronchiolitis. *Pediatrics*. 2015;136(4):782.
Shaker MS, Wallace DV, Golden DBK, et al. Anaphylaxis-a 2020 practice parameter update, systematic review, and Grading of Recommendations, Assessment, Development and Evaluation (GRADE) analysis. *J Allergy Clin Immunol*. 2020;145(4):1082–1123.

CHAPTER 6

HEADACHE AND NEUROLOGIC COMPLAINTS

Scott Goldstein, DO, FACEP, FAEMS, EMT-PHP

TOP SECRETS

1. All headaches can be treated with oxygen.
2. Bell's Palsy never involves the arms or legs, but it does involve the forehead.
3. Continuous nonpositional dizziness can be a posterior stroke.

MIGRAINE

1. **What are the typical pain characteristics of migraine headaches?**
   - The typical pain characteristics of migraine headaches are that they are unilateral and pulsatile or throbbing.
   - Migraines are usually worsened by physical activity, bright lights (photophobia), and loud noises (phonophobia). Migraines are usually associated with nausea/vomiting.

2. **What is an aura?**
   - An aura is a reversible cerebral dysfunction (abnormal smells, flashing lights, halos, etc.) that develops over 5 (or more) minutes and lasts less than an hour. Migraine headache usually presents after the aura.

3. **What is the treatment for migraine headaches?**
   See Table 6.1.

4. **What is the treatment of choice for migraine headaches?**
   - Migraine-specific medications are the triptans. These can be given orally, subcutaneously, nasally, or intravenously. These work well alone or in conjunction with symptomatic control of associated symptoms.

5. **What are the seven different types of migraine headaches?**
   - Hemiplegic, basilar, childhood periodic syndromes, retinal, ophthalmologic, vertiginous, and nocturnal.

TENSION TYPE HEADACHE

6. **What is the most common type of headache?**
   Most common type of headache is tension headache.
       The main causes of tension headaches:
   - Any stressor.
   - Any other factor that can cause muscle spasm of the neck and head, like poor posture, weak neck extensors (e.g., from sitting at a desk all day), anxiety, or depression.

Table 6.1 Treatment for Migraine Headaches

SEVERITY	W/O N/V	WITH N/V	MISC.
Mild	NSAIDs Acetaminophen	Metoclopramide chlorpromazine	Oxygen
Moderate	NSAIDs Acetaminophen	Metoclopramide chlorpromazine	IV hydration IV/IM dopamine antagonist Oxygen
Severe	Triptans NSAIDs Acetaminophen	Triptans Ketorolac Metoclopramide	IV Hydration Oxygen IV dopamine antagonist IV/IM/SQ Triptans

- Mild-to-moderate (without nausea/vomiting) oral NSAIDs and/or acetaminophen is sufficient.
- Other agents that can be used are dopamine antagonists (like metoclopramide or chlorpromazine). Their greatest effect is in the treatment nausea/vomiting to maintain oral hydration and medication compliance.
- The use of high-flow oxygen can be a great adjunct to any treatment decision.

7. What is the best way to treat tension headaches?
   - Pharmacological and stress reduction therapies work well together. Unfortunately, in the fast-paced world of urgent care, stress reduction techniques are not a viable option.
   - In the urgent care setting the use of NSAIDs (IV, IM, or PO), acetaminophen, hydration (IV or PO), and oxygen would be your best option for rapid relief.
   - Consideration of a small dose of benzodiazepine if muscle spasm is a contributing factor.

8. How can I differentiate a tension headache from other headaches?
   - If you were to guess the type of headache as tension, you would be right most of the time (almost 70% of the time).
   - Before deciding this, one must make sure it's not a life-threatening headache like an intracranial hemorrhage or meningitis.

CLUSTER HEADACHE

9. What is the classic presentation of a cluster headache?
   - Unilateral pain around the eye and temporal area with cranial nerve autonomic dysfunction (presenting as tearing and/or facial pain).
   - Headaches usually lasts 45–90 minutes and are cyclic in nature. Cluster headaches can last as long as 1 week!

10. What is the best treatment for a cluster headache?
   - The fastest and easiest medicine to relieve cluster headaches is high-flow (greater than 15 liters/minute) oxygen for ~30 minutes.
       The best adjunct medication being the triptans, along with symptomatic control.

FACIAL DROOP/BELL'S PALSY (FIG. 6.1)

11. How can I differentiate Bell's Palsy from a stroke?
   - Bell's palsy is an acute, unilateral facial nerve paralysis. This results in weakness of the muscles of facial expression, including the forehead, and never involves any extremity.
   - Any extremity involvement should be a concern for a stroke.

12. What is the treatment for Bell's Palsy?
   - All patients should be provided symptomatic pain control with NSAIDs.
   - Eye lubricant to keep the eye moist (as the eyelid doesn't usually close all the way).
   - Eye shield for sleep (so the patient doesn't inadvertently scratch their cornea while sleeping due to inadequate eyelid closure and dryness).
   - Oral corticosteroids (usually prednisone is prescribed in a 10-day tapering course starting at 60 mg).
   - Based on current literature, antivirals are currently not recommended, but if you want to give them, it's best to do so within 3 days of symptom presentation.

13. How long does Bell's Palsy last?
   - It usually lasts for a couple of weeks but can range from months to years. Most recover completely within 2 months.

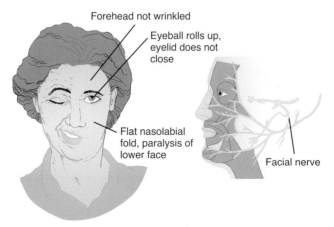

Forehead not wrinkled

Eyeball rolls up, eyelid does not close

Flat nasolabial fold, paralysis of lower face

Facial nerve

Fig. 6.1 Physical exam findings of Bell's Palsy.

VERTIGO

14. **What is benign positional vertigo (BPV)?**
    - It is a peripheral vestibular disorder involving the semicircular canals.
    - There is no brain or central component.

15. **How can I differentiate benign vertigo from central (CNS) causes?**
    - BPV is episodic in nature, and there are no symptoms during a quiescent period; patients prefer to lay still so as not to elicit the vertigo.
    - An adjunct for diagnosis (and treatment!) is position testing, like the Dix-Hallpike maneuver. This helps establish this as a peripheral, not central, disorder.
    - Cerebellar signs/symptoms of vertigo and imbalance don't wax/wain during strokes.

16. **What is the Dix-Hallpike maneuver and how does one do it?**
    The patient starts in sitting position, facing forward with eyes open.
    Rapidly lie patient backward with their head turned 45 degrees to the right and their neck extended over the end of the table for about 30 seconds. This is repeated on the left side.

17. **Why would I want to do the Dix-Hallpike maneuver?**
    - A few things will happen here; some good, some bad, some ugly.
    - Good: You will see nystagmus and symptoms and, if they stay with it, this test is also the treatment! This movement repositions the otolith in the semicircular canal, and they will feel (and be) better after!
    - Bad: You will reproduce the vertiginous symptoms, which can lead to nausea/vomiting, and this will make the patient want to get themselves out of the position. If they want to get out of the position, then you are doing it right!
    - Ugly: they may vomit!

18. **What is the initial workup/evaluation of vertigo?**
    - If there is still uncertainty of central versus peripheral nature, further testing may be needed.
    - These tests can include CAT scans, MRIs, EKGs, and bloodwork. These types of patients should be referred to the emergency department.

VASOVAGAL SYNCOPE

19. **What is the definition of syncope?**
    - Transient loss of consciousness due to hypoperfusion of the brain.
    - The characteristics are:
      1. Rapid onset
      2. Brief duration
      3. Spontaneous recovery

20. **What are the causes of vasovagal syncope?**
    - Almost anything!
    - The main ones are:
      1. Pain
      2. Prolonged standing
      3. Being in hot and/or crowded areas
      4. Emotional stress
      5. Urination or defecation
      6. Seeing blood (if this is you, you may be in the wrong field)

21. **Is there a prodrome to vasovagal syncope?**
    - Yes.
      They can be:
      1. Yawning
      2. Lightheadedness
      3. Nausea
      4. Sweating
      5. Ringing in the ears
      6. Visual changes
         - This is important, because if there is no prodrome, then a cardiac cause should be sought, and the patient needs to go to the hospital!

22. **How do you treat vasovagal syncope?**
    - The main goal is to prevent injury from the actual physical event of falling, which you probably won't be there for, unless it's from the sight of blood or needles—then you may be the cause.

- Most (if not all) will have completely resolved by the time you evaluate them, which makes your job even tougher!
- The key is to find out what the prodromal symptoms were to help decide if the episode was vasovagal or cardiovascular/neurological in nature.

23. **What tests should I order?**
    1. EKG to evaluate for dysthymia, infarct, or pauses.
    2. HCG to evaluate for pregnancy status, which can cause lead to hypovolemia.
    3. Urine dipstick to evaluate for ketones due to dehydration or infection.
    4. Blood glucose to evaluate for new-onset diabetes or hypoglycemia.

NEUROPRAXIA/NUMBNESS

1. Numbness/tingling of an isolated upper extremity is usually cervical (peripheral) radiculopathy.
2. Numbness/tingling of an isolated lower extremity with radiation of pain into the buttocks or back is usually sciatica.
   a. Any of the above can be an isolated stroke in the homunculus area of the brain. This is extremely rare, since there are usually associated sensory deficit and motor deficit. Isolated sensory or motor infarcts are even rarer.

KEY POINTS

1. Migraine headaches are usually unilateral and pulsatile in nature.
2. Oxygen is a great adjunct to treat all types of headaches.
3. Bell's Palsy never involves the arms or legs.
4. Tension headaches are the most common type of headaches.
5. Any concern for a stroke should be evaluated completely.

BIBLIOGRAPHY

Becker WJ. Acute Migraine Treatment in Adults. *Headache*. 2015;55(6):778–793. doi:10.1111/head.12550. Epub 2015 Apr 15.
Dancy, J, PA-C, MPAS, Evaluation of headaches in urgent care part: non-emergent headaches. Journal of Urgent Care Medicine. https://www.JUCM.com/evaluation-of-headaches-in-urgent-care-part-2-non-emergent-headaches/. Accessed on March 28 2022.
Headache Classification Committee of the International Headache Society (IHS). The International Classification of Headache Disorders, 3rd ed. *Cephalalgia*. 2018;38(1):1–211. doi:10.1177/0333102417738202. PMID: 29368949.
Long, B., Koyfman, A., emDocs Cases: Headache Management in the ED, Nov 20, 2017, practice updates. Accessed: emdocs.net/emdocs-cases-headache-management-ed.
Malu O, Bailey J. Cluster headache: rapid evidence review. *Am Fam Physician. Jan;*. 2022;105(1):24–32. https://fpnotebook.com/neuro/exam/HdchRdFlg.htm.
Mayans L, Walling A. Acute migraine headache: treatment strategies. *Am Fam Physician*. 2018;97(4):243–251. PMID: 29671521.
Muhammet A, Tushar S, Wilke I, Willems S. Management and therapy of vasovagal syncope: a review. *World J Cardiol*. 2010;2(10):308–315.
Mullen M, Loomis C. Differentiating facial weakness caused by Bell's palsy vs acute stroke. *JEMS*. March 2014.
Muncie H, Sirmans S. Dizziness: approach to evaluation and management. *Am Fam Physician*. 2017;95(3):154–162.
Nguyen JD, Duong H. Neurosurgery, sensory homunculus. [Updated 2021 Jul 26]. *StatPearls [Internet]*. Treasure Island, FL: StatPearls Publishing; 2022. https://www.ncbi.nlm.nih.gov/books/NBK549841/.
Ozkurt B, Cinar O, Cevik E. Efficacy of high-flow oxygen therapy in all types of headache: a prospective, randomized, placebo-controlled trial. *Am J Emerg Med*. 2012;30(9):1760–1764. doi:10.1016/j.ajem.2012.02.010. Epub 2012 May 3. http://www.uptodate.com/contents/acute-treatment-of-migraine-in-adults.
Runser L, Gauer R, Houser A. Syncope: evaluation and differential diagnosis. *Am Fam Physician*. 2017;95(5):303–312B.
Schwedt, T. Garza, I. Acute treatment of migraine in adults. https://www.uptodate.com/contents/acute-treatment-of-migraine-in-adults. Literature review current through: Feb 2022. | This topic last updated: Oct 20, 2021.
Shukla GJ. Syncope. *Circulation*. 2006;113(16) n. pag.
Talmud JD, Coffey R, Edemekong PF. Dix Hallpike maneuver. [Updated 2021 Dec 19]. StatPearls [Internet]. Treasure Island, FL: StatPearls Publishing; 2022. https://www.ncbi.nlm.nih.gov/books/NBK459307/.
Warner MJ, Hutchison J, Varacallo M. Bell palsy. [Updated 2022 Feb 12]. StatPearls [Internet]. Treasure Island, FL: StatPearls Publishing; 2022. https://www.ncbi.nlm.nih.gov/books/NBK482290.
Wei DY, Khalil M, Goadsby PJ. Managing cluster headache. *Practical Neurology*. 2019;19:521–528.

CHAPTER 7

RED EYE, EYE PAIN, AND VISION LOSS

Jeff Cloyd, MD

1. **How should the eye be examined?**
   Start with an examination of the soft tissue around the eye looking for swelling and redness that might indicate a soft-tissue condition. Examine the eye using an ophthalmoscope and UV light (i.e., Wood lamp) or a slit lamp if available. Additional tools for the exam include fluorescein stain, visual acuity, and tonometry.

2. **How can you differentiate between periorbital and orbital cellulitis?**
   Periorbital cellulitis causes redness and swelling of the soft tissues around the eye but does not cause pain with eye movement and is treated with outpatient oral antibiotic therapy. Orbital cellulitis causes pain with eye movement and requires intravenous antibiotic therapy and close monitoring.

3. **What is the treatment for a chalazion (cyst) and a hordeolum (stye) (Fig. 7.1)?**
   Both present with swelling, pain, and erythema of the affected eyelid. Neither require antibiotic treatment. Both are best treated with frequent warm compresses and antiinflammatory pain medication.

4. **What is blepharitis and how is management different from that of chalazion and hordeolum?**
   Blepharitis is an infection of the eyelash and can extend into the eyelid; it should be treated with topical antibiotic drops or ointment. Oral antibiotics are typically not indicated.

5. **Which method should be used to examine the underside of the eyelid for a foreign body?**
   Place a cotton-tip swab against the skin along the margin between the orbit and the superior orbital bone. Holding the patient's upper eyelashes, the lid can then be everted by rolling the skin over the cotton-tip swab. Repeat on the lower lid.

6. **How many places can a contact lens hide?**
   Careful examination of the cornea and sclera of a patient who has "lost" a contact lens in the eye may not reveal the missing contact. Evert the eyelid and sweep the upper fornix while the patient is looking down. Fluorescein stain can be used to help locate a missing lens in the eye, but keep in mind staining of the contact lens is permanent. The conjunctiva and mucosal membrane of the eyelid are confluent, and a contact lens cannot migrate around to the back of the orbit.

7. **What are the characteristics of different corneal injuries with examination using fluorescein stain?**
   See Fig. 7.2 for the different characteristics.

8. **What options exist for removing a splinter caused by metal grinding?**
   After anesthesia, a cotton-tip swab typically removes most foreign bodies. However, a metal splinter can be removed using an electric burr drill. Iron-containing foreign bodies will produce a rust ring within several hours and should be removed using a cotton-tip swab or burr drill. Topical antibiotics should be provided, and tetanus vaccine status should be considered.

9. **When is an appropriate time to use topical antibiotics with corneal injuries?**
   Most injuries to the cornea caused by a foreign body should be treated with topical antibiotics. Antibiotics should be considered in simple corneal abrasions but are not always required. Drops and ointment have similar efficacy; treatments for injuries in patients wearing contact lenses should be chosen with *Pseudomonas* species in mind (e.g., ciprofloxacin).

10. **Should conjunctivitis be treated with antibiotics?**
    Antibiotic therapy is not recommended in the treatment of acute conjunctivitis, as the most common cause is viral. Allergic inflammation is another common cause of conjunctivitis; this should be treated with standard allergy medications (e.g., histamine blockers). Bacterial conjunctivitis treatment with antibiotics has not been shown to significantly reduce the number of days of symptoms, and most infections are self-limited; however, antibiotics should be considered in infants and immunocompromised patients.

11. **How does iritis present differently from conjunctivitis?**
    Iritis is not improved with topical anesthetics, and vision in the affected eye is often affected by inflammatory proteins in the aqueous humor of the anterior chamber ("cell and flare"). Conjunctival injection of iritis is typically adjacent to the iris, versus conjunctivitis, where the erythema is predominantly peripheral and peri-limbic sparing is noted.

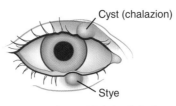

Fig. 7.1 Chalazion vs. hordeolum. (Adapted from Image 2. Styes and Chalazions Guide: Causes, Symptoms, and Treatment Options. [n.d.]. Available at: https://www.drugs.com/health-guide/styes-and-chalazions.html. Accessed July 15, 2016.)

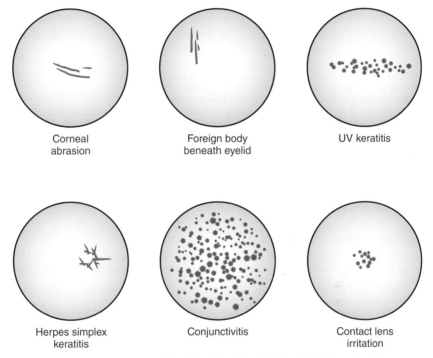

Fig. 7.2 Pattern of fluorescein stain uptake in corneal pain. (Adapted from Roberts J, Hedges K. Clinical Procedures in Emergency Medicine. Saunders Elsevier; 2010:1149, Fig. 63.11. Reprinted with permission.)

12. **Why is iritis painful? How is it treated?**
    Iritis causes inflammation of the ciliary muscles of the iris, and when light stimulates pupillary constriction, pain is worsened. This inflammation can sometimes cause transient paralysis of the muscle, causing an asymmetric pupil. Iritis is treated with cycloplegic/parasympatholytic drops, which are always found in bottles with red caps (e.g., atropine, homatropine, cyclopentolate).

13. **Do any studies need to be performed on a patient with a subconjunctival hemorrhage?**
    The condition is most commonly caused by a sudden increase in globe pressure that occurs with coughing, sneezing, vomiting, or straining; the hemorrhage is painless, does not require treatment, and typically resolves in 10–20 days. Patients taking warfarin should have their levels checked.

14. **What is a hyphema?**
    Hyphema is bleeding into the anterior chamber, typically caused by trauma to the globe. The blood collection in the anterior chamber will form a fluid level that can be seen anterior to the iris. Patients with hyphema should remain in the sitting position. Patients with a hyphema that is greater than 33% of the iris—or features any elevation of intraocular pressure—should be referred to an ophthalmologist, as red blood cells can obstruct flow through the trabecular meshwork and elevate intraocular pressure.

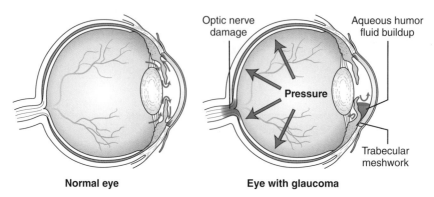

Fig. 7.3 Acute angle glaucoma. (From Glaucoma, Garden City Eye Care. Available at: http://gardencityeyecare.com/glaucoma/. Accessed July 15, 2016.)

15. **Why is acute angle glaucoma made worse by the dark?**
   In patients with glaucoma, pupil dilation (mydriasis) blocks the canal of Schlemm, which drains the aqueous humor from the orbit. In turn, the pressure increase within the posterior chamber elicits pain (Fig. 7.3). Vision loss occurs when pressure from the fluid compresses the blood vessels surrounding the optic nerve, causing ischemia. Treatment of acute angle glaucoma should focus first on constricting the pupil (meiosis).

KEY POINTS

1. "Eye pain" should be carefully examined to determine if the problem is in the soft tissue or the orbit.
2. Visual acuity should be part of every eye exam.
3. Fluorescein staining is a helpful tool in most eye exams.

BIBLIOGRAPHY

Acute Angle Glaucoma.Glaucoma. Garden City Eye Care. <http://gardencityeyecare.com/glaucoma/>; Accessed 14.07.16.
Conjunctivitis Preferred Practice Patterns–2015. American Academy of Ophthalmology. <http://www.aao.org/summary-benchmark-detail/conjunctivitis-summary-benchmark–october-2012>; Accessed 23.05.16.
Garrity J: *Blepharitis.* Merck Manual Online, Professional Version. <http://www.merckmanuals.com/professional/eye-disorders/eyelid-and-lacrimal-disorders/blepharitis>; Accessed 15.06.16.
Garrity J: *Chalazion and hordeolum (stye).* Merck Manual Online, Professional Version. <http://www.merckmanuals.com/professional/eye-disorders/eyelid-and-lacrimal-disorders/chalazion-and-hordeolum-stye>; Accessed 15.06.16.
Garrity J: *Preseptal and orbital cellulitis.* Merck Manual Online, Professional Version. <http://www.merckmanuals.com/professional/eye-disorders/orbital-diseases/preseptal-and-orbital-cellulitis>; Accessed 01.07.16.
Knoop K, Dennis W, Hedges J. Ophthalmologic, otolaryngologic, and dental procedures. In: *Roberts and Hedges: Clinical Procedures in Emergency Medicine.* Saunders Elsevier; 2010:1141–1177.
Oldham G: Hyphema. American Academy of Ophthalmology, EyeWiki. <http://eyewiki.aao.org/Hyphema>; Accessed 03.07.16.
Primary Angle Closure Summary Benchmark–2016. American Academy of Ophthalmology. <http://www.aao.org/summary-benchmark-detail/primary-angle-closure-summary-benchmark-october-2>; Accessed 12.07.16.
Styes and Chalazions Guide: Causes, Symptoms, and Treatment Options. <Drugs.com.https://www.drugs.com/health-guide/styes-and-chalazions.html>; Accessed 14.07.16.

CHAPTER 8

EAR, NOSE, AND THROAT

Joseph Ash, MD, Jacob Silverman, MD

1. **What are the common causes of otalgia?**
   Common causes are otitis media, cerumen impaction, and otitis externa, as well as referred pain from the throat or temporal bone. Less common causes include foreign bodies in the ear canal, mastoiditis, perichondritis, external ear dermatitis/cellulitis, or ear tumors (such as eosinophilic granulomas or rhabdomyosarcomas).

2. **How does otitis media typically present?**
   Ear pain associated upper respiratory infection symptoms (including rhinitis and cough), constitutional symptoms (such as irritability and difficulty sleeping), and fever.

3. **What are the common tympanic membrane findings with otitis media?**
   The tympanic membrane (TM) may be cloudy and opacified or appear red. There is often bulging of the TM, loss of landmarks (inability to see the umbo), and absent light reflex.

4. **Which organisms typically cause otitis media?**
   Bacterial causes include *Streptococcus pneumoniae, Haemophilus influenzae,* and *Moraxella catarrhalis.* Viruses (including respiratory syncytial virus [RSV], adenovirus, rhinovirus, or influenza) account for less than 10% of otitis media.

5. **What is the recommended treatment for otitis media?**
   Duration on first-line treatment may be 5–7 days; if recurrent otitis media, duration is recommended to be 7–10 days (Table 8.1) and may require follow-up with an otolaryngologist. Azithromycin and trimethoprim/sulfamethoxazole are no longer recommended for routine use for acute otitis media due to increased antibiotic resistance.

6. **What is mastoiditis?**
   A complication of acute otitis media, where the infection causes inflammation of the mastoid bone, is subdivided into two categories: osteitis within the mastoid air-cell system and periostitis of the mastoid process.

7. **How does mastoiditis present?**
   Pain located over the mastoid. Patients often complain of pain deep within the ear or behind the ear, with associated tenderness over the mastoid process. There may be a persistent fever (despite adequate antibiotic treatment for acute otitis media), mastoid erythema, or proptosis of the auricle.

8. **What are the complications of mastoiditis?**
   Hearing loss, facial nerve palsy, cranial nerve involvement, osteomyelitis, labyrinthitis, sigmoid sinus thrombosis, and abscess formation.

Table 8.1 Treatment of Otitis Media

RECOMMENDED FIRST-LINE TREATMENT	RECOMMENDED FIRST-LINE TREATMENT IF PENICILLIN ALLERGIC	SECOND-LINE TREATMENT, AFTER FAILURE TO FIRST-LINE ANTIBIOTIC
Amoxicillin (875 mg po bid)	Cefdinir (300 mg po bid)	Clindamycin (300 mg po tid)
Amoxicillin/clavulanate if patient received amoxicillin within 30 days (875 mg/125 mg po bid)	Cefuroxime (500 mg po bid)	May use amoxicillin/clavulanate or ceftriaxone IM/IV, if not used previously
	Cefpodoxime (200 mg po bid)	
	Ceftriaxone (1–2 g IV qd or 1 g IM qd for 3 days)	

Adapted from Harmes KM, Blackwood RA, Burrows HL, et al. Otitis media: diagnosis and treatment. *Am Fam Physician.* 2014;89(5):318. Available at: http://www.aafp.org/afp/2013/1001/p435.html. Accessed April 18, 2023; Natal BA: Acute Otitis Media Empiric Therapy. Medscape. Available at: http://emedicine.medscape.com/article/2012609-overview. Accessed April 18, 2023.

9. What are the treatment recommendations for mastoiditis?
   Subacute mastoiditis (mastoiditis without osteitis or periostitis) may be treated with purely medical management. Patients should be prescribed antibiotic coverage similar to otitis media with close follow-up. If worsening of pain or no significant improvement in 48 hours, patients should be referred to ENT, as they will most likely require tympanoplasty (treatment and diagnostic for bacterial culture), imaging (CT scan or MRI for evaluation of extension of disease), and/or mastoidectomy.

10. What are the most common causes of a perforated tympanic membrane?
    Trauma (including physical abuse, foreign body, or forceful ear irrigation), infection, and middle ear barotrauma (such as a blast trauma, scuba diving injury, or airplane ascent/descent).

11. How is a perforated tympanic membrane best managed in the urgent care setting?
    The ear canal may be cleaned using gentle suction; do not irrigate the ear canal, as water in the middle ear may introduce bacteria and cause infection. Treat concurrent otitis media with oral antibiotics. Regarding antibiotic ear drops, avoid gentamicin, neomycin sulfate, or tobramycin, as they carry the risk of ototoxicity. Prophylactic antibiotics (for perforated tympanic membrane in the absence of acute infection) are only advised if the injury involved contamination with lake water, seawater, or a dirty object such as a tree branch. Advise patient to keep ear dry by using ear plugs for showering and avoid submerging head underwater. Recommend appropriate analgesia; oral nonsteroidal antiinflammatory drugs (NSAIDs) typically are sufficient.

12. What symptoms or physical exam findings warrant referral to an otolaryngologist?
    The majority (80–90%) of tympanic membrane perforations will heal spontaneously in 4–6 weeks. Referral to an otolaryngologist is advised for large or marginal perforations (as they may require surgery) and for patients with nystagmus, vertigo, profound hearing loss, or disruption of the ossicles.

13. How does otitis externa typically present?
    Patients with otitis externa will often complain of ear pain, pruritus, otorrhea, and hearing loss. Pain may be exacerbated by chewing and other auricle movement. Inspection of otorrhea can function as a diagnostic indicator of the cause of otitis externa, as acute bacterial otitis externa will often have a white purulent drainage, whereas fungal otitis externa (otomycosis) will have a fluffy cottonlike grayish or black material.

14. What are the most common bacterial causes of otitis externa?
    Staphylococcus aureus, Streptococcus pyogenes, Pseudomonas aeruginosa, and *Vibrio alginolyticus* are the bacteria most often associated with otitis externa.

15. How is otitis externa best treated?
    Otitis externa is treated first with removal of the debris/purulent drainage with ear canal suctioning or ear irrigation, second with prescription ear drops specific to the causative agent (Table 8.2), and third with management of pain either using topical analgesic agents such as Auralgan or tetracaine or oral analgesic agents such as NSAIDs. Often otitis externa will require placement of an ear wick to allow for medication penetration.

16. What are the recommendations for swimmers in regard to returning to the water?
    Otitis externa is five times more common in swimmers than in nonswimmers. The conservative recommendation would be to avoid submersion for 7–10 days. To help prevent reoccurrence, advising use of ear plugs is a good idea.

17. How can otitis externa be prevented?
    Otitis externa is primarily caused by moisture and warmth in the ear canal, creating an environment conducive to bacterial growth. Preventative techniques include preventing moisture from entering the canal (with a tight-fitting swimming cap, ear plugs, etc.), drying the ear canal (e.g., with a hair dryer on the lowest setting after bathing or swimming), or instilling one to two drops of otic acetic acid or aluminum acetate (Burrow solution) after bathing or swimming.

Table 8.2 Treatment of Otitis Externa

UNCOMPLICATED BACTERIAL INFECTION	UNCOMPLICATED FUNGAL INFECTION
Neomycin-polymyxin B-hydrocortisone otic 4 drops in the affected ear tid or qid for 7 days	Clotrimazole 1% otic 4 drops in the affected ear qid for 7 days
Ofloxacin 0.3% otic 5 drops in the affected ear bid for 7 days	
Ciprofloxacin-hydrocortisone otic 3 drops in the affected ear bid for 7 days	

18. **What causes cerumen impaction?**
Cerumen, or earwax, is a naturally occurring substance in the ear canal, composed of secretions, sloughed epithelial cells, and hair. Typically, cerumen is naturally extruded, although sometimes it can accumulate and occlude the canal. Cerumen impaction can present with otalgia, hearing loss, clogged sensation, tinnitus, dizziness, and chronic cough (due to irritation of the auricular branch of the vagus nerve).

19. **How is cerumen impaction treated?**
Removal of cerumen can be performed with the use of cerumenolytic agents (acetic acid, hydrogen peroxide, carbamide peroxide, or mineral oil), manual removal (using ear curette or forceps for large clumps of cerumen), and/or ear irrigation. Studies have shown no significant difference between the effectiveness of varying cerumenolytic agents. Approximately 40% of patients with cerumen impaction can clear ear wax with use of a cerumenolytic agent alone (without irrigation).

20. **What are the most common ear/nose foreign bodies?**
Common ear foreign bodies include insects, plastic toys/beads, cotton such as tip from cotton swab/Q-tip, organic material such as popcorn kernels or candy, and small batteries. Organic material increases the risk of bacterial infection, and batteries (especially button batteries) can be caustic.

21. **How do ear/nose foreign bodies typically present?**
Ear foreign bodies often present with ear pain, foreign body sensation, hearing loss/muffled hearing, and/or malodorous otorrhea. Nose foreign bodies often present with nasal pain, malodorous unilateral rhinorrhea, and/or epistaxis.

22. **Where is the most common location for an ear foreign body to become lodged/stuck?**
The narrowest portion of the external auditory canal is at the bony cartilaginous junction, which is the most common place for a foreign body.

23. **Where is the most common location for a nasal foreign body to become lodged/stuck?**
Nasal foreign bodies are most often located on the floor of the nasal passage just below the inferior turbinate or in the upper nasal fossa anterior to the middle turbinate.

24. **What is the best way to remove a foreign body from the ear?**
There are multiple techniques, and the choice is best determined by the clinical situation: type of foreign body, compliance of the patient, and associated factors (e.g., amount of associated edema/pain or concern for perforated TM). Options include ear irrigation, use of forceps (bayonet or alligator), cerumen loop, suction catheters, or magnet (for metal foreign bodies). Live insects should be killed prior to removal; you may place several drops of alcohol, 2% lidocaine, or mineral oil into the ear canal. Irrigation should not be used if the foreign body is a battery due to concern for electrical current and/or battery contents causing tissue necrosis.

25. **What is the best way to remove a foreign body from the nose?**
As with ear foreign bodies, there are multiple techniques that can be utilized for nasal foreign body removal. Often before attempting removal, 0.5% phenylephrine or topical lidocaine can be used to reduce mucosal edema and to provide analgesia, respectively. First-line treatment should be to encourage the patient to expel the foreign body by blowing the nose while obstructing/blocking the opposite nostril. For easily visualized and easily grasped foreign bodies, direct instrumentation (e.g., forceps, hook) is often preferred. Another technique is placing a thin lubricated balloon-tip catheter beyond the foreign body and inflating the balloon, then pulling the inflated catheter balloon forward. Gentle suction can also be utilized for foreign body removal. Sedation is typically not advised due to decreasing gag reflex and glottis closure, therefore increasing risk of choking/aspiration.

26. **When should a patient with an ear/nose foreign body be referred to an otolaryngologist?**
Success rates for removing the foreign body significantly decline after the first attempt; also, multiple attempts cause complications of increased pain and bleeding, thus limiting visualization and causing the foreign body to extend further into the canal. A patient should be referred to an otolaryngologist if there have been multiple unsuccessful attempts or if there is concern for trauma to the TM. Additionally, if there are already symptoms present, such as bleeding, infection, difficulty bleeding, or considerable pain, an otolaryngologist should be considered.

27. **What are common causes of epistaxis?**
Most cases of epistaxis are caused by direct trauma; however, epistaxis can also be caused by repetitive nasal mucosa irritation (such as with rhinitis), corticosteroid nasal sprays (such as Flonase or Nasonex), anticoagulant therapy (such as warfarin, Xarelto, Pradaxa), coagulopathy disorder, and arteriovenous malformation, among others. Additionally, things as simple as dry air, allergies, or anatomical abnormalities such as deviated septum can be the cause of nasal bleeding. A good history of present illness and medical history can help determine if the epistaxis is benign or an indicator of a more serious condition.

28. **What is the most common site of bleeding for epistaxis?**
Anterior epistaxis is the most common etiology for nasal bleeds, accounting for more than 90% of bleeds. The most common site of anterior epistaxis is Little area, also known as Kiesselbach plexus.

29. **How is epistaxis best managed in the urgent care setting?**
Direct visualization of the bleed is beneficial; however, it can be difficult initially. Have the patient blow their nose and/or use suction to expel clots. Use phenylephrine or oxymetazoline nasal spray, or soak a cotton ball in topical tetracaine, epinephrine (adrenaline) solution and place in naris for 10–15 minutes with associated concurrent 10–15 minutes of digital pressure. This pressure should be anterior to the nasal bone (cartilaginous area) occluding both nares and may assist in stopping the nasal bleeding. The patient must lean forward to avoid draining down the nasopharynx. If hemostasis is achieved with digital pressure and the site of bleeding can be visualized, further measures should be considered to prevent rebleeding. Options include electrocautery, silver nitrate cautery, and tranexamic acid-soaked pledgets. Be sure to cauterize just proximal to the bleeding site and never apply to both sides of the septum to avoid septal perforation. Pledgets soaked in tranexamic acid have also been shown to be effective in stopping bleeding and decreasing rebleeding at 1 week. Packing is considered only if the above solutions have failed. Patients who receive nasal packing have traditionally been placed on prophylactic antibiotics to avoid toxic shock syndrome, although there is no robust evidence indicating benefit. Packing should be removed 48 hours after placement.

30. **Which patients with epistaxis should not be managed in an outpatient setting?**
Patients who are not hemodynamically stable, have a coagulopathy disorder, have respiratory or cardiac compromise from nasal bleeding, or have failed hemostasis attempts should be referred to the emergency department.

31. **How does rhinitis typically present?**
Rhinitis, inflammation of the nasal membranes, most commonly presents with nasal congestion, rhinorrhea, sneezing, nasal pruritus, postnasal drip, facial pain or pressure, anosmia, and potentially cough. Acute rhinitis is most commonly allergic.

32. **How is rhinitis treated?**
Simple solutions include avoiding triggers if it is caused by an allergen or an irritant. Also, saline nasal irrigation can be used to rinse the nasal passages, which helps reduce congestion and remove mucus. Oral antihistamines (such as first-generation H1 blockers [diphenhydramine] or nonsedating/less sedation second-generation H1 blockers [loratadine, fexofenadine, cetirizine]) along with intranasal corticosteroids (fluticasone or mometasone) can be used. Patients who fail to respond to first-line treatment can be referred to an allergist for consideration for immunotherapy.

33. **How does sinusitis typically present?**
Acute sinusitis or acute rhinosinusitis is one of the most common conditions that medical providers treat in the urgent care setting. Patients may complain of congestion, rhinorrhea, pain overlying frontal or maxillary sinuses, radiating pain to teeth, and/or pain exacerbated by bending down. Fatigue is also commonly associated with sinusitis. Symptoms typically last less than 4 weeks and are often accompanied by fever and other signs of infection, while chronic sinusitis can last for several months or longer.

34. **What are the most common causes of rhinosinusitis?**
Rhinosinusitis episodes are most commonly viral in origin, including rhinovirus, influenza, and parainfluenza. Viral upper respiratory tract infections (URIs) are the number-one risk factor for development of acute bacterial sinusitis. Approximately 90% of patients with a viral URI have sinus involvement, and 5–10% of these patients have bacterial superinfection requiring antibiotic treatment. The most common bacterial causes of rhinosinusitis are *Streptococcus pneumoniae*, *Haemophilus influenzae*, *Moraxella catarrhalis*, and *Staphylococcus aureus*. Fungal sinusitis is rare, but the most common fungal species associated with sinusitis are Aspergillus and Alternaria, and usually only occur in patients with weakened immune systems or those who have had previous nasal surgery.

35. **What are the indications that acute sinusitis is bacterial in origin and warrants antibiotic treatment?**
Double sickening (initially got better but then worsened), purulent rhinorrhea, purulent secretion in the nasal cavity, and elevated erythrocyte sedimentation rate increase the likelihood of bacterial etiology. Guidelines also suggest prescribing a patient an antibiotic if symptoms fail to improve within 7–10 days. Radiography is not recommended for evaluation of uncomplicated acute rhinosinusitis.

36. **What are some alternative/adjunctive treatment options for sinusitis?**
Patients may have symptom improvement with analgesics, oral decongestants, topical decongestants, mucolytics, intranasal corticosteroids, saline nasal irrigation, or oral antihistamines. There is limited evidence to suggest significant benefits from the aforementioned therapies.

37. **What is the best antibiotic treatment for acute rhinosinusitis?**
Antibiotic course should be prescribed for 10 days (Table 8.3). Continued symptoms despite second-line treatment typically warrant computerized tomography (CT) of the sinuses (without contrast) for evaluation of possible complications or anatomic abnormalities and/or referral to an otolaryngologist.

Table 8.3 Treatment of Rhinosinusitis

FIRST-LINE TREATMENT	SECOND-LINE TREATMENT
Amoxicillin/clavulanate	Amoxicillin/clavulanate (high dose)
Amoxicillin	Levofloxacin
Azithromycin (extended release)	Clindamycin

38. **How does pharyngitis typically present?**
    Pharyngitis most commonly presents with sore throat. Patients may also have low-grade fever, dysphagia, odyno-phagia, or hoarseness.

39. **What are the red flags associated with a sore throat?**
    Red flags with pharyngitis include associated unilateral sore throat pain, drooling and/or inability to swallow, trismus, muffled/"hot potato" voice, stridor/respiratory distress, or high fever.

40. **What are the causes of pharyngitis?**
    The most common cause is a viral or bacterial illness (including streptococcal pharyngitis). Sore throat can also be due to postnasal drip associated with upper respiratory infection or seasonal allergies or recurrent irritation from gastroesophageal reflux disease. Patients would then present with associated rhinorrhea, sneezing, nasal congestion, cough or eructation, epigastric discomfort, bloating, and so forth, respective to the disease process. Concerning causes of pharyngitis include peritonsillar abscess, Ludwig angina, foreign body, malignancy, epiglot-titis, and diphtheria, among others.

41. **How is streptococcal pharyngitis diagnosed?**
    On physical examination, a practitioner can use the modified Centor Criteria: tonsillar exudate or erythema, anterior cervical lymphadenopathy, absent cough, present fever, and differential based on age (+1 point if age 3–14, 0 points if age 15–45, and −1 point if over age 45). A strep score of 4–5 warrants empiric treatment with antibiotics. Controversy exists regarding empiric treatment. Rapid streptococcal antigen tests are frequently used for diagnostic purposes. Specificity and sensitivity vary based on the test manufacturer; however, the tests are generally high in positive predictive values (90–98%) but show insufficient sensitivity to rule out group A beta-hemolytic streptococci (GABHS) infection (79–95%). Negative rapid streptococcal antigen tests should be confirmed with culture. Culture for GABHS is 90–95% sensitive and 94–100% specific. The gold standard in diagnosing strep throat is a throat culture. The test is highly accurate, but it can take up to 2 days to get the results.

42. **What are some caveats to streptococcal pharyngitis testing?**
    An estimated 15–20% of the population are GABHS carriers, which will give a positive result on both the rapid streptococcal antigen tests and throat cultures, as neither test is specific for active infection. This results in over-treatment of a significant portion of patients. Also, an estimated 33% of patients with infectious mononucleosis and diphtheria have positive GABHS cultures, leading to misdiagnoses.

43. **Does streptococcal pharyngitis require antibiotic treatment?**
    GABHS infection is a self-limited disease, often resolving in 3–5 days without treatment. However, streptococcal pharyngitis is treated for prevention of serious sequelae including rheumatic fever and glomerulonephritis.

44. **What is the recommended treatment for streptococcal pharyngitis?**
    First-line treatment for GABHS is penicillin, amoxicillin, or (for patients allergic to penicillin) first-generation cephalosporin, clindamycin, or macrolide antibiotics. Other causes of pharyngitis, such as candidal or herpetic, should be treated appropriately based on causative agents such as oral fluconazole, itraconazole or acyclovir, and famciclovir, respectively.

45. **What is a peritonsillar abscess?**
    A peritonsillar abscess is the progression of a bacterial infection: exudative tonsillitis, to cellulitis, to abscess. The abscess generally forms in the Weber glands (a group of salivary glands in the supratonsillar fossa). Pre-senting symptoms are similar to pharyngitis (fever, sore throat, dysphagia, odynophagia); however, on physical examination, there may be trismus and/or a muffled/"hot potato" voice. Inspection of the oropharynx reveals edema and erythema of the anterior tonsillar pillar with tonsil displacement and contralateral deviation of the uvula.

46. **What are the complications/concerns with a peritonsillar abscess?**
    The primary concern with a peritonsillar abscess is airway obstruction. However, there are also possibilities of aspiration pneumonitis, hemorrhage from erosion or septic necrosis into carotid sheath, or extension of the infec-tion into the soft tissues of the deep neck or posterior mediastinum.

47. **How is a peritonsillar abscess treated?**
Treatment of choice for a peritonsillar abscess is needle aspiration or incision and drainage. Patients should then be placed on a broad-spectrum antibiotic. In the outpatient setting, oral options include amoxicillin/clavulanate (875 mg/125 mg bid), clindamycin (600 mg bid or 300 mg qid), or penicillin (500 mg qid) plus metronidazole (500 mg qid). Recent studies suggest an adjunctive corticosteroid can speed recovery. Patients with a peritonsillar abscess require close follow-up and should be reseen in 1–2 days. The decision for more intensive medical management will depend on several factors including the severity of the infection, the patient's overall health, and the presence of other medical conditions that may increase the risk of complications.

48. **How does mononucleosis present?**
Mononucleosis, or Epstein-Barr virus, typically presents initially with mild flulike symptoms for a few days. Patients will then develop fever, sore throat, and lymphadenopathy; exudate tonsillitis and prominent cervical lymphadenopathy present in 97% of patients. Other common associated symptoms include fatigue, malaise, myalgias, and headache. Mononucleosis has the highest incidence in the 15- to 24-year-old age group and increased frequency on college campuses and among military recruits (due to congested, confined spaces).

49. **What are some diagnostic testing options for mononucleosis?**
One of the most common tests is the mononuclear spot (monospot) test, which tests for heterophile antibodies (Paul-Bunnell IgM). The monospot test has a high false-negative rate in the first week of symptoms (25%). Antibodies peak between weeks 2 and 5. The monospot test has a low false-negative rate by the third week of symptoms (5%). The benefits of the test are that it is relatively inexpensive and produces results quickly. Other testing includes a complete blood count (CBC) for reevaluation of lymphocyte count and predominance as well as lymphocyte atypia. Liver function tests are abnormal in 80% of mononucleosis patients. An Epstein-Barr virus antibody test can also be ordered; however, this is expensive in an urgent care center and is typically sent out to a lab, so it should only be ordered if the results would change the management of the disease.

50. **What is the best treatment for mononucleosis?**
Most of the treatment for mononucleosis is symptomatic: rest (important for supporting the immune system) and analgesic agents (NSAIDs or acetaminophen) can be used to help manage symptoms such as headache, fever, and sore throat. Oral corticosteroids (such as prednisone or dexamethasone) have not proven to be effective in reducing the clinical course of the illness. However, they should be reserved for patients with airway compromise. Approximately 75% of patients with mononucleosis have splenomegaly and should be advised limited exercise/athletics and no contact sports (due to risk of splenic rupture) for 4 weeks minimum, or longer if splenomegaly has not resolved.

KEY POINTS

1. Of tympanic membrane perforations, 80–90% will heal spontaneously in 4–6 weeks.
2. Acute rhinitis is most commonly allergic.

Acknowledgments
We would like to thank the previous author, Samantha F. Singer, PA-C, for her contributions to the previous edition of this chapter.

BIBLIOGRAPHY
Andrejko K, Ratnasiri B, Hausdorff WP, Laxminarayan R, Lewnard JA. Antimicrobial resistance in paediatric Streptococcus pneumoniae isolates amid global implementation of pneumococcal conjugate vaccines: a systematic review and meta-regression analysis. *The Lancet Microbe.* 2021;2(9):e450–e460.
Aring AM, Chan MM. Current concepts in adult acute rhinosinusitis. *Am Fam Physician.* 2016;94(2):97–105.
Bousquet J, Anto JM, Bachert C, et al. Allergic rhinitis. *Nat Rev Dis Primers.* 2020;6:95.
Brook I. Acute sinusitis. http://emedicine.medscape.com/article/232670; accessed April 18, 2023.
Caglar D, Kwun R. Mouth and throat disorders in infants and children. In: Tintinalli JE, Ma O, Yealy DM, Meckler GD, Stapczynski J, Cline DM, Thomas SH, eds. *Tintinalli's Emergency Medicine: A Comprehensive Study Guide, 9e.* McGraw Hill; 2020.
Chow AW, Benninger MS, Brook I, Brozek JL, Goldstein EJ, Hicks LA, et al. IDSA clinical practice guideline for acute bacterial rhinosinusitis in children and adults. *Clin Infect Dis.* 2012;54(8):e72–e112.
Cohen JS, Agrawal D. Nose and sinus disorders in infants and children. In: Tintinalli JE, Ma O, Yealy DM, Meckler GD, Stapczynski J, Cline DM, Thomas SH, eds. *Tintinalli's Emergency Medicine: A Comprehensive Study Guide, 9e.* McGraw Hill; 2020.
D'Aguanno V, Ralli M, Greco A, de Vincentiis M. Clinical recommendations for epistaxis management during the COVID-19 pandemic. *Otolaryngol Head Neck Surg.* 2020;163:75–77.
Devan PP. Mastoiditis. Medscape. http://emedicine.medscape.com/article/2056657; accessed April 18, 2023.
Domino FJ, Baldor RA, Grimes JA, et al. *Griffith's 5 Minute Clinical Consult.* Philadelphia: Lippincott Williams & Wilkins; 2014:740.
Earwood JS, Rogers TS, Rathjen NA. Ear pain: diagnosing common and uncommon causes. *Am Fam Physician.* 2018;97(1):20–27.
Fischer JI. Nasal foreign bodies. Medscape. http://emedicine.medscape.com/article/763767; accessed April 18, 2023.
Galioto NJ. Peritonsillar abscess. *Am Fam Physician.* 2017;95(8):501–506.
Hayashi T, Kitamura K, Hashimoto S, et al. Clinical practice guidelines for the diagnosis and management of acute otitis media in children—2018 update. *Auris Nasus Larynx.* 2020;47:493–526.
Hom D. *Essential Tissue Healing of the Face and Neck.* Shelton, CT: PMPH-USA; 2009:150.

Kalra MK, Higgins KE, Perez ED. Common questions about streptococcal pharyngitis. *Am Fam Physician*. 2016;94(1):24–31. http://www.aafp.org/afp/2016/0701/p24.html; accessed October 24, 2016.

Kawaguchi R, Matsui S, Hayashi T, et al. Characteristics of pediatric nasal foreign body cases that required multiple removal procedures: a single tertiary medical center cross-sectional study. *Pediatr Emerg Care*. 2022;38:E1606–E1612.

Lieberthal AS, Carroll AE, Chonmaitree T, Ganiats TG, Hoberman A, Jackson MA, et al. The diagnosis and management of acute otitis media. *Pediatrics*. 2013;131(3):e964–e999.

Mahadevan SV, Garmel GM. *An Introduction to Clinical Emergency Medicine*. Cambridge, MA: Cambridge University Press; 2012:332.

Matz G, Rybak L, Roland PS, et al. Ototoxicity of ototopical antibiotic drops in humans. *Otolaryngol Head Neck Surg*. 2004;130(suppl 3):S79–S82.

Moses S: Mononucleosis. Family Practice Notebook. Mononucleosis (fpnotebook.com); accessed October 24, 2016.

Oyama LC. Foreign bodies of the ear, nose and throat. *Emerg Med Clin*. 2019;37(1):121–130.

Prasad N, Harley E. The aural foreign body space: a review of pediatric ear foreign bodies and a management paradigm. *Int J Pediatr Otorhinolaryngol*. 2020;132:109871.

Rosenfeld RM, Piccirillo JF, Chandrasekhar SS, Brook I, Kumar Ashok K, Kramper M, et al. Clinical practice guideline (update) adult sinusitis executive summary. *Otolaryngol Head Neck Surg*. 2015;152(4):598–609.

Rutter P, Newby D. *Community Pharmacy ANZ: Symptoms, Diagnosis and Treatment*. Cambridge, MA: Elsevier Health Sciences; 2015:78.

Schilder AGM, Chonmaitree T, Cripps AW, et al. Otitis media. *Nat Rev Dis Primers*. 2016;2:16063.

Schwartz SR, Magit AE, Rosenfeld RM, Ballachanda BB, Hackell JM, Krouse HJ, et al. Clinical practice guideline (update): earwax (cerumen impaction). *Otolaryngol Head Neck Surg*. 2017;156:S1–S29.

Smith MA, Schrager SB, WinklerPrins V. *Essentials of Family Medicine*. 7th ed. Philadelphia: Wolters Kluwer; 2019.

Wiegand S, Berner R, Schneider A, Lundershausen E, Dietz A. Otitis externa investigation and evidence-based treatment. *Deutsches Ärzteblatt international*. 2019;116:224–234.

Wolfson AB, Cloutier RL, Hendey GW, et al. *Harwood-Nuss' Clinical Practice of Emergency Medicine*. 7th ed. Philadelphia, PA: Wolters Kluwer; 2020.

Womack J, Jimenez M. Common questions about infectious mononucleosis. *Am Fam Physician*. 2015;91(6):372–376.

Zahed R, Mousavi Jazayeri MH, Naderi A, Naderpour Z, Saeedi M. Topical tranexamic acid compared with anterior nasal packing for treatment of epistaxis in patients taking antiplatelet drugs: randomized controlled trial. *Acad Emerg Med*. 2018;25(3):261–266.

CHAPTER 9

DENTAL AND MOUTH PAIN

Spencer Adoff, MD, FACEP

1. **What is the anatomy of a tooth?**
   The crown is the visible portion of the tooth, which consists of three layers. The pulp (neurovascular supply of the tooth) is surrounded by dentin, which is covered by enamel. The root is the portion of the tooth that extends into the bone. It is covered by cementum, which adheres to the periodontal ligament.

2. **How are teeth numbered? (Fig. 9.1)**

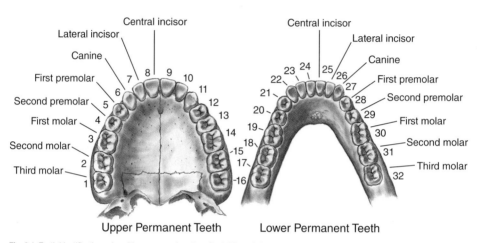

Fig. 9.1 Tooth identification using either name or American Dental Association numbering system; letters for deciduous teeth, numbers for permanent teeth. (From Mosby's Guide to Physical Examination, 2006.)

3. **Describe the types of dental fractures.**
   Ellis type I is a fracture of the enamel only and does not require treatment. Ellis type II fractures to the dentin are most common, and the tooth is usually sensitive to changes in temperature. Ellis type III (blood exposure) fractures expose the pulp. Types II and III require placement of a protective covering, such as calcium hydroxide base, as a delay in treatment increases the likelihood of pulpal necrosis. Patients require urgent referral to a dentist. Root fractures will have mobility of the crown (with or without Ellis fractures); radiographs will confirm. Alveolar fractures will allow multiple teeth to move together with palpation (Fig. 9.2).

4. **Describe and define the different types of dental trauma.**
   See Table 9.1.

5. **What is the treatment for an avulsed tooth?**
   The best way to transport the tooth is in the patient's tooth socket. Gently rinse (to remove debris) and replace it (only primary teeth should be reimplanted). Handle the tooth by the crown so as not to damage the periodontal ligament. It should be reimplanted within 2 hours and stabilized with a dental dressing paste. If it cannot be reimplanted, use Hank salt-based solution or cold milk. The patient's saliva is less ideal, and do not place the tooth in the mouth due to risk of aspiration.

6. **Which gum lacerations need to be sutured?**
   Gum lacerations that require suturing are those that are large, have flaps, or expose bone.

7. **Describe the types of dental infections.**
   With dental caries, instruct patients to use fluoride mouth rinses and toothpaste to reduce occurrences. Irreversible pulpitis causes acute, severe pain and is a common cause for patients to seek nondental care. Gingivitis commonly causes the gums to bleed; treatment consists of good brushing, flossing, warm saltwater rinses five times per day,

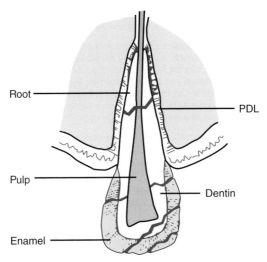

Fig. 9.2 Dental Tooth Fracture. (From Curtis, Emergency and Trauma Care for Nurses and Paramedics, 2011.)

Table 9.1 Types of Dental Trauma	
Concussion	Normal appearance, but will have pain with pressure (biting)
Subluxation	Loose tooth, without displacement; bleeding at the gumline
Intrusion	Tooth is driven upwards into the socket; bleeding at the gumline
Extrusion	Tooth is dislocated from the socket; bleeding at the gumline
Luxation	Tooth is displaced lateral, labial (toward lip), lingual (toward back/tongue)
Avulsion	Tooth is completely displaced from the socket

and chlorhexidine (0.12%) rinses twice per day. Acute necrotizing ulcerative gingivitis (ANUG) consists of diffuse mouth pain, halitosis, and pain with chewing. Patients will have bleeding gums and sloughing of the gingiva with gray-white pseudomembrane, which will bleed when removed. Treatment consists of chlorhexidine or hydrogen peroxide rinses, pain control, debridement of the pseudomembrane (gauze), and antibiotics if extensive/systemic or lymphadenopathic. Periodontitis is a severe progression of gingival inflammation, loss of tooth attachment, and tooth loss/mobility. It generally affects young adults. Treat with chlorhexidine rinses and systemic antibiotics. Periapical abscesses have painful swelling at the buccal and gingival mucosa. The teeth may be sensitive and have pain with chewing. Treatment consists of incision, drainage, and antibiotics.

8. **Which antibiotics should I use for the dental infections described above?**
   Penicillin VK, amoxicillin-clavulanate, erythromycin, clindamycin, metronidazole. Beta-lactamase production within oral bacteria is becoming increasingly common; penicillin monotherapy may no longer be enough.

9. **What are aphthous ulcers (canker sores)?**
   Canker sores are a chronic inflammatory and ulcerative disorder of unknown etiology. Patients will have painful, single, small, circular ulcerations. They are treated with topical anesthetics and cleansing rinses. They can be distinguished from oral herpes simplex virus 1 (HSV-1), which are small, painful, clustered vesicles. HSV-1 can be treated with topical acyclovir early in its course.

10. **What are the three main salivary glands that form stones?**
    Parotid, submandibular, and sublingual salivary glands form stones.

11. **What are the clinical features that suggest a patient may have sialolithiasis?**
    Patients typically present with pain and swelling of the affected gland, which will be exaggerated by anything that stimulates salivation. They may also present with painless swelling of the gland. Symptoms may be persistent or intermittent over days to weeks due to complete versus incomplete obstruction. You may be able to palpate stones within the Wharton duct by palpating on the floor of the mouth from a lingual to labial direction. Parotid gland

stones may be palpated within the Stenson duct along the buccal mucosa within the mouth and along the face from the earlobe along the mandible (place one finger within the mouth at the same time).

12. **When should you suspect sialadenitis and how should you treat it?**
Patients may have systemic symptoms such as fevers and chills in conjunction with pain, swelling, and erythema around the affected gland. Viral infections are typically bilateral, as compared to bacterial infections, which are unilateral. You may see purulent drainage from the respective duct. Treatment consists of antibiotics, sialagogues, gentle heat, massage, and pain control. Consider clindamycin, amoxicillin-clavulanate, or cephalexin with metronidazole; 7 to 10 days should be effective. Lack of improvement or worsening of the patient's condition may suggest abscess formation and will require further evaluation.

13. **What are the most common presenting signs and symptoms of temporal mandibular disorder (TMD)?**
Facial pain triggered by jaw motions (chewing and speaking), limitation of jaw movements, temporal mandibular joint tenderness, popping sounds with jaw function, headaches, ear pain, neck stiffness, and pain.

14. **What treatment recommendations are there for TMD?**
Pharmacologic (NSAIDs and muscle relaxers for 14 days) and nonpharmacologic (patient education and behavioral modification) treatments are recommended.

15. **What does oral candidiasis look like?**
It is a white-cream, curd-like exudate; it can be scraped off, leaving raw or bleeding mucosa. It is most commonly on the tongue but may be present on the buccal mucosa, soft palate, and hypopharynx.

16. **What are the symptoms?**
Asymptomatic, pain with eating, loss of taste, and change of sensation within the oral cavity.

17. **What patients are at risk for oral candidiasis?**
Infants, patients who wear dentures, patients on antibiotics or receiving chemotherapy, those getting radiation to the head/neck, and all patients who are immunocompromised.

18. **What are the preferred treatment regimens for non-HIV- and HIV-induced oral candidiasis?**
Clotrimazole troches, miconazole buccal tablets, nystatin swish and swallow for 7 to 14 days. Failure of local therapy may require oral fluconazole. If patients wear dentures, they should remove them nightly, brush them, and soak them in chlorhexidine in addition to the local or oral therapies. If patients have HIV, you may try the above for mild disease, but for more serious or recurrent episodes, utilize fluconazole as the first-line treatment.

KEY POINTS

1. The best way to transport an avulsed tooth is in the patient's tooth socket.
2. Gum lacerations that need to be repaired include large lacerations, flaps, and exposed bone.
3. Canker sores are treated with topical anesthetics and cleansing rinses.

BIBLIOGRAPHY

Andreasen JO, Andreasen FM. *Textbook and Color Atlas of Traumatic Injuries to the Teeth*. 4th ed. Munksgaard, Copenhagen: Wiley-Blackwell; 2007.

Cooper BC, Kleinberg I. Examination of a large patient population for the presence of symptoms and signs of temporomandibular disorders. *Cranio*. 2007;25:114.

Elluru RG. Inflammatory disorders of the salivary glands. In: Flint PW, Haughey BH et al., eds. *Cummings Otolaryngology: Head and Neck Surgery*. 6th ed. Philadelphia: Mosby Elsevier; 2015.

Jackson NM, Mitchell JL, Walvekar RR. Inflammatory disorders of the salivary glands. In: Flint PW, Haughey BH et al., eds. *Cummings Otolaryngology: Head and Neck Surgery*. 6th ed. Philadelphia: Mosby Elsevier; 2015.

Keels MA. Section on Oral Health, American Academy of Pediatrics: management of dental trauma in a primary care setting. *Pediatrics*. 2014;133:e466.

Malmgren B, Andreasen JO, Flores MT, et al. International Association of Dental Traumatology guidelines for the management of traumatic dental injuries: 3. Injuries to primary dentition. *Dent Traumatol*. 2012;28:174.

Mujakperuo HR, Watson M, Morrison R, Macfarlane TV. Pharmacological interventions for pain in patients with temporomandibular disorders. *Cochrane Database Syst Rev*. 2010.

Pappas PG, et al. Clinical practice guideline for the management of candidiasis: 2016 update by the Infectious Diseases Society of America. *Clin Infect Dis*. 2016.

Selwitz RH, Ismail AI, Pitts NB. Dental caries. *Lancet*. 2007;369:51.

Slots J, Ting M. Systemic antibiotics in the treatment of periodontal disease. *Periodontol*. 2000-2002;28:106.

CHAPTER 10

COUGH, SHORTNESS OF BREATH, AND CHEST PAIN

David A. Sanchez, MSPAS, PA-C

TOP SECRETS

1. The history of present illness is extremely important! There are multiple ways patients can characterize their chest pain, and this usually can help in determining a diagnosis. Pay close attention to descriptive terms such as sharp, crushing, pressure, and burning. Ask questions about what makes the pain worse. Perform a thorough review of systems to help differentiate between cardiac, pulmonary, and other sources of chest pain.
2. Certain cardiac workup is not available in the urgent care setting. Any patient presenting with chest pain of concern for cardiac etiology will need referred to the emergency department for evaluation.

1. **What are the most common triggers for cough?**
   Viruses! Most cases of acute cough are due to viral upper respiratory infections that lead to increased nasal secretions and subsequent postnasal drip. Other common triggers include asthma, chronic obstructive pulmonary disease, environmental or occupational exposures, gastroesophageal reflux disease, and congestive heart failure.

2. **What is the best way to treat a cough?**
   The best management strategy depends on the specific problem that triggers the cough. For example, bronchospasm caused by asthma is best treated with corticosteroids and inhaled beta-agonists. For cough associated with postnasal drip or viral bronchitis, symptomatic treatment may be achieved with over-the-counter antihistamines, decongestants, antitussives, or expectorants. Prescriptive antitussives such as benzonatate (Tessalon) can also help alleviate cough.

3. **What are some complications that may accompany severe or prolonged coughing?**
   Common complaints in patients with persistent cough include musculoskeletal chest pain, pleurisy, posttussive emesis, sore throat, and headache. Rarely, more serious complications such as rib fractures, pneumothorax, or pneumomediastinum can occur with severe or prolonged bronchospasm.

4. **A patient presents with shortness of breath. What are the most important parts of the history?**
   Age and history of known cardiac or pulmonary disease. Other key features of the history include associated symptoms such as diaphoresis or chest pain, presence of fever or cough, and status as a current or former smoker.

5. **What physical exam finding would be most concerning in a patient complaining of shortness of breath?**
   Work of breathing! Vital signs and overall appearance are critical in determining how to manage these patients. Abnormal vital signs, accessory muscle use, and decreasing mental status are likely to have a more serious etiology as a cause of their difficulty breathing. Auscultating lung sounds, checking for lower extremity edema, and evaluating the nasopharynx, throat, and ears for signs of infection/inflammation are also important pieces of the clinical puzzle.

6. **Describe the relevance of wheezing, rales, rhonchi, and diminished breath sounds.**
   Wheezing is generally associated with reactive airway diseases such as COPD or asthma. It can also be heard in acute bronchitis, foreign body aspiration, or CHF. Rhonchi are generally coarse sounds heard in specific lobes that tend to correspond to underlying infection. Rales or crackles are wet sounds often heard at lung bases that usually are due to fluid accumulation. Diminished breath sounds can be due to diminished air movement, pleural effusion, pneumothorax, or prohibitive body habitus.

7. **What features of the history favor noncardiac etiology of chest pain?**
   Younger patients without known cardiac risk factors are unlikely to have chest pain due to occlusive coronary artery disease. Pain that is very brief in duration, described as sharp or burning, does not radiate, is not associated with shortness of breath, nausea/vomiting (N/V), or diaphoresis, and is not made worse with exertion or improved with rest, all decrease the chances of serious underlying disease as the cause of their symptoms.

8. **What are some common causes of chest pain in patients presenting to urgent care?**
   Rib strains, costochondritis, pectoral muscle injury, and other variations of musculoskeletal pain are commonly found to be the cause of chest pain. GERD or chest discomfort associated with gastrointestinal (GI) illness, pleuritic

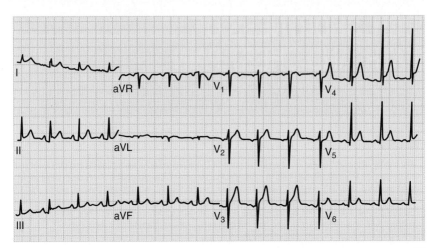

Fig. 10.1 Early EKG changes in pericarditis. This EKG shows typical EKG findings in early pericarditis, with J point changes and PR depression. Also noted are pronounced ST segment increases in II, aVF, V_2-V_6. (Reprinted from Mann D. *Braunwald's Heart Disease: A Textbook of Cardiovascular Medicine*. 10th ed. Saunders; 2014:1639. Overview of community-acquired pneumonia in adults. Available at https://www.uptodate.com/contents/overview-of-community-acquired-pneumonia-in-adults?search=communicty%20acquired%20pneumonia&source=search_result&selectedTitle=2~150&usage_type=default&display_rank=2#H1488131322. Published 2022. Accessed September 9, 2022. Overview of acute pulmonary embolism in adults. Available at https://www.uptodate.com/contents/overview-of-acute-pulmonary-embolism-in-adults?search=pulmonary%20embolism&source=search_result&selectedTitle=1~150&usage_type=default&display_rank=1#H86227218. Published 2022. Accessed September 9, 2022.)

discomfort in smokers or those suffering from acute bronchitis, and skin irritation (including zoster rash in a thoracic dermatome) can all present as a chief complaint of chest pain.

9. **What tools are available in most urgent care settings that can help with your workup of chest pain or shortness of breath?**
   Electrocardiogram (EKG) and chest x-ray.

10. **What features of the history favor cardiac etiology of chest pain?**
    History of prior coronary artery disease, diabetes, hypertension, hypercholesterolemia, and family history. Pressure, a squeezing feeling in the chest, and diaphoresis with chest pain should also raise the degree of suspicion of cardiac etiology. Additionally, radiating chest pain to other areas such as the arm, jaw, neck, or back should increase suspicion for cardiac etiology.

11. **If you are concerned that a patient is having cardiac chest pain, what should you do?**
    Call 911. The patient should be transported by ambulance to the nearest emergency department.

12. **What is the treatment for patients with acute exacerbations of asthma or COPD?**
    Inhaled bronchodilators! These can be given as inhaled puffs from a metered dose inhaler or as a nebulized solution. Patients may need to use these medications every 4 hours or even more frequently during an acute exacerbation. For moderate to severe symptoms, a course of steroids is generally recommended; either a short 5-day burst course without a taper or a more prolonged course of 7–10 days with a taper is prescribed.

13. **What is the typical presentation of acute pericarditis and the expected EKG findings?**
    Of patients who present, 95% will report chest pain. Usually, the pain is described as "sharp and pleuritic," and sitting up and leaning forward tends to improve the pain. Rarely, an audible pericardial friction rub can be appreciated. In the acute phase of disease, typical EKG findings include diffuse ST segment elevation that is usually concave upward (Fig. 10.1). The PR segment may also be depressed below baseline, which is a more specific, though less sensitive, finding in acute pericarditis. These typical EKG changes may become much subtler or even normalize after the acute phase of the disease is over, typically within 1 week.

14. **How does one define an acute exacerbation of COPD?**
    This is defined as "an acute event characterized by a worsening of the patient's respiratory symptoms that is beyond normal day-to-day variations and leads to a change in medication." There are generally three areas that may be affected: increased severity/frequency of cough, change in volume/character of sputum production, and increased shortness of breath beyond baseline. Generally, at least one of these criteria, and often all three, is seen during acute exacerbations of COPD.

15. What are common historical complaints of and major risk factors for pulmonary embolism?
    Common complaints could include lower extremity edema, shortness of breath, chest pain, cough, and palpitations/rapid heart rate. Hemoptysis is an unusual presenting symptom. Major risk factors for a PE include genetic predisposition, history of prior PE/DVT, active oncologic disease, hormone therapy, smoking history, trauma, and history of recent immobilization (surgery/travel).

16. A 23-year-old otherwise healthy male patient comes into urgent care complaining of sudden onset left-sided chest pain and shortness of breath that started while he was rock climbing. Pain is pleuritic in nature. He has no risk factors concerning for cardiac etiology. Physical exam reveals no reproducible chest wall tenderness, O_2 saturation of 92%, and lung sounds are diminished throughout on the left. What should your next step be?
    Order a chest x-ray. The patient's history and exam are clinically concerning for a spontaneous pneumothorax. He will likely require emergency evaluation for treatment if the x-ray reveals a compromised lung.

17. What is the most common causative organism of community-acquired pneumonia (CAP)?
    Streptococcus pneumoniae and respiratory viruses.

18. How is CAP treated in the outpatient setting for an otherwise healthy patient under the age of 65?
    A recommended treatment is oral amoxicillin (1 g) three times daily with a macrolide (azithromycin/clarithromycin) or doxycycline. The American Thoracic Society (ATS)/Infectious Diseases Society of America (IDSA) recommends initial monotherapy with only amoxicillin as first-line therapy barring contraindication.

KEY POINTS

1. Viral upper respiratory infections and bronchitis are the most common overall causes of cough and shortness of breath, and treatment is often directed at symptom control.
2. Be vigilant about not overprescribing antibiotics to otherwise healthy, well-appearing patients with clear viral etiology of symptoms.
3. All chest pain of concern for cardiac etiology, regardless of whether or not there are EKG abnormalities, should be referred to the emergency department for further workup.

Acknowledgments

The authors would like to thank Dr. Jeffrey Waskin, DO, for their contributions to this chapter in the previous edition.

BIBLIOGRAPHY

Anderson JL, Adams CD, Antman EM, et al. 2012 ACCF/AHA focused update incorporated into the ACCF/AHA 2007 guidelines for the management of patients with unstable angina/non-ST-elevation myocardial infarction: a report of the American College of Cardiology Foundation/American Heart Association Task Force on Practice Guidelines. *J Am Coll Cardiol.* 2013;61(23):e179.
Bohadana A, Izbicki G, Kraman SS. Fundamentals of lung auscultation. *N Engl J Med.* 2014;370(8):744.
Dave BR, Sharma A, Kalva SP, Wicky S. Nine-year single-center experience with transcatheter arterial embolization for hemoptysis: medium-term outcomes. *Vasc Endovascular Surg.* 2011;45(3):258–268.
Fine MJ, Auble TE, Yealy DM, et al. A prediction rule to identify low-risk patients with community-acquired pneumonia. *N Engl J Med.* 1997;336(4):243.
Global Strategy for the Diagnosis, Management and Prevention of COPD, Global Initiative for Chronic Obstructive Lung Disease (GOLD). http://www.goldcopd.org; Accessed March 17, 2016.
Irwin RS, Boulet LP, Cloutier MM, et al. Managing a cough as a defense mechanism and as a symptom. A consensus panel report of the American College of Chest Physicians. *Chest.* 1998;114(suppl 2):133S.
Kwon NH, Oh MJ, Min TH, Lee BJ, Choi DC. Causes and clinical features of subacute cough. *Chest.* 2006;129(5):1142.
Troughton RW, Asher CR, Klein AL. Pericarditis. *Lancet.* 2004;363(9410):717.

CHAPTER 11

ABDOMINAL PAIN, NAUSEA, VOMITING, AND DIARRHEA

Bradley Chappell, DO, MHA, FACOEP, FACEP

1. **Why is abdominal pain so difficult to diagnose?**
   Pain in the abdomen is often referred based on the embryological development of the organs. There are two types of pain: visceral (diffuse crampy and achy pain from distention of the hollow organs) and somatic (localized constant pain from the parietal peritoneum).

2. **How should I approach a patient with right upper quadrant (RUQ) pain?**
   Taking an adequate history will often help narrow your differential diagnosis. There are three main considerations:
   • Gallbladder (biliary colic, cholecystitis, choledocholithiasis, cholangitis)
   • Liver (hepatitis, Fitz-Hugh-Curtis syndrome)
   • Referred pain (renal colic, pyelonephritis, lower lobe pneumonia, colitis near hepatic flexure, duodenal ulcer)

3. **What workup is helpful in evaluating RUQ pain in the urgent care setting?**
   • Urinalysis (to look for pyelonephritis and assess pregnancy status when indicated)
   • Chest x-ray (if indicated to evaluate for RLL pneumonia)
   • Outpatient labs (complete blood count [CBC], metabolic panels [including liver function panel and lipase]) and a scheduled RUQ ultrasound (Note: If a patient appears ill or in severe pain, these would need to be done acutely in an emergency department.)

4. **Why does the patient with abdominal pain also have pain in the shoulder?**
   This pain is called Kehr sign, an example of referred pain from diaphragmatic irritation that is transmitted through the phrenic nerve.

5. **Should I order an outpatient CT for my patient with RUQ pain?**
   Typically not. Ultrasound is the initial test of choice for gallbladder-related pathologies. There is no radiation exposure, computed tomography (CT) will often have an exaggerated appearance of gallbladder wall thickening, and other tests such as a hepatobiliary iminodiacetic acid (HIDA) scan for gallbladder dysfunction or magnetic resonance cholangiopancreatography/endoscopic retrograde cholangiopancreatography (MRCP/ERCP) for intra-ductal stone confirmation and extraction are more appropriate. If there is concern for hepatic or biliary mass, a thin-slice CT may be indicated.

6. **My patient had a recent cholecystectomy and now is presenting with RUQ pain. What testing should I perform?**
   This patient will likely need to be evaluated in the emergency department. It is wise to have early consultation with the surgeon for postoperative management. Fever raises suspicion of complications, but local preference will vary between HIDA and CT to evaluate for postoperative biliary leak and abscess.

7. **What are commonly encountered causes of epigastric pain?**
   Esophagitis, esophageal foreign body, gastroesophageal reflux disease (GERD), peptic ulcer disease, and pancreatitis.

8. **My patient has classic symptoms of peptic ulcer disease (PUD): gnawing, burning pain starting after eating. How do I differentiate between gastric and duodenal ulcers?**
   Gastric ulcers tend to worsen immediately after eating, whereas duodenal ulcers tend to immediately improve after eating due to the bicarbonate production and ultimately cause pain several hours after a meal.

9. **What are some lifestyle modifications I can recommend to my patients with presumed PUD?**
   Avoid contributing factors such as nonsteroidal antiinflammatory drugs (NSAIDs) or anything specific that worsens the pain, and limit alcohol consumption.

10. **What is the medication regimen of choice for patients with PUD?**
    • Use proton pump inhibitors (PPIs) for 4–8 weeks.
    • Histamine H_2-receptor antagonists (H_2 blockers) are less effective than PPIs and do not have significant additive effects when combined with PPIs.
    • Sucralfate is most effective with duodenal ulcers.

11. **What are some potential complications of PUD?**
Hemorrhage (vomiting bright red blood or coffee-ground emesis, melena), perforation, scarring (resulting in gastric outlet obstruction).

12. **Should I order an electrocardiogram (EKG) on patients with epigastric pain?**
Patients with "atypical" chest pain often present with vague symptoms including nausea and epigastric pain. It is reasonable to use this as a screening exam for low-risk cardiac patients for patients over age 30 with vague symptoms or other risk factors (dyslipidemia, hypertension [HTN], diabetes mellitus [DM], smoking, family history, obesity)?

13. **What are some common causes of pancreatitis?**
Alcohol use (acute and chronic), biliary disease, triglyceridemia, medications, viral infections, and pregnancy.

14. **What should be considered when evaluating left upper quadrant (LUQ) pain?**
Referred pain from myocardial infarction, lower lobe pneumonia, gastritis, splenomegaly, splenic infarct, splenic laceration in the setting of trauma, renal infarction, or pyelonephritis.

15. **What does mononucleosis (mono) have to do with abdominal pain?**
Because mono can cause splenomegaly, patients need to avoid contact sports or be evaluated after minor trauma for a minimum of 4 weeks after onset of illness. Mono can be confirmed using a monospot test or a CBC showing a lymphocytic predominance (>50%).

16. **How are patients with traumatic injury to the LUQ and stable vital signs managed?**
These patients should be referred to a trauma center for evaluation.

17. **What are some of the splenic complications associated with sickle cell anemia?**
Splenomegaly, sequestration crisis, splenic infarction, and abscesses.

18. **What common disease processes present with flank pain?**
   - Herpes zoster: often presents with a superficial burning sensation several days prior to the onset of rash. Be sure to carefully inspect for any lesions along a dermatomal distribution.
   - Nephrolithiasis: renal colic is typically severe and intermittent in nature. Posterior pain is associated with stones near the kidney, pain along the flank is typically referred as the stone transcends the ureter, and pelvic or scrotal pain is more prominent as the stone approaches the bladder.
   - Pyelonephritis: these patients often appear ill, have constant pain, and have had preceding urinary tract infections that may have been partially treated or untreated.

19. **What are significant causes of right lower quadrant (RLQ) pain?**
   - Appendicitis
   - Cecal diverticulitis
   - Referred renal pain and pelvic causes such as ovarian cyst, ectopic pregnancy, ovarian or testicular torsion, sexually transmitted infections/pelvic inflammatory disease, or tubo-ovarian abscess (TOA)

20. **How should RLQ pain be approached?**
History and physical exams are key. Clinical components such as fever, anorexia, migration of pain to the RLQ, and leukocytosis increase the suspicion for appendicitis. A bimanual exam should be performed to help differentiate between RLQ and right pelvic pain in females. If the majority of pain appears to be in the pelvic region, ultrasound (US) to evaluate for torsion, cyst, or tubo-ovarian abscess is a reasonable first step. If the pain is mainly in the RLQ, then CT is the test of choice. Depending on the degree of pain and what diagnosis you are expecting, the patient may need to be referred to the emergency department.

21. **My patient states her last menstrual period (LMP) was 2 weeks ago. Do I really need a pregnancy test?**
All females of childbearing age should receive a pregnancy test to rule out ectopic pregnancy.

22. **What causes should be considered in lower left quadrant (LLQ) pain?**
Diverticulitis, sigmoid volvulus, referred renal and pelvic causes (same as RLQ).

23. **What are common symptoms that raise suspicion for diverticulitis?**
Patients with diverticulitis often present with recurrent episodes and previous diagnoses made by colonoscopy or CT. They are able to relate the current symptoms to previous ones, increasing the index of suspicion. Common symptoms include LLQ pain (often worsened by food), change in bowel pattern (typically diarrhea), and occasional fever. Rectal bleeding can be seen with diverticulitis, but frank bleeding (not occult, guaiac positive) is not typical with diverticulitis.

24. **What are the current treatment recommendations for diverticulitis?**
The current guidelines by the American Gastroenterological Association recommend selective use of antibiotics, as the current understanding is the disease is more inflammatory mediated than infectious. When antibiotics are used, several options exist, including ciprofloxacin plus metronidazole, amoxicillin-clavulanate, or moxifloxacin for 7–10 days.

25. **Are there dietary changes for patients with diverticulosis?**
Traditional teaching has been to avoid seeds, nuts, and popcorn; however, there is no statistically significant data to support the claims that this will decrease the incidence of flares through food avoidance. Current recommendations include diets rich in fibrous foods, but there is little evidence that supplements such as probiotics alter the course of disease.

26. **How should pelvic tenderness be approached?**
For females of childbearing age, pregnancy should be ruled out first. If there is a history of unprotected sex or vaginal discharge, the patient may need treatment for bacterial vaginosis or sexually transmitted infections. If significant pain is present on bimanual exam, the patient may need empiric treatment for pelvic inflammatory disease. When patients complain of severe intermittent or waxing/waning pain, consideration should be given to torsion (ovarian or testicular). For females with cyclical (monthly) ovarian pain, referral to gynecology may be warranted for fibroid or endometrial management. Although epididymitis is a clinical diagnosis, US should be performed to rule out torsion.

27. **This patient has dysuria but clean urine. What else could be the cause?**
Be aware that dysuria may be the major presenting symptom of chlamydia.

28. **Is there a role for observation in patients with abdominal pain?**
There should be an effort toward shared decision making, especially given the potential cumulative effects of ionizing radiation. It is reasonable to have a patient with nonfocal abdominal pain of unclear etiology return for reevaluation in 8–12 hours. The concern for possible diagnoses and a clear follow-up plan should be discussed with the patient and documented. The patient should be tolerating oral intake, and vital signs must be stable.

29. **What is the treatment of choice for pregnancy-induced vomiting?**
   - Eat small, frequent meals; avoid spicy, fatty, or other nausea-triggering foods
   - Ginger chews or in diet
   - Pyridoxine (12.5 mg q6 hours)
   - Doxylamine (12.5 mg q12 hours)
   - Metoclopramide (10 mg q6 hours)
   - Ondansetron (4 mg q4 hours)

30. **Which pregnant patients with hyperemesis need IV fluids?**
When the urinalysis shows 3+ ketones or the patient has lost greater than 5% of her weight, administer IV fluids. If the patient has greater than 10% weight loss, she will likely require admission.

31. **What are the best treatment options for patients with acute vomiting?**
There is little evidence to suggest the efficacy of one antiemetic over another. Multiple classes of medications including antihistamines (e.g., diphenhydramine, promethazine), dopamine receptor antagonists (e.g., prochlorperazine, metoclopramide), serotonin receptor antagonists (e.g., ondansetron), and glucocorticoids (e.g., dexamethasone, which is used in conjunction with chemotherapy) are used to treat nausea.

32. **Should Gatorade be used for rehydration of patients with acute gastroenteritis?**
The World Health Organization's (WHO's) recommended oral rehydration solution (ORS) varies significantly from most commercial athletic-targeted beverages. The excessive carbohydrate load may actually lead to osmotic diuresis, equating to increased diarrhea and further dehydration. The closest commercial product to the WHO-ORS available in the United States is Pedialyte.

33. **How is hyperemesis from cannabis treated?**
Discontinue all use of cannabis products for 1–2 weeks. Symptoms may temporarily improve with hot showers, and medications including topical capsaicin and haloperidol have been shown to be effective in reducing symptoms. If symptoms persist after 2 weeks of no cannabis use, the diagnosis of cyclical vomiting syndrome should be reconsidered.

34. **How should patients with chronic nausea from diabetic gastroparesis be managed?**
   - Dietary changes: blend food, tight glucose control
   - Promotility agents
     - Metoclopramide (10 mg three times daily before meals)
     - Erythromycin (125 mg three times daily before meals)
   - Antiemetics
     - Diphenhydramine
     - Ondansetron
     - Prochlorperazine

35. **The patient is presenting with severe chest pain after multiple episodes of retching and vomiting. How should this be evaluated?**
Patients with severe vomiting will often have small Mallory-Weiss tears, resulting in blood-tinged sputum. Sometimes, there can be rupture of the esophagus resulting in irritating and life-threatening mediastinitis. These have a high mortality rate, so clinical suspicion and early detection are essential. Approximately 90% of patients will have abnormalities on the chest x-ray.

36. **What are common pathogens and sources of diarrhea?**
    - Bacillus cereus: reheated rice
    - Staphylococcus aureus: mayonnaise
    - *Salmonella*: eggs, poultry, pet reptiles
    - *Shigella*: poor sanitation
    - Escherichia coli: ground beef
    - *Campylobacter*: untreated water
    - Vibrio parahaemolyticus: shellfish
    - Yersinia: pork
    - Clostridium botulinum: honey

37. **Do stool cultures need to be routinely sent for patients with diarrhea?**
    No. Cultures are expensive and have a low diagnostic yield (less than 5%). Antibiotics are not needed in most cases as the symptoms tend to be self-limited. However high-risk populations such as the elderly, immunocompromised, those with fever, and those who travel to high-risk countries (refer to CDC website for guidance), have blood or mucus in the stool, or have greater than 10 stools in a 24-hour period may benefit from stool cultures.

38. **What patients with diarrhea should receive antibiotics?**
    Empiric antibiotics (ciprofloxacin [500 mg] twice daily for 3 days) may be considered for traveler's diarrhea in patients with associated fever or symptoms greater than 2 weeks. In patients with recent hospitalization, consideration for *Clostridium difficile* should be given. Otherwise, antibiotics should be tailored to culture results. Those patients with bloody diarrhea should not receive antibiotics until cultures demonstrate it is not *E. coli O157:H7* due to the risk of precipitating hemolytic uremic syndrome. In either case, bismuth subsalicylate can be safely taken per label instructions, with caution to avoid use in HIV patients or overdose causing salicylate toxicity.

39. **My patient states he feels a fishbone stuck in his throat. How quickly does he need to be seen by a gastroenterologist?**
    This patient should be referred for emergent endoscopy. Any sharp foreign body or button battery above the lower esophageal sphincter, or any patient with a foreign body who is unable to handle their secretions, should have it removed immediately due to risk of perforation. All other ingestions should be evaluated by endoscopy within 24 hours. Most objects that make it to the stomach will pass without intervention.

40. **Can you clarify the terminology of gastrointestinal bleeding?**
    - Hematemesis: bright red blood or coffee-ground emesis
    - Hematochezia: bright or dark red blood in stool; most commonly from lower gastrointestinal (GI) bleed but can occasionally be from a massive upper GI bleed
    - Melena: black tarry stool, most frequently originates from the stomach or duodenum

41. **A healthy young adult presents with reported small blood in their stool or on toilet paper. Do I need to transfer this patient to the emergency department for evaluation?**
    If the heart rate and blood pressure are normal, and the patient has normal appearing conjunctiva (no pallor) or a normal hemoglobin, then the patient is likely stable for outpatient follow-up with gastroenterology. Be sure to perform a rectal exam looking for fissures or hemorrhoids.

42. **A patient with atrial fibrillation had a colonoscopy last week and is now presenting with diffuse, severe abdominal pain. The abdominal x-ray did not show any free air, so perforation is less likely. What diagnosis should I be concerned about?**
    This is a classic presentation for mesenteric ischemia. The patient was likely off anticoagulants for the procedure and may have formed a clot with resultant bowel ischemia. These patients will appear ill (tachycardic, hypotensive), have nonfocal and unrelenting pain, and often have very abnormal labs (high leukocytosis, anion gap, lactic acidosis, and base deficit). They should be transferred immediately for surgical evaluation and CT angiogram. Although free air is not visualized on an x-ray, a CT should be obtained if there is significant pain, as small pockets of air from a microperforation may be missed on plain films.

43. **An elderly patient was brought in by family members for evaluation of a syncopal episode that was preceded by severe abdominal pain. The patient says the pain is tolerable and is declining analgesics but occasionally reports severe bouts of pain. There was blood in the UA, so is it safe to send the patient home with a presumptive diagnosis of kidney stones?**
    First episodes of kidney stones should be imaged to confirm diagnosis. It is imperative to be mindful of other causes of painful hematuria (especially in elderly patients), including critical items such as abdominal aneurysms. Unruptured abdominal aortic aneurysms are largely asymptomatic; however, once rupture occurs, the pain is often severe and can radiate to the back and groin. The classic pulsatile mass may not be appreciated in patients with a higher body mass index (BMI). Intermittent bouts of pain can be indicative of active shearing and enlargement of the rupture. This is a truly time-sensitive surgical emergency.

44. **What recommendations can I give to the patient who is constipated?**
    - Increase daily fluid intake.
    - Ingest adequate dietary fiber (fruits, vegetables, legumes, nuts, grains).
    - Take bulk-forming laxatives (psyllium or methylcellulose).
    - Short-term use of osmotic agents such as polyethylene glycol to increase stool frequency.
    - If related to short-term narcotic use or recent initiation of iron supplementation, an emollient laxative such as docusate should be utilized, and stimulant laxatives such as bisacodyl and senna may be considered to improve bowel function.

45. **A patient presents with a large ventral hernia that had been intermittently protuberant for years but today does not slide back in. Does the patient require emergent surgery?**
    If it is truly incarcerated, the patient will require surgical evaluation. However, with patience and proper positioning, the majority of hernias are reducible in most cases. The first step is to have the patient lie in a supine or Trendelenburg position. Next, provide adequate analgesia and apply firm, direct pressure to the hernia. If this does not relieve the incarcerated hernia, the patient must be transferred. Incarcerated hernias can become strangulated, causing compromised blood supply to the herniated tissue, resulting in an ischemic bowel. This can be diagnosed on CT or intraoperatively, but severe intractable pain is a clue toward this diagnosis.

46. **How can I best manage the patient with painful hemorrhoids?**
    - Corticosteroids: topical or rectal suppositories
    - Vasoactive agents (topical phenylephrine)
    - Protectants: zinc oxide paste
    - Bulk-forming laxatives (psyllium or methylcellulose)
    - Emollient laxatives (docusate)

KEY POINTS

1. Patients with an acute abdomen (guarding, rebound, or rigidity) need immediate transfer to an emergency department for surgical evaluation. Do not delay for lab testing or results.
2. Any female of childbearing age should have a pregnancy test performed.
3. Patients with abdominal trauma should be referred to a local trauma center to be evaluated for intraabdominal pathology, which can be present despite stable vital signs.
4. Elderly patients rarely have benign presentations of abdominal pain or vomiting. Have a high degree of suspicion for diagnoses such as bowel obstruction, cholangitis, ruptured appendicitis, abdominal aortic aneurysm, and mesenteric ischemia.

BIBLIOGRAPHY

Acute Colonic Diverticulitis. Medical Management. Available at: https://www.uptodate.com/contents/acute-colonic-diverticulitis-medical-management. Accessed November 15, 2022.

AH Al-Salem. Splenic Complications of Sickle Cell Anemia and the Role of Splenectomy. *ISRN Hematology.* 2011;864257.

Anderson BA, et al. A Systematic Review of Whether Oral Contrast is Necessary for the Computed Tomography Diagnosis of Appendicitis in Adults. *Am J Surg.* 2005;190(3):474.

Atilla R, Oktay C. Pancreatitis and Cholecystitis. In: Tintinalli J, ed. *Tintinalli's Emergency Medicine: A Comprehensive Study Guide.* 7th ed. The McGraw-Hill Companies, Inc; 2011:558–566.

Boerhaave Syndrome. Available at: http://emedicine.medscape.com/article/171683-overview. Accessed November 15, 2022.

Burgess BE. Anorectal Disorders. In: Tintinalli J, ed. *Tintinalli's Emergency Medicine: A Comprehensive Study Guide.* 7th ed. The McGraw-Hill Companies, Inc; 2011:587–601.

Chohan N. *Nursing: Interpreting Signs and Symptoms.* 1st ed. Lippincott, Williams, and Wilkins; 2007:355.

Cyclical Vomiting Syndromes. Available at: https://www.uptodate.com/contents/cyclic-vomiting-syndrome. Accessed November 15, 2022.

Egerton-Warburton D, Meek R, Mee MJ, Braitberg G. Antiemetic Use for Vomiting in Adult Emergency Department Patients: Randomized Controlled Trial Comparing Ondansetron, Metoclopramide, and Placebo. *Ann Emerg Med.* 2014;64(5):526.

Freedman SB, Thull-Freedman JD. Vomiting, Diarrhea, and Dehydration in Children. In: Tintinalli J, ed. *Tintinalli's Emergency Medicine: A Comprehensive Study Guide.* 7th ed. The McGraw-Hill Companies, Inc; 2011:830–839.

Graham A. Diverticulitis. In: Tintinalli J, ed. *Tintinalli's Emergency Medicine: A Comprehensive Study Guide.* 7th ed. The McGraw-Hill Companies, Inc; 2011:579–581.

Haines EJ, Thompson H. Liver and Biliary Tract Disorders. In: Marx JA, ed. *Rosen's Emergency Medicine: Concepts and Clinical Practice.* 10th ed. Philadelphia: Elsevier; 2023:1058–1083.

Hlibczuk V, et al. Diagnostic Accuracy of Non-contrast Computed Tomography for Appendicitis in Adults: A Systematic Review. *Ann Emerg Med.* 2010;55(1):51.

Kman NE, Werman HA. Disorders Presenting Primarily with Diarrhea. In: Tintinalli J, ed. *Tintinalli's Emergency Medicine: A Comprehensive Study Guide.* 7th ed. The McGraw-Hill Companies, Inc; 2011:531–540.

Management of Chronic Constipation in Adults. Available at: https://www.uptodate.com/contents/management-of-chronic-constipation-in-adults. Accessed November 15, 2022.

McDonald, et al. Clinical Practice Guidelines for Clostridium Difficile Infection in Adults and Children: 2017 Update by the Infectious Disease Society of America (IDSA) and Society for Healthcare Epidemiology of America (SHEA). *Clin Infect Dis.* 2018;66(7):1–48.

O'Brien MC. Acute Abdominal Pain. In: Tintinalli J, ed. *Tintinalli's Emergency Medicine: A Comprehensive Study Guide.* 7th ed. The McGraw-Hill Companies, Inc; 2011:519–527.

Peptic Ulcer Disease: Management. Available at: https://www.uptodate.com/contents/peptic-ulcer-disease-management?source=search_result&search=peptic+ulcer+disease%3A+management &selectedTitle=1%7E150. Accessed: November 15, 2022.

Salo JA, et al. Hematuria is an Indication of Rupture of an Abdominal Aortic Aneurysm into the Vena Cava. *J Vasc Surg.* 1990;12(1):41–44.

Selective Non-operative Management of Blunt Splenic Injuries. Available at: https://www.east.org/Content/documents/practicemanage-mentguidelines/Selective_nonoperative_management_of_blunt_splenic.4.pdf. Accessed November 15, 2022.

Stollman N, Smalley W, Hirano I. American Gastroenterological Association Institute Guideline on the Management of Acute Diverticulitis. *Gastroenterology.* 2015;149(7):1944–1949.

Treatment and Outcome of Nausea and Vomiting of Pregnancy. Available at: https://www.uptodate.com/contents/treatment-and-out-come-of-nausea-and-vomiting-of-pregnancy. Accessed November 15, 2022.

Treatment of Gastroparesis. Available at: https://www.uptodate.com/contents/treatment-of-gastroparesis. Accessed November 15, 2022.

Treatment of Hemorrhoids. Available at: https://www.uptodate.com/contents/treatment-of-hemorrhoids. Accessed November 15, 2022.

CHAPTER 12

GENITOURINARY COMPLAINTS

Jessica J. Kirby, DO, FACEP, Ryan P. Kirby, MD, FAAEM, FACEP

1. **Which organisms commonly cause epididymitis?**
   Sexually transmitted infections (*Neisseria gonorrhoeae* and *Chlamydia trachomatis*) are the most common in 16- to 30-year-old men, but *Escherichia coli, Klebsiella pneumoniae, Proteus mirabilis,* and *Pseudomonas aeruginosa* are a prevalent cause in the 51- to 70-year-old age group. Noninfectious inflammation of the epididymis is far less common, occurring mostly in prepubertal boys.

2. **How does acute epididymitis typically present?**
   Insidious onset. Several days to weeks of progressive dull aching pain of the epididymis and testes, often with swelling. Associated abdominal pain and fever are common, and urinary tract infection symptoms, such as dysuria, frequency, and hematuria, may also be present.

3. **Are there risk factors associated with developing epididymitis?**
   Yes. Unprotected sexual activity, trauma from strenuous exercise, prolonged sitting, prostatic hypertrophy, and urologic instrumentation are potential risk factors for epididymitis.

4. **What other urologic conditions can mimic epididymitis?**
   Trauma, inguinal hernia, testicular torsion, torsion of the appendix epididymis (most common in prepubertal boys), Fournier gangrene, and testicular cancer may all cause genital pain and swelling of the scrotal contents.

5. **What is the best exam approach to assess for scrotal pain?**
   A standing exam is helpful to differentiate epididymitis. Patients with epididymitis have palpable tenderness and swelling of the epididymis. They may have a positive Prehn sign, pain relief with elevation of the scrotum. Your exam should also include the cremasteric reflex. The presence of an ipsilateral cremasteric reflex is reassuring that testicular torsion is not as likely, though ultrasound should be considered to truly assess for torsion. A mass within the testes is not consistent with epididymitis and warrants further investigation. Supine abdominal examination is also integral to assess for an intraabdominal process radiating pain to the external genitalia.

6. **What testing is indicated in the evaluation of suspected epididymitis?**
   Testing for sexually transmitted infections (STIs), especially *N. gonorrhoeae* and *C. trachomatis*, should be done for sexually active men, at least those under 35 years of age. A urine analysis with culture is indicated, particularly for older men and younger adolescents, as coliform bacteria are more likely causative in these age groups.

7. **When is scrotal ultrasound indicated for a patient presenting with a scrotal complaint?**
   The loss of cremasteric reflex, a painless mass, uncertain diagnosis, or unexplained pain warrants further evaluation with an ultrasound.

8. **With such variable bacterial causes, what treatment should be started for presumed epididymitis?**
   Treatment should be tailored to likely pathogens. Because sexually transmitted infection is the most common cause of epididymitis in younger men, standard treatment for *N. gonorrhoeae* and *C. trachomatis* should be given while studies are pending. For older men, the same treatment may be appropriate given the clinical presentation, but coverage for typical urinary pathogens may be more appropriate. See Table 12.1 for drug and dosage details.

9. **What are the adjunctive treatments for epididymitis?**
   Scrotal support and elevation, cold compresses, and antiinflammatory pain medication are helpful.

10. **What tests should be considered for patients presenting with genital vesicles and/or ulcers?**
    By far the most common cause of such genital lesions is herpes simplex virus (HSV), with or without systemic prodromal symptoms. Other vesicle/ulcer-causing infectious agents include chancroid, granuloma inguinale, lymphogranuloma venereum, syphilis, and monkeypox. There are less common noninfectious etiologies, including Behçet syndrome and trauma.

Table 12.1 CDC STI Treatment Guidelines, 2021

Recommended Regimens for Epididymitis

For acute epididymitis most likely caused by chlamydia or gonorrhea:

Ceftriaxone 500 mg* IM in a single dose

Plus

Doxycycline 100 mg orally 2 times/days for 10 days

For acute epididymitis most likely caused by chlamydia, gonorrhea, or enteric organisms (men who practice insertive sex):

Ceftriaxone 500 mg* IM in a single dose

Plus

Levofloxacin 500 mg orally once daily for 10 days

For acute epididymitis most likely caused by enteric organisms only:

Levofloxacin 500 mg orally once daily for 10 days

Recommended Regimens for First Clinical Episode of Genital Herpes[†]

Acyclovir[‡] 400 mg orally 3 times/day for 7–10 days

or

Famciclovir 250 mg orally 3 times/day for 7–10 days

or

Valacyclovir 1 g orally 2 times/day for 7–10 days

Recommended Regimens for Episodic Therapy for Recurrent HSV-2 Genital Herpes[§]

Acyclovir 800 mg orally 2 times/day for 5 days

or

Acyclovir 800 mg orally 3 times/day for 2 days

or

Famciclovir 1 g orally 2 times/day for 1 day

or

Famciclovir 500 mg orally once, followed by 250 mg 2 times/day for 2 days

or

Famciclovir 125 mg orally 2 times/day for 5 days

or

Valacyclovir 500 mg orally 2 times/day for 3 days

or

Valacyclovir 1 g orally once daily for 5 days

Recommended Regimens for Urethritis

Gonoccal urethritis (GU) treat as you would *N. gonorrhoeae* above

Nongonoccal urethritis (NGU) treat per below:

Recommended Regimen for Nongonococcal Urethritis

Doxycycline 100 mg orally 2 times/day for 7 days

Alternative Regimens

Azithromycin 1 g orally in a single dose

Or

Azithromycin 500 mg orally in a single dose; then 250 mg orally daily for 4 days

*For persons weighing ≥ 150 kg, 1 g of ceftriaxone should be administered.

[†]Treatment can be extended if healing is incomplete after 10 days of therapy.

[‡]Acyclovir 200 mg orally 5 times/day is also effective but is not recommended because of the frequency of dosing.

[§]Acyclovir 400 mg orally 3 times/day for 5 days is also effective but is not recommended because of frequency of dosing.

Adapted from the Centers for Disease Control and Prevention, Sexually Transmitted Infections Treatment Guidelines, 2021. Available at: https://www.cdc.gov/std/treatment-guidelines/STI-Guidelines-2021.pdf. Accessed September 28, 2022.

11. **Is viral culture better than polymerase chain reaction (PCR) testing, and better than serologic testing for genital herpes simplex?**

Viral culture is the diagnostic standard of care for genital infection. PCR testing currently has a higher rate of detection and may replace culture at some time. Serologic testing (antigen detection) by enzyme-linked immuno-sorbent assay (ELISA) and Western blot assays have high sensitivity and specificity for herpes simplex; that is, 96–100% and 97–100%, respectively.

12. Should the diagnosis be confirmed before initiating treatment?

No. Treat presumptively while cultures are pending. In addition to antiviral medication, pain management is impor-tant. Burow solution cool compresses (1 tsp to 1 quart of cool water) applied locally may provide significant relief. Sitz baths may also be soothing.

13. How long is genital herpes contagious?

There is no clear-cut answer, as asymptomatic viral shedding is quite common and the patient should be appro-priately counseled. Abstinence from sexual contact during any prodromal symptoms or while there are active lesions should be maintained until there is complete healing. A barrier contraceptive method may be appropriate even when asymptomatic.

14. What are the antiviral treatment options for genital herpes?

See Table 12.1.

15. How is acute urethritis in men diagnosed?

History of penile discharge (with or without dysuria), urgency, or other typical urinary tract infection (UTI) symp-toms with examination findings of urethral discharge, positive leukocyte esterase, or greater than 10 white blood cells (WBCs) per high-power field on urine analysis are diagnostic of acute urethritis.

16. Is acute urethritis in men always due to STIs?

Essentially yes. For clinical purposes, urethritis can be categorized as gonococcal (GU) and nongonococcal (NGU). *N. gonorrhoeae* and *C. trachomatis* are the most prevalent STIs. *Trichomonas* and *Ureaplasma urealyticum* are also common. *Mycoplasma genitalium* is a potential cause of NGU; however, specific testing for this is not cur-rently available. Other, less common causes include *Haemophilus influenzae,* adenovirus, and herpes simplex.

17. Do all patients with urethritis require diagnostic tests?

Remember that STIs are frequently coincidental. For this reason, testing should be done uniformly in addition to symptomatic relief, preventing complications in the patient and sexual partner, and identifying and limiting transmission of additional STIs. For men who have sex with men, partake in other high-risk sexual behavior, or use IV drugs, hepatitis B, hepatitis C, human immunodeficiency virus (HIV), herpes (HSV), and syphilis should also be assessed.

18. What treatment is appropriate for urethritis?

Treatment should be given at the point of access to care (see Table 12.1). Expedited partner treatment, as advocated by the Centers for Disease Control and Prevention (CDC) and approved in many US states, may be considered. Guidelines and legal status are available online through the CDC.

19. What populations get urinary tract infections (UTI)?

UTIs are most common in women of childbearing age, but they are common in children with various urologic ana-tomic and functional problems. UTIs are less common in men, but with the onset of prostatic enlargement around age 50, they increase in frequency to equal the incidence in postmenopausal women.

20. What are the risk factors for getting a UTI?

Common risk factors include inadequate hydration and delayed or infrequent emptying of the bladder, all of which allow the infection to establish in the bladder epithelium. Coitus is another risk factor for women, as bacteria may be mechanically introduced into the distal urethra. Adequate hydration, regular emptying, and voiding shortly after coitus help decrease the opportunity for infection. Anatomic abnormalities, including prostatic enlargement, increase the risk of UTI.

21. What defines a UTI as complicated?

There is some variation in definition, but practically, in the outpatient setting, pregnancy, urologic instrumentation (e.g., ureteral stent), and urolithiasis are complicating factors. A patient with a single kidney or other abnormal urologic anatomy requires careful management and follow-up. A UTI in the setting of an obstructing ureteral stone is a urologic emergency, as sepsis can commonly occur.

22. What are the most common symptoms of UTI?

Dysuria, frequency, and small amounts of urine voided are quite common. Dysuria alone is associated with UTI about 50% of the time; dysuria with another symptom (e.g., frequency) increases the likelihood of infection to 96%. Additional symptoms are commonly hematuria, nocturia, hesitancy, suprapubic pain, and mild nausea. Fever, vomiting, and back pain associated with dysuria are suggestive of upper tract infection. Dysuria as an isolated symptom has a high prevalence of STI in sexually active young adults.

23. What are the physical examination findings?

There may be minimal or no remarkable exam findings with an uncomplicated UTI. Mild suprapubic tenderness (or mild periumbilical tenderness) is common; however, the presence of moderate to severe unilateral periumbilical pain on palpation or flank tenderness on percussion (Lloyd sign) should raise concern for pyelonephritis.

24. **What findings on urine analysis confirm UTI?**
The confirmatory test for a UTI is a urine culture. The presence of leukocyte esterase on urine analysis has the best sensitivity and specificity. In the presence of leukocyte esterase and a high pretest probability, this may also be considered confirmatory. The presence of nitrite may support the diagnosis of UTI, but its absence does not rule out UTI because not all urinary pathogens form nitrite from nitrate.

25. **What may commonly cause false-positive or false-negative findings on urine analysis?**
A false-positive leukocyte esterase is frequently caused by phenazopyridine and contamination (e.g., due to vaginal discharge, balanitis, urethritis, foreign body). A false-positive nitrite may be due to contamination, exposure to air, and phenazopyridine. A false-negative nitrite may be due to dilution secondary to aggressive hydration and frequent voiding.

26. **Under what circumstances is it reasonable to treat for UTI based on history and exam alone?**
A nonpregnant woman with urinary symptoms without gynecologic symptoms and a consistent examination may be treated presumptively. A urine analysis may be omitted in this case.

27. **Who should be cultured?**
Patients who have dysuria with unrevealing dipstick, children, pregnant women, postmenopausal women, men, those with history of recurrent UTI, and those with single kidney/urologic anatomic problems all warrant urine culture with sensitivities.

28. **Which antibiotics are not first-line for empiric treatment of acute uncomplicated cystitis?**
Due to the development of significant bacterial resistance, fluoroquinolones and beta-lactam antibiotics are better held for complicated, resistant, or culture-proven infection if there is treatment failure on a targeted antibiotic.

29. **Does the absence of fever rule out pyelonephritis?**
No, treat based on the presentation and physical findings, with supportive lab studies and probability assessment.

30. **What are the recommended treatments for UTI?**
See Table 12.2 for treatment of uncomplicated UTI/pyelonephritis in the outpatient setting.

31. **What causes prostatitis?**
Acute bacterial prostatitis (ABP) is thought to be caused by retrograde seeding of the prostate by bacteria and occurs in 2–5% of episodes of diagnosed prostatitis. It occurs predominantly in men ages 20–40 years, often by typical gram-negative urinary tract pathogens, most often *E. coli. N. gonorrhoeae, C. trachomatis,* and *Trichomonas* are not uncommon pathogens, especially in younger sexually active men, although those more commonly present as urethritis.

32. **What differentiates acute from chronic prostatitis?**
Chronic bacterial prostatitis (CBP) is a diagnosis made over time, involving repeated examinations for recurrent or persistent urologic symptoms of urogenital pain, dysuria, and urinary culture with the same organism. It accounts for about 10% of chronic prostatitis and is to be distinguished from nonbacterial prostatitis/chronic pelvic pain syndrome (NBP/CPPS).

33. **What is nonbacterial prostatitis/chronic pelvic pain syndrome (NBP/CPPS)?**
Defining features of this condition are a chronic urologic condition with symptoms of UTI; and without, response to antibiotic treatment, variable organisms on culture, and often with associated sexual dysfunction and psychological symptoms.

34. **What is the differential diagnosis of ABP?**
Additional diagnoses include other urologic problems, such as acute cystitis, interstitial cystitis, STI, and gastrointestinal (GI) disease, including diverticulitis and proctitis. Prostate cancer may also cause outlet obstructive symptoms and should be considered.

35. **How is ABP diagnosed?**
A good history and examination are key in diagnosing ABP and should include abdominal, genital, and digital rectal examinations. The diagnosis of ABP is clinical, and based on the findings of an enlarged, boggy, and tender prostate. Always obtain a urinalysis when considering ABP.

36. **What is the treatment for ABP?**
For ABP in the outpatient setting without risk factors for admission, treat with 10–14 days of levofloxacin (superior penetration of the prostate). Consider ceftriaxone and doxycycline if STI is a high probability. For CBP, initial levofloxacin (and guidance with culture) for 6 weeks is a good choice but may need to be repeated if symptoms recur. Reculture pre- and postprostatic massage to match the pathogen and confirm chronic infection may be appropriate.

Table 12.2 Antimicrobial Agents for the Management of Acute Uncomplicated Cystitis

TIER	DRUG	DOSAGE	COST OF GENERIC (BRAND)	PREGNANCY CATEGORY
First	Fosfomycin (Monurol)	3-g single dose	NA ($51)*	B
	Nitrofurantoin (macrocrystals)	100 mg twice per day for five days.	$55 ($64)*	B
	Trimethoprim/ Sulfamethoxazole (Bactrim, Septra)	160/800 mg twice per day for three days.	$17 ($34)*†	C
Second	Ciprofloxacin (Cipro)	250 mg twice per day for three days	$26 ($30)†‡	C
	Ciprofloxacin, extended release (Cipro XR)	500 mg per day for three days	$57 ($76)*	C
		NA ($86)*		C
	Levofloxacin (Levaquin)	250 mg per day for three days	$14 (NA)‡	C
	Ofloxacin	200 mg per day for three days *or* 400-mg single dose	$10 (NA)‡	C
Third§	Amoxicillin/clavulanate (Augmentin)	500/125 mg twice per day for seven days	$32 ($98)*	B
	Cefdinir (Omnicef)	300 mg twice per day for 10 days	$40 ($119)*	B
	Cefpodoxime	100 mg twice per day for seven days	$71 (NA)‡	B

NA = not available.

*Estimated retail price of one course of treatment based on information obtained at http://www.drugstore.com (accessed May 11, 2011)

†May be available at discount prices ($10 or less for one month's treatment) at one or more national retail chains.

‡Estimated cost to the pharmacist based on average wholesale prices in Red Book. Montvale, N.J.: Medical Economics Data; 2010. Cost to the patient will be higher, depending on prescription filling fee.

§Not generally recommended because of relatively high rates of resistance. Third-tier options include beta-lactam antibiotics.

Reformat Screenshot from https://www.aafp.org/pubs/afp/issues/2011/1001/p771.html.

37. What requires hospital care?

For patients with apparent prostatitis, reasons for hospital referral include urinary obstruction, inability to take oral medication, history of recent transurethral instrumentation, and systemic symptoms such as fever, chills, or signs of sepsis; all likely will require admission with urologic consultation.

38. How is NBP/CPPS treated?

Antibiotics are appropriate initial treatment; however, with failed treatment, urology referral is appropriate. This will provide for diagnostic confirmation and additional treatment options, which may include alpha$_1$ blockers, pain management, urology physical therapy modalities, and psychological care.

39. What causes kidney stones?

Usually soluble mineral compounds, which precipitate when the saturation point is reached in the urine.

40. What kind of stone is most common?

Calcium compounds are most frequent at about 80%, along with uric acid and struvite as the most common noninfectious stones. Stones formed due to genetic disorders include cysteine, xanthine, and 2,8-dihydroxyadenine. Stones associated with infectious etiology include magnesium ammonium phosphate, carbonate apatite, and ammonium urate.

41. Who gets kidney stones?

Urinary tract stones are common, occurring in up to 10% of the population. They occur predominantly in men. Causes are multifactorial, including nutritional and fluid issues, medical conditions, genetic predisposition, and less frequent causes, including infection and crystallized medication or supplements (e.g., vitamin C).

42. What medical conditions predispose a patient to develop stones?

Inadequate hydration, high dietary calcium, parathyroidism, and altered bone metabolism are frequently related. Gastrointestinal diseases such as malabsorption, chronic inflammatory bowel disease, and intestinal bypass surgery also have higher incidence of urinary stone formation. Common diseases including diabetes mellitus, hypertension, obesity, osteoporosis, gout, and chronic kidney diseases are also frequently associated.

43. **What is the typical presentation for a kidney stone?**
A stone in the ureter is generally quite symptomatic. When a stone dislodges from the renal collecting system and enters the ureter, it causes severe unilateral flank pain. There is often radiation into the abdomen or groin, associated nausea/vomiting, and urinary frequency may occur with a distal ureteral stone. Note that stones that remain in the kidney may not be symptomatic and usually require no treatment or intervention.

44. **What causes the pain?**
The average stone is 2.5–3 mm, which is larger than the lumen of the ureter. Scraping the lining of or obstructing the ureter causes the abrupt onset of symptoms. The pain is severe, independent of position or activity.

45. **What are the physical findings?**
The patient has severe pain and therefore cannot find a comfortable position and may be restless. There is often associated nausea and vomiting. The abdominal exam is generally soft without tenderness, but there may be flank or abdominal tenderness with longer duration of symptoms. The presence of fever with this presentation is concerning, and the patient must be thoroughly evaluated.

46. **What finding on urinalysis supports the diagnosis of a stone?**
Microscopic hematuria is usually present. The presence of leukocyte esterase or nitrates would suggest infection but does not rule out the possibility of a stone. Always consider a stone when hematuria is present.

47. **Does ureterolithiasis always cause hematuria?**
No; while it is most common to have microscopic hematuria, an impacted stone may not permit passage of urine or blood. Still consider ureterolithiasis if the clinical presentation suggests it, even if no hematuria is present.

48. **What imaging study is best for initial assessment of suspected ureterolithiasis?**
If available, an urgent retroperitoneal ultrasound is currently thought to be the best imaging study because it can confirm ureteral obstruction and may detect a stone without subjecting the patient to a large radiation dose. In the right clinical picture, hydronephrosis on ultrasound even without a visible stone likely suggests stone. Patient may benefit from CT. If available, an abdominal plain film (kidney, ureter, and bladder [KUB]) may be helpful, but many ureteral stones are not radiopaque, and hydronephrosis is not detectable.

49. **When is noncontrast CT (NCCT) indicated for apparent renal colic?**
A NCCT of the abdomen and pelvis is appropriate when there is a presentation suggestive of ureterolithiasis but with a negative ultrasound, a fever, a history of a solitary kidney, or if the diagnosis is in question. One NCCT has the equivalent of about 30 times the radiation dose of one KUB.

50. **For a confirmed ureteral stone, what are the priorities in management?**
Immediate pain relief is the priority. Nonsteroidal antiinflammatory drugs are more effective and have less side effects that opiates and should be first-line pain management. Then consider if the patient can be managed at home or needs ED or urology referral.

51. **Which patients may be treated as outpatients?**
Patients with a ureteral stone 4 mm or smaller and who have adequate pain control on oral medication and no infection or impairment of renal function may be given a chance to pass the stone. Pushing fluids, maintaining physical activity, and pain management promote stone passage, usually within several weeks.

52. **Do alpha$_1$ blockers help with passing a stone in the short term?**
Tamsulosin (0.4 mg) has the most evidence and does show benefit with increased percentage of stones passed and passed sooner than with placebo (one of three patients passed an average of 3 days sooner).

53. **Of what value is stone analysis?**
Recovery of a stone is important, and straining the urine should be done for the first diagnosed episode. Identification of the stone helps with prognosis, as recurrent stones are quite common. Additional metabolic evaluation of blood and urine tests (complete blood count [CBC], renal function, electrolytes, parathyroid hormone, calcium and urine creatinine, sodium, pH, oxalate, and citrate) should be considered to assess for underlying conditions.

54. **What are the referral criteria?**
Nonurgent urology referral would be appropriate for a large stone that may require lithotripsy or instrumentation, for a small stone that is not passed after a reasonable time as an outpatient, and if other concurrent urologic concerns are discovered.

KEY POINTS

1. Treat acute epididymitis for STIs in men 35 years or younger and for typical urinary pathogens in older men.
2. Ultrasound is the preferred initial advanced imaging for suspected ureterolithiasis.
3. Absence of hematuria does not preclude the presence of urolithiasis.

Acknowledgment

The authors would like to thank Vernne W. Greiner, DO, FAAFP for her contributions to this chapter in the previous edition.

BIBLIOGRAPHY

Bultitude M, Smith D, Thomas K. Contemporary management of stone disease: the new EAU guidelines for 2015. *Eur Urol.* 2016;69(3):483–484. http://dx.doi.org/10.1016/jeurouro2015.08.010.

Campschroer T, Zhu Y, Duijvesz D, Grobbee DE, Lock MT. Alpha blockers as medical expulsive therapy for ureteral stones. *Cochran Database Syst Rev.* 2014;4:CD008509. pub2. http://dx.doi.org/10.1002/14651858.

Centers for Disease Control and Prevention. Guidance on the Use of Expedited Partner Therapy in the Treatment of Gonorrhea. http://www.cdc.gov/std/EPT/default.htm; accessed October 4, 2016.

Crawford P, Crop J. Evaluation of scrotal masses. *Am Fam Physician.* 2014;89:723–727.

Curhan C. Nephrolithiasis. In: Kapser DL, Fauci AS, Jauser SL, Longo DL, Jameson JL, Loscalzo J, eds. *Harrison's Principles of Internal Medicine.* 19th ed. McGraw-Hill; 2016:1866–1871.

Fontenelle LF, Sarti TD. Kidney stones: treatment and prevention. *Am Fam Physician.* 2019;99(8):491–496.

Groves MJ. Genital herpes: a review. *Am Fam Physician.* 2016;93(11):928–934.

Gupta K, Trautner BW. Urinary tract infections, pyelonephritis and prostatitis. In: Kapser DL, Fauci AS, Jauser SL, Longo DL, Jameson JL, Loscalzo J, eds. *Harrison's Principles of Internal Medicine.* 19th ed. McGraw-Hill; 2016:861–868.

Hanno PM. Lower urinary tract infections in women and management. In: Hanno PM, Guzzo TJ, Malkowicz SB, Wein AJ, eds. *Penn Clinical Manual of Urology.* 2nd ed. Saunders, an imprint of Elsevier, Inc.; 2014:114–116.

Ito S, Honaoka N, Shimata K, et al. Male non-gonococcal urethritis: from microbiological etiologies to demographic and clinical features. *Int J Urol.* 2016;23(4):325–331.

Kodner C. Sexually transmitted infections in men. In: Heidelbaugh JJ, ed. *Men's Health in Primary Care (electronic resource).* Springer International Publishing; 2015:165–196.

Krieger JN. Bacterial infections of the male urinary tract. In: Bope E, Kellerman RD, eds. *Conn's Current Therapy.* Elsevier; 2016:1005–1007.

Legoff I, Pere H, Belec L. Diagnosis of genital herpes simplex virus infection in the clinical laboratory. *Virol J.* 2014;11:83.

Limpkin MW, Ferradino MN, Preminger GM. Evaluation and medical management of urinary lithiasis. In: McDougal WS, Wein A, Kavoussi LR, Partin AW, Peters CA, eds. *Campbell-Walsh Urology.* 11th ed. Elsevier, 52; 2016:1200–1234.e7.

Malone M, Shiraz A. Testicular, scrotal & penile disorders. In: Heidelbaugh JJ, ed. *Men's Health in Primary Care (electronic resource).* Springer International Publishing; 2015:225–248.

Meng MV. Infections of the upper urinary tract. In: Wessels H, ed. *Urologic Emergencies: A Practical Approach (electronic resource).* 2nd ed. Springer Science & Business Media; 2013:105–109. http://dx.doi.org/10.1007/978-1-62703-423-4_8.

Middlekoop SJ, van Pelt LJ, Kampinga GA, ter Maaten JC, Stegeman CA. Routine tests and automated urinalysis in patients with suspected urinary tract infection at the ED. *Am J Emerg Med.* 2016;16:30112–30117. pii:S0735–S6757. http://dx.doi.org/10.1016/j.ajem.2016.05.005.

Rakel R, Rakel D, eds. *Textbook of Family Medicine.* 9th ed. Saunders; 2015:213–215.

Ramakrishnan K, Salinas R. Prostatitis: acute and chronic. *Prim Care.* 2010;37(3):547–563.

Rees J, Abraham M, Doble A, Cooper A. Prostatitis Expert Reference Group (PERG). Diagnosis and treatment of chronic bacterial prostatitis and chronic prostatitis/chronic pelvic pain syndrome: a consensus guideline. *BJU Int.* 2015;116(4):509–525.

Smith-Bindman R, Aubin C, Bailitz J, et al. Ultrasonography versus computed tomography for suspected nephrolithiasis. *N Engl J Med.* 2014;71(12):1100–1110.

Turk C, Petrik A, Sarica K, et al. EAU guidelines on diagnosis and conservative management of urolithiasis. *Eur Urol.* 2016;69(3):468–474. http://dx.doi.org/10.1016/jeurouro.2015.07.040.

Walker NA, Challacombe B. Managing epididymo-orchitis in general practice. *Practitioner.* 2013;257(1760):21–25. https://www.cdc.gov/std/treatment-guidelines/STI-Guidelines-2021.pdf.

CHAPTER 13

GYNECOLOGIC COMPLAINTS

Toral Bhakta, DO, Harsh Bhakta, DO

1. **What is vaginitis?**
   Vaginitis is the inflammation of vulvar and vaginal tissues. Its variety of possible etiologies include infection, irritants, foreign bodies, and atrophy.

2. **What are common organisms that cause infectious vaginitis?**
   Infectious vaginitis can be caused by *Trichomonas vaginalis, Candida albicans, Gardnerella vaginalis,* and overgrowth of anaerobes.

3. **How does vaginitis present clinically?**
   The most common presenting symptoms of vaginitis are foul-smelling vaginal discharge and pruritus; however, depending on the cause, patients can also present with dysuria, dyspareunia, and pelvic pain.

4. **What are the CDC criteria for treatment of bacterial vaginosis?**
   Bacterial vaginosis can be diagnosed in the presence of three of the following four criteria: vaginal discharge, pH >4.5, positive amine test (emittance of a fishy odor upon addition of KOH to the vaginal discharge), and presence of clue cells on wet prep.

5. **How can vaginitis be treated?**
   The treatment of vaginitis involves treating the underlying etiology. Bacterial vaginosis is treated with antibiotics such as metronidazole (500 mg po bid for 7 days) or clindamycin (300 mg po bid for 7 days). For treatment of trichomoniasis, metronidazole (500 mg po bid for 7 days or a one-time 2-g dose) is indicated. Similarly, fungal (*Candida*) vaginitis can be treated with fluconazole (one dose, 150 mg po) or topical clotrimazole. Contact vaginitis is treated by removal of the foreign body or offending agent, whereas atrophic vaginitis is treated with topical estrogen creams.

6. **What is pelvic inflammatory disease?**
   Pelvic inflammatory disease (PID) is an ascending infection from the lower genital tract. It is a female disease and can include a variety of diseases such as salpingitis, endometritis, tubo-ovarian abscesses, and peritonitis.

7. **What are the risk factors for PID?**
   Multiple sexual partners, previous PID, adolescence, intrauterine device (IUD) use, recent menses, douching, and cigarette smoking.

8. **What are the most common presenting signs and symptoms of PID?**
   The most common presentation of PID is lower abdominal pain. Other signs and symptoms include vaginal discharge, fever, nausea, vomiting, and dyspareunia. As the signs and symptoms are very nonspecific, PID should be considered in any female presenting with complaints of lower abdominal pain.

9. **How can PID be diagnosed?**
   In the urgent care setting, PID is a clinical diagnosis. The triad of minimal criteria for diagnosing PID includes lower abdominal tenderness, adnexal tenderness (usually bilateral), and cervical motion tenderness.

10. **What testing can diagnosis PID?**
    Wet prep, urine analysis, urine pregnancy test, elevated C-reactive protein (CRP) and erythrocyte sedimentation rate (ESR), leukocytosis, and laboratory evidence of gonococcal/chlamydia infection. If there is suspicion for tubo-ovarian abscess, pelvic sonography can be used as a definitive imaging study. Laparoscopy remains the most accurate test and the gold-standard imaging test for diagnosing PID; however, it is not very useful in the urgent care setting.

11. **What is the treatment for PID?**
    There are multiple outpatient regimens recommended by the CDC for the treatment of mild to moderate PID in patients that can tolerate PO. These are outlined in Box 13.1.

12. **When is it indicated to transfer for parenteral treatment and hospitalization?**
    Severe clinical illness (e.g., high fever, nausea/vomiting preventing oral intake, severe abdominal pain), suspected pelvic abscess, pregnancy, or a possible alternative diagnosis that could warrant surgery (e.g., appendicitis).

13. **What is defined as "normal" vaginal bleeding?**
    "Normal" vaginal bleeding can be defined as menses lasting less than 7 days, losing less than 60 mL of blood, and having greater than 21-day recurrence cycle.

> **Box 13.1** IM/Oral Treatment Regimens for Mild/Moderate PID
>
> 1. Ceftriaxone 250 mg IM in a single dose PLUS doxycycline 100 mg orally twice a day for 14 days WITH metronidazole 500 mg orally twice a day for 14 days
>   OR
> 2. Cefoxitin 2 g IM in a single dose and probenecid 1 g orally administered concurrently in a single dose PLUS doxycycline 100 mg orally twice a day for 14 days WITH metronidazole 500 mg orally twice a day for 14 days
>   OR
> 3. Other parenteral third-generation cephalosporin (e.g., ceftizoxime or cefotaxime) PLUS doxycycline 100 mg orally twice a day for 14 days WITH metronidazole 500 mg orally twice a day for 14 days

Adapted from CDC.gov.

14. **What is abnormal vaginal bleeding?**
    Abnormal vaginal bleeding can be defined as any bleeding that does not fall into the following criteria: bleeding in between periods, bleeding after sex, spotting at any time in the menstrual cycle, bleeding heavier or for more days than normal, and bleeding after menopause.

15. **Name some causes of abnormal vaginal bleeding.**
    Abnormal vaginal bleeding can have multiple etiologies. Some of the more common etiologies include:
    - Alterations in the endocrine system causing hormonal imbalance
    - Drugs: anticonvulsants and antibiotics (penicillin, tetracycline, trimethoprim/sulfamethoxazole [TMP-SMX]) are the most common causes of breakthrough bleeding
    - Pelvic infections
    - Neoplasm
    - Trauma
    - Bleeding dyscrasia

16. **What is the management of abnormal vaginal bleeding?**
    Treatment of abnormal vaginal bleeding in the urgent care setting is dictated by the patient's hemodynamic stability.
    - In the acute care setting, the provider's first responsibility is to rule out life-threatening hemorrhage and pregnancy. If the patient has unstable vital signs, the first step is to stabilize the patient with intravenous (IV) fluids such as normal saline (NS) or lactated Ringer and blood products. Once the patient is stabilized, the next step is to initiate transfer immediately.
    - If the patient is hemodynamically stable, evaluation includes complete blood count (CBC), coagulation studies, pregnancy test, and pelvic ultrasound (US). Once the underlying cause is identified, a referral to gynecology is appropriate to provide further definitive treatment.

17. **What are condyloma acuminata?**
    Genital warts that start as flesh-colored papules or cauliflower-like projections, caused by human papillomavirus (DNA virus) transmitted by direct contact.

18. **How are they diagnosed and what is the treatment?**
    The diagnosis of genital warts is clinical. They can be treated with topical podofilox 0.5% applied bid for 3 days, followed by 4 days off and then repeating the cycle for up to four times. Alternatively, imiquimod 5% cream can be applied nightly at bedtime three times a week for 16 weeks.

19. **What is the treatment for cases of condyloma acuminata that are resistant to topical therapy?**
    For those patients who fail topical treatment, cryotherapy in their physician's office is the best option.

20. **What is a Bartholin abscess?**
    Bartholin glands are pea-sized glands located on the labia minora. This gland can sometimes form a fluid-filled cyst. When the cyst or the gland itself gets infected, it forms a Bartholin abscess.

21. **What are the signs and symptoms of a Bartholin abscess?**
    A Bartholin abscess is most commonly present as a golf-ball-sized swelling on the lateral aspect of the labia majora. It is extremely painful, especially with walking and sitting.

22. **Name the most common organisms that cause a Bartholin abscess.**
    Most common organisms are *Escherichia coli, Neisseria gonorrhoeae, Chlamydia,* or mixed organisms from the genital tract.

23. **What is the treatment of a Bartholin gland abscess?**
    - Incision and drainage with Word catheter placement is the standard treatment of a Bartholin cyst or abscess. The Word catheter should subsequently be left in the wound for 2 to 4 weeks. If there is accompanying cellulitis, antibiotics are indicated.

- Marsupialization is the definitive treatment. It involves opening the abscess or cyst and suturing the edges, creating an open tract. This procedure is best performed by a gynecologist and is out of the scope of urgent care practice.

24. **What is dysmenorrhea?**
Dysmenorrhea can be defined as painful menses. About 55% of the women in the United States experience some degree of dysmenorrhea.

25. **What is the difference between primary and secondary dysmenorrhea?**
- Primary dysmenorrhea has no pelvic pathology. It is also known as spasmodic dysmenorrhea and is caused by an increase in prostaglandins.
- Secondary dysmenorrhea has pelvic pathology such as endometriosis or uterine fibroids. It is also known as congestive dysmenorrhea.

26. **What are common risk factors associated with severe dysmenorrhea?**
Early age at menarche, prolonged menses, heavy menses, smoking, family history.

27. **How can dysmenorrhea be evaluated in the urgent care setting?**
By abnormal findings on pelvic exam, and with the aid of ancillary tests such as a pelvic sonography.

28. **What is the management of dysmenorrhea?**
Mild to moderate dysmenorrhea can be managed with over-the-counter or prescription nonsteroidal antiin-flammatory drugs (NSAIDs). For more severe cases, oral therapy with estrogens or progestins can also be implemented.

29. **What is the most common age group that typically presents with a vaginal foreign body?**
Vaginal foreign bodies are a common presentation across all age groups. Children may insert any object and not tell parents secondary to fear of being disciplined, whereas adults usually tend to forget objects such as tampons or pessaries.

30. **How does a patient with a vaginal foreign body typically present?**
Patients with a retained vaginal foreign body can complain of pelvic pain and/or foul-smelling vaginal discharge. In more severe and rare cases of retained tampons, patients may also have fever, rash, and leukocytosis from toxic shock syndrome.

31. **How can you treat a vaginal foreign body?**
Treatment of a vaginal foreign body involves removal of the foreign body itself, followed by a Betadine douche and outpatient follow-up with a gynecologist. In severe cases of toxic shock syndrome, treatment will also include IV antibiotics, IV fluids, and hospitalization.

KEY POINTS

1. The most common cause of vaginal discharge or malodor is bacterial vaginosis.
2. PID during the first trimester may cause fetal loss; it is therefore imperative to diagnose and treat during pregnancy.
3. In postmenopausal women, the most common causes of vaginal bleeding are exogenous estrogens, atrophic vaginitis, and endometrial lesions (including cancers).

BIBLIOGRAPHY

American College of Obstetrics and Gynecology. https://www.acog.org.
Centers for Disease Control. https://www.cdc.gov/std/treatment-guidelines/pid.htm.
Dysmenorrhea Clinical Presentation. http://emedicine.medscape.com/article/253812-clinical.
Ma O, Cline D, Tintinalli J, Kelen G, Stapczynski O, eds. *Emergency Medicine: Just the Facts.* 2nd ed. McGraw Hill Medical Publishing; 2005:207–212, 223–228.
Rivers C, Howell J, Barkin R, eds. *Preparing for the Written Board Exam in Emergency Medicine.* 5th ed. Emergency Medicine Educational Enterprises Inc; 2006:534–549.
Tintinalli J, Kelen G, Stapczynski O, eds. *Emergency Medicine: A Comprehensive Study Guide.* 6th ed. McGraw Hill Medical Publishing; 2004:647–653, 691–700.

CHAPTER 14

RASHES AND SKIN INFECTIONS

Nathan J. Morrison, DO, M.Eng, Alexander Lee, MD

Primary skin lesions are evaluated utilizing a detailed history including timing, location, characteristics, exposures, occupation, and recent drug use. Physical examination should incorporate inspection and palpation of the skin lesions, mucous membranes, and eyes. Internationally agreed descriptive terms for the skin lesions are used to describe any findings (Table 14.1).

Commonly encountered dermatologic issues in the outpatient setting will be outlined throughout the chapter. Prior to review, it is of the utmost importance to consider the dermatologic emergencies outlined in Table 14.2. Any of the aforementioned cases are associated with severe morbidity or mortality and typically require emergent referral to a burn center or intensive care unit.

ERYTHEMA MULTIFORME (EM), DRUG REACTION WITH EOSINOPHILIA AND SYSTEMIC SYMPTOMS (DRESS) SYNDROME, STEVEN-JOHNSON SYNDROME (SJS), AND TOXIC EPIDERMAL NECROLYSIS (TEN)

1. **What is the difference between EM, DRESS syndrome, and SJS and TEN?**
   EM is described as a target-like skin lesion and may be isolated, recurrent, or persistent. The management of EM is with topical steroids, antihistamines, and treating the underlying etiology (if identified). EM can be confused with SJS and TEN, although SJS usually contains widespread erythematous targetoid lesions. SJS is defined by targetoid cutaneous lesions involving 10% or less of the patient's total body surface area and involvement of mucous membranes in most cases. The inciting factors of SJS include infection, systemic diseases, physical agents, foods, and various drugs. SJS and TEN overlap in pathophysiology, onset, and clinical manifestation and are recognized as variants of the same condition with differing severities. TEN is more severe than SJS, involving 30% or more of the patient's total body surface area, and has a worse prognosis with a mortality rate of around 30%, regardless of initiation of treatment. DRESS syndrome is often confused with SJS and TEN but with distinct differences.

Table 14.1 Internationally Agreed-Upon Descriptive Terms for Skin Lesions

TERM	DEFINITION
Macule	Flat, circumscribed, nonpalpable lesion that differs in color from the surrounding skin; it can be any color or shape (≤1 cm); referred to as a patch if >1 cm
Papule	Elevated, solid, palpable lesion ≤1 cm in diameter
Plaque	Circumscribed, palpable lesion >1 cm in diameter; most plaques are elevated; may result from a coalescence of papules
Nodule	Elevated, solid, palpable lesion >1 cm usually located primarily in the dermis or subcutis; the greatest portion of the lesion may be exophytic or beneath the skin surface
Weal	Transient elevation of the skin caused by dermal edema; often centrally pale with an erythematous rim
Vesicle	Circumscribed lesion ≤1 cm in diameter that contains liquid (clear, serous, or hemorrhagic)
Bulla	Circumscribed lesion ≤1 cm in diameter that contains liquid (clear, serous, or hemorrhagic)
Pustule	Circumscribed lesion that contains pus
Scale	Visible accumulation of keratin, forming a flat plate or flake
Crust	Dried serum, blood, or pus on the surface of the skin
Erosion	Loss of either a portion of or the entire epidermis
Excoriation	Loss of the epidermis and a portion of the dermis caused by scratching or an exogenous injury
Ulcer	Full-thickness loss of the epidermis plus at least portion of the dermis; may extend into the subcutaneous tissue

From Life-threatening skin conditions presenting to critical care. *BJA Educ.* 2021;376–383. Table 2.

Table 14.2 Life-Threatening Skin Conditions

PRIMARY SKIN INFECTIONS	DRUG-RELATED CONDITIONS	IMMUNE-RELATED CONDITIONS	INFLAMMATORY DERMATOSES
Necrotizing Fasciitis (NF)	Stevens-Johnson Syndrome (SJS) & Toxic Epidermal Necrolysis	Pemphigus Vulgaris (PV)	Acute Generalized Pustular Psoriasis (AGPP)
Toxic Shock Syndrome (TSS)	Drug Rash Eosinophilia and Systemic Symptoms Syndrome (DRESS Syndrome)	Widespread Erythema Multiforme (EM)	Erythroderma (Exfoliative Dermatitis)
Severe Cellulitis			

Table 14.3 EM, DRESS Syndrome, SJS and TEN Characteristics

	SJS	TEN	DRESS SYNDROME
Onset	4–28 days	4–28 days	2–6 weeks
Symptoms	Fever >38.0°C Malaise Flu-like symptoms	Fever >38.0°C Malaise Flu-like symptoms	Facial edema Lymphadenopathy
Skin Lesion	Target-like skin lesion <10% TSA	Target-like skin lesion <30% TSA	No particular rash by definition Often exfoliative dermatitis or maculopapular rash
Pathophysiology	CD8+ cytotoxic T Lymphocytes	CD8+ cytotoxic T Lymphocytes	T-cells Eosinophils
Organs involved	Oropharynx Nasopharynx Genitalia Anus	Oropharynx Nasopharynx Genitalia Anus	Liver (most common) Kidneys Lungs Heart
Treatment	Identification (if possible) and discontinuation of causative agent Supportive care	Identification (if possible) and discontinuation of causative agent Supportive care	Identification (if possible) and discontinuation of causative agent Topical or systematic corticosteroids

DRESS syndrome is characterized by a triad of fever, dermatitis, and internal organ involvement, often presenting 2 to 6 weeks after the first treatment with the responsible drug agent. Notably, mucosal lesions and eosinophilia are present in all three diagnoses, although DRESS syndrome is not defined by a particular rash. Elevated liver enzymes have most often been reported in cases of DRESS syndrome (Table 14.3).

CONTACT DERMATITIS

2. Describe allergic contact dermatitis.
   Allergic contact dermatitis is a very itchy eczematous rash with varying sizes of papules, vesicles, and bullae (Fig. 14.1). It affects skin exposure sites and is associated with erythema and edema that can be oozing or crusting depending on the timing of presentation. These are immune-mediated, delayed hypersensitivity reactions and typically present 1–2 days after the exposure.

3. What are some common precipitants of allergic contact dermatitis?
   Cosmetics, plants (poison ivy), detergents, soaps, lotions, antibiotic ointments and creams, metals, plastics, latex, rubber, various chemicals, and tapes. Specifically, nickel, balsam of Peru, chromium, neomycin, formaldehyde, thiomersal, fragrance mix, cobalt, and parthenium have been identified as common allergens.

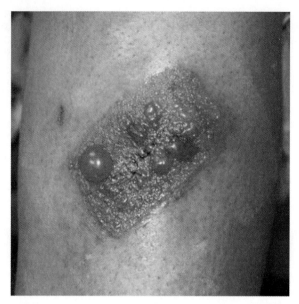

Fig. 14.1 Contact dermatitis. (From Nelson Essentials of Pediatrics, 2011. Fig. 191.2.)

4. Describe the treatment for allergic contact dermatitis.
   Avoidance or removal of identified allergen. Clean and wash skin with hypoallergenic soap. Symptom management with cold compresses and antihistamines. It is generally accepted that the mainstay of treatment is topical steroids for mild reactions and systemic steroids for severe reactions. It is key to appreciate any secondary infection and treat it with appropriate antibiotics; however, antibiotics are only indicated if an infection is present.

5. What is a common cause of treatment failure in contact dermatitis?
   Short courses of steroids. Systemic corticosteroids such as prednisone or triamcinolone should usually consist of a higher dose for at least 5 days and then a prolonged taper in an effort to prevent rebound dermatitis. It is not necessary to provide both topical and systemic steroids.
   It should be noted that very potent topical steroids should be avoided for use on the face and genitals, and fluorinated corticosteroids should be limited to 10–14 days, specifically on the face.

6. Poison ivy, oak, and sumac all cause forms of allergic contact dermatitis. What is the typical duration of symptoms?
   Typical duration is 2 weeks untreated. If treated with topical or oral steroids, duration may be shorter. However, treatment usually needs to be continued for 2 more weeks after resolution of symptoms; otherwise, dermatitis may reappear.

7. A patient with small linear vesicles after exposure to poison ivy presents with severe itching that does not resolve with Benadryl cream or tablets. Why?
   This is a delayed immune-mediated reaction and not related to histamine release. Because of this, antihistamines may not provide much relief of symptoms. Initial treatment should include cool compresses and tepid baths with oatmeal colloid or baking soda. Small areas of involvement can be treated with topical steroids. Severe involvement or involvement of face, eyes, and genitalia may require oral steroids. This needs to be over a 2- to 3-week period or the patient will have rebound dermatitis.

8. How can you tell the difference between allergic contact dermatitis and irritant contact dermatitis?
   In many cases, it is impossible to tell the difference by appearance, although symptomatology may help distinguish the two with key parts of the history and timing of onset. Irritant contact dermatitis often presents with burning, itching, stinging, soreness, and pain, particularly at the beginning of the clinical course, while allergic contact dermatitis more often presents with pruritus. Irritant contact dermatitis does not require previous sensitization and is not a delayed immune reaction, but it is a skin barrier disruption and may present within a few hours of exposure to an irritant. Through exposure, irritant contact dermatitis is more likely to develop with increased duration, intensity, or concentration of the substance.

9. **List some common irritants for irritant contact dermatitis and describe initial treatment.**
   Anything that can cause a skin barrier disruption can lead to irritant contact dermatitis (ICD). This includes (but is not limited to) water, soaps, detergents, or repetitive trauma. Query of the patient's occupation, hobbies, or other exposures is important in diagnosing irritant contact dermatitis. Initial treatment is avoidance of the irritant and frequent moisturization of the skin. Since this is a barrier breakdown process and not related to an immune-mediated response, steroids are not always indicated. Topical steroids may be used to help with local inflammation, but only if necessary.

CUTANEOUS ABSCESSES

10. **What is the most accepted management for a simple cutaneous abscess?**
    Simple abscess management is typically a bedside incision and drainage. The use of warm compresses or antibiotic use alone without incision and drainage has not been proven effective. Additionally, needle aspiration has been shown to be an inferior method of treatment and is not recommended as a management technique. The use of topical povidone-iodine antiseptic solutions or copious abscess cavity irrigation is common practice but has not been shown to decrease rates of subsequent intervention and treatment.

11. **Why do people presenting with a cutaneous abscess think they have been bitten by a spider?**
    Many abscesses will present with a central area of skin thinning with a dark necrotic center that looks similar to the erythematous lesion of a spider bite. Spider bites can be differentiated by a thorough history and detailed physical examination. A careful history can determine the patient's risk for a spider bite, although a confirmed bite typically requires a captured or recovered spider. If a bite is suspected, treatment is generally supportive care with immobilization, elevation, and cold compresses (avoid heat). Early excision or debridement is not recommended but should be delayed until the wound has stabilized. Other treatment strategies should be based on the type of spider involved.

12. **Should all cutaneous abscesses be incised and drained?**
    In general, the standard treatment of an abscess is to drain it. There are times when a patient may present early in the formation of a simple abscess and the cavity may not be identified or yet present. The use of bedside ultrasound to identify the abscess cavity is appropriate in these settings if available. An abscess will appear as a clearly demarcated, hypoechoic area with surrounding hyperemia. Color Doppler ultrasound can be utilized to differentiate the abscess from a vascular structure (Fig. 14.2). Small pustules do not need large incisions but can be unroofed with an 18-gauge needle with an aseptic technique and many times do not require any anesthesia.

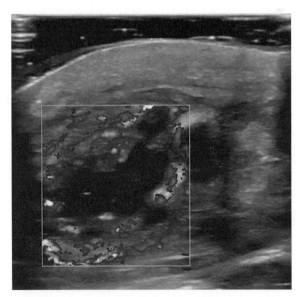

Fig. 14.2 Ultrasonographic appearance of an abscess showing a hypoechoic fluid filled pocket with lack of color doppler in the abscess cavity. (From Infectious Disease/Expert Clinical Management. 2021;78(1):44–48. Figure 2.)

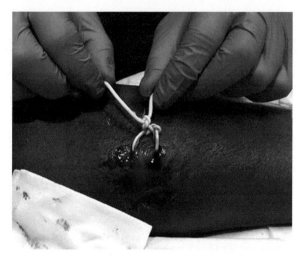

Fig. 14.3 Loop drainage technique for cutaneous abscess management. (From Infectious Disease/Expert Clinical Management. 2021;78(1):44–48. Figure 4.)

13. **After incision and drainage of an abscess, should the cavity be packed with sterile or iodoform gauze?**
Recent literature has not shown a benefit to wound packing for simple cutaneous abscesses. It is now accepted that simple abscesses (not immunocompromised, smaller abscess size, nondiabetic patient) can be left unpacked. All drained abscesses should receive close follow-up as well as daily wound care with soap and water. Also, new commercially available products can be used to help keep an incision open for drainage. Recent studies have shown that the loop drainage technique has a lower failure rate (8.3% versus 14.2%), and improved cosmetic outcomes compared with incision and drainage (Fig. 14.3).

14. **Who should receive antibiotics after incision and drainage?**
This is also a controversial question and continues to be debated. Based on recent literature, incision and drainage alone is adequate for management of simple abscesses (small size, nondiabetic, immunocompetent patients without surrounding cellulitis or systemic symptoms). When antibiotics are indicated, they should be targeted to cover community-acquired methicillin-resistant Staphylococcus aureus (CA-MRSA) due to its increased prevalence. The provider should incorporate shared decision making, local antibiotic resistance patterns, as well as stay current with the Infectious Diseases Society of America (IDSA) guidelines on management of skin and soft tissue infections.

15. **Who would be considered higher risk or described as a complicated case in the management of a cutaneous abscess?**
Immunocompromised patients, diabetic patients, large abscess size (>5 cm), patients who present toxic and febrile, significant associated cellulitis, infections on the hands or face.

16. **What is the difference between a folliculitis, a furuncle, and a carbuncle?**
Folliculitis is a superficial infection of a hair follicle that can initially be treated with daily cleansing using soap and water, warm compresses, and topical mupirocin ointment (Fig. 14.4). A furuncle is an extension of a folliculitis to subcutaneous tissue. Large furuncles require CA-MRSA antimicrobials and abscess drainage if indicated. A carbuncle represents interconnected furuncles, which are essentially multiseptate abscesses that require drainage with blunt dissection and antibiotic treatment.

CELLULITIS AND ERYSIPELAS

17. **What is the difference between erysipelas and cellulitis?**
Both are soft tissue skin infections; however, cellulitis involves the deeper subcutaneous connective tissue. Erysipelas is typically bright red with very distinct, demarcated borders (Fig. 14.5). Cellulitis is also erythematous and red but has indistinctive borders and is more associated with systemic symptoms (Fig. 14.6). Cellulitis can often be diagnosed by ultrasound with the appearance of a characteristic "cobblestoning" appearance (Fig. 14.7). Both are warm to touch and tender upon palpation.

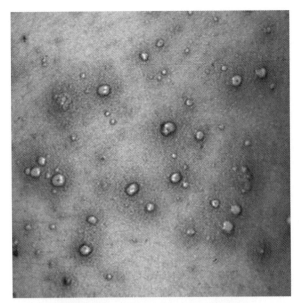

Fig. 14.4 Folliculitis. (From Clinical Dermatology, 2010, 1–74.)

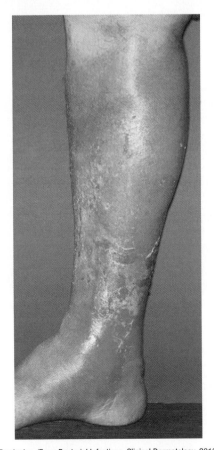

Fig. 14.5 Erysipelas. (From Bacterial Infections. Clinical Dermatology, 2010. Fig. 9.13.)

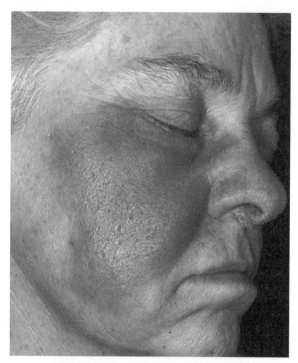

Fig. 14.6 Cellulitis. (From Bacterial Infections. Andrews' Diseases of the Skin: Clinical Dermatology. Philadelphia: Saunders; 2011:247–286. Fig. 14.17.)

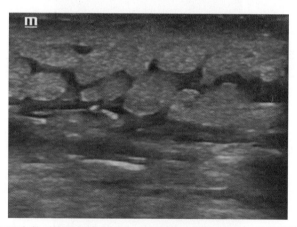

Fig. 14.7 Cellulitis on ultrasound with cobblestoning. (From Infectious Disease/Expert Clinical Management. 2021;78(1):44–48. 3.)

18. What is the best antibiotic choice for a patient with cellulitis?

A patient presenting with cellulitis who does not appear to be toxic or systemically ill and does not have any history to suggest immunocompromise usually can be treated as an outpatient. Due to the recent increased prevalence of CA-MRSA, all patients should be evaluated for risk for MRSA infection, and the infection should be evaluated for any purulent drainage. If either is present, the patient should be treated empirically with antibiotics that target MRSA infection. The provider should also take into account local resistance patterns and tailor therapy appropriately. The IDSA has provided clinical guidelines for antibiotic therapy as seen in Fig. 14.8. These are guaranteed to change in the future, and the provider should attempt to stay current in order to prevent antibiotic resistance.

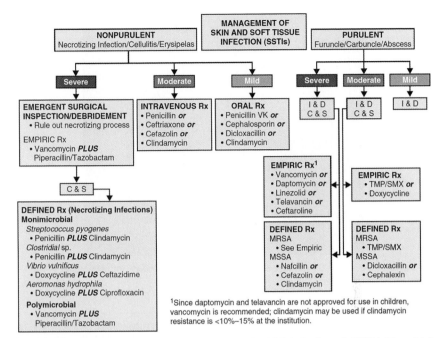

Fig. 14.8 Management of SSTIs. Purulent skin and soft tissue infections (SSTIs). Mild infection: for purulent SSTI, incision and drainage is indicated. Moderate infection: patients with purulent infection with systemic signs of infection. Severe infection: patients who have failed incision and drainage plus oral antibiotics or those with systemic signs of infection, such as temperature >38°C, tachycardia (heart rate >90 beats per minute), tachypnea (respiratory rate >24 breaths per minute), abnormal white blood cell count (>12 000 or <400 cells/μL), or immunocompromised patients. Nonpurulent SSTIs. Mild infection: typical cellulitis/erysipelas with no focus of purulence. Moderate infection: typical cellulitis/erysipelas with systemic signs of infection. Severe infection: patients who have failed oral antibiotic treatment or those with systemic signs of infection (as defined above under purulent infection), or those who are immunocompromised, or those with clinical signs of deeper infection, such as bullae, skin sloughing, hypotension, or evidence of organ dysfunction. Two newer agents, tedizolid and dalbavancin, are also effective agents in SSTIs, including those caused by methicillin-resistant Staphylococcus aureus, and may be approved for this indication by June 2014.C & S, Culture and sensitivity; I & D, incision and drainage; MRSA, methicillin-resistant Staphylococcus aureus; Rx, treatment; TMP/SMX, trimethoprim-sulfamethoxazole. (From Stevens DL, et al. Practice guidelines for the diagnosis and management of skin and soft tissue infections: 2014 update by the infectious diseases society of America. *Clin Infect Dis.* 2014;59(2):e10–e52. http://dx.doi.org/10.1093/cid/ciu296.)

19. Should you obtain blood cultures for uncomplicated cases of cellulitis?
    No. Cultures are not indicated for uncomplicated cases of cellulitis, because they are of low yield and are very costly.

20. Who should be referred to a higher level of care for evaluation and possible admission for management of cellulitis?
    Immunocompromised patients, diabetic patients, patients who appear sick or those where concern exists for systemic infection or early sepsis, involvement of >50% of a limb or torso, rapidly advancing edge, failure of initial outpatient treatment, or concern exists for possible necrotizing fasciitis, myonecrosis, or pyomyositis.

21. What are the key elements to outpatient management of cellulitis?
    Early and appropriate antibiotic regimen, pain control, removal of any infectious source or nidus, daily wound management and cleaning, elevation of any infected and edematous extremity, skin marking of cellulitic border in order to aid in tracking of spread, and close follow-up in 24–48 hours.

SHINGLES

22. A 68-year-old patient presents with a unilateral skin eruption that stays in a single dermatome with small vesicles on an erythematous base.
    The rash is described as burning and very painful, sharp, and stabbing. It was associated with 2–3 days of general malaise, low-grade fever, and pain at the site where the rash appeared. The patient wants to know if she is contagious. This presentation is consistent with herpes zoster (shingles) and is a reactivation of latent *varicella-zoster* (chickenpox). She is contagious only to those who have not previously had varicella or have not received

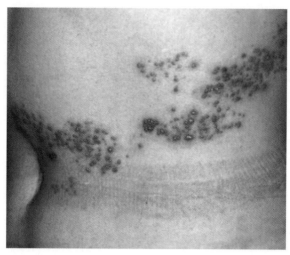

Fig. 14.9 Shingles. (From Exploring Medical Language: A Student-Directed Approach, 2012;694–749. Fig. 15.11.)

the varicella vaccine. For this reason, the patient should avoid contact with unvaccinated children, infants, and pregnant women as well as any individual who has not previously been vaccinated or had the chickenpox virus. See Fig. 14.9.

23. **How long is a typical shingles infection and what is the most common complication related to the infection?**
A typical infection will last 3–4 weeks. If a patient presents within 72 hours of rash onset, an antiviral prescription can shorten the duration of viral replication, reduce formation of new lesions, help with healing, and reduce pain. Valacyclovir 1000 mg TID for 7 days is recommended as the most economical treatment option. Immunocompromised patients and patients presenting with new lesions may also benefit from therapy outside of the 72-hour window. Patients severely immunocompromised, or those unable to tolerate oral medications, may require the use of IV acyclovir. In addition to antivirals, pain should be managed with nonsteroidal antiinflammatory drugs (NSAIDs), opiates, gabapentin, or pregabalin—they are the most promising treatments to reduce postherpetic neuralgia, which is the most common complication of herpes zoster. Corticosteroids do not reduce the risk of postherpetic neuralgia as previously thought and are no longer recommended. Postherpetic neuralgia should be controlled until pain resolves, which is typically self-limited. This can be managed topically with capsaicin cream or a lidocaine patch, and/or orally with tricyclic antidepressants or anticonvulsants in conjunction with NSAIDs.

24. **What is Hutchinson sign?**
The eponym refers to the extension of a rash in the trigeminal nerve distribution to the tip of the nose (Fig. 14.10). This implies possible ocular lesions, and the patient should be evaluated for ocular involvement. If ocular lesions or concern for ocular involvement is noted, the patient should be referred to an ophthalmologist for close follow-up and may need ophthalmic corticosteroids.

ERYTHEMA MIGRANS AND LYME DISEASE

25. **What is erythema migrans (EM) and what does it look like?**
EM is the characteristic clinical manifestation of early localized (single lesion) or early disseminated (multiple lesions) Lyme disease. It is a flat, red rash that develops 3–30 days following infection of Lyme disease (Fig. 14.11). It usually begins at the site of a tick bite and can spread to multiple areas of distribution. It is often warm to touch. Patients do not complain of itching or pain. Sometimes a clearing occurs as the rash enlarges, causing a "bullseye" appearance.

26. **How many patients with Lyme disease will develop erythema migrans?**
70–80%.

27. **What is the treatment for erythema migrans?**
All patients with EM should be treated for Lyme disease as seen in Table 14.4.

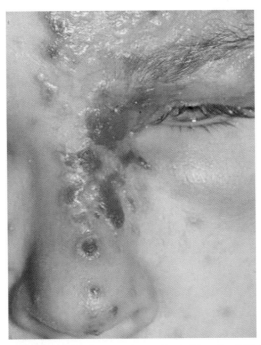

Fig. 14.10 Hutchinson sign. (From Krachmer JH, Palay DA. Corneal abnormalities. In: *Primary Care Ophthalmology*, 2nd ed. N.p.: Mosby; 2005:103–117.)

TICK BITE AND REMOVAL

28. **What is the proper method for removing a tick?**
    Using fine-tipped forceps, the tick is grasped close to the skin and pulled upward with constant motion (Fig. 14.12). It is important not to twist the tick, as this may cause parts to break off and remain embedded in the skin. Do not squeeze the body of the tick, as fluid may be expelled, increasing the possibility of infection. If the tick's mouthparts remain in the skin, wait for the parts to fall out spontaneously; digging them out may increase the risk of soft tissue infection. The bite site should be observed for 30 days. Components of tick saliva can cause transient erythema that should not be confused with erythema migrans.

29. **What are the indications for antimicrobial prophylaxis following tick removal?**
    Antibiotic prophylaxis is indicated for nonpregnant adults and children who meet **all** the following criteria:
    1. The attached tick is identified as an adult or nymphal *I. scapularis* tick (deer tick).
    2. The tick is estimated to have been attached for ≥36 hours based on the degree of engorgement or time of exposure.
    3. Prophylaxis is begun within 72 hours of tick removal.

TINEA

30. **What is tinea?**
    This is an infection of the skin, hair, and nails caused by a group of fungi called dermatophytes. It is classified according to which portion of the body is affected: tinea capitis (scalp), tinea manuum/pedis (palms, soles), tinea corporis (body), tinea cruris (groin), tinea faciale (face), tinea unguium (nailbed, also known as onychomycosis). See Fig. 14.13.

31. **How is tinea treated?**
    Tinea corporis is typically treated with topical antifungal agents (ketoconazole, clotrimazole, terbinafine), but oral antifungals (fluconazole) can be considered in extensive disease. For tinea capitis and tinea involving the nailbeds, oral therapy is required. Use of extensive oral antifungal treatment regimens requires baseline liver function testing and must be repeated halfway through the course of treatment. Prescribing combination steroid/antifungal creams is common; however, it is not recommended. Typical oral antifungal regimens include:
    - Terbinafine: 250 mg/day for 2 weeks
    - Itraconazole: 200 mg twice daily for 1 week

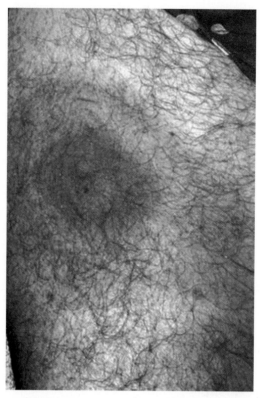

Fig. 14.11 Erythema migrans. (From Tick-Related Infections. Current Clinical Medicine. Philadelphia: Saunders; 2010:785–791. Figure 2.)

Table 14.4 Treatment Regimens of Erythema Migrans

DRUG	ADULT DOSE	PEDIATRIC DOSE	COMMENTS
Doxycycline	100 mg orally twice daily for 10 days	4.4 mg/kg/day orally divided twice daily (maximum 100 mg per dose) for 14 days	**1.** Patients with early disseminated disease who present with multiple EM lesions are treated the same as those with a single EM lesion
OR Amoxicillin	500 mg orally three times daily for 14 days	50 mg/kg/day orally divided three times daily (maximum 500 mg per dose) for 14 days	**2.** For patients unable to tolerate the preferred regimens, alternative treatments include: **2a.** Azithromycin (in adults 500 mg orally once daily; in children: 10 mg/kg/day ([maximum 500 mg per dose]) for 7 days (range 5–10 days) **OR**
OR Cefuroxime	500 mg orally twice daily for 14 days	30 mg/kg/day orally divided twice daily (maximum 500 mg per dose) for 14 days	**2b.** Clarithromycin (in adults: 500 mg orally twice daily; in children:15 mg/kg/day divided twice daily ([maximum 500 mg per dose]) for 14–21 days.

- Fluconazole: 150 mg once weekly for 2–6 weeks
- Griseofulvin (frequent used for Tinea capitis): 1000 mg/day of griseofulvin microsize for 4–8 weeks or 750 mg/day of griseofulvin ultra microsize for 4–8 weeks

32. **What is a kerion?**
    Severe manifestation of tinea capitis resulting from an intense immune response to a superimposed bacterial infection (Fig. 14.14). It is treated similarly to tinea capitis, with the possible addition of an oral course of antibiotics.

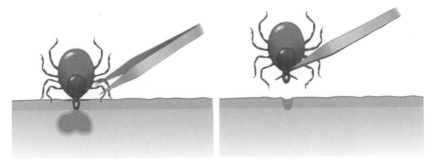

Fig. 14.12 Tick removal. (From Goldman L, Ausiello D. Cecil Medicine. 23rd ed. Philadelphia: Saunders; 2007.)

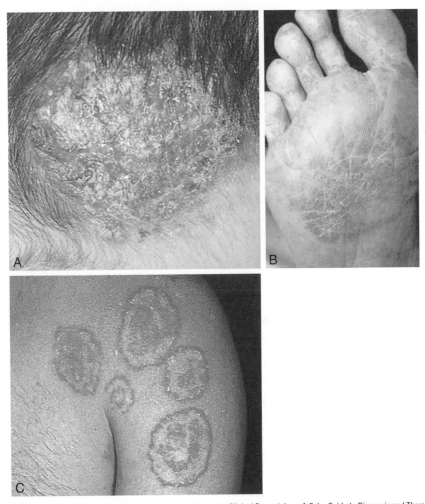

Fig. 14.13 A. Tinea capitis. (From Principles of Diagnosis and Anatomy. Clinical Dermatology: A Color Guide to Diagnosis and Therapy. Philadelphia: Mosby; 2010:1–74.) B. Tinea pedis. (From Goldstein BG, Goldstein AO. Practical Dermatology. 2nd ed. St Louis: Mosby; 1997.) C. Tinea corporis. (From Care of the Patient with an Integumentary Disorder. Foundations and Adult Health Nursing. Philadelphia: Mosby; 2011:1295–1344. Fig. 43.8.)

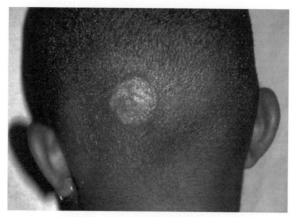

Fig. 14.14 Kerion. (From Training Room Management of Medical Conditions: Sports Dermatology. *Clin Sports Med.* 2005. Figure 3.)

WARTS

33. What is a wart?

    Benign skin eruptions caused by human papillomavirus. Warts can occur at any age and can occur at any anatomic location. Common warts are those most often treated in urgent care settings. They appear as rough, raised irregular projections that can be as large as 1 cm. They occur most commonly on the hands, knees, and feet.

34. What percentage of warts resolve spontaneously in 2 years?

    65%. "Benign neglect" is an accepted treatment option; however, treatment is recommended if the wart is extensive or symptomatic.

35. What is the treatment for warts?

    Salicylic acid is the first-line therapy. This is bought over the counter and has a cure rate of 70–80%. Cryotherapy has been shown to be an effective treatment option. Liquid nitrogen is applied with a cotton applicator to destroy the lesion. This needs to be repeated every 3 weeks for up to 3 months for complete resolution. Alternatively, electrodesiccation (oftentimes with a hyfrecator) has also been shown to be effective; however, it is more likely to scar.

NECROTIZING FASCIITIS

36. What is necrotizing fasciitis?

    Necrotizing fasciitis (NF) is an aggressive and rapidly proliferating skin and soft tissue infection that causes necrosis of the muscle, fascia, and subcutaneous tissue. These infections often spread quickly, within hours, and are associated with severe morbidity and mortality (Table 14.2 and Fig. 14.15).

37. What predisposes a patient to necrotizing fasciitis?

    Patients with diabetes, a history of alcohol use disorder, and liver cirrhosis are more likely to develop NF.

38. How is necrotizing fasciitis recognized and diagnosed?

    NF commonly presents with severe "pain out of proportion to exam" and signs of systemic illness. When palpated, these patients will often display extreme discomfort, seemingly more severe than the appearance of the primary skin lesion. Other findings include tenderness beyond the erythematous skin lesion border, crepitus, subcutaneous emphysema, or cellulitis. Patients may begin to display anesthesia, dysesthesia, or paresthesia as the deeper fascia, nerve fibers, and muscle becomes involved. The Laboratory Risk Indicator for Necrotizing Infection (LRINEC) Score can be utilized to help distinguish necrotizing from nonnecrotizing skin infections. The scoring tool incorporates C-reactive protein (CRP), total white cell count (WBC), hemoglobin (Hg), serum sodium, creatinine, and glucose.

39. How is necrotizing fasciitis treated?

    Early surgical consultation is needed in cases of high suspicion. Patients have improved outcomes with early surgical treatment. These infections are often polymicrobial and require broad antibiotic coverage as soon as they are identified. Three accepted regimens can be used as an adjunct to manage NF along with surgical intervention:

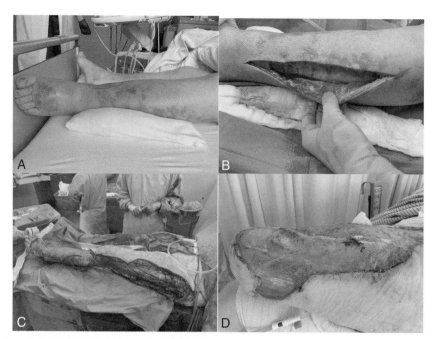

Fig. 14.15 Necrotizing fasciitis. A. Landscape-like necrosis, B. Intraoperative findings, C. Postradical debridement, and D. Postamputation and skin grafting. (From Necrotizing fasciitis caused by mono-bacterial gram-negative infection with E. coli–the deadliest of them all: A case series and review of the literature, 2021. Figure 1.)

1. Imipenem, 1 gram IV every 6–8 hours, AND daptomycin, 6 mg/kg IV daily, AND clindamycin, 600–900 IV mg four times per day.
2. Piperacillin/tazobactam, 3.375 g IV every 6 hours OR 4.5 g IV every 8 hours AND daptomycin, 6 mg/kg IV daily, AND clindamycin, 600–900 mg IV four times per day.
3. Meropenem, 1 g IV every 8 hours AND vancomycin, 15–20 mg/kg/dose IV every 8–12 hours AND clindamycin, 600–900 mg IV four times per day.

MONKEYPOX

40. **What is Monkeypox?**

    A viral zoonotic infection that is caused by the Monkeypox virus and results in a rash similar to that of smallpox. However, person-to-person spread and mortality are significantly less than for smallpox. The rash can also be similar in appearance to those observed in secondary syphilis, herpes simplex infection, and varicella zoster virus infection. On July 23, 2022, the World Health Organization (WHO) declared a global outbreak of Monkeypox a public health emergency of international concern.

41. **How is Monkeypox transmitted?**

    Spread of Monkeypox occurs primarily through direct contact with infectious sores, scabs, or body fluids. Activities that involve close personal contact with an infected individual increase the risk of transmission. Monkeypox can also be acquired through contact with an infected animal's bodily fluids, through a bite, or preparation of raw or minimally processed meat that comes from wild animals in certain endemic regions. Additionally, transmission can occur through percutaneous inoculation, contact with materials or fomites that have become contaminated, as well as through respiratory secretions (although prolonged face-to-face contact may be required for transmission to occur via this route).

42. **How is Monkeypox recognized and diagnosed?**

    The generalized disease usually manifests as fevers, chills, and myalgias, with a characteristic rash. The skin eruption usually occurs between 1 to 2 days before and 3 to 4 days after the onset of the systemic symptoms and progresses through several stages:

    1. Typically begins as 2–5 mm in diameter macules.
    2. Lesions subsequently evolve into papules, vesicles, and then pseudopustules. Lesions are well circumscribed, deep seated, and often develop umbilication.

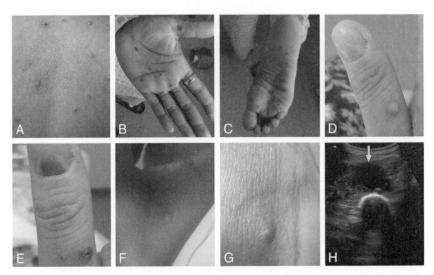

Fig. 14.16 Skin and soft tissue Monkeypox lesions. A. & D. Vesicular or pustular lesions, B & C. Macular lesions involving the palms and soles. D. & E. A subungual lesion. F & G. More subtle papules and smaller vesicles. H. A deep abscess (arrow, image obtained during ultrasound-guided drainage). (From Adler H, Gould S, Hine P, et al. Clinical features and management of human monkeypox: a retrospective observational study in the UK. *Lancet Infect Dis.* 2022;22(8):1153–1162. Figure 2.)

3. Lesions eventually crust over, and these crusts dry up and then fall off. This typically occurs 7–14 days after the rash begins.
   Lesions often occur in the genital and anorectal areas or in the mouth. The rash is often described as painful but can become itchy in the healing phase. The number of lesions varies from a few to 100. Most commonly, there are 1–20 lesions on the skin. Sometimes, coalescing lesions result in large plaques, ulcerations, or crusts. Some severe complications include the evolution of genital, perianal, or facial lesions into a coalescing large plaque, ulceration, or crust and superimposed cellulitis. Clinical suspicion of a diagnosis of Monkeypox should be followed by viral or serologic testing. See Fig. 14.16.

43. **How long is a person with Monkeypox contagious?**
    A person is considered infectious from the onset of clinical manifestations until all skin lesions have scabbed over and reepithelialization has occurred.

44. **How is Monkeypox treated?**
    Mild disease is treated supportively without medical intervention. Some may require analgesics for pain-related proctitis or tonsillitis. Antiviral therapy with tecovirimat is indicated for individuals at risk for severe disease and those with lesions involving the eyes, mouth, or anogenital area. There are vaccines available for postexposure prophylaxis, and the decision for administration is dependent primarily on the risk type of exposure, defined by the United States Centers for Disease Control and Prevention.

Acknowledgements

The authors would like to thank Dr. Brian Kipe, MD for their contributions to this chapter in the previous edition.

KEY POINTS

1. Treatment failure is common in allergic contact dermatitis if the course of steroids is not long enough.
2. In general, simple cutaneous abscesses require incision and drainage for treatment, but not all abscesses require antibiotics. Utilization of the loop drainage technique may improve cosmetic outcomes and prevent subsequent intervention. Adjuncts such as ultrasound can help identify a drainable pocket of fluid.
3. Antiviral treatment should be initiated within 72 hours of rash onset to be most effective in cases of herpes zoster.
4. Life-threatening conditions with widespread involvement or systemic symptoms require referral to an emergency department or burn center.
5. On July 23, 2022, the WHO declared a global outbreak of Monkeypox a public health emergency of international concern.

BIBLIOGRAPHY

Adler H, Gould S, Hine P, et al. Clinical features and management of human monkeypox: a retrospective observational study in the UK [published correction appears in Lancet Infect Dis. 2022 Jul;22(7):e177] [published correction appears in Lancet Infect Dis. 2022 Jul;22(7):e177]. *Lancet Infect Dis.* 2022;22(8):1153–1162. doi:10.1016/S1473-3099(22)00228-6.

Albrecht M. Treatment of herpes zoster in the immunocompromised host. In: Mitty J, ed. *UpToDate.* Accessed October 28, 2016.

Antinori A, Mazzotta V, Vita S, et al. Epidemiological, clinical and virological characteristics of four cases of monkeypox support transmission through sexual contact, May 2022. *Euro Surveill.* 2022;27(22):2200421.

Ali S, Graham TA, Forgie SE. The assessment and management of tinea capitis in children. *Pediatr Emerg Care.* 2007;23(9):662–665.

American Academy of Pediatrics. Lyme disease. In: Kimberlin DW, Brady MT, Jackson MA, Long SS, eds. *Red Book: 2018 Report of the Committee on Infectious Diseases.* 31st ed. American Academy of Pediatrics; 2018:515.

Bayard IPE, Grobbelaar AO, Constantinescu MA. Necrotizing fasciitis caused by mono-bacterial gram-negative infection with E. coli - the deadliest of them all: A case series and review of the literature. *JPRAS Open.* 2021;29:99–105. doi:10.1016/j.jpra.2021.04.007 Published 2021 May 14.

Buttaravoli P. *Minor emergencies: splinters to fractures.* 2nd ed. Elsevier; 2007.

Baddour LM. Cellulitis and erysipelas. In: Baron EL, ed. *UpToDate.* (Accessed October 25, 2016.)

Baddour LM. Impetigo. In: Ofori AO, ed. *UpToDate,* Waltham, MA. (Accessed October 14, 2016.)

Baddour LM. Skin abscesses, furuncles, and carbuncles. In: Baron EL, ed. *UpToDate,* Waltham, MA. (Accessed October 23, 2016.)

Centers for Disease Control and Prevention. Lyme. Available at <https://www.cdc.gov/lyme/signs_symptoms>; Accessed November 8, 2016.

Centers for Disease Control and Prevention. Parasites. Scabies. Available at <http://www.cdc.gov/parasites/scabies/index.html>; Accessed November 9, 2016.

Clinical Practice Guidelines by the Infectious Diseases Society of America (IDSA), American Academy of Neurology (AAN), and American College of Rheumatology (ACR): 2020 Guidelines for the Prevention, Diagnosis, and Treatment of Lyme Disease.

Gammons M, Salam G. Tick removal. *Am Fam Physician.* 2002;66(4):643–645.

Gupta AK, Cooper EA. Update in antifungal therapy of dermatophytosis. *Mycopathologia.* 2008;166(5-6):353–367.

Goldfarb MT, Gupta AK, Gupta MA, Sawchuk WS. Office therapy for human papillomavirus infection in nongenital sites. *Dermatol Clin.* 1991;9(2):287–296.

González LM, Allen R, Janniger CK, Schwartz RA. Pityriasis rosea: an important papulosquamous disorder. *Int J Dermatol.* 2005;44(9):757–764.

Jeffrey B, Robert JF, Spider B (eds.). In: Lynn CG, Jeffrey MK, Cynthia C. *Pediatric Clinical Advisor* (Second Edition), Mosby, 2007, pp 535–536. ISBN 9780323035064, https://doi.org/10.1016/B978-032303506-4.10307-4. https://www.sciencedirect.com/science/article/pii/B9780323035064103074.

Jeung YJ, Lee JY, Oh MJ, Choi DC, Lee BJ. Comparison of the causes and clinical features of drug rash with eosinophilia and systemic symptoms and stevens-johnson syndrome. *Allergy Asthma Immunol Res.* 2010;2(2):123–126. doi:10.4168/aair.2010.2.2.123.

Kano Y, Shiohara T. Long-term outcome of patients with severe cutaneous adverse reactions. *Dermatologica Sinica.* 2013;31(4):211–216. doi:10.1016/j.dsi.2013.09.004.

Kwok CS, Gibbs S, Bennett C, Holland R, Abbott R. Topical treatments for cutaneous warts. *Cochrane Database Syst Rev.* 2012;9:CD001781.

Lantos PM, Rumbaugh J, Bockenstedt LK, et al. Clinical Practice Guidelines by the Infectious Diseases Society of America (IDSA), American Academy of Neurology (AAN), and American College of Rheumatology (ACR): 2020 Guidelines for the Prevention, Diagnosis, and Treatment of Lyme Disease. *Arthritis Rheumatol.* 2021;73:12.

Litchman G, Nair PA, Atwater AR, et al. Contact Dermatitis. [Updated 2023 Feb 9]. In: StatPearls [Internet]. Treasure Island (FL): StatPearls Publishing; 2023 Jan-. Available from: https://www.ncbi.nlm.nih.gov/books/NBK459230/.

Lloyd ECO, Rodgers BC, Michener MS, Williams MS. Outpatient burns: prevention and care. *Am Fam Physician.* 2012;1(1):25–32 85.

Palaiologou A, Crum P, Owens J. Managing severe delayed cutaneous allergic drug reactions. Decisions in Dentistry. https://decisionsindentistry.com/article/managing-severe-delayed-cutaneous-allergic-drug-reactions/. Published September 3, 2019. Accessed April 14, 2023.

Prok L, McGovern T. Poison Ivy (Toxicodendron) dermatitis. In: Corona R, ed. *UpToDate,* Waltham, MA. Accessed 17.10.2016.

Sanchez E, Vannier E, Wormser GP, Hu LT, et al. Diagnosis, treatment, and prevention of Lyme disease, human granulocytic anaplasmosis, and babesiosis: a review. *JAMA.* 2016;315:1767.

Schmitz GR, Gottlieb M. Managing a Cutaneous Abscess in the Emergency Department. *Ann Emerg Med.* 2021;78(1):44–48. doi:10.1016/j.annemergmed.2020.12.003.

Stankus SJ, Dlugopolski M, Packer D. Management of herpes zoster (shingles) and postherpetic neuralgia. *Am Fam Physician.* 2000;61(8):2437–2448.

Sterling JC, Gibbs S, Haque Hussain SS, Mohd Mustapa MF, Handfield-Jones SE. British Association of Dermatologists' guidelines for the management of cutaneous warts 2014. *Br J Dermatol.* 2014;171(4):696–712.

Stevens DL, Bisno AL, Chambers HF, et al. Practice guidelines for the diagnosis and management of skin and soft tissue infections: 2014 update by the Infectious Disease Society of America. *Clin Infect Dis.* 2014;59:147–159.

Tarín-Vicente EJ, Alemany A, Agud-Dios M, et al. Clinical presentation and virological assessment of confirmed human monkeypox virus cases in Spain: a prospective observational cohort study [published correction appears in Lancet. 2022 Dec 10;400(10368):2048]. *Lancet.* 2022;400(10353):661–669.

Trayes KP, Love G, Studdiford JS. Erythema Multiforme: Recognition and Management. *Am Fam Physician.* 2019;100(2):82–88.

United States Centers for Disease Control and Prevention. Interim clinical guidance for the treatment of monkeypox. https://www.cdc.gov/poxvirus/monkeypox/clinicians/treatment.html#anchor_1655488137245.

United States Centers for Disease Control and Prevention. Monkeypox: transmission. https://www.cdc.gov/poxvirus/monkeypox/transmission.html.

Weston WL, Howe W. Overview of dermatitis. In: Corona R, ed. *UpToDate,* Waltham, MA. Accessed 28.09.2016.

Wolf R, Matz H, Marcos B, Orion E. Drug rash with eosinophilia and systemic symptoms vs toxic epidermal necrolysis: the dilemma of classification. *Clin Dermatol.* 2005;23(3):311–314. doi:10.1016/j.clindermatol.2005.02.001.

World Health Organization. Second meeting of the International Health Regulations (2005) (IHR) Emergency Committee regarding the multi-country outbreak of monkeypox. https://www.who.int/news/item/23-07-2022-second-meeting-of-the-international-health-regulations-(2005)-(ihr)-emergency-committee-regarding-the-multi-country-outbreak-of-monkeypox.

CHAPTER 15

HEAD AND NECK TRAUMA

J. Elizabeth Allen, DO, FACEP, Monica Corsetti, MD

TOP SECRETS

1. The Canadian Head CT Rule, the Canadian Cervical-Spine Rule (CCR), and the National Emergency X-Radiography Utilization Study (NEXUS) can help clinicians decide which patients require head or cervical spine imaging.
2. For a suspected globe rupture, avoid direct pressure to the injured eye. Instead, apply a rigid shield or a cup, tape the uninjured eye, control pain and nausea, and elevate the patient's head to 30 degrees.

1. **What anatomical features of the head should be considered when evaluating a patient with head and neck trauma?**

   Understanding the anatomy of the head and neck can allow the clinician to better evaluate a patient for injury. The brain is contained within the skull, which is in essence a rigid container with a fixed volume. Trauma that causes intracranial bleeding or cerebral edema introduces additional mass without room to expand and thus will increase intracranial pressure. This increase in pressure can compromise blood flow to the brain, and if left untreated, can progress to herniation of the brain through the base of the skull. This can lead to a loss of physiologic control of breathing, blood pressure, and heart rate. It is lethal without intervention.

2. **What anatomic features of the cervical spine should be considered when evaluating a patient with head and neck trauma?**

   There are seven cervical vertebrae that protect the spinal cord within the spinal canal. These vertebrae are separated by intervertebral disks and held in place by the anterior and posterior longitudinal ligaments. When the ring-like structure of these vertebrae is disrupted via traumatic injury, spinal cord damage can result. The spinal canal, which is wider from the base of the skull to the inferior portion of C2, narrows at C3, increasing the likelihood of injury at C3 and distally. The phrenic nerves that innervate the diaphragm originate at the levels of C3–C5; a complete spinal cord injury at this level may lead to apnea and death.

3. **What first steps should I take when evaluating a patient with head or neck trauma?**

   As with any other kind of trauma, always start by evaluating the "ABCs": Airway, Breathing, and Circulation. You should ensure that the patient's airway is patent, that the patient is breathing normally, and that they have adequate perfusion with no major hemorrhage. The scalp is well-perfused and can bleed profusely even with seemingly minor trauma; it is possible for patients to exsanguinate from scalp wounds. Hemorrhage control is critical. Remember that while evaluating the ABCs, cervical spinal precautions should be maintained either manually or with a hard cervical collar.

4. **How can I assess for airway compromise in a patient with head and neck trauma?**

   Although unlikely to encounter major trauma at an urgent care center, you should always perform a standard airway assessment for obvious direct injury or airway distress/compromise and lack of ability to protect the airway. You should also evaluate your patient for neck and upper airway hemorrhage/hematoma, voice change (including stridor), and subcutaneous emphysema around the face, upper chest, or neck. This may signal damage to the airway, digestive, and/or neurovascular structures of the neck. Remember that airway compromise in neck trauma may be delayed from the time of injury. Neck trauma may initially appear deceptively benign.

5. **What are the hard signs of penetrating neck trauma?**

   Remember that any injury that violates the platysma has potentially serious complications and requires stabilization and transfer to a trauma center. It is important to recognize physical exam signs that necessitate emergent surgical intervention (hard signs) and those that mandate further investigation and observation (soft signs). Hard signs include expanding/pulsatile neck hematoma, active hemorrhage, shock, airway compromise, massive subcutaneous emphysema or air bubbling through the wound, hematemesis, and neurologic deficit. Soft signs include hemoptysis (including undifferentiated blood in the oropharynx), the "3 Ds" (dyspnea, dysphagia, and dysphonia), a neck hematoma that is not expanding nor pulsatile, any vascular bruit or thrill, any brachial or radial pulse deficits, an air leak on the patient's chest tube (if one is placed), and nonmassive subcutaneous or mediastinal/prevertebral air (including crepitus).

6. **How do I assess a patient's mental status?**

   The Glasgow Coma Scale (GCS) provides a standardized and objective method of assessing a patient's mental status. The 10th edition of the *Advanced Trauma Life Support Student Course Manual* reflects the revised GCS (outlined in Table 15.1), which allows for an area that cannot be assessed. (Remember that a low GCS score may have other etiologies, such as acute intoxication and medication overdose, and a low GCS does not always imply a

Table 15.1 Revised GCS Score

EYE OPENING (E)	SPONTANEOUS	4
	To sound	3
	To pressure	2
	None	1
	Not testable	NT
Verbal response (V)	Oriented	5
	Confused	4
	Words	3
	Sounds	2
	None	1
	Not testable	NT
Best motor response (M)	Obeys commands	6
5	Localizing	5
	Normal flexion	4
	Abnormal flexion	3
	Extension	2
	None	1
	Not testable	NT

*Normal flexion–withdrawal to pain in the original GCS.

severe brain injury.) You should also ask about confusion or amnesia after the event. Any patient with an abnormal mental status after trauma requires further evaluation including but not limited to further observation or imaging and may necessitate transfer to a trauma center.

7. **How do I assess the need for further imaging to detect intracranial hemorrhage in a patient with minor head trauma?**
   Deciding whether to refer a patient for further imaging and evaluation can be a challenge for the urgent care physician. There are several clinical decision rules that can supplement a clinician's clinical judgment in determining need for CT scan after minor head trauma. The Canadian CT Head Rule, as shown in Table 15.2, has been shown to have 100% sensitivity for identifying clinically important brain injury requiring neurosurgical intervention. This tool may be applied to patients who had a loss of consciousness, amnesia to the event, or disorientation. If they do not meet the exclusion criteria, high or medium risk criteria below, discharge without a CT scan is generally supported by the literature as safe.

8. **How do I assess the need for further imaging to detect cervical spine injuries?**
   In alert, stable patients younger than 65 years, two well-validated rules exist to help clinicians determine the need for cervical spine imaging in trauma: the Canadian Cervical-Spine Rule (CCR) and the National Emergency X-Radiography Utilization Study (NEXUS). In these patients, NEXUS may rule out cervical spine injury if these are absent: focal neurological deficit, midline spinal tenderness, altered level of consciousness, intoxication, or distracting injury. The CCR excludes patients who have extremity paresthesias or dangerous mechanisms (fall >= 3 feet or 5 stairs, axial load, high speed or rollover MVC, ejection from MVC, MVC vs. bicycle, or recreational motor vehicle accident). Patients then must be able to actively rotate their neck 45 degrees in both directions and have any one of the following low-risk factors: sitting upright in the ED, being ambulatory at any time, delayed presentation of neck pain, no midline tenderness, and simple rear-end MVC. Discharge of patients who meet these criteria without further spinal imaging is supported by the literature as safe practice.

9. **How can I achieve hemorrhage control for a patient with a scalp laceration?**
   As previously mentioned, the scalp is highly vascularized and exsanguination secondary to scalp laceration is possible. Any hemorrhage should be rapidly addressed. Direct pressure and local infiltration of lidocaine with

Table 15.2. Canadian CT Head Rule

Canadian CT Head Rule–High and Medium Risk Criteria		
HIGH-RISK CRITERIA	**MEDIUM-RISK CRITERIA**	**EXCLUSION CRITERIA**
• 2 hours postinjury; GCS <15 • Suspected open or depressed skull fracture • Basilar skull fracture signs on exam (hemotympanum, raccoon eyes, Battle sign, CSF otorrhea or rhinorrhea) • 2 or more episodes of vomiting • Age 65 or older	• Retrograde amnesia to the event that lasts 30 minutes or longer • Dangerous mechanism (pedestrian vs. motor vehicle, occupant ejected from motor vehicle, fall from 3 feet [or 5 stairs] or higher)	• Age <16 • Anticoagulant use or bleeding disorder • Seizure after the event • GCS <13 • Unclear if trauma was the inciting event • Penetrating or depressed skull fracture • Acute focal neurological deficit • Unstable vital signs • Return ED visit for the same injury • Pregnancy

Adapted from Stiell I, et al. The Canadian CT Head Rule for patients with minor head injury. *Lancet.* 2001 PMID: 11356436.

epinephrine may combat hemorrhage by local vessel constriction. If a bleeding vessel is identified, manual compression of the vessel against the skull or clamping of the vessel may be a temporary solution. However, Lammers notes in *Clinical Procedures in Emergency Medicine* that unless the vessels are "large or few," this is usually ineffective. Everting the edges of the wound over the skin edge with a hemostat and suturing the wound may provide hemostasis in these cases.

10. **How should I evaluate my patient if I suspect traumatic injury to the eye or orbits?**
    Orbital blow-out fracture, globe rupture, retrobulbar hematoma, hyphema, and corneal abrasion from a foreign body are all potential complications of trauma. In addition to visual inspection of the eye, pupillary exam, visual acuity, extraocular motion, and a fluorescein examination can aid in diagnosis. CT, if available, may aid in the diagnosis of globe rupture or orbital fracture. Common symptoms of these include (but are not limited to):
    • Orbital fractures: enophthalmos or abnormalities of extraocular motion
      • An orbital blow-out fracture may cause inferior rectus entrapment resulting in upward gaze diplopia and paralysis
    • Globe rupture: decreased visual acuity, pupil asymmetry, pupillary defect, flattened anterior chamber, prolapse of ocular structures
    • Retrobulbar hematoma: proptosis, pain, pupillary defect, decreased visual acuity, diffuse subconjunctival hemorrhage
    • Hyphema: red blood cells in the anterior chamber on visual inspection, decreased visual acuity
    • Corneal abrasions: pain, abnormal fluorescein examination

11. **How can I initiate management of a traumatic globe rupture?**
    For a suspected globe rupture, avoid anything that could potentially increase pressure in the eye, and never apply direct pressure to the injured eye. Protect the injured eye using a rigid shield or a cup. Taping the uninjured eye can help minimize movement of the injured eye. Elevating the patient's head to 30 degrees if there is no concern for spine injury may help decrease intraocular pressure. The patient with a globe rupture requires emergent management by ophthalmology. The patient should be made NPO, tetanus prophylaxis and antibiotics should be administered, and pain and nausea should be controlled.

12. **How can I classify and initiate treatment of a tooth fracture or avulsion?**
    Dental injury is a common urgent care complaint. Patients may complain of a traumatic avulsion, which is a complete displacement of the tooth out of the socket and severing of the periodontal ligament. Avulsed teeth should be immediately replanted by grasping the tooth at the crown, removing debris gently and quickly with cold water, and replacing it. Patients may also complain of a "cracked" tooth, often an infraction (simple crack of the enamel surface) or crown fracture. Crown fractures are classified as "uncomplicated" if they only involve the enamel or only enamel and dentin. Crown fractures are classified as "complicated" if they involve exposure of the pulp, which is often visualized as a pink or red center within the fracture surface. Emergent referral to a dentist is warranted in complicated crown fractures, usually for endodontic therapy.

13. **A 25-year-old female presents to urgent care with a headache and some neck soreness after a car accident. The patient was rear-ended by a vehicle traveling 15 mph while she was at a stop sign. Although she was wearing a seatbelt, her head struck the back of the seat, and she was briefly disoriented. She has no abnormalities on physical examination as well as the full neck range of motion and no midline tenderness. Does this patient require advanced imaging of her head or neck?**
    This patient is presenting to your urgent care with a case of blunt head trauma. She should be evaluated using ATLS protocol and the ABCDEs of trauma but ultimately has a mechanism that is not high-risk according to the

Canadian CT Head Rule and the CCR. As long you find no other concerning signs or symptoms during the patient's history and physical evaluation, she meets inclusion criteria for Canadian Head CT Rule, as well as CCR and NEXUS, and based on these clinical decision rules, can be safely discharged without need for advanced imaging.

Decision rules are designed to supplement and not replace clinician judgment. You should obtain imaging if you have reason to believe that doing so is in the patient's best interests.

KEY POINTS

1. Always start by evaluating the "ABCs": Airway, Breathing, and Circulation. In head trauma, "circulation" frequently encompasses control of hemorrhage from scalp lacerations.
2. Globe rupture is an ophthalmologic emergency. In addition to emergency ophthalmology consultation, take measures to avoid any increase in intraocular pressure, and apply a shield to the affected eye.
3. The Canadian Head CT Rule, Canadian Cervical-Spine Rule (CCR), and the National Emergency X-Radiography Utilization Study (NEXUS) are all well-validated decision tools that can help the urgent care clinician safely discharge trauma patients without the need for advanced imaging.
4. Avulsed teeth should be immediately replanted in the socket and referred to a dentist. Complicated crown fractures require emergency dental referral.

BIBLIOGRAPHY

Advanced Trauma Life Support Student Course Manual. 10th ed. American College of Surgeons; 2018:129–145.
Burgess CA, et al. An Evidence Based Review of the Assessment and Management of Penetrating Neck Trauma. *Clinical Otolaryngology.* 2012;37(1):44–52. https://doi.org/10.1111/j.1749-4486.2011.02422.x.
Hoffman JR, Mower WR, Wolfson AB, Todd KH, Zucker MI. Validity of a set of clinical criteria to rule out injury to the cervical spine in patients with blunt trauma. National Emergency X-Radiography Utilization Study Group. *N Engl J Med.* 2000;343(2):94–99.
Keels MA. Section on Oral Health, American Academy of Pediatrics. Management of dental trauma in a primary care setting. *Pediatrics.* 2014;133(2):e466–e476. doi:10.1542/peds.2013-3792.
Kman, Nicholas E. Neck Trauma. Edited by Nur-Ain Nadir and Chris Fowler, Nov. 2019. https://www.saem.org/about-saem/academies-interest-groups-affiliates2/cdem/for-students/online-education/m4-curriculum/group-m4-trauma/neck-trauma.
Kroesen CF, Snider M, Bailey J, Buchanan A, Karesh JW, La Piana F, Seefeldt E, Egan JA, Mazzoli RA. The ABCs of Ocular Trauma: Adapting a Familiar Mnemonic for Rapid Eye Exam in the Pre-Ophthalmic Zone of Care. *Mil Med.* 2020;185(Suppl 1):448–453. doi:10.1093/milmed/usz262. PMID: 32074325.
Lammers RL. Methods of wound closure. In: Roberts JR, Hedges JR, eds. *Clinical Procedures in Emergency Medicine.* 5th ed. Saunders Elsevier; 2010:592.
Olympia R, et al. Chapter 26: Head Injuries and Facial Trauma. *Prehospital Emergency Medicine Secrets.* Elsevier; 2022.
Olympia R, et al. Chapter 27: Cervical Spine and Spinal Cord Injuries. *Prehospital Emergency Medicine Secrets.* Elsevier; 2022.
Stiell I, et al. The Canadian CT Head Rule for patients with minor head injury. *Lancet.* 2001. PMID: 11356436.
Stiell IG, Wells GA, Vandemheen KL, Clement CM, Lesiuk H, De Maio VJ, Laupacis A, Schull M, McKnight RD, Verbeek R, Brison R, Cass D, Dreyer J, Eisenhauer MA, Greenberg GH, MacPhail I, Morrison L, Reardon M, Worthington J. The Canadian C-spine rule for radiography in alert and stable trauma patients. *JAMA.* 2001;286(15):1841–1848.
Walls Ron, et al. *Rosen's Emergency Medicine - Concepts and Clinical Practice E-Book.* 9th ed. Elsevier - OHCE; 2017. Available from: Elsevier eBooks+.

CHAPTER 16

CHEST AND ABDOMINAL TRAUMA

Michael Mesisca, D.O., M.B.A., M.S., C.C.H.P.-P.

TOP SECRETS: (1–2)

X-rays—2-view or rib series—can miss rib fractures. The "occult" rib fractures are unlikely to be clinically significant if there are no signs of pleural injury (PTX or HTX) or underlying lung injury (contusion) seen on the x-ray. Most stable patients can be managed with x-rays alone but require education that a negative x-ray does not rule out rib fractures.

Major blunt chest and abdominal trauma patients presenting to the ER with a significant trauma mechanism, seat belt or handlebar bruising, on anticoagulation, pregnant or elderly, or any patient with hemodynamic instability should be rapidly transferred to a trauma center or emergency department with trauma capability. Transfer should NOT be delayed to obtain imaging or labs. Predetermined workflows with the accepting facility and EMS transporting agencies to expedite care will save lives.

1. **What potential significant injuries can occur following blunt chest trauma?**
   Critical injuries can include airway obstruction/injury, laryngeal injury, chest wall injuries (rib, clavicle, sternum, manubrium, and scapular fractures), tension pneumothorax (PTX), open pneumothorax, massive hemothorax (HTX), and cardiac tamponade.

   Initial assessment of any blunt or penetrating trauma patient should include?

   Rapid assessment of the airway, breathing, and circulation. Any concern for hemodynamic instability or potential for significant injuries described above should prompt immediate ambulance transfer to a local emergency department. Optimal patient care comes from understanding regional EMS trauma resources and having workflows established in advance to expedite transport to trauma-capable facilities and transfer of care. Obtaining labs, x-rays, and EKGs should not be done if that will delay the transport of a major trauma patient.

2. **What is the most common, serious complication of blunt chest trauma?**
   Hypoxemia is the most serious complication of blunt chest trauma. This can be the result of lung or pleural injury. Early intervention is aimed at airway support (basic life support measures of oxygen supplementation) and immediate treatment of a tension pneumothorax.

3. **What physical exam findings may suggest injury to the upper airway from thoracic trauma?**
   Signs of respiratory distress with increased work of breathing and accessory muscle use, stridor, muffled voice, crepitus in the neck, hemoptysis, and/or posterior displacement, and pain of the clavicular head would suggest a potential for serious airway injury.

4. **What is subcutaneous emphysema and how does it present clinically?**
   Subcutaneous emphysema is the collection of air in the skin. Chest wall or neck crepitus is appreciated by palpation and feels like pushing on crunchy rice-crispy cereal under the skin. The presence of crepitus on exam suggests an injury to the airway with air leakage into the pleural spaces and subsequently into the soft tissues. This finding is highly sensitive for the presence of pneumothorax, pneumomediastinum, or injury to the upper airway.

5. **What are the clinical symptoms of a tension pneumothorax?**
   Tension pneumothorax may present with some or all of the following: decreased breath sounds, tracheal deviation away from the side of injury, distended neck veins, hypoxemia, hyper-resonance on percussion, crepitus of the chest wall, and eventually hypotension.

6. **What is the best way to diagnose a tension pneumothorax?**
   This is a clinical diagnosis and intervention with a needle, finger, or chest tube thoracostomy should not be delayed for medical imaging in a hemodynamically unstable patient. Other thoracic injuries can present similarly to a tension PTX in the setting of major trauma, such as a large pulmonary contusion or diaphragmatic rupture.

7. **What radiographic tools are available to diagnose a pneumothorax?**
   Bedside ultrasound through an extended-Focused Assessment with Sonography in Trauma (e-FAST) examination can be very sensitive in the diagnosis of a PTX. CXR is often used to assess for PTX and optimal imaging is obtained with an upright and inspiratory film; however, a chest x-ray is much less sensitive than ultrasound, and CT scan and may miss a PTX. The x-ray in Fig. 16.1 demonstrates a tension PTX.

8. **What is an open pneumothorax and how is it treated?**
   An open PTX occurs when a large penetrating chest wound allows air into the chest wall with each breath and causes the lung to collapse. This is treated with a three-sided dressing that allows air to flow out of the chest and

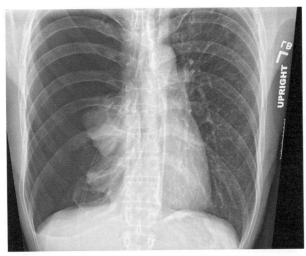

Fig. 16.1 Tension PTX. The right lung is completely collapsed and none of the heart border is on the right side of the chest suggesting that the air expanding inside the pleural space is pushing on the heart into the left side of the chest cavity and likely compressing the venous return.

limits the amount of air flowing into the chest with each breath. Placing a four-sided dressing and occluding the wound completely can potentially convert the injury from an open PTX to a closed PTX and result in a tension PTX.

9. **What is a traumatic asymptomatic PTX and how is it treated?**
A traumatic asymptomatic PTX is one that is found on CXR, ultrasound, or CT scan and does not result in hypoxemia or respiratory distress. These are often small. The management decision should be made in consultation with trauma or pulmonary specialists. Multiple factors are weighed, including the size of the PTX (rated as a percentage of the lung collapsed), presence of other injuries, age of the patient, and presence and size of a hemothorax in determining if chest tube placement is necessary.

10. **What clinical signs suggest an HTX and how is it treated?**
An HTX can present on exam as decreased breath sounds and dullness to percussion. A CXR may show blunting of the costophrenic angles (similar to a pleural effusion) and e-FAST may also detect the presence of fluid in the pleural space. Treatment includes airway and oxygen support and rapid emergency department transport with anticipated chest tube placement for drainage.

11. **What mechanisms contribute to blunt cardiac injuries? How are they diagnosed?**
Direct chest trauma, most commonly from major mechanisms such as motor vehicle accidents and falls above 6 feet, can result in blunt cardiac injury. That can include myocardial injury-producing tachycardia, EKG changes, and/or troponin elevations. It can also result in pericardial effusions that can progress to cardiac tamponade. Early use of point-of-care ultrasound (FAST scan) is highly sensitive at detecting pericardial effusions and tamponade. Concern for cardiac injury should be referred immediately to the Emergency department. Persistent tachycardia in a trauma patient should elevate concern for blood loss from hemorrhage and cardiac injury and prompt transfer to a higher level of care.

12. **What are 2 ways that significant thoracic and abdominal traumatic injuries might be missed?**
    (1) Failing to fully expose the area. Care must be taken when evaluating a fully dressed patient with chest or abdominal trauma. Significant injury may be missed, such as significant bruising of the abdominal wall or a puncture wound in the axilla, by failing to examine under the clothing.
    (2) The second less obvious injury is often missed in a trauma patient. Consider a patient who presents with a displaced open forearm fracture after a fall and also has a pneumothorax from a rib fracture. Both the patient and the doctor focus entirely on the open forearm and fail to appreciate the other injuries.

13. **Are there any clinical decision tools that can be used to determine who needs a CXR and/or CT scan?**
The NEXUS chest decision instrument for blunt chest trauma can be used to determine if a CXR or CT is indicated. This tool combines age, mechanism, and other risk factors. The NEXUS chest CT decision instrument can be used to determine which patients benefit from a chest CT.

14. **What percentage of rib fractures are missed on a CXR but can be detected on CT scan?**
    A 2-view CXR can miss up to two-thirds of rib fractures that are detectable on a CT scan. Yet, those not seen on CXR are rarely clinically significant.

15. **Is a rib series helpful in detecting rib fractures?**
    A rib series does NOT increase the sensitivity of rib fractures when both are read by a radiologist; however, it may aid in increasing the sensitivity of identifying a rib fracture/s when images are read by Urgent Care providers.

16. **Can bedside ultrasound detect rib fractures?**
    The sensitivity of point-of-care ultrasound (POCUS) in detecting rib fractures is quite high. The sensitivity increases with the level of experience of the provider.

17. **What is the significance of first and second rib, scapular, and sternal fractures?**
    The impact required to fracture these particular bones is significant. As such, these fractures are often associated with other significant and potentially life-threatening injuries to the underlying vascular and neurologic structures. The presence of these injuries should prompt a very thorough physical assessment, close monitoring, and consideration of the potential for other injuries.

18. **What is the significance of lower rib fractures?**
    Lower rib fractures can be associated with intraabdominal injury, including liver, kidney, and splenic lacerations.

19. **Where do clavicle fractures most commonly occur? How are they managed?**
    The middle 1/3 of the clavicle is the most common fracture site. Most clavicle fractures are treated with pain control and a sling. Consult ortho if severely displaced, more than one fracture, open fracture, or skin tenting. Skin tenting can progress to an open fracture if not managed immediately or with very close follow-up.

20. **In the presence of 3 or more rib fractures, what factors increase the potential for increased morbidity and mortality?**
    (1) Additional underlying injury, including a pulmonary contusion. The presence of 3 or more rib fractures increases the potential of underlying serious injury. Pulmonary contusions can develop over time (up to 6 hours) and lead to delayed hypoxemia and respiratory failure, particularly in elderly patients.
    (2) Uncontrolled pain. Rib fractures can be extremely painful, and some patients will require hospitalization for pain management.
    (3) Hypoventilation due to pain. Incentive spirometry is encouraged in patients with risk fractures.

CASE 1

A 16-year-old male presents after being tackled while playing football. An opponent's helmet hit his left side. He has focal rib pain laterally around rib 6 on his left. His vitals are all normal. He has equal breath sounds, no noted bruising or skin changes, no crepitus, and is in no respiratory distress but has sharp pain with movement, deep inspiration, and palpation. What is the most likely injury? Diagnostic test? Treatment?
    (1) The patient clinically likely has a rib fracture, given his symptoms and exam.
    (2) A chest x-ray should be obtained, mainly to assess for any pulmonary injury (e.g., PTX, HTX, or contusion). A rib series may increase the sensitivity of detecting the rib fracture but does not likely enhance the diagnostic yield of underlying injuries.
    (3) Treatment: Initial treatment in an adolescent should include NSAIDs, acetaminophen, rest, and consideration of topical lidocaine and/or NSAIDs as well.
    (4) Education: the player and parents should be aware that, even if the x-ray is normal, it can miss one or more rib fractures. Return precautions should be provided and anticipated removal from contact sports for 4–6 weeks to prevent further injury.

ABDOMINAL TRAUMA

21. **What is the significance of an abdominal seat belt sign?**
    A seat belt sign is a bruise across the lower or midabdomen from a seat belt. This sign is associated with an increase in serious injuries including hollow viscus (bowel) injury, chance fractures of the spine, and bowel ischemia from mesenteric artery injury. The association with injury is present when the seat belt sign is located above the anterior superior iliac spine (ASIS).

22. **What is the significance of a handlebar sign?**
    Circular bruising at the chest-abdominal wall from the impact of a bicycle handlebar is also associated with an increased risk of significant intraabdominal injuries.

23. **What is the role of ultrasound in abdominal trauma?**
    FAST is highly sensitive in detecting the presence of free fluid or bleeding in the abdomen. It cannot detect retroperitoneal, diaphragmatic, pancreatic, or hollow viscus injuries. It cannot differentiate traumatic hemorrhage from ascites or free fluid from an ovarian cyst. Ultrasound can also miss solid organ injuries that have not resulted

in hemoperitoneum. A negative FAST does NOT exclude serious traumatic injury. A positive FAST should be treated as hemodynamic instability and prompt immediate transfer to a trauma center.

24. **What type of CT scan should be performed in the setting of abdominal trauma?**
If the decision is made to perform a CT scan in an advanced urgent care setting or rural setting, the CT scan should include both the abdomen and pelvis and should utilize IV contrast. Oral contrast is not indicated. In the setting of trauma, CT should NOT be delayed for baseline labs (e.g., creatinine). Any CT scan for trauma obtained in an urgent care should be done after carefully weighing the risks to benefits of transferring the patient to an emergency department/trauma center prior to diagnostic studies.

25. **After blunt abdominal trauma, what physical exam findings are most associated with an intraabdominal injury?**
A seat belt sign, handlebar sign, rebound tenderness, hypotension, abdominal distention or guarding, gross hematuria, and associated long bone fractures are all highly predictive of major and potentially time-sensitive life-threatening injuries and warrant immediate intervention.

26. **What physical exam finding can suggest a urethral injury and how is it assessed?**
The presence of blood at the urethral meatus can suggest urethral injury and is investigated with a retrograde urethrogram.

27. **What patients are at great risk of significant injury intraabdominal injury from lower mechanism blunt trauma, including ground-level falls?**
The following patients are at a high risk of serious injury even with minor mechanisms of injury, including ground or low-level falls and slow-moderate speed motor vehicle collisions:
Pregnant patients, elderly (age over 60 years old), those on anticoagulants (including aspirin), acutely intoxicated patients, chronic alcoholics, patients with chronic severe liver and renal disease, patients with dementia, patients with distracting injuries, and/or those with coagulopathies (e.g., hemophilia).

28. **Which patients may present with a reported injury from a mechanical fall but may have experienced more serious physical trauma?**
Pregnant patients are at an increased risk of domestic violence which is often directed at the abdomen. Significant abdominal trauma may be masked by a reported fall. The treatment team should carefully assess for domestic violence. Social and physiologic changes place these patients at a high risk of morbidity and mortality from trauma.

CASE 2

A 22-year-old male was running toward his BBQ at college when he was injured. He was carrying a plate of skewers when he turned into a wall and a skewer was inadvertently jammed into his abdomen. He thinks about 4 inches of the skewer went into his right abdominal wall before he quickly pulled it out. He has a small puncture wound without active bleeding. He has minimal tenderness at the site and his vitals are normal. What is the best course of action for this patient?

The patient should be sent immediately by ambulance transport to the local emergency department/trauma center. Any potential penetrating traumatic wound to the chest or abdomen should undergo immediate evaluation at a trauma center. Seemingly small puncture wounds can induce significant internal injuries requiring time-sensitive specialty intervention.

KEY POINTS

1. Chest x-rays can miss a majority of nondisplaced rib fractures; although, most undetected fractures are not clinically significant.
2. After a major mechanism of trauma with suspicion of serious injury, medical imaging or labs should NOT be obtained if it will delay transfer to a major medical center.
3. Mechanisms of injury, elderly age, pregnancy, underlying health conditions, and patients taking anticoagulants including aspiring should all be considered in the management decisions of a trauma patient.
4. The presence of 3 or more rib fractures is associated with a higher incidence of underlying organ injury and potential for complications.
5. Even seemingly small puncture wounds to the chest or abdomen can have severe underlying injuries; therefore, careful consideration and a low threshold for an immediate transfer to a major medical center are required.
6. A seat belt sign, handlebar sign, rebound tenderness, hypotension, abdominal distention or guarding, gross hematuria, and associated long bone fractures are all highly predictive of major injuries and warrant immediate intervention.

BIBLIOGRAPHY

Jiang O, Asha SE, Keady J, Curtis K. Position of the abdominal seat belt sign and its predictive utility for abdominal trauma. *Emerg Med Australas*. 2019;31(1):112–116. doi:10.1111/1742-6723.13187. Epub 2018 Oct 16.

McVaney Kevin, Haamid Ameera. Blunt Abdominal Trauma. In: Mattu A and Swadron S, ed. CorePendium. Burbank, CA: CorePendium, LLC. https://www.emrap.org/corependium/chapter/reccY0ETe97XUuID8/Blunt-Abdominal-Trauma. Updated January 28, 2021. Accessed September 30, 2022.

Raja, A., Mason, J. *Imaging of rib fractures*. EM. January 2022. https://www.emrap.org/episode/emrap2022/imagingofrib.

Rodriguez RM, Anglin D, Langdorf MI, et al. NEXUS chest: validation of a decision instrument for selective chest imaging in blunt trauma. *JAMA Surg*. 2013;148(10):940–946. doi:10.1001/jamasurg.2013.2757. Erratum in: JAMA Surg. 2013 Dec;148(12):1086.

Stewart RM (2018). *Atls: Advanced trauma life support: Student course manual*. American College of Surgeons.

Wang RC, Niedzwiecki MJ, Nishijima D, Rodriguez RM. An impact analysis of the NEXUS Chest CT clinical decision rule. *Am J Emerg Med*. 2020;38(5):906–910. doi:10.1016/j.ajem.2019.07.010. Epub 2019 Jul 8. PMID: 31303535.

Wright Angela, Wolf Stephen. Blunt Thoracic Trauma. In: Mattu A and Swadron S, ed. CorePendium. Burbank, CA: CorePendium, LLC. https://www.emrap.org/corependium/chapter/recwp71YmuzjjxT8P/Blunt-Thoracic-Trauma. Updated September 23, 2022. Accessed September 30, 2022.

CHAPTER 17

MUSCULOSKELETAL PRESENTATIONS

Jessica Deitrick, DO, Tori Beth L. Snoad, MD

THE UPPER EXTREMITY

CASE #1

A 56-year-old obese male with arthritis and diabetes presents with left upper extremity pain after a mechanical fall where he tried to catch himself with his left arm out. His pain and swelling have not resolved despite conservative measures. There are no injuries below the level of the shoulder.

1. **What is included in a complete physical exam of the shoulder?**
   Inspection and Comparison: Compare both shoulders looking for asymmetry or anatomical differences.
   Palpation: palpate on and around the three bones that make up the shoulder: the scapula, the clavicle, and the proximal humerus.
   Cervical spine exam to assess for cervical spine pathology as a possible cause of referred shoulder pain.
   Range of motion: flexion, extension, abduction, adduction, external rotation, internal rotation
   Neurovascular exam distal to the injury bilaterally

2. **What specific x-ray views make up a complete shoulder series?**
   Complete radiographic views of the shoulder include AP, lateral (in the plane of the scapula), and axillary views

3. **What are the most common acute shoulder injuries, and which need to be sent quickly to the ER?**
   Rotator cuff injuries <u>are</u> the most common cause of shoulder pain. The rotator cuff consists of four muscles that can be remembered by the mnemonic "SItS": Supraspinatus, Infraspinatus, teres minor, and Subscapularis muscles, where the teres minor is in all lowercase to remember it's the teres minor muscle and not the Teres Major. Patients will report "aching" in the anterolateral shoulder pain that typically persists at night.
   - Pain or weakness with shoulder abduction
   - Drop arm test: inability to withstand downward pressure while the shoulder is abducted at 90 degrees, indicative of a supraspinatus tear
   - The supraspinatus is the most commonly injured part of the rotator cuff.
   - Radiographs cannot diagnose rotator cuff injuries unless the tear is very large.
   - Rotator cuff injuries are largely a diagnosis of exclusion.
   - Conservative measures and outpatient setting follow-up are part of an appropriate management plan.
     Shoulder dislocations: anterior dislocations are the most common type and make up >95%. Shoulder dislocations in general make up about 50% of all large joint dislocations.
   - A history of prior shoulder injuries or dislocations is a common risk factor.
   - Patients will report "popping" or feeling their shoulder "rolled out of place."
   - Holding the injured arm extended in abduction and external rotation is an indication of dislocation and limitations of adduction and internal rotation.
   - They are easily spotted on x-rays. Further imaging may be required via CT scan or MRI.
     Fractures: the proximal humerus and clavicle are most commonly fractured. Scapular fractures are rare and can be associated with seizures in the right clinical setting.

CASE #2

A 56-year-old obese male with arthritis and diabetes presents with left upper extremity pain after a mechanical fall where he tried to catch himself with his left arm out. His pain and swelling have not resolved despite conservative measures. The patient plays golf frequently and uses a computer daily for work.

4. **What radiographic views are required for complete visualization of the elbow? What about the wrist?**
   Three views are required: AP, lateral, and oblique.
   For the wrist, AP and lateral are appropriate.

5. **What is the most common mechanism of acute upper extremity injury?**
   "FOOSH" injuries (fall on outstretched hand)

Table 17.1 Common Chronic Elbow and Wrist Injuries

DIAGNOSIS	MECHANISM OF INJURY	TREATMENT
Lateral epicondylitis	aka "tennis elbow," the most common overuse injury of the elbow due to repetitive wrist *extension*	Conservative measures are successful 90% of the time Rest, therapy, NSAIDs, bracing/splinting, or corticosteroid injections
Medial epicondylitis	aka "golfer's elbow," overuse injury that occurs due to repetitive wrist *flexion*	Conservative treatment as with lateral epicondylitis
Carpal tunnel	Compression of the median nerve at the level of the wrist	Early treatment includes wearing a splint at night, exercises or therapy, avoiding exacerbating symptoms, or corticosteroid injections Persistent symptoms are surgical candidates
DeQuarvian tenosynovitis	Irritation and/or inflammation of the flexor and extensor tendons of the thumb due to entrapment caused by trauma or repetitive motions	Can be self-limited Persistent symptoms are treated conservatively with rest, therapy, NSAIDs, bracing/splinting, or corticosteroid injections

6. What direction do most elbow dislocations occur? Are fractures commonly associated?
   Elbow dislocation: >90% occur in the posterolateral direction
   - Patients will hold their elbow at 45 degrees of flexion with the olecranon prominent posteriorly.
   - Easily spotted on x-ray
   - Radial head fractures can commonly occur with elbow dislocations.
       Common fractures to be aware of:
   - Olecranon fracture
   - Radial head fracture
   - Distal radius Fracture
   - Distal ulnar Fracture
   - Colles fracture

7. What are common chronic elbow or wrist injuries that could be the hidden culprit occurring prior to the patient's fall in Case #2?
   See Table 17.1.

THE LOWER EXTREMITY

CASE #8

A 24-year-old female presents for 2 weeks of foot and ankle pain. Two weeks ago, she attended a wedding where she accidentally fell while walking to her friend's car. She doesn't remember exactly how she fell, since she was drinking some that night. Conservative measures haven't helped. She plays club soccer and has picked up distance running for extra conditioning in the past 3–4 weeks.

8. What is included in the physical exam?
   Inspection, palpation, range of motion, neurovascular comparison, examination of nearby structures, in addition to ambulation and weight-bearing trial. Depending on the injury, there are specific exams that should be performed. If there is an obvious deformity, an intense amount of pain and swelling, or the practitioner feels it is unsafe, ambulation and weight-bearing trials should be deferred until imaging is complete. Because the injury in this case is acute in onset and conservative measures have not improved the patient's condition, extra precautions should be practiced.
       (https://stanfordmedicine25.stanford.edu/the25/Ankleandfootexam.html)

9. What other differentials might you consider in this case?
   - Distal fibular fracture
   - Bimalleolar and trimalleolar fractures
   - Ankle sprains or syndesmosis injury
   - Lisfranc fracture
   - Cuneiform or midfoot fractures
   - Metatarsal fractures
       (https://www.orthobullets.com/trauma/1047/ankle-fractures) See Table 17.2.

Table 17.2 Common Acute Isolated Distal Fibular Fractures

WEBER CLASSIFICATION	DESCRIPTION	DISPOSITION
Weber A	Below the level of the syndesmosis	• CAM boot or three-sided short-leg splint • Crutches WBAT • Outpatient ortho referral • No surgery required
Weber B	At the level of the syndesmosis Can have associated ligament damage	• CAM Boot or three-sided short-leg splint • Crutches • Non-weight-bearing • Outpatient ortho follow-up within 3–5 days • May require surgical repair
Weber C	Above the level of the syndesmosis	• CAM boot or three-sided short-leg splint • Crutches • Non-weight-bearing • Outpatient ortho follow-up within 3–5 days

10. **What is the difference between bimalleolar and trimalleolar fractures?**
Bimalleolar fracture: involves two malleoli (bi means two)
Trimalleolar fracture: involves three malleoli (tri means three)
These fractures should be placed in a well-padded, three-sided, short-leg splint. A short-leg splint goes from the toes to below the knee. It has a sugar tong and a posterior slab component.

11. **Are bimalleolar and trimalleolar fractures stable or unstable?**
Unstable. They are managed with surgery and ultimately need to be seen by an orthopedic surgeon. Bimalleolar fractures can be seen in the outpatient setting with follow-up if they are mildly displaced, but patients should be placed in support and given crutches with non-weight-bearing instructions. Trimalleolar fractures should be referred to the ER, especially if grossly displaced.

CUNEIFORM FRACTURES

12. **Are fracture lines always evident on x-ray?**
No; when in doubt, immobilize the patient and have them follow up with orthopedics.

13. **What type of splint is indicated?**
A well-padded, three-sided splint or a CAM boot. The patient should be non-weight-bearing with crutches.
Lisfranc fracture: tarsometatarsal fracture dislocation caused by disruption of the ligament between the second metatarsal base and medial cuneiform. Always be on the lookout for these. X-rays of the affected foot alone may not demonstrate the injury. Bilateral weight-bearing x-rays or CT non-con of the feet may be needed for diagnosis. If this injury is suspected and these forms of imaging are not available, refer to the local ER.
• The splint of choice is a Bulky Jones splint. The management plan includes strict non-weight-bearing with crutches and quick ortho follow-up for surgery.

METATARSAL FRACTURES

14. **What is the most commonly fractured metatarsal?**
The base of the fifth metatarsal is also known as a Jones or pseudo-Jones fracture depending on the location. A pseudo-Jones fracture is an avulsion of the proximal tubercle of the fifth metatarsal that does not interfere with the fourth and fifth metatarsal articulation. A Jones fracture appears distal to where a Pseudo-Jones fracture would occur and interferes with fourth and fifth metatarsal articulation. See Table 17.3.
For other metatarsal fractures, they have a high potential of remodeling if not appropriately treated. Use a stiff-soled shoe, WBAT, and crutches if needed to help with pain. Quick reference: https://www.orthobullets.com/foot-and-ankle/7031/5th-metatarsal-base-fracture

ACUTE ACHILLES' TENDON RUPTURE

15. **What is the most common description of injury by the patient?**
It felt like someone kicked me in the back of the ankle, but no one was there, and I felt and heard a "pop."

16. **What is the physical exam finding associated with an acute Achilles' tendon rupture, and what specific exam can confirm the diagnosis?**
Tenderness to palpation and a palpable defect directly over the Achilles' insertion. A positive Thompson test will reveal no movement of the foot when the calf muscle is squeezed.

Table 17.3 Jones vs. Pseudo-Jones Fracture Management

	SPLINT	DISPOSITION
Jones fracture	• Three-sided short-leg • NWB and crutches	• May be surgical • Quick ortho follow-up as outpatient
Pseudo-Jones fracture	• Stiff sole shoe • WBAT	• Nonsurgical • Outpatient ortho follow-up

Adapted from 5th Metatarsal Base Fracture – Foot & Ankle – Orthobullets: https://www.orthobullets.com/foot-and-ankle/7031/5th-metatarsal-base-fracture.

Table 17.4 Differential Diagnoses for Atraumatic Foot Pain

DIAGNOSIS	LOCATION AND QUALITY OF PAIN	TREATMENT	DISPOSITION
Plantar fasciitis	• Bottom of foot • Worse with first few steps	• Arch support in shoes	• Follow-up with primary care provider (PCP) or referral to podiatry or ortho if severe
Heel spur	• Pain on bottom of heel	• NSAIDs, ice	• Follow-up with podiatry or ortho foot and ankle
Achilles' tendonitis	• Pain over Achilles' near insertion site	• RICE therapy, can consider short period of immobilization for soft tissue rest if severe	• Follow-up with PCP, podiatry, or ortho depending on severity

Adapted from www.physio-pedia.com/Achilles_Tendinopathy.

17. **What is the disposition for an acute Achilles' tendon rupture?**
The patient needs to be non-weight-bearing in a Equinus splint and have expedited orthopedic outpatient follow-up. Many can be managed nonoperatively.
    See Table 17.4.

MUSCULAR PAIN

CASE #9

A 37-year-old male presents for 2 days of leg pain after he started working out again. He hasn't performed any exercise in the past 6 months, but he decided to lift heavier weights to get in better shape. The patient denies any particular injury. He was sore as expected, but his soreness has progressed in both legs over the past 2 days. His physical exam demonstrates soft compartments that are neurovascularly intact bilaterally, but he has diffuse pain with palpation over both of his legs. He had a 3-day weekend from work so he has been resting at home without much activity but feels, with the weekend ending, he can't go back to work.

18. **What are some common differential diagnoses based on this case?**
Muscle soreness, muscle strain, rhabdomyolysis.

19. **What potential complication should be considered with acute rhabdomyolysis?**
   • Compartment syndrome is a very dangerous complication, presenting with the six Ps: pain out of proportion, pallor, paresthesias, pulselessness, paralysis, and poikilothermia. Remember that all six are not necessary to make the diagnosis. Send these patients to the nearest ER for emergent orthopedic evaluation.
   • Acute kidney injury is another complication. Patients will not likely experience symptoms, but it is a devastating injury to the kidneys. Blood work will show an elevated creatinine level and indicate the patient needs immediate IV fluids and ER evaluation.

CASE #10

A 37-year-old male presents for 2 days of leg pain after he started working out again. He hasn't performed any exercise in the past 6 months, but he decided to lift heavier weights to get in better shape faster. While exercising, the patient felt a "pop" in his right thigh with subsequent acute-onset pain, so he stopped working out. He barely made it home due to difficulty with ambulation. The swelling and pain in his thigh have worsened. He had a 3-day weekend from work so he has been resting at home without much activity but feels, with the weekend ending, he can't go back to work.

20. What differentials are there to consider in this patient's case?
    - Acute quad tendon rupture
    - Acute patellar tendon rupture
    - Quadriceps muscle tear
    - Quadriceps muscle strain
    - Myositis
        See Table 17.5.

CASE #5, PART 1

A 68-year-old male presents with concerns of progressive right lower extremity pain. Over the past month, his pain has worsened and now he is having trouble with ambulation, requiring assistance. On inspection and comparison of both legs, there are noticeable discoloration and edema from the ankle to the mid-shin. His past medical history includes atrial fibrillation on Xarelto, hypertension, type 2 diabetes, and obesity.

21. At this point, what other key information from Case #5, Part 1, must be known to move forward?
    There are a variety of questions to ask a patient; however, it is important to begin to think broadly and sift through the information received quickly to come up with the most important decision of a patient encounter: benign or life-threatening?
    - Always check the patient's vital signs and repeat them if they are concerning or if the patient feels or looks unwell. Always clinically correlate vital signs with the patient's appearance.

Table 17.5 Differential Diagnoses for Acute-Onset Thigh Pain

PATHOLOGY	EXAM FINDINGS	IMAGING	TREATMENT	DISPOSITION
Acute quadriceps tendon rupture	• Palpable defect over quad tendon • Cannot do straight leg raise • Patella sitting lower on affected limb	• X-rays to rule out bony pathology	• Knee immobilizer • Crutches • NWB	• Emergent orthopedic evaluation
Acute patellar tendon rupture	• Palpable defect over patellar tendon • Cannot do straight leg raise • Patella sitting higher up on affected limb	• X-rays to rule out bony pathology	• Knee immobilizer • Crutches • NWB	• Emergent orthopedic evaluation
Quadriceps muscle tear	• Pain over quad muscle • Bruising over muscle • Intact tendons • Extreme pain with movement • Amount of quad function depending on degree of tear	• X-rays to rule out bony pathology	• Crutches	• Outpatient follow-up
Quadriceps muscle strain	• Tenderness over muscle • Full, active ROM • Intact quad tendons • No bruising/no large amount of swelling	• None required unless associated trauma	• NSAIDs • Light stretching • Heat/ice	• Follow-up with PCP
Myositis	• Mild pain with palpation over muscle • History of recent viral illness before muscle pain developed • Both limbs affected	• None required, can obtain lab work	• NSAIDs • Tylenol	• Follow-up with PCP • Usually self-resolves

www.orthoinfo.org/en/diseases--conditions/quadriceps-tendon-tear/; www.orthoinfo.org/en/diseases--conditions/common-knee-injuries/.

- Transport the patient as quickly as possible if their pathology is life-threatening. If the patient decompensates, follow the typical BLS and ACLS protocols if necessary.

Next, inquire about the longevity and a more detailed history of symptoms. In Case #5, the patient has had progressing symptoms for 1 month; however, questions about surrounding factors should be asked to help narrow the diagnosis.

- For example, ask if the patient has been hiking, spends time outdoors, or about where they live to investigate Lyme arthritis as a possibility. If the patient reports he went hiking 6 months ago and had a rash soon after, that's a great clue into a more specific diagnosis. If the patient told you his symptoms started after an injury 20 years ago, that may steer questioning and evaluation in a different direction.

Now, ask about associated or specific symptoms at present. For this case, it's essential to ask about the following:

- Fever or systemic infectious versus inflammatory symptoms
- History of "clots" (thrombi or emboli)
- Symptoms localized to a joint (monoarthralgias) versus symptoms within multiple joints (polyarthralgias).

22. **What positive physical exam finding would aid in the diagnosis of deep vein thrombosis (DVT) for the patient in Case #5?**
    The Homan sign is the best-known specific physical exam test to assess for DVT, also known as the dorsiflexion sign. Here are the steps on how to perform the Homan test to assess *for* DVT:
    - Have the patient sitting down or lying supine.
    - Ask the patient to fully extend their knee.
    - The examiner passively raises the patient's leg to approximately 10 degrees.
    - Once raised, the examiner rapidly dorsiflexes the patient's foot and simultaneously squeezes their calf.

        Calf pain and/or tenderness would indicate a *positive* test and would suggest engaging in DVT evaluation and diagnostic tests.
    - Notice the question says *"aid"* in diagnosis. Remember, before performing specific physical exam tests, always perform a thorough general exam that includes body systems outside of the patient's chief concern to be all-inclusive. Use specific tests to help guide workup and differential diagnosis. Homan test is *not* specific and should be used on a case-by-case basis.

CASE #5, PART 2

While interviewing the patient, you decide to open his chart and notice the following vital signs:
Temperature 38.6 C, heart rate 112 bpm, respiration rate 19, blood pressure 114/84 with MAP 94, and 98% oxygen saturation on room air.

23. **For Case #5, what are some current differential diagnoses?**
    Hopefully, infectious etiologies are the first to come to mind. Infection would definitely be the most life-threatening diagnosis, and this is what the workup will evolve around. However, it is important to keep an open mind and consider other etiologies (e.g., inflammatory or rheumatological etiologies, though these will not be discussed fully in detail in this chapter).

24. **What is the difference between cellulitis and erysipelas? When do you refer a patient to the ER?**
    Skin infections are very common. Cellulitis is a bacterial infection of the skin, usually including the epidermis and dermis. Erysipelas is a form of cellulitis, but it typically spreads quicker than cellulitis and just includes the epidermis. Patients will report erythema, pain, and warmth of the infected region. Patients with skin infections that are otherwise healthy and superficial can be discharged with home antibiotic therapy. If the infection persists or worsens beyond 3 days, the patient should be referred to the ER for further management. If the infection is large, surpasses a superficial level, or the patient has systemic symptoms, refer the patient to the local ER for evaluation and likely IV antibiotic treatment.
    - Front Line ER's website is a great source for quick reference: https://frontlineer.com/when-to-go-to-urgent-care-for-skin-infections/
    - Additionally, if the decision is made to refer the patient to the local ER, use a skin marker to mark the borders of the infection prior to transport.

25. **Why is cellulitis different from chronic venous stasis?**
    Chronic venous stasis changes most commonly occur bilaterally, and patients will report itchiness rather than erythema and pain. This is why it is *very* important to include comparison in the inspection portion of the physical exam.

26. Explain the differences between osteoarthritis, rheumatoid arthritis, and septic arthritis. How is each diagnosed?

See Table 17.6.

Table 17.6 Differential Diagnoses, Presentations, and Management of the Most Common Types of Arthritis

ARTHRITIS TYPE, PATHOPHYSIOLOGY, RISK FACTORS	PRESENTATION	DIAGNOSIS	TREATMENT & DISPOSITION
Osteoarthritis (OA) occurs due to degradation of cartilage and subsequent bone remodeling over time Most common risk factors: • Older age • Obesity • Prior injury • Females > males	• Chronic pain • Worsens as the day goes on • Relieved with rest • Tender joint • Bilateral joint involvement	Diagnosis of exclusion Radiographs are best initial test May need blood work or MRI Be wary of patients who are elderly with a history of injury, trauma, or new acute to subacute onset of pain Obtain new images for these patients due to their higher risk of fractures	• Conservative treatment • Outpatient PCP follow-up Can escalate to orthopedic referral, if necessary, in the outpatient setting
Rheumatoid arthritis (RA) is an autoimmune disorder in which the body's immune system attacks the joint lining and joint destruction over time Risk factors: • Older age • Females > males • Smoking • Other autoimmune conditions	• Chronic pain • Worse in the morning with improvement throughout the day • Reduced ROM • Tender joint • Asymmetric Check patient's hands for rheumatoid, Heberden, and/or Bouchard nodules for diagnostic aid	Even if RA is the most likely diagnosis, all patients should receive radiographs Blood work includes rheumatoid factor, anticyclic citrullinated peptide (CCP) antibodies, and antinuclear antibody test If evaluation is obscure, perform arthrocentesis to evaluate and rule out septic arthritis	• NSAIDs for initial treatment • If single joint, consider glucocorticoid injection • If multiple joints, can try systemic glucocorticoids • Opiates are not effective and should be avoided • Outpatient follow-up with PCP and likely rheumatology
Septic arthritis is caused by infection, usually from urinary, pulmonary, or cutaneous infections, then hematogenous spread or direct inoculation Most common risk factors: • Artificial joint(s) • Immunosuppression • Trauma • IV drug abuse	• Warm • Erythematous • Very painful • Edematous • Usually singular joint • Minimal active and passive ROM • Systemic symptoms typically present	If there is any suspicion of septic joint at all, perform arthrocentesis Assess this patient for sepsis and/or septic shock Blood work must include CBC, blood culture, ESR, and CRP	• Transfer for immediate ER evaluation

Aletaha D, Smolen JS. Diagnosis and management of rheumatoid arthritis. *JAMA*. 2018;320(13):1360–1372. jamanetwork.com/journals/jama/article-abstract/2705192; Abramoff B, Caldera FE. Osteoarthritis: pathology, diagnosis, and treatment options. *Med Clin North Am.* 2020;104(2):293–311. doi:10.1016/j.mcna.2019.10.007. Epub 2019 Dec 18. PMID: 32035570; Ross JJ. Septic arthritis of native joints. *Infect Dis Clin North Am.* 2017;31(2):203–218. doi:10.1016/j.idc.2017.01.001. Epub 2017 Mar 30. PMID: 28366221.

KEY POINTS

1. Clinical history is important with musculoskeletal complaints. Consider traumatic causes, but also consider nontraumatic etiologies.
2. With musculoskeletal complaints that involve the upper and lower extremities, always conduct a proper neurovascular examination, and consider compartment syndrome (the six Ps: pain out of proportion, pallor, paresthesias, pulselessness, paralysis, and poikilothermia, and remember that all six are not necessary to make the diagnosis).
3. There are six parts to the physical exam of an extremity: inspection, palpation, range of motion, neurovascular comparison, and examination of nearby structures. For lower extremities, include ambulation and weight-bearing.
4. Conservative therapy to treat extremity injuries includes "R.I.C.E": Rest, Ice therapy, Compression to help with swelling, and Elevation above the heart to eliminate swelling from the area of injury and return it back into normal circulation.
5. X-rays are the initial diagnostic test of choice for musculoskeletal injuries. MRI may be considered if conservative therapy does not improve symptoms after 3–5 days.

BIBLIOGRAPHY

Abbasi D. Medial Epicondylitis (Golfer's Elbow). *Orthobullets.* www.orthobullets.com/shoulder-and-elbow/3083/medial-epicondylitis-golfers-elbow. Accessed 1 June 2023.

Abramoff B, Caldera FE. Osteoarthritis: pathology, diagnosis, and treatment options. *Med Clin North Am.* 2020;104(2):293–311. doi:10.1016/j.mcna.2019.10.007. Epub 2019 Dec 18. PMID: 32035570.

Achilles Tendinopathy. *Physiopedia.* www.physio-pedia.com/Achilles_Tendinopathy. Accessed 1 May 2023.

Alaia MJ, Williams R. Quadriceps tendon tear - orthoinfo - aaos. *OrthoInfo.* 2021. www.orthoinfo.org/en/diseases–conditions/quadriceps-tendon-tear/.

Aletaha D. Diagnosis and management of rheumatoid arthritis. *JAMA.* 2018. https://jamanetwork.com/journals/jama/fullarticle/2705192.

Allen D. Distal Radial Ulnar Joint (DRUJ) Injuries. *Orthobullets.* 2023. www.orthobullets.com/trauma/1028/distal-radial-ulnar-joint-druj-injuries.

Cadogan M. Posterior Shoulder Dislocation. *Life in the Fast Lane.* 2022. litfl.com/posterior-shoulder-dislocation/.

Common Knee Injuries - Orthoinfo - Aaos. *OrthoInfo.* 2022. www.orthoinfo.org/en/diseases–conditions/common-knee-injuries/.

Frank R, Cohen M. Elbow Dislocation. *Orthobullets.* 2023. www.orthobullets.com/trauma/1018/elbow-dislocation?hideLeftMenu=true.

Haghighat SS, et al. *EMRA Ortho Guide.* Emergency Medicine Residents' Association, Medical Student Committee; 2019.

Hooper M. When to go to urgent care for skin infections. *Emergency Room.* 2021. http://www.orthoinfo.org/en/diseases–conditions/quadriceps-tendon-tear/.

Ross JJ. Septic arthritis of native joints. *Infect Dis Clin North Am.* 2017;31(2):203–218. doi:10.1016/j.idc.2017.01.001. Epub 2017 Mar 30. PMID: 28366221.

Sharareh B. Radius and Ulnar Shaft Fractures. *Orthobullets.* 2023. www.orthobullets.com/trauma/1025/radius-and-ulnar-shaft-fractures?hideLeftMenu=true.

Steffes MJ, Weatherford B. 5th Metatarsal Base Fracture. *Orthobullets.* 2023. www.orthobullets.com/foot-and-ankle/7031/5th-metatarsal-base-fracture.

Taylor BC, Tarazona D. Ankle Fractures. *Orthobullets.* 2023. www.orthobullets.com/trauma/1047/ankle-fractures.

Tintinalli JE, et al. Section 22 Orthopedics. In: Garth MD, et al., ed. *Tintinalli's Emergency Medicine: A Comprehensive Study Guide.* 9th ed. New York Etc: McGraw-Hill Education; 2020:1767–1879.

Triplet J. Proximal Humerus Fractures. *Orthobullets.* 2023. www.orthobullets.com/trauma/1015/proximal-humerus-fractures?hideLeftMenu=true.

Verghese A, Elder A, Ozdalga E, Chi J, Zaman J, Kugler J, Osterberg L, Artandi M, Hosamani P, Wang S, Ong'uti S, Thadaney S. Ankle and Foot Exam. *Stanford Medicine 25,* 2023. https://stanfordmedicine25.stanford.edu/the25/Ankleandfootexam.html.

CHAPTER 18

INFECTIOUS DISEASE ISSUES

Rory O'Neill, DO, MBA

TOP SECRETS

1. Erythema migrans, if identified, is an indicator for antibiotic treatment without laboratory confirmation.
2. No one has ever contracted rabies from a dog, cat, or ferret who was able to be observed for 10 days.

TUBERCULOSIS (TB)

1. **How does TB spread from one person to another?**
   TB, which is caused by *Mycobacterium tuberculosis,* is spread via respiratory droplets from one person to another. It is not spread by contact.

2. **How does latent TB differ from active TB?**
   Latent TB occurs when patients are infected with TB but do not become ill, and they exhibit no symptoms. Patients with latent TB are not contagious and therefore are not at risk for transmission to others.

3. **What clinical symptoms would a patient with active TB exhibit?**
   Cough (lasting several weeks), chest pain, night sweats, weakness, weight loss, fever, chills.

4. **What parts of the world are considered at highest risk for TB?**
   India, China, Indonesia, the Philippines, Pakistan, Nigeria, Bangladesh, and South Africa.

5. **What past medical/social history in a patient would increase your suspicion for TB?**
   HIV, drug/alcohol abuse, prior TB infection, immunosuppression, homelessness, incarceration, recent immigration, or travel from high-risk areas.

6. **What constitutes a positive TB purified protein derivative (PPD) test?**
   See Table 18.1.

7. **Would you recommend any treatment for patients with latent TB?**
   Yes. Treatment of latent TB is recommended, as there is a risk of progression of latent to active TB.

8. **Is there a vaccination for TB?**
   Yes, many countries with large numbers of TB patients give bacille Calmette-Guérin (BCG); however, in the United States, it is not routinely administered secondary to the low risk. Note that patients who have had BCG may have a false-positive reaction to a TB test.

9. **How should I interpret a PPD test in a patient with a prior BCG vaccine?**
   The reaction to PPD testing can vary in patients with prior BCG; therefore, the recommendation is to interpret the same (see Table 18.1) and treat based on risk factors.

LYME DISEASE

10. **How does a patient get Lyme disease?**
    The spirochete *Borrelia burgdorferi* is transmitted to humans by infected ticks who bite their skin.

11. **What clinical sign of Lyme disease can be used to make the diagnosis without laboratory confirmation?**
    Erythema migrans – a rash that develops on average 1 week following the tick bite. It is an erythematous circular rash, typically a single lesion, but also can present as multiple lesions.

12. **What percentage of patients with Lyme disease develop at least one episode of erythema migrans?**
    Up to 80%.

13. **What is the recommended laboratory testing for Lyme disease?**
    Step 1: Enzyme immunoassay (EIA) or immunofluorescence assay (IFA) – total Lyme titer or IgG and IgM titers.
    Step 2: Western blot (only done if step 1 results are positive or equivocal).

Table 18.1 Positive PPD Measurements

INDURATION	>5 MM	>10 MM	>15 MM
Positive in a patient with…	• HIV • Recent contact with TB patient • CXR findings • Transplant patient • Immunosuppressed	• Immigrants and travelers from high-risk regions • IV drug users • Children <4 years • Residents or employees in high-risk settings • Pediatric patients at high risk	• No risk factors

Conrad Stoppler M. *Tuberculosis Skin Test (PPD Skin Test)*. https://www.medicinenet.com/tuberculosis_skin_test_ppd_skin_test/article. htm. Last reviewed Mar 30, 2022.
Tuberculosis (TB). https://www.cdc.gov/tb/default.htm.

14. **What are the clinical stages and symptoms of Lyme disease?**
    See Table 18.2.

15. **What is the treatment for Lyme disease?**
    See Table 18.3.

16. **What is posttreatment Lyme disease syndrome?**
    Some people may experience persistent symptoms (joint/muscle aches, fatigue) despite appropriate antibiotic treatment. This is also known as "chronic Lyme disease." No controlled studies have shown benefits of antibiotic therapy. In fact, guidelines recommend against additional antibiotic therapy for patients who have recurring nonspecific symptoms.

17. **How do I remove a tick?**
    Using forceps, grab the tick at the base of the attachment to the skin surface. Pull upward steadily; do not twist. See Fig. 18.1.

RABIES

18. **What animals cause the majority of diagnosed human rabies cases in North America?**
    Bats.

19. **A patient wakes up and notices a bat in the room in which he was sleeping. What do you recommend?**
    Postexposure prophylaxis is recommended for any contact between a human and a bat unless the bat can be tested and is negative for rabies. Prophylaxis is recommended in situations of unknown exposure/risk.

20. **What are the Centers for Disease Control and Prevention (CDC) recommendations on animals that can be observed?**
    No rabies prophylaxis is recommended if the animal can be observed for 10 days. If signs suggestive of rabies develop in the animal during this observation period, postexposure prophylaxis should be administered.

21. **According to the CDC, how many people in the United States have ever contracted rabies from a dog, cat, or ferret that was observed for 10 days?**
    Zero.

22. **What are the CDC rabies postexposure prophylaxis recommendations?**
    See Table 18.4.

Table 18.2 Stages of Lyme Disease

STAGE	SYMPTOMS
Early localized	Erythema migrans, fever, chills, myalgias, fatigue, headache
Early disseminated	Multiple erythema migrans, facial nerve palsy, meningitis, encephalitis, atrioventricular block
Late	Arthritis, peripheral neuropathy

Table 18.3 Symptoms and Treatment of Lyme Disease

STAGE	CLINICAL SYMPTOMS	ROUTE	ANTIBIOTIC DOSING AND DURATION
Early localized	Erythema migrans	Oral	Doxycycline 100 mg BID *Peds*: 4 mg/kg (max 100 mg) BID x 10 days Amoxicillin 500 mg TID *Peds*: 50 mg/kg/day (up to 500 mg, divided into three doses) x 14 days Cefuroxime 500 mg BID *Peds*: 30 mg/kg/day (max 500 mg) x 14 days Azithromycin 500 mg daily peds: 50–100 mg/kg/day divided in three doses) x 7 days
Early disseminated	Multiple erythema migrans	Oral	Same as above; 14 days
	Isolated cranial nerve palsy	Oral	Same as above; 14–21 days
	Meningitis	IV or Oral	Oral: same as above IV: dosed inpatient
Late	Arthritis	Oral	Same as above for 28 days
	Recurrent arthritis after oral therapy	Oral or IV	Oral: 28 days IV: dosed by specialists
	Encephalitis	IV	IV: dosed inpatient

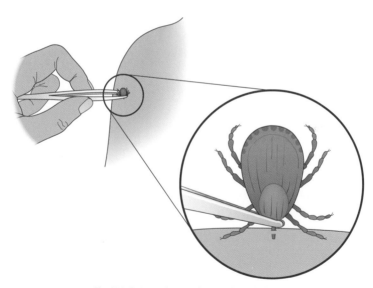

Fig. 18.1 Technique for removing an embedded tick.

MEASLES

23. **When should you consider a diagnosis of measles?**
    Unvaccinated child, usually under the age of 5, fever, cough, runny nose, and conjunctivitis for several days, followed by maculopapular rash beginning on the face and upper neck.

24. **What are complications of measles?**
    While usually a mild illness, it can be associated with pneumonia, seizures, encephalitis, diarrhea, and even death.

Table 18.4 Rabies Vaccine Scheduling

PATIENT IS	VACCINE	IMMUNOGLOBULIN (20 IU/KG) LOCAL ADMIN, THEN MUSCLE
Unvaccinated, immunocompetent	4-dose—Day 0, 3, 7, 14	Yes
Unvaccinated, immunocompromised	5-dose—Day 0, 3, 7, 14, 28	Yes
Previously vaccinated	2-dose—Day 0, 3	No

Rabies. Centers for Disease Control and Prevention (CDC). https://www.cdc.gov/rabies/index.html. Last updated May 4, 2022.

KEY POINTS

1. A positive PPD test indicates that a person at some point in time has been infected with tuberculosis.
2. Lyme disease is the most common tickborne disease in the United States, and there is no rash in up to 20% of cases.
3. Postexposure rabies vaccination is recommended in any human–bat interaction.

BIBLIOGRAPHY

Lyme Disease. https://emedicine.medscape.com/article/330178-overview. Last updated Apr 5, 2021
Gastanaduy, MD, Haber P, Rota PA, Patel M. *Epidemiology and Prevention of Vaccine-Preventable Diseases: Measles*. https://www.cdc.gov/vaccines/pubs/pinkbook/meas.html.

FEVER

Ariella Nadler, MD, Jeffrey R. Avner, MD, FAAP

CHAPTER 19

TOP SECRETS

1. Fever itself is not dangerous to an otherwise healthy child, and the specific temperature value (as opposed to its presence or absence) is generally not important.
2. The height of fever has limited use in determining management; other clinical features, especially the child's clinical appearance, are better predictors.

1. **What causes fever?**
   The body has a "central thermostat" comprised of a specialized group of neurons in the hypothalamus that act to maintain the body at a physiologic "set point." This set point changes when pyrogens (endogenous or exogenous substances that produce fever) stimulate an inflammatory response that increases the production of prostaglandin E, which in turn acts on the hypothalamus to raise the set point. When the body's temperature is lower than the set point, various mechanisms are employed to increase heat production and raise the body's temperature to be in balance with the new set point, resulting in fever.

2. **What are the different phases of the febrile response?**
   The first phase of the febrile response is the "chill" phase. Various mechanisms, including increasing cellular metabolism, increasing skeletal muscle activity through involuntary shivering, peripheral vasoconstriction, and seeking a warmer environment are employed in order to raise the body's temperature to a new set point. The "flush" phase occurs as the set point is lowered back toward normal body temperature with illness resolution or administration of antipyretics. This phase is characterized by peripheral vasodilation, sweating, and seeking a cooler environment as the body seeks to lower its temperature to the new set point.

3. **A child is noted to be pale and shivering, yet the oral temperature taken at that time is normal; why is that?**
   When children are in the *early* stage of the "chill" phase of fever, their body temperature may not yet be elevated at a peripheral site (e.g., rectal, oral) as it lags behind changes in core body temperature. However, children may manifest symptoms of the febrile response such as shivering, cool skin, tachycardia, tachypnea, and decreased appetite. Fever will likely occur 20–30 minutes after the development of these systemic symptoms.

4. **Is there a difference between fever and hyperthermia?**
   Yes; *fever* is a physiologic response, while *hyperthermia* is not. *Fever* is an elevation of body temperature that is regulated by the body's internal thermoregulatory center in the hypothalamus, whereas *hyperthermia* represents elevation of body temperature due to either internal factors or an external environmental source that overwhelms the body's normal thermoregulatory mechanisms. Temperature elevation secondary to hyperthermia is dangerous, as the thermoregulatory center does not stimulate vasodilation and sweating to lower the temperature as it would in the case of fever. Because the thermoregulatory system is dysfunctional in *hyperthermia* (as opposed to a normal febrile response), management usually requires aggressive attempts at cooling.

5. **What circumstances may cause hyperthermia?**
   Hyperthermia may result from disorders of excessive heat production (exertional heatstroke, thyrotoxicosis, cocaine intoxication), disorders of diminished heat dissipation (classic heatstroke, severe dehydration, autonomic dysfunction), or disorders of hypothalamic function (cerebrovascular accidents, trauma).

6. **Is normal body temperature 98.6°F (37°C)?**
   There is no single normal value for body temperature. Rather, there is a range of normal that can vary in each person by as much as 0.5°C from the mean, based on various factors. These include time of day (lowest in the morning and highest in the evening), age (higher in infants), sex, physical activity, and ambient temperature.

7. **So where did the value 98.6°F come from?**
   The value 98.6°F is attributed to Carl Wunderlich, who published, in 1868, a study in which he used a foot-long axillary thermometer to take 1 million temperature readings in more than 25,000 patients and found 98.6°F to be the mean temperature; hardly accurate by today's standards.

8. **What body temperature is considered to be a fever?**
   In general, most consider a fever to be higher than 38.0–38.2°C (rectally) [100.4–100.8°F] in an appropriately dressed infant and higher than 37.2–37.7°C (orally) [100.0°F] in an older child or adult.

9. Which method of temperature measurement (rectal, oral, tympanic, skin) is best to use, or does it really matter?

Rectal temperature is generally used as the standard measurement to indirectly measure core body temperature. Digital axillary and oral thermometry tend to underestimate rectal temperature by about 0.5–1.0°C. Infrared tympanic and temporal thermometry are popular methods used in urgent care settings, and studies show that, at least in older children and adults, the results are reasonably accurate, achieving high specificity. It should be noted that there are inherent limitations in temperature measurement and that the specific temperature determination by peripheral thermometry should be complemented by additional clinical elements (e.g., history, vital signs, physical exam findings) when assessing children. It is also important to use a consistent form of measurement to monitor changes in body temperature.

10. Is there a value that is considered a "high" fever (or how high is too high)?

There is no specific value considered too "high" for a *fever* (as opposed to hyperthermia). Fever increases a child's metabolic rate and catabolism, making him or her more prone to heat loss. Most healthy children can accommodate these stresses through normal physiologic processes; however, children with chronic illnesses and those who are immunosuppressed or have cardiopulmonary disease may not be able to adjust to this increased demand and are at higher risk for systemic effects.

11. Does the height of fever predict the risk of serious bacterial illness (SBI) or mortality?

While the presence of fever is usually indicative of an ongoing infectious process, the height of the temperature is not an accurate marker of SBI or mortality in otherwise healthy children. Thus the height of fever has limited use in determining management. Other clinical features, especially the child's clinical appearance, are better predictors. This does not mean that a thorough evaluation of a child with a high fever is unnecessary; rather, *any child with a fever, regardless of the height of the temperature, should receive a thorough evaluation.*

12. Do parents pay too much attention to taking their child's temperature?

Parents often exhibit "fever phobia," displaying excessive concern about fever and its potential effects on their child with heightened concern at higher temperatures. This often leads to frequently taking the child's temperature. It is important to educate parents that fever is a *symptom* of their child's illness that will persist until the underlying illness has resolved. Fever itself is not dangerous to an otherwise healthy child, and the specific temperature value (as opposed to its presence or absence) is generally not important.

13. Should I make the parents focus on preventing fever in their child?

Trying to prevent or "control" fever is generally futile and will likely increase fever phobia. Parents should be directed to focus on the child's comfort and clinical appearance until the resolution of the underlying illness. Antipyretics can be used for comfort. A change in clinical appearance should prompt reassessment by a health care provider.

14. Does high fever cause brain damage or death?

There is no evidence that high fever itself (*as opposed to hyperthermia*) causes brain damage or death in otherwise healthy children. Although excessive heat (>107°F) may denature proteins in vitro, fever likely affects protein expression, allowing them to adapt to high temperatures in vivo. When brain damage does occur in association with fever, it is usually due to sequelae of the underlying disease (such as meningitis) rather than the fever itself. Nevertheless, over 25% of parents believe fever causes brain damage.

15. Can I trust parents who say their child is "burning up"?

Parents' tactile assessment of their child's fever has a moderate sensitivity (75–93%) but lower specificity (48–86%), suggesting that parents' assessment is more reliable at ruling out a fever rather than ruling one in. When the height of fever is critical for determining management (e.g., immunocompromised host or infants <2 months old), an accurately measured temperature should be obtained.

16. Is alternating antipyretics more beneficial than monotherapy?

There is no conclusive proof that alternating antipyretics is more efficacious than single-drug therapy. Although there is some evidence that the antipyretic combination results in slightly lower temperatures at 4–6 hours, there is no evidence of overall improvement in other clinical outcomes. Conversely, there is a risk that parents will be confused with the different doses and time intervals of each antipyretic, leading to incorrect dosing and increased risk for toxicity. Additionally, ibuprofen inhibits glutathione production, which binds acetaminophen to prevent hepatic and renal toxicity. It is therefore generally safer to reinforce monotherapy and caution against alternating antipyretics.

17. Does a failure to respond to antipyretics predict serious illness?

In general, fevers due to serious infections are as responsive to antipyretics as those due to benign illness. The child's appearance after fever reduction is a more useful predictor of the clinical condition; a child with a serious illness often remains ill-appearing even after fever reduction, whereas a child with a more benign illness usually improves clinically.

18. Do antipyretics prevent febrile seizures?

No studies have demonstrated that antipyretics, in the absence of anticonvulsants, reduce the recurrence risk of simple febrile seizures in otherwise healthy children.

19. **Is there a way to calculate the increase in heart rate and/or respiratory rate with fever?**
Although somewhat dependent on age, the heart rate generally increases by 10–15 beats/min/°C and the respiratory rate rises by about 5 breaths/min/°C.

20. **Do I need to refer all febrile infants less than 8 weeks old to the emergency department?**
In general, yes. Assuming the fever is not due to environmental factors, such as bundling, most studies recommend some laboratory evaluation for serious bacterial infection (SBI) for any febrile infant less than 8 weeks old, as these infants have an immature immune response and a relatively high rate of SBI (about 10%), with about 8% having urinary tract infection, 1.8% bacteremia, and 0.5% bacterial meningitis. Due to their developmental inability to show clinical signs of illness (e.g., no social smile), neonates (age <3–4 weeks) in particular should undergo a complete evaluation for SBI. For infants less than 21 days old, this includes testing the urine, blood, and cerebrospinal fluid (CSF) for bacterial infection. Infants 22–28 days old have a lower risk of meningitis, and therefore some clinicians may defer the lumbar puncture based on clinical findings and inflammatory markers. Evaluation of febrile infants 29–60 days is more variable and depends on clinical judgment, benefit–harm assessment, and shared decision making (Table 19.1.)

21. **How should I manage a neonate who has a reported fever at home but is afebrile on presentation?**
A neonate who has a documented fever at home but is afebrile on presentation should be managed as a febrile neonate and referred to the emergency department.

22. **Does risk stratification work for febrile young infants?**
Yes. In 2021, the AAP released updated guidelines for evaluating and managing febrile infants. Their recommendations are constructed on three age-based algorithms: (1) infants 8–21 days old; (2) infants 22–28 days old; and (3) infants 29–60 days old. Infants 29–60 days old who are considered low risk for SBI may be managed as an outpatient, sometimes without antibiotic therapy, as long as there is reliable outpatient follow-up. Table 19.1 is a summary of these guidelines. It is important to note that any approach should consider the clinician's experience, the nature of their relationship with the patient's family, the reliability of follow-up, and the parents' comfort level and observational skills.

23. **What's the chance the infant who tests positive for a virus also has a serious bacterial infection?**
Confirmed viral infection (e.g., RSV, influenza, enterovirus, SARS-CoV-2) in febrile infants <60 days of age is associated with a decreased *but not negligible* SBI risk, compared with non-viral-infected febrile infants. Additionally, although the frequency of bacterial meningitis is very low overall, there is no difference between febrile infants with and without viral infection. Thus in a well-appearing febrile infant, clinicians should exercise caution, especially in the first month of life, regarding comprehensiveness of evaluation, including performance of lumbar puncture, regardless of virus infection status. At a minimum, an evaluation for UTI should be strongly considered for infants 4–8 weeks old, and a more extensive evaluation considered for infants less than 29 days old.

24. **Do I need to get lab tests for the evaluation of well-appearing febrile toddlers and children?**
A well-appearing, healthy child who has a fever but no source of infection on physical examination does not need routine lab tests as part of their evaluation. A thorough history and physical exam are generally sufficient in

Table 19.1 Management Options for Well-Appearing Febrile Young Infants

AGE	8–21 DAYS	22–28 DAYS	29–60 DAYS
Urine	Yes	Yes	Yes
Blood culture	Yes	Yes	Yes
Inflammatory markers*	Optional	Yes	Yes
CSF	Yes	Maybe	Maybe
Antibiotics	Yes	Maybe	Maybe
Disposition	Hospitalize	Hospital vs. home	Hospital vs. home

*Inflammatory markers: temperature >38.5°C, procalcitonin >0.5 ng/mL, CRP >20 mg/L, and ANC >4000 or >5200 mm^3.
Adapted from: Pantell RH, Roberts KB, Adams WG, Dreyer BP, Kuppermann N, O'Leary ST, Okechukwu K, Woods CR Jr. Subcommittee on febrile infants. Evaluation and management of well-appearing febrile infants 8–60 days old. *Pediatrics.* 2021;148(2):e2021052228. doi: 10.1542/peds.2021-052228. Epub 2021 Jul 19. Erratum in: Pediatrics. 2021;148(5): PMID: 34281996.
Reprinted from: Avner JR. Fever. Pediatric Emergency Medicine Secrets, 4th Edition, Selbst S, Savage J (eds), Hanley and Belfus, 2022.

determining care. In some children under 2 years, depending on their risk factors, a urinalysis and urine culture may be useful. Children who are immunosuppressed or have underlying chronic illness are at higher risk for developing serious illness and sepsis and therefore may need individualized management including selected lab studies and possibly empiric antibiotics.

25. **Has pneumococcal conjugate vaccine (PCV13) changed the incidence of serious bacterial illness in febrile children?**
Since the introduction of PCV13 in 2010, the rate of invasive pneumococcal disease (IPD) declined significantly. According to the CDC (https://www.cdc.gov/pneumococcal/surveillance.html, accessed January 1, 2023), from 1998 through 2019, overall IPD rates among children less than 5 years old decreased by 93%. Pneumonia cases have also decreased. Children with comorbidities remain at increased risk of invasive disease.

26. **Can biomarkers distinguish febrile children with SBI from those with self-limited nonbacterial infections?**
A variety of inflammatory markers have been suggested as possible predictors of SBI in febrile children, and although they have moderate sensitivity for SBI, their usefulness in the acute care setting is limited by generally low positive predictive values. Procalcitonin (PCT), at a level >0.5 ng/ml, appears to be a more accurate predictor than C-reactive protein (CRP), white blood cell count (WBC), or absolute neutrophil count (ANC), particularly early in the disease course. Importantly, if meningitis is being considered, the decision to perform a lumbar puncture should be based primarily on history and physical exam findings rather than solely on nonspecific inflammatory markers.

27. **When should a febrile child be tested for UTI?**
The overall prevalence of UTIs in 2- to 24-month-old febrile children without another source of infection is 5–7%. Girls and uncircumcised boys have an increased likelihood of having a UTI, and one should use a lower threshold to test these groups. Individual risk factors for children 2–23 months old, which form the basis for a recently developed UTI calculator (https://uticalc.pitt.edu/, accessed January 2023), are listed in Table 19.2. Additionally, older children with dysuria, frequency, abdominal pain, suprapubic pain, or back pain should be evaluated for UTI.

28. **How should urine be obtained for urinalysis and/or culture?**
Urethral catheterization is the preferred method of obtaining a urine specimen in children who are not toilet trained. A clean bagged urine specimen is an option in children older than 6 months for urinalysis; but if positive, only urine obtained by catheterization should be sent for culture. A clean-catch specimen is generally acceptable for children who are toilet trained.

29. **Can a febrile child have pneumonia without respiratory symptoms?**
While many children with pneumonia present with respiratory symptoms such as abnormal breath sounds, tachypnea, hypoxia, or increased work of breathing, there is also an increased likelihood of pneumonia in children with prolonged fever (>5 days), prolonged cough (>10 days), or leukocytosis (WBC >20,000) despite an absence of other respiratory symptoms.

30. **Is a CXR necessary to confirm pneumonia?**
No. Routine CXRs are not necessary to confirm a diagnosis of community-acquired pneumonia. CXRs may be useful if the child has hypoxemia, significant respiratory distress, or failure to improve 48 hours after initiation of antibiotics.

31. **How many days of fever require further evaluation and/or referral to a specialist?**
When a child has a daily fever for more than 7–9 days without an identifiable source, it is considered a "fever of unknown origin" (FUO) and often warrants further evaluation. It is important to differentiate FUO from two short febrile illnesses that are temporally related.

Table 19.2 Risk Factors for UTIs in Febrile Children 2–23 Months Old

- Age <12 months
- Maximum temperature ≥39°C (i.e., 102.2°F)
- History of UTI
- Female or uncircumcised male
- No other fever source
- Duration of fever ≥48 hrs

Adapted from: Shaikh N, Hoberman A, Hum SW, et al. Development and validation of a calculator for estimating the probability of urinary tract Infection in young febrile children. *JAMA Pediatr.* 2018;172(6):550–556. doi: 10.1001/jamapediatrics.2018.0217.

32. **What is the initial workup for an FUO?**
Workup starts with a history and physical exam and proceeds in a stepwise, focused approach. Factors that affect the patient's evaluation include duration of fever, age, clinical appearance, and the patient's exposure. While 50% of cases of FUO are infectious, a longer duration of fever is associated with noninfectious etiologies including rheumatologic or oncologic. In many cases, a definitive diagnosis is not made.

33. **What is the best way for parents to keep their febrile child comfortable?**
Because children lose water and nutrients due to the increased metabolic demand during fever onset, it is important to keep them well hydrated, adjust their activity level, and lessen their amount of clothing. While sponging or bathing with tepid water may help reduce the child's temperature, it may also cause shivering and discomfort. Cold water and rubbing alcohol should be avoided, as both cause vasoconstriction, which will prevent vasodilation needed for heat dissipation and fever reduction. Rubbing alcohol can also be toxic when inhaled or absorbed through the skin. Antipyretics such as acetaminophen and ibuprofen can reduce body temperature, adding to the child's comfort.

34. **Does teething cause fever?**
Although some studies show that eruption of primary teeth is associated with a slight rise in body temperature, it is not characterized as having a fever (temperature $>38°C$).

35. **Does management of a child change if he or she presents with a fever after receiving immunizations?**
Children may develop fever after receiving immunizations (Table 19.3). Since the first set of vaccines is generally given at 2 months of age, this will not affect the workup of a patient younger than that. Older patients should have the same evaluation as a patient who has not just been vaccinated, with a thorough history, physical exam, and any ancillary tests that are necessary based on the clinical situation.

36. **Are there any other reasons why a child would require referral to an emergency department/inpatient hospital setting for fever?**
One should refer a febrile child to the emergency department or inpatient hospital if he or she requires a specific therapy or subspecialty expertise that is only available in this setting, such as intravenous antibiotics for invasive bacterial illness, or if the child has symptoms related to appendicitis or a septic joint that may require surgical evaluation and potential intervention. Patients who are febrile and dehydrated or unable to tolerate fluid intake may require intravenous fluids. Patients with fever for more than 5 days with other signs related to Kawasaki disease should also be referred.

Table 19.3 Febrile Side Effects of Common Vaccinations in Children

VACCINE	FEBRILE REACTION
COVID-19 (mRNA)	Mild fever (1–7%) within 1–2 days lasting 1–3 days, more commonly reported after the second dose than after the first dose; generally less frequent in younger children.
Chickenpox vaccine	Mild fever lasting 1–3 days begins 17–28 days after the vaccine (in 14% of children)
DTaP or DT vaccine	Fever (in 25% of children) and lasts <48 hours
Hepatitis (A or B) vaccine	Usually no fever
Influenza vaccine	Mild fever <103°F (<39.5°C) occurs in 18% of children
Measles vaccine	Mild fever <103°F (<39.5°C) in 10% and lasts 2–3 days; 103°F (39.4°C) or higher in 5–15%, usually lasts 1–2 days but can last up to 5 days
Meningococcal vaccine	Mild fever occurs in 4% of children
Mumps or Rubella vaccine	Usually no fever
Papillomavirus vaccine	Fever >100.4°F (38°C) in 10% and fever >102°F (39°C) in 1–2% of children
Pneumococcus vaccine	Mild fever <102°F (39°C) in 15% for 1–2 days
Polio vaccine	No fever
Rotavirus vaccine	No fever

37. **Do doctors sometimes get pressured into prescribing unnecessary antibiotics?**
Studies of ambulatory care practices have consistently shown widespread inappropriate antibiotic prescribing. In a recent study (Butler 2022), 9% to as many as 70% of children diagnosed with typical viral illnesses (bronchitis, nonsuppurative otitis media, viral URI, and bronchiolitis) received unnecessary antibiotics. Additionally, over 30% of children with bacterial infections received non-guideline-concordant antibiotics. Furthermore, inappropriate antibiotic prescriptions were associated with increased risk of adverse drug events including *C. difficile* infection, severe allergic reaction, and skin rash.

KEY POINTS

1. *Fever* is an elevation of body temperature that is regulated by the body's internal thermoregulatory center in the hypothalamus, whereas *hyperthermia* represents an elevation of body temperature due to an external environmental source, with no input from the body's thermoregulatory center, and is therefore more dangerous than fever.
2. There is no evidence that high fever itself (*as opposed to hyperthermia*) causes brain damage or death in otherwise healthy children.
3. The height of fever has limited use in determining management; other clinical features, especially the child's clinical appearance, are better predictors.
4. There is no conclusive proof that alternating antipyretics is more efficacious than single-drug therapy.
5. No studies have demonstrated that antipyretics, in the absence of anticonvulsants, reduce the recurrence risk of simple febrile seizures.

BIBLIOGRAPHY

Avner JR. The Febrile or Septic Appearing Infant or Child. In: Schafermeyer R, Tenenbein M, Macias C, Sharieff G, Yamomoto L, (eds). *Strange and Schafermeyer's Pediatric Emergency Medicine*. 5th ed. McGraw-Hill Professional; 2019.

Avner JR. Fever. In: Selbst S, Savage J, eds. *Pediatric Emergency Medicine Secrets*. 4th ed. Hanley and Belfus nc; 2022.

Butler AM, Brown DS, Durkin MJ, et al. Association of inappropriate outpatient pediatric antibiotic prescriptions with adverse drug events and health care expenditures. *JAMA Netw Open*. 2022;5(5):e2214153. doi:10.1001/jamanetworkopen.2022.14153.

Chiappini E, Bortone B, Galli L, de Martino M. Guidelines for the symptomatic management of fever in children: systematic review of the literature and quality appraisal with AGREE II. *BMJ Open*. 2017;7(7):e015404.

Edwards G, Fleming S, Verbakel JY, et al. Accuracy of parents' subjective assessment of paediatric fever with thermometer measured fever in a primary care setting. *BMC Prim Care*. 2022;23(1):30.

Fever in under 5s: assessment and initial management. National Institute for Health and Care Excellence (NICE); 2021.

Hubert-Dibon G, Danjou L, Feildel-Fournial C, Vrignaud B, Masson D, Launay E, Gras-Le Guen C. Procalcitonin and C-reactive protein may help to detect invasive bacterial infections in children who have fever without source. *Acta Paediatr*. 2018;107(7):1262–1269.

Mahajan P, Browne LR, Levine DA, et al. Risk of bacterial coinfections in febrile infants 60 days old and younger with documented viral infections. *J Pediatr*. 2018;203:86–91.e2.

Pantell RH, Roberts KB, Adams WG, Dreyer BP, Kuppermann N, O'Leary ST, Okechukwu K, Woods CR Jr; Subcommittee on Febrile Infants. Evaluation and management of well-appearing febrile infants 8–60 days old. *Pediatrics*. 2021;148(2): e2021052228. doi:10.1542/peds.2021-052228. Epub 2021 Jul 19. Erratum in: Pediatrics. 2021;148(5): PMID: 34281996.

Pecoraro V, Petri D, Costantino G, Squizzato A, Moja L, Virgili G, Lucenteforte E. The diagnostic accuracy of digital, infrared and mercury-in-glass thermometers in measuring body temperature: a systematic review and network meta-analysis. *Intern Emerg Med*. 2021;16(4):1071–1083.

Shaikh N, Hoberman A, Hum SW, et al. Development and validation of a calculator for estimating the probability of urinary tract infection in young febrile children. *JAMA Pediatr*. 2018;172(6):550–556. doi:10.1001/jamapediatrics.2018.0217.

Vicens-Blanes F, Miró-Bonet R, Molina-Mula J. Analysis of nurses' and physicians' attitudes, knowledge, and perceptions toward fever in children: a systematic review with meta-analysis. *Int J Environ Res Public Health*. 2021;18(23):12444.

CHAPTER 20

HEADACHE

Sixtine Valdelièvre Herold, MD, MS, Richard G. Bachur, MD

1. **An 8-year-old boy presents to your urgent care center with a 3-day history of frontal headache associated with fever, sore throat, nausea, and vomiting. What is the basic differential for a nontraumatic pediatric headache?**
   - Primary headache: migraine, tension, cluster (in order of prevalence).
   - Secondary headache: infections (such as meningitis, upper respiratory infection [URI], pharyngitis, sinusitis, otitis media, mastoiditis), medications, idiopathic intracranial hypertension, systemic hypertension, brain tumor, nontraumatic intracranial bleed (e.g., arteriovenous [A-V] malformation), and posttraumatic headache (covered separately). Infections of the head and neck can also be complicated by sinus venous thrombosis and associated increased ICP.

2. **How is the timing of a headache important?**
   - A headache may be acute, acute-recurrent, chronic-progressive, or chronic-nonprogressive.
   - Chronic-progressive headaches are those that may be indicative of a gradual increase in intracranial pressure and warrant concern of space-occupying lesions.

3. **What is the appropriate physical exam for a headache?**
   - Neurologic exam is essential. Six critical findings with headache are papilledema, ataxia, hemiparesis, abnormal eye movements, depressed reflexes, and altered mental status.
   - Exam to support secondary headache:
     - Vital signs: fever, tachycardia or bradycardia, hypertension, orthostatic changes.
     - General: findings to suggest dehydration (tacky or dry mucous membranes, decreased or absent tears, delayed capillary refill, reduced perfusion, decreased skin turgor).
     - Head, ears, eyes, nose, and throat (HEENT): findings supporting URI, otitis media, sinusitis, streptococcal pharyngitis, dental etiology; mydriasis or nystagmus to support toxicologic etiology; papilledema or anisocoria, or cranial nerve palsy suggesting increased intracranial pressure; scalp hematoma to suggest trauma.
     - Neck: meningismus, thyromegaly, carotid bruit, torticollis.
     - Skin: neurocutaneous disorders (e.g., café-au-lait spots), Lyme disease (erythema migrans), petechiae, or purpura (invasive bacterial infection).

4. **A 15-year-old girl presents to your urgent care center with right-sided, pulsating headache intermittently for 3 days that worsens with bright lights and loud sounds. What constitutes a migraine headache without aura?**
   - Lasts 2–72 hours.
   - Usually frontal, pulsating, moderate to severe in pain intensity, aggravated by routine physical activity.
   - Usually bilateral in childhood, may transition to unilateral in adolescents/adults.
   - Nausea/vomiting, photo- or phonophobia.

5. **What is a migraine with aura?**
   A fully reversible focal visual, sensory, speech, motor, brainstem, or retinal attack that lasts for 5–60 minutes and is accompanied by or followed by a headache within 60 minutes of onset.

6. **What is a tension headache?**
   A headache that is mild to moderate in intensity and usually bilateral. It may be associated with photo- or phonophobia but not usually with vomiting.

7. **What constitutes a cluster headache (trigeminal cephalalgia)?**
   - Severe unilateral, orbital, supraorbital, and/or temporal pain lasting up to 3 hours.
   - Ipsilateral conjunctival injection or lacrimation, congestion/rhinorrhea, eyelid edema, forehead/facial sweating or flushing, fullness sensation in ear, miosis, or ptosis.

8. **What is the recommended acute management of primary headaches?**
   There are multiple options available depending on the severity of the headache. Not to forget: "simple" po medications! See Table 20.1 for medical management details.

9. **What should immediately put meningitis at the top of my list in the pediatric patient?**
   - The acute onset of fever, headache, nausea/vomiting, neck pain, or meningismus.
   - In neonates, meningitis may present with fever or hypothermia, a bulging fontanel, seizures, or subtler signs of poor feeding or lethargy.

Table 20.1 Treatment of Primary Headaches

PRIMARY HEADACHE TYPE	TREATMENT

Migraine	Mild headache:
	  Oral acetaminophen (10–15 mg/kg q4h, limit daily dose to ≤ 75 mg/kg/day not to exceed 4,000 mg in 24 hours)
	  Rectal acetaminophen 10–20 mg/kg/dose, for a maximum of 75 mg/kg/day not to exceed 1,625 mg/day.
	  Ibuprofen (10 mg/kg, q6h, max of 40 mg/kg in 24 hours)
	  Sumatriptan (25–50 mg po or 20 mg IN single nostril)
	Moderate to severe headache:
	  Combination therapy of NS fluid bolus, IV ketorolac (0.5 mg/kg IV, max of 30 mg), prochlorperazine
	  Consider dexamethasone, valproate IV, dihydroergotamine

Tension	Acetaminophen/ibuprofen, po Risk of medication overuse headache from regular use of ibuprofen
Cluster	Intranasal triptan High flow (6–12 L/min) O_2 for minimum 15 minutes

10. What symptoms should raise suspicion for nontraumatic raised intracranial pressure and thus possibly lead to the need for referral to an emergency department for acute imaging?
    - Headache and/or vomiting, if present, is worse in the morning and with cough, urination, or defecation.
    - Occipital location.
    - Inability to describe the pain.
    - Change in gait (ataxia or falling to one side), limb weakness.
    - Diplopia.
    - Confusion or depressed mental status.
    - Seizure.

11. What physical exam signs should raise suspicion for nontraumatic intracranial pressure and thus possibly lead to the need for acute imaging?
    - Vital signs: bradycardia, hypertension, irregular respirations ("Cushing triad").
    - Abnormal neurologic exam
      - Altered mental status (irritability, coma).
      - Eyes: papilledema, unilateral pupil dilatation, restricted lateral gaze.
      - Ataxia, hemiparesis, hypertonia, dysarthria.
    - Not responding to typical analgesia medications may be an indication for further workup/disposition.

12. You consider sending a child with a headache to your local emergency department for diagnostic imaging. What should you obtain?
    - A head computerized tomography (CT) should be obtained if the description of the headache warrants suspicion for sudden increased intracranial pressure or stroke. Magnetic resonance imaging (MRI) may also be required in the presence of acute neurologic changes but is not the initial modality if critically ill or there is suspected acute hemorrhage. Rapid, limited MRI has significant limitations.
    - Otherwise, routine neuroimaging in the child or adolescent with headache and a normal neurologic examination is rarely warranted, and clinical follow-up is a reliable alternative.

13. What lab work is useful to aid in the diagnosis of a nontraumatic headache?
    - For primary headaches, laboratory studies are generally not helpful.
    - A lumbar puncture with an opening pressure aids in the diagnosis of idiopathic intracranial hypertension and meningitis.

14. In conclusion, what should be the disposition of a child being evaluated in your urgent care center with acute, nontraumatic headaches?
    - Immediate referral to your local emergency department should occur when the child presents with signs of Cushing triad or evidence of increased intracranial pressure, altered mental status, acute neurologic findings, rapid-onset severe headache, signs of moderate to severe dehydration, or signs of life-threatening infection (meningitis, encephalitis, orbital cellulitis).
    - Consider outpatient follow-up with pediatric neurology for a diagnosis of chronic headaches or migraine.
    - Return precautions include a brief discussion of signs of increased intracranial pressure.
    - Close follow-up with a primary care provider.

KEY POINTS

1. Most acute headaches in the pediatric patient are due to viral infections, mostly upper respiratory infections.
2. Migraines, when mild, can be treated with appropriate doses of PO acetaminophen/ibuprofen.
3. With a normal neurologic exam, pediatric headaches rarely warrant emergent imaging.
4. Head CT is the preferred initial imaging modality for headaches with acute neurologic findings or in the presence of a rapid-onset severe headache.

BIBLIOGRAPHY

Brousseau DC, et al. Treatment of pediatric migraine headaches: a randomized, double-blind trial of prochlorperazine versus ketorolac. *Ann Emerg Med.* 2004;43:256–262.

Gilles F. The Childhood Brain Tumor Consortium, the epidemiology of headache among children with brain tumor. *Journal Neuroonc.* 1991;10:31–46.

Headache Classification Committee of the International Headache Society (IHS). The International Classification of Headache Disorders, ed 3 (beta version). *Cephalalgia.* 2013;33(9):629–808.

Leung S, et al. Effectiveness of standardized combination therapy for migraine treatment in the pediatric emergency department. *Headache.* 2013;53:491–497.

Lewis DW, Koch T. Headache evaluation in children and adolescents: when to worry? When to scan? *Pediatr Ann.* 2010;39(7):399–406.

Lewis DW, et al. Acute headache in children and adolescents presenting to the emergency department. *Headache.* 2000;40:200–203.

Lewis DW, et al. The utility of neuroimaging in the evaluation of children with migraine or chronic daily headache who have normal neurological examinations. *Headache.* 2000;40:629–632.

Seupaul R, Wilbur L. Do triptans effectively treat acute cluster headache in the emergency department? *Ann Emerg Med.* 2011;58:284–285.

UpToDate. Headaches in children: approach to evaluation and general management strategies. www.utdol.com; Accessed July 15, 2016.

CHAPTER 21

EYE COMPLAINTS

Kaynan Doctor, MD, MBBS, BSc, Tabassum F. Ali, MD

TOP SECRETS

- The red, painful eye in a contact lens wearer is an ominous sign and warrants immediate referral for ophthalmological evaluation to assess for sight-threatening corneal ulcers
- Child abuse should be suspected in a non-neonatal *child* presenting with symptoms concerning for *N. gonorrhoeae*-associated conjunctivitis.

1. **What are the important historical questions in the setting of pediatric eye complaints?**
   Think of "D.O.C.T.O.R. D.U.V.S."
   Duration of symptoms
   Onset of symptoms
   Contact lens wear and comorbid systemic conditions (e.g., rheumatoid arthritis or inflammatory bowel disease)
   Trauma to the eye or recent treatments (medications, surgeries)
   Ocular pain and photophobia
   Redness
   Discharge
   Unilateral or bilateral symptoms
   Vision change
   Sensation of foreign body

2. **A shy 3-year-old female presents with concerns for blurry vision. Name one technique that could be used to evaluate her visual acuity.**
   It can be challenging to evaluate visual acuity in a young patient. As with any pediatric examination, be opportunistic with the patient and utilize imaginative methods to make the assessment a game or challenge.
   Use a matching picture acuity chart system: the child looks at pictures or letters on a visual acuity chart held 20 feet away and is asked to point to the corresponding picture or letter on a handheld chart to indicate that she sees that picture. Each eye is evaluated individually by completely occluding the other eye with tape or by asking the parent to cover the eye. It is best to start near the 20/20 line to ensure cooperation, as the child may lose interest in a long test that begins with the largest-sized letters or pictures.

3. **A patient whom you examined for corneal abrasion reported miraculous improvement in her eye pain symptoms after receiving topical anesthetic drops. Her mother asks if you can prescribe this medication for use at home. Would this be a good idea?**
   Never! Topical ophthalmic anesthetic (e.g., tetracaine or proparacaine drops) use is only indicated in the office to assist in the performance of the eye exam. Chronic use damages the corneal nerves, resulting in poor reepithelialization and impaired healing with a substantial risk of corneal ulceration, scarring, and vision loss.

4. **What are systemic causes or conditions associated with red eye in children?**
   - **Rheumatologic:** Collagen vascular disease, juvenile idiopathic rheumatoid arthritis, systemic lupus erythematosus, Kawasaki disease
   - **Gastrointestinal/dietary:** Vitamin A deficiency, inflammatory bowel disease
   - **Pulmonary:** Cystic fibrosis
   - **Oncologic:** Radiation, leukemia, bone marrow transplantation
   - **Genetic:** Trisomy 21, Cornelia de Lange syndrome
   - **Dermatologic:** Rosacea, Stevens-Johnson syndrome, toxic epidermal necrolysis
   - **Infectious:** Varicella zoster, herpes simplex virus infections, adenovirus, SARS-CoV-2, otitis media

5. **What are the classic signs and symptoms of viral conjunctivitis and how can it be distinguished from bacterial conjunctivitis?**
   (See Table 21.1)

6. **How can you differentiate between the causes of ophthalmia neonatorum (neonatal conjunctivitis)?**
   (See Table 21.2)
   ***N. gonorrhoeae*-associated conjunctivitis:** Patients usually present with sudden, severe, and grossly purulent discharge between 2–5 days of life. This disease is vision-threatening due to the considerable risk of ulceration and globe perforation. Gonococcal meningitis is an associated disease. Treatment involves hospital admission and systemic antibiotic treatment covering both *N. gonorrhoeae* and *C. trachomatis*.

TABLE 21.1 Comparison of Viral and Bacterial Conjunctivitis

	VIRAL CONJUNCTIVITIS	**BACTERIAL CONJUNCTIVITIS**
Discharge	Commonly nonpurulent	Purulent
Conjunctival injection and chemosis	+	+
Foreign body sensation, tearing, and photophobia	+	+
Unilateral or bilateral	Unilateral but can become bilaterally	Commonly unilateral
Common etiologies and variants	• Adenovirus (most common) • Pharyngoconjunctival fever • COVID-19 infection (since 2019)	• *S. aureus, S. epidermidis, S. pneumococcus, S. viridans, H. influenza, S. pneumonia, M. catarrhalis* • *N. gonorrhoeae* (hyperacute presentation over 12–24 hours, severe purulent discharge)
Duration	Up to 2–3 weeks	Less than 3 weeks' duration
Additional Features	• Concomitant viral upper respiratory infection, sore throat, and/or preauricular lymphadenopathy • Follicular ("dome-shaped") conjunctival reaction	• Less common than viral conjunctivitis • Papillary conjunctival reaction ("cobble stoning")
Important considerations for immediate referral	• Epidemic keratoconjunctivitis • Acute hemorrhagic conjunctivitis: associated with large subconjunctival hemorrhages and enterovirus infection	• Suspected gonococcal conjunctivitis *If Neisseria or chlamydia conjunctivitis is suspected in a *child* a workup for abuse is indicated
Treatment and supportive management	• Self-limited • Cool compresses, artificial tears. Antibiotics do not hasten resolution. • Avoid school or daycare until resolution; can be contagious for 10–21 days • Hand hygiene	• Topical antibiotics (see corneal abrasions) • Systemic therapy indicated for gonococcal or chlamydial conjunctivitis

+ indicates present.

Adapted from Gervasio KA, Friedberg MA, Rapuano CJ. Conjunctiva/Sclera/Iris/External Disease; 5.1 Acute Conjunctivitis. In: Gervasio KA, Peck TJ, Fathy CA, Sivalingam MD, eds. The Wills Eye Manual Office and Emergency Room Diagnosis and Treatment of Eye Disease. 8th ed. Wolters Kluwer; 2022:240–255.

C. trachomatis-associated conjunctivitis: Commonly begins within 1–2 weeks of life (but suspect in infants <30 days old) with beefy red conjunctiva and mucoid "ropy" discharge. This disease can cause permanent scarring and is associated with chlamydial pneumonitis. Treatment involves systemic antibiotics with concurrent treatment for *N. gonorrhoeae.* As with *N. gonorrhoeae*-associated conjunctivitis, the patient's mother and her sexual partner(s) also require treatment.

Pseudomonas conjunctivitis: This can cause sight-threatening infection in preterm infants.

Nasolacrimal duct obstruction/dacryostenosis: Only half of all nasolacrimal ducts are patent at birth. Obstruction causes tearing and discharge without redness. Treatment of this condition involves digital massage over the lacrimal sac. Most cases resolve spontaneously by 1 year of age. Persistent cases may require surgical correction by ophthalmology.

7. A 3-year-old male patient presents with a 2-day history of fevers in the setting of right otalgia and right eye discharge. You prescribe a 10-day course of high-dose amoxicillin at 80–90 mg/kg divided twice daily with erythromycin eye ointment after diagnosing a right-sided otitis media with concurrent right-sided conjunctivitis. The patient returns 3 days later with worsening symptoms. What should have been prescribed and why?
This patient likely has conjunctivitis-otitis syndrome, which is usually caused by nontypeable *H. influenzae* and, less commonly, *S. pneumoniae.* Due to the high frequency of β-lactamase production in *H. influenzae,*

TABLE 21.2 Infectious Neonatal Ophthalmia

FEATURES	CHLAMYDIA TRACHOMATIS	NEISSERIA GONORRHOEAE	HERPES SIMPLEX VIRUS	PSEUDOMONAS AERUGINOSA
Proportion of cases	2–40%	<1%	<1%	<1%
Presentation/ incubation period	First 1–2 weeks of life	72–96 hours after birth	6–14 days	5–28 days
Distinctive clinical features	Initially mild swelling, hyperemia, tearing, mucopurulent discharge with pseudomembrane formation with possible bloody discharge Unilateral or bilateral	Initially mild conjunctival hyperemia but can progress to severe chemosis with purulent conjunctival discharge with marked eyelid edema	Cloudy cornea, conjunctival injection, and tearing Classic herpetic vesicles may not be seen in the newborn A corneal dendrite may be seen on fluorescein staining	Seen in preterm infants Eyelid edema, erythema, purulent drainage, and pannus formation
Severity of conjunctivitis	Mild	Severe	Mild	Severe
Potential complications	Self-limited Rarely conjunctival or corneal scarring Potential development of upper and lower respiratory tract infections	Corneal ulceration and perforation Septicemia, meningitis, or arthritis	Ulceration, keratitis Disseminated infection Meningoencephalitis	Corneal perforation Endophthalmitis Sepsis Meningitis
Diagnosis	ELISA, EIA, Direct antibody tests, PCR, DNA-hybridization probe	Gram-negative diplococci seen on gram stain	Viral culture/PCR Multinucleated giant cells seen on Giemsa stain	Gram stain and culture of exudate to identify gram-negative bacilli
Treatment	Oral erythromycin elixir for 2 weeks with erythromycin ointment	Assess for systemic complications (e.g., blood and CSF studies as needed) Parenteral ceftriaxone or Cefotaxime Also treat for concurrent suspected chlamydial infection	Assess for systemic complications (e.g., blood and CSF studies as needed) Parenteral acyclovir coupled with vidarabine, ganciclovir, or trifluridine Ophthalmic preparations	Topical and systemic (parenteral) antipseudomonal antibiotic therapy

amoxicillin-clavulanate (90 mg/kg/day of amoxicillin and 6.4 mg/kg/day of clavulanate divided twice daily) or cefdinir (14 mg/kg/day divided twice daily) for 10 days is the recommended first-line therapy.

8. What is the classic conjunctivitis that is seen with Kawasaki disease?
   The conjunctivitis of Kawasaki disease is often not associated with discharge. It only involves the bulbar conjunctiva and displays limbic sparing (sparing of the vessels immediately surrounding the cornea).

9. Describe the initial presentation and management of herpetic eye disease.
   - Think of herpes simplex virus or varicella zoster virus infections causing conjunctivitis if you see vesicular lesions near the eyelid margin or along the tip of the nose (due to involvement of the nasociliary branch of the trigeminal nerve).

- Presentation is often initially unilateral.
- Confirm findings by performing fluorescein corneal staining which may show a branching dendritic pattern.
- If there is high suspicion, the patient should be started on acyclovir immediately and referred to ophthalmology.
- If seen in neonates, transfer directly to the emergency department.

10. Indications to culture and Gram stain eye discharge.
    - Marked purulence
    - Hyperacute onset of symptoms (over 12–24 hours)
    - Immunocompromised state
    - Suspicion of N gonorrhea or C trachomatis

11. How does allergic conjunctivitis present and what are treatment options?
    - Bilateral itchy eyes
    - "Allergic shiners," eyelid edema and erythema, conjunctival chemosis, and papillary conjunctivitis
    - Dennie-Morgan lines (small creases forming along the lower eyelids)
    - Concomitant allergic rhinitis or asthma
    - Treatment includes avoidance of allergens, frequent artificial tears, and cool compresses. Moderate disease may be treated with olopatadine 0.2% (over the counter) or 0.7%, ketotifen 0.025% (over the counter), azelastine 0.05%, or epinastine 0.05% as first-line treatments.
    - Oral antihistamines, such as diphenhydramine and loratadine, can often be helpful.
    - Topical steroids/immunomodulators should only be prescribed by an ophthalmologist.

12. Describe the typical presentation and management of a spontaneous subconjunctival hemorrhage.
    - Painless red eye
    - Sharply circumscribed redness without conjunctival inflammation due to rupture of small conjunctival capillaries, often localized to one sector of the eye. There is usually no associated corneal pathology.
    - Etiology: birth trauma, frequent eye rubbing, and Valsalva maneuver (e.g., vomiting and coughing). Subconjunctival hemorrhages can be associated with pertussis infection due to coughing.
    - Resolution usually occurs without treatment and within weeks with no effect on vision.
    - Referral is only indicated with frequent recurrence; suspected bleeding disorders; large, extensive hemorrhages, and/or in the case of trauma or nonaccidental trauma.

13. What are indications to refer a pediatric patient presenting with red eye to the emergency department or urgently to see an ophthalmologist?
    - Vision loss
    - Severe red eye and photophobia in a contact lens wearer
    - Copious purulent discharge
    - Vesicles or ulcers
    - Trauma or noxious chemical exposure
    - Recent ophthalmological surgery
    - Abnormal pupil shape or blood in anterior chamber
    - Recurrent/ongoing eye infections or systemic inflammatory conditions
    - Aggressive neonatal conjunctivitis and/or concerns for *N. gonorrhea*

14. A 9-year-old female presents with a painful nodule over the right upper eyelid for the last 3 days. What is your differential diagnosis and how would you manage her care?
    - Chalazion: local, tender, or nontender eyelid inflammation secondary to obstruction of the eyelid margin gland (meibomian gland or gland of Zeis)
    - Hordeolum: acute, tender bacterial infection of eyelid margin gland that may evolve into preseptal cellulitis
    - Initial management typically involves warm compresses and gentle massage to the affected eye for 10 minutes QID +/– topical antibiotic therapy (e.g., erythromycin ointment). If the lesion fails to improve after 3–4 weeks of conservative therapy, referral is indicated for incision and curettage.

15. How do you distinguish between preseptal and orbital cellulitis?
    (See Table 21.3)

16. What is the outpatient management of preseptal cellulitis?
    Amoxicillin/Clavulanate 25–40 mg/kg/day, Cefpodoxime 10 mg/kg/day, or Cefdinir 14 mg/kg/day, all divided twice daily.
    If MRSA is suspected or if penicillin allergic: Trimethoprim-Sulfamethoxazole; 8–12 mg/kg/day trimethoprim with 40–60 mg/kg/day Sulfamethoxazole in two divided doses *or* Clindamycin 20–30 mg/kg/day divided every 6–8 hours are treatment modalities. All antibiotics should be given orally for 10 days.

17. What are indications for referring a patient with preseptal cellultis?
    - Age <5 years
    - Moderate to severe preseptal cellulitis
    - Inability to rule out orbital cellulitis

TABLE 21.3 Preseptal Versus Orbital Cellulitis in Children

FEATURE	PRESEPTAL CELLULITIS	ORBITAL CELLULITIS
Location	Infection of the eyelids and periorbital soft tissues anterior to the orbital septum	Infection posterior to the orbital septum involving the tissues within the orbit (eye, orbital fat, extraocular muscles, optic nerve)
Etiology	• Adjacent infection (i.e., hordeolum, sinusitis) • Trauma (i.e., insect bite, local skin abrasions)	• Direct spread from adjacent sinus infection (i.e., ethmoid sinusitis); most common • Direct inoculation from penetrating trauma or surgery • Vascular seeding from systemic bacteremia or local facial cellulitis
Clinical presentation		
• Fever/malaise	+/− (usually mild if present)	Usually +
• Orbital/eye pain	+/−	+
• Conjunctival hyperemia or chemosis	+/−	+
• Upper-/lower-eyelid edema or erythema	+	+
• Signs of external trauma (insect bite, etc.)	+/−	+/−
• Fluctuance	+/−	+/−
• Photophobia	−	+/−
• Proptosis*	−	+
• Orbital pain	−	+
• Pain on eye movement	−	+
• Normal movement of eye*	+	−
• Visual loss or abnormal pupillary reactivity*	−	+ (if severe: relative afferent pupillary defect, loss of color vision)
• Signs of cavernous sinus thrombosis, meningitis, or intracranial abscess formation	−	+ (if severe)

+ indicates present, - indicates absent.
*The three most important features.
Adapted from Gervasio KA, Friedberg MA, Rapuano CJ. Orbit; 7.3.1 Orbital Cellulitis. In: Gervasio KA, Peck TJ, Fathy CA, Sivalingam MD, eds. The Wills Eye Manual Office and Emergency Room Diagnosis and Treatment of Eye Disease. 8th ed. Wolters Kluwer; 2022:343–350.
Also adapted from Gervasio KA, Friedberg MA, Rapuano CJ. Eyelid; 6.10 Preseptal Cellulitis. In: Gervasio KA, Peck TJ, Fathy CA, Sivalingam MD, eds. The Wills Eye Manual Office and Emergency Room Diagnosis and Treatment of Eye Disease. 8th ed. Wolters Kluwer; 2022:318–323.

- Incomplete vaccination against *H. influenzae* type b (HIB)
- Toxic appearance and/or signs of meningitis
- Anorexia and/or inability to tolerate oral medications/antibiotics
- Presence of subcutaneous abscess
- Failure of outpatient management (no improvement within 24–48 hours of oral antibiotics)

18. **Describe the classic presentation and management of blepharitis.**
    - Patients may complain of ocular itching, burning, foreign body sensation, and eyelid margin crusting or erythema.
    - Management involves frequent warm compresses and twice-daily eyelid cleansing with commercial eyelid cleansers or dilute baby shampoo. Topical erythromycin ointment may also be used for more severe cases. Referral is indicated if these treatments fail to improve symptoms.

19. A 5-year-old child presents with acute foreign body sensation, photophobia, and redness after being poked in the eye by her younger sister. Fluorescein staining reveals a corneal abrasion. What is your management?
    - Treat with topical antibiotic drops or ointment (bacitracin/polymyxin B, ciprofloxacin, moxifloxacin, or erythromycin ophthalmic).
    - A fluoroquinolone should be used in the setting of injuries involving fingernails or vegetable matter.
    - If the abrasion is large, the patient should be seen by an ophthalmologist within 24 hours.
    - Contact lens wearers should be referred immediately to rule out sight-threatening corneal infection.

20. How do vertical linear corneal abrasions most commonly arise and how are they treated?
    The most common etiology is a retained foreign body within the upper eyelid, which causes a vertical abrasion pattern due to movement of the eyelid with blinking. The abrasions can be seen with fluorescein staining and a Wood lamp.
    Management typically involves anesthetizing the painful eye, followed by eversion of the eyelid using a cotton-tipped applicator to identify and remove the foreign body (using a wet cotton-tipped applicator). The eye should then be irrigated with saline. Topical antibiotics are then applied to the eye.
    Follow-up with ophthalmology within 48 hours is recommended if there is no improvement or sooner in the presence of a large corneal abrasion. An embedded corneal foreign body requires urgent referral.

21. What examination features suggest a penetrating eye injury or globe rupture and warrant immediate referral?
    - History of trauma, fall, or injury to the eye with a sharp object
    - Visual disturbance or loss
    - The appearance of an abnormally shaped or "peaked" pupil
    - Prolapsing brown material or fluid drainage from the eye
    - Presence of a hyphema (blood within the anterior chamber of the eye)
    - Subconjunctival hemorrhages that encircle 360 degrees around the cornea
    - The extent of injury may be difficult to assess in young children and may require a sedated exam. If in doubt, refer!

22. What steps should you take when preparing a patient with penetrating eye trauma for transfer/referral?
    - Avoid any eye manipulation or inspection once the penetrating eye trauma is confirmed.
    - Keep the patient NPO.
    - Consider administering an antiemetic or pain medications.
    - The patient should be on bed rest with avoidance of any strenuous activity or bending.
    - Apply a shield to the affected eye.
    - If no shield is available, a cut-down plastic foam or paper cup taped over the affected eye is an adequate substitute. The shield should not apply any pressure to the globe. Do not apply a patch.
    - Consider tetanus prophylaxis.
    - Contact the ophthalmology team/emergency department at the time of transfer.

KEY POINTS

Eye Examination Tips

1. Assess extraocular movements by getting the child to focus on a toy; both eyes should move equally in all directions as they follow the toy. There are multiple smartphone applications that can aid in this assessment by showing a moving shape with or without sound.
2. Determine the patient's gross visual acuity in each eye. This is an essential yet often forgotten component of the eye exam. Again, smartphone applications may be used to assess visual acuity and can help identify significant changes in vision that warrant urgent referral. However, these are often less accurate than traditional methods of assessing acuity used by optometrists/ophthalmologists.
3. Apply proparacaine or tetracaine drops to a fluorescein strip when staining a painful eye to avoid excessive discomfort from the drops and to successfully visualize ocular surface abrasions under a Wood lamp.
4. A cotton-tipped applicator can be used to evert a nontraumatized upper eyelid to look for embedded foreign bodies.

The Red Eye

1. The most common cause of pediatric acute conjunctivitis is a viral infection. COVID-19 infection can also present as acute conjunctivitis.
2. In the newborn, purulent conjunctivitis presenting from 2 days to 2 weeks of life must be investigated and treated for *N. gonorrhoeae* with cotreatment of *C. trachomatis*. Between the first 5–28 days of life, *Pseudomonas* infection can also be a causative agent.

3. Periocular vesicular lesions +/− a dendritic pattern seen on fluorescein staining of the cornea are signs of herpetic eye disease and warrant urgent initiation of an antiviral and referral to an ophthalmologist.
4. Vertical corneal abrasions are commonly caused by eyelid foreign bodies which may be identified and removed by eyelid eversion and irrigation in the nontraumatized eye.

Preseptal and Orbital Cellulitis

1. A hordeolum, insect bite, or eyelid trauma are predisposing factors for preseptal cellulitis.
2. Preseptal cellulitis can be treated with outpatient oral antibiotics. If there are concerns for orbital cellulitis, urgent referral to the emergency department is warranted for imaging and intravenous antibiotics.
3. Preseptal and orbital cellulitis are distinguished by the involvement of the orbital contents (globe, extraocular muscles, optic nerve) in the latter.

BIBLIOGRAPHY

Beal C, Giordano B. Clinical evaluation of red eyes in pediatric patients. *J Pediatr Health Care*. 2016. doi:10.1016/j.pedhc.2016.02.001.
Delaney AC, Levin AV. Eye: Red Eye. In: Shaw KN, Bachur RG, Chamberlain JM, Lavelle J, Nagler J, Shook JE, eds. *Fleisher & Ludwig's Textbook of Pediatric Emergency Medicine*. 7th ed. Wolters Kluwer; 2016:153–157.
Gervasio KA, Gervasio KA, Peck TJ, et al. In: Gervasio KA, Peck TJ, Fathy CA, Sivalingam MD, eds. *The Wills Eye Manual Office and Emergency Room Diagnosis and Treatment of Eye Disease*. 8th ed. Wolters Kluwer; 2022.
Kimberlin DW, Barnett ED, Lynfield R, Sawyer MH. Red Book: 2021–2024 Report of the Committee on Infectious Diseases, Committee on Infectious Diseases, American Academy of Pediatrics. *Neonatal Ophthalmia*. 2021.
Klein JO, Pelton S. Acute otitis media in children: Epidemiology, microbiology, clinical manifestations, and complications. UpToDate; 2016 Retrieved from UpToDate website.
Seth D, Khan FI. Causes and management of red eye in pediatric ophthalmology. *Curr Allergy Asthma Rep*. 2011;11(3):212–219. doi:10.1007/s11882-011-0186-7.
Teoh DL, Reynolds S. Diagnosis and management of pediatric conjunctivitis. *Pediatr Emerg Care*. 2003;19(1):48–55.
Upshaw JE, Brenkert TE, Losek JD. Ocular foreign bodies in children. *Pediatr Emerg Care*. 2008;24(6):409–414; quiz 415–407. doi:10.1097/PEC.0b013e318177a806.
Wald ER. Acute otitis media in children: Clinical manifestations and diagnosis. UpToDate; 2022. Retrieved from UpToDate website.
Wong MM, Anninger W. The pediatric red eye. *Pediatr Clin North Am*. 2014;61(3):591–606. doi:10.1016/j.pcl.2014.03.011.

CHAPTER 22

EAR PAIN, NASAL CONGESTION, AND SORE THROAT

Kaitlyn R. Swimmer, MD, Robert P. Olympia, MD

TOP SECRETS

1. With unilateral or bilateral purulent nasal discharge, always consider a foreign body.
2. The treatment of choice for otitis media, bacterial sinusitis, and GABHS pharyngitis is amoxicillin.

EAR PAIN

1. **A 3-year-old female patient presents to your urgent care center with a 2-day history of fever and right ear pain. What are the most likely etiologies and treatment recommendations for otalgia in a child?**
Acute Otitis Media
   - The second most common diagnosis in children after URIs.
   - Peak incidence of AOM occurs in the first 2 years.
   - Diagnosis: Infants with AOM may present with fever, upper respiratory symptoms (nasal congestion and cough), irritability, decreased appetite, and vomiting, while children and adolescents present with similar symptoms and complaints of significant unilateral or bilateral ear pain.
   - AOM should be diagnosed in children who present with:
      - Moderate to severe bulging of tympanic membrane (TM).
      - New onset otorrhea not due to otitis externa.
      - Decreased TM mobility observed on pneumatic insufflation.
   - AOM may be diagnosed in children who present with:
      - Mild bulging of the TM and <48 hours of otalgia (holding, tugging, or rubbing of the ear in a nonverbal child) or intense erythema of the TM.
   - Treatment: Antibiotics vs. watchful waiting (see Table 22.1 for treatment recommendations)
   - If tympanic membrane perforation or patent tympanostomy tube, otic topical antibiotic drops are recommended.
   Acute Otitis Externa, AKA "Swimmer's Ear"
   - Defining characteristics: tender, erythematous, and edematous ear canal; tenderness with pulling and pressure on the pinna; ear discharge, from clear, odorless to seropurulent, foul-smelling
   - The vast majority of AOE is caused by bacteria, with a mix of gram-positive and gram-negative microorganisms. Fungi is rarely the cause of AOE. Therefore, treatment should be geared toward covering for these, including pseudomonas (i.e., ofloxacin ear drops).
   - First-line treatment: Ofloxacin ear drop
   Acute Mastoiditis
   - Defining characteristics: postauricular swelling, erythema, and tenderness; the involved pinna is deviated outward and rotated forward.
   - Diagnosis is made by computed tomography (CT) scan of the head showing destruction of mastoid air cells, with or without abscess.
   - Requires inpatient admission for IV antibiotics
   Foreign body
      Treatment: Removal of foreign body

2. **How should I treat cerumen impaction?**
   - If asymptomatic, no need to disimpact.
   - If symptomatic, can disimpact in the ED or give instructions for earwax cleanout at home.

NASAL CONGESTION

3. **What are the diagnostic criteria for bacterial sinusitis?**
   - Persistent nasal discharge (of any quality) or daytime cough >10 days without improvement (+/− fever) ("persistent acute bacterial sinusitis"), or
   - Worsening or new onset of discharge, daytime cough, or fever after initial improvement ("worsening acute bacterial sinusitis"), or
   - Concurrent fever >39°C and purulent nasal discharge for at least 3 days ("severe acute bacterial sinusitis").

123

Table 22.1 Acute Otitis Media Treatment by Age and Severity

AGE	SEVERITY	SIGNS/ SYMPTOMS	TREATMENT RECOMMENDATIONS	LENGTH OF TREATMENT
6–23 months	Mild to moderate	Unilateral mild to moderate otalgia Otalgia <48 hrs Temp <39°C	Watchful waiting with close follow-up	
>24 months	Mild to moderate	Mild to moderate otalgia Otalgia <48 hrs Temp <39°C	Watchful waiting with close follow-up	
6–23 months	Moderate to severe	Moderate to severe otalgia Otalgia >48 hours Temp >39°C	1st line: Amoxicillin (90 mg/kg/day divided BID) *2nd line: Augmentin (90 mg/kg/day divided BID) **3rd line: Cefdinir (14 mg/kg/day QD) vs Ceftriaxone (50 mg/kg IM QD X 1–3 days)	10 days
>24 months	Moderate to severe	Moderate to severe otalgia Otalgia >48 hours Temp >39°C	1st line: Amoxicillin (90 mg/kg/day divided BID) *2nd line: Augmentin (90 mg/kg/day divided BID) **3rd line: Cefdinir(14 mg/kg/day QD) vs Ceftriaxone (50 mg/kg IM QD X 1–3 days)	5–7 days

*Indicated if amoxicillin within prior 30 days, concomitant purulent conjunctivitis, hx of recurrent AOM unresponsive to amoxicillin.
**Indicated if no improvement after 48–72 hrs on initial antibiotics.
Table created by Kaitlyn Swimmer. Data from: (McCormick et al., 2005) (Lieberthal et al., 2013).

4. How common is bacterial sinusitis in infants and children?
   Bacterial sinusitis is not a common diagnosis. Only approximately 6–7% of children with respiratory symptoms will develop clinical bacterial sinusitis as defined above. Since infants are born with maxillary and ethmoid sinuses, sinusitis can technically be diagnosed early in infancy. Sphenoid and frontal sinuses typically begin formation during school age and early adolescence.

5. What are the guidelines for treatment of bacterial sinusitis?
   - First line: Amoxicillin (90 mg/kg/day divided BID) x 10–14 days
   - Second line: Augmentin, cefdinir, cefuroxime, cefpodoxime, clarithromycin, azithromycin, clindamycin, and levofloxacin
   - If complicated sinusitis: Consider IV vancomycin + third-generation cephalosporin + metronidazole

6. What other treatment/symptom management options should be considered in a child with a diagnosis of bacterial or nonbacterial sinusitis?
   - Intranasal steroids (budesonide, flunisolide, fluticasone, mometasone)
   - Saline irrigation
   - Nasal decongestants
   - Mucolytics
   - Antihistamines

7. When should you send a child or adolescent with suspected sinusitis to the emergency department for diagnostic imaging, intravenous antibiotics, and/or hospitalization?
   - Diagnostic imaging studies should *not* be routinely used to distinguish acute bacterial sinusitis from a viral URI.
   - A contrast-enhanced CT scan of the sinuses is indicated if:
     a. There are signs of complicated sinusitis (concerns for orbital abscess, optic neuritis, epidural or subdural empyema, cavernous or sagittal sinus thrombosis, meningitis, brain abscess, osteomyelitis)
     b. Numerous recurrences
     c. Protracted or unresponsive course
     d. Anticipated surgical drainage (failure to respond to multiple courses of antibiotics, severe facial pain, orbital or intracranial complications, immunocompromised child or adolescent).
   - Other indications for referral include evidence of sepsis, significant dehydration, or inability to tolerate oral antibiotics.

8. You have ruled out bacterial sinusitis and other bacterial infections (AOM or pneumonia). Should an infant, child, or adolescent with nasal congestion, with or without cough, ever be treated with antibiotics?

   No. There are many recent studies documenting the overuse of antibiotics for viral infections. This practice may lead to resistance of bacterial organisms to common antibiotics later in life.

9. In addition to URI or sinusitis, what should be on your differential diagnosis in a child with persistent nasal congestion?
   - With unilateral or bilateral purulent nasal discharge, always consider a foreign body.
   - With persistent clear nasal discharge, consider seasonal allergies (allergic rhinitis). Symptoms of allergic rhinitis may include paroxysms of sneezing, rhinorrhea, nasal obstruction, nasal itching, postnasal drip, cough, irritability, and fatigue.
   - Treatment includes:
     (a) Children under 2 years: cromolyn sodium nasal spray, second-generation oral antihistamines (cetirizine and fexofenadine approved for children over 6 months of age)
     (b) Children over 2 years: second-generation oral antihistamine, antihistamine nasal spray (azelastine approved for >5 years, olopatadine for >12 years of age), glucocorticoid nasal spray (mometasone, fluticasone, triamcinolone approved for >2 years of age).

10. A child presents to your urgent care center after getting elbowed in the face and has significant nasal swelling and epistaxis. Should you order an x-ray of the nasal bones?

    Despite a fracture to the nasal bone, most pediatric otolaryngologists do not recommend acute management of the fracture, regardless of displacement. Therefore, delayed imaging and otolaryngology referral is recommended (after 3–4 days) if the patient has difficulty breathing through his nostrils or if significant deformity persists.

11. How should you treat epistaxis in your urgent care center?

    Ask the child or guardian to pinch the tip of the nose for several minutes, holding the head forward, as most nosebleeds arise anteriorly. If the bleeding persists, consider inserting a roll of cotton saturated with a topical decongestant (oxymetazoline or adrenaline) in the affected side and squeezing the nose gently for 5 minutes. If the bleeding is visible, cauterize it with silver nitrate. For persistent bleeding >15 minutes or suspicion for a posterior nosebleed (no obvious site is visible anteriorly, bleeding from both nostrils, blood in the posterior pharynx), pack the nose and send the child to an emergency department to see otolaryngology.

12. What is a nasal septal hematoma?

    Nasal septal hematomas are bluish "grapelike" protrusions from the nasal septum associated with trauma. These hematomas should be immediately drained and packed if detected; failure to drain these hematomas may lead to cosmetic deformities.

SORE THROAT

13. What are the most likely etiologies and recommended treatments for sore throat in a child?
    - Viral pharyngitis accounts for 40% of cases of tonsillopharyngitis and is most common in children <5 years old.
      a. Typically self-limiting
    - Bacterial pharyngitis accounts for 15–30% of cases of tonsillopharyngitis. Most common in children 5–15 years old. Very uncommon in children <3 years old! The most common organism is GABHS.
      a. Antibiotic (recommendations in Table 22.2)
      b. Symptomatic management: one dose of oral dexamethasone (0.6 mg/kg)
    - Other: 30–45% of cases of tonsillopharyngitis. Often irritation from postnasal drip. Commonly, this type of sore throat is worse in the morning and gets better throughout the day. Treatment should be geared towards preventing postnasal drip (antihistamine, fluticasone nasal spray).

Table 22.2 Therapeutic Options for GABHS Pharyngitis

PREFERENCE	MEDICATION	DOSAGE	DURATION
1st Line	Amoxicillin	50 mg/kg/dose QD	10 days
2nd Line	Cephalexin	20 mg/kg/dose BID	10 days
3rd Line	Azithromycin	12 mg/kg/dose QD	5 days
	Clindamycin	7 mg/kg/dose TID	10 days
	Clarithromycin	7.5 mg/kg/dose BID	10 days

Table created by Kaitlyn Swimmer. Data from: (Shulman, Bisno, & Clegg, 2012).

14. How do I decide whether to test for and/or treat GABHS pharyngitis?
    - Centor Criteria
        a. Absence of cough (1 point)
        b. Swollen/tender anterior cervical adenopathy (1 point)
        c. Temp >100.4°F (1 point)
        d. Tonsillar exudate/swelling (1 point)
        e. Age 3–14 (1 point)
    - See Fig. 22.1 for recommendations based on total centor criteria points.

15. In a child with suspected GABHS pharyngitis, what are some other common physical exam findings?
    - Scarlatiniform rash is the most common. It appears as a generalized erythema with scattered papules, "sandpaper-like," increased in the folds of the neck, axilla, antecubital, popliteal, and inguinal regions, with subsequent desquamation.
    - Generalized petechiae or urticaria
    - Abdominal pain due to mesenteric adenitis. Enlargement of lymph nodes in the abdominal cavity (can be in RLQ, mimicking appendicitis).

16. Why should I treat GABHS Pharyngitis?
    Antibiotic treatment for GABHS is only to reduce the risk of rheumatic fever; antibiotic therapy does not affect the duration of symptoms, nor does it prevent poststreptococcal glomerulonephritis.

17. When should you refer a child or adolescent with "sore throat" to the emergency department?
    - Concern for meningitis, retropharyngeal abscess (school-age child with fever, stiff neck, "hot potato" voice, sore throat, drooling, dysphagia), or peritonsillar abscess (older child or adolescent with fever, severe unilateral sore throat, drooling, trismus, dysphagia, deviated uvula)
    - Severe dehydration requiring IV fluids
    - Trauma, burns, or foreign body–associated sore throat
    - Concerns for rheumatic fever

18. How long are GABHS patients contagious after starting antibiotics?
    24 hours

19. How do you make the diagnosis of rheumatic fever?
    Jones criteria. Two major criteria, or one major and two minor criteria, PLUS evidence of an antecedent streptococcal pharyngitis (throat culture, RADT, antistreptolysin O, anti-deoxyribonuclease B).
    Major criteria: carditis, migratory polyarthritis, chorea, erythema marginatum, subcutaneous nodules.
    Minor criteria: fever, arthralgias, elevated acute phase reactants (sedimentation rate, C-reactive protein), prolonged PR interval.

20. Why should you care about infectious mononucleosis?
    Children and adolescents who have infectious mononucleosis (fever and other constitutional symptoms, severe sore throat, enlarged tonsils with exudates) may develop splenomegaly. Therefore, a clinical suspicion for infectious mononucleosis in a child or adolescent who is physically active or participates in sports should be tested. If positive, the child should have frequent subsequent examinations to rule out splenomegaly.

21. Is the Monospot always positive in infectious mononucleosis?
    The heterophile antibody test (Monospot) is not always positive during early infectious mononucleosis (first 2 weeks of symptoms) and in young children. Therefore, Epstein-Barr virus (EBV) titers should be ordered in these two scenarios.

22. What is hand, foot, and mouth disease?
    Hand, foot, and mouth disease presents with oral ulcerations (located frequently in the posterior oropharynx in contrast to herpes simplex virus [HSV], which tends to present with vesicles in a more anterior location) along with small erythematous macules, papules, or vesicles on an erythematous base, commonly on hands, feet, and buttocks, but also generalized in infants. Systemic symptoms such as fever, URI, vomiting, or diarrhea may also occur. Since coxsackievirus A16 is the most common cause, presentations often occur during late summer and early fall. Treatment is symptomatic.

23. When should I be concerned for airway obstruction in a child?
    - Signs of respiratory distress include tachypnea, retractions, nasal flaring, tripoding, head bobbing, inability to lay down, and stridor.
    - Stridor at rest: if inspiratory stridor, think extrathoracic or upper airway obstruction (can be due to croup/laryngotracheitis, laryngomalacia, epiglottitis, anaphylaxis, or foreign body ingestion). If expiratory stridor, think intrathoracic or lower airway obstruction.
    - Suspect foreign body aspiration in a child who is between toddler and preschool age; was last seen with a small, hard object; and has sudden onset of cough, choke, or wheeze.
    - Stabilize with supplemental oxygen, positional changes, racemic epinephrine, and nasal/OP suctioning.

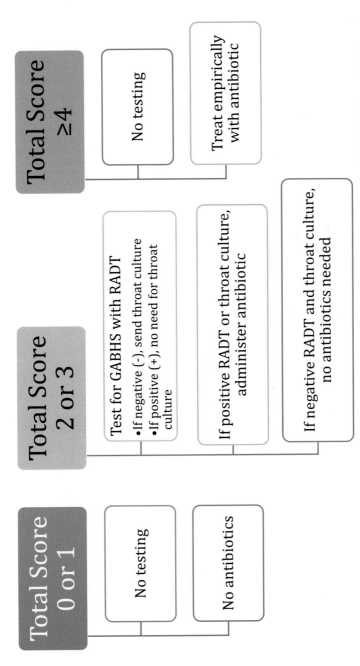

Fig. 22.1 Flowchart for guiding decisions regarding testing and treatment for GABHS pharyngitis based on Centor Criteria scores. (Figure created by Kaitlyn Swimmer. Data from Shulman, Bisno, & Clegg, 2012.)

KEY POINTS

1. Consider watchful waiting for mild AOM in children >6 months old.
2. With unilateral or bilateral purulent nasal discharge, always consider a foreign body.
3. Bacterial sinusitis is rare in children; more likely allergic/viral and likely does not need antibiotics.
4. Rheumatic fever does not occur in children less than 3 years of age; therefore, young children in this age group should not be tested or treated for GABHS pharyngitis.
5. The treatment of choice for otitis media, bacterial sinusitis, and GABHS pharyngitis is amoxicillin.

BIBLIOGRAPHY

Acosta R. Rhinosinusitis. In *Pediatric Emergency Medicine*. Philadelphia: Saunders Elsevier; 2008:405–408.

Bartlett A, Williams R, Hilton M. Splenic rupture in infectious mononucleosis: a systematic review of published case reports. *Injury*. 2016;47(3):531–538. https://doi.org/10.1016/j.injury.2015.10.071.

Gao L, Zou G, Liao Q, Zhou Y, Liu F, Dai B, et al. Spectrum of enterovirus serotypes causing uncomplicated hand, foot, and mouth disease and enteroviral diagnostic yield of different clinical samples. *Clin. Iinfect. Diseas.* 2018;67(11):1729–1735. https://doi.org/10.1093/cid/ciy341.

Gewitz MH, Baltimore RS, Tani LY, Sable CA, Shulman ST, Carapetis J, et al. American Heart Association Committee on Rheumatic Fever, Endocarditis, and Kawasaki Disease of the Council on Cardiovascular Disease in the Young. Revision of the Jones Criteria for the diagnosis of acute rheumatic fever in the era of Doppler echocardiography: a scientific statement from the American Heart Association. *Circulation*. 2015;131(20):1806–1818. https://doi.org/10.1161/CIR.0000000000000205.

Ida JB, Thompson DM. Pediatric stridor. *Otolaryngologic Clinics of North America*. 47 (5):795–819.

Jalaludin MA. Nasal septal abscess: retrospective analysis of 14 cases from University Hospital, Kuala Lumpur. *Singapore Medical Journal*. 1993;34(5):435–437.

Kalan A, Tariq M. Foreign bodies in the nasal cavities: a comprehensive review of the aetiology, diagnostic pointers, and therapeutic measures. *Postgraduate Medical Journal*. 2000;76(898):484–487. https://doi.org/10.1136/pmj.76.898.484.

King BR. An evidence-based approach to the evaluation and treatment of pharyngitis in children. *Pediatric Emerg Med Pract*. 2007;4:1.

Lieberthal AS, Carroll AE, Chonmaitree T, et al. The diagnosis and management of acute otitis media. *Pediatrics*. 2013;131(3):964–999.

Marshall-Andon T, Heinz P. How to use ... the Monospot and other heterophile antibody tests. *Archives of Disease in Childhood*. 2017;102(4):188–193. https://doi.org/10.1136/archdischild-2016-311526.

McCormick DP, Chonmaitree T, Pittman C, et al. Nonsevere acute otitis media: a clinical trial comparing outcomes of watchful waiting versus immediate antibiotic treatment. *Pediatrics*. 2005;115(6):1455–1465.

Olympia RP, Khine H, Avner JR. The effectiveness of oral dexamethasone in the treatment of moderate to severe pharyngitis in children and young adults. *Archives of Pediatrics and Adolescent Medicine*. 2005:278–282.

Rosenfeld RM, Schwartz SR, Cannon CR, et al. Clinical practice guidelines: acute otitis externa. *Otolaryngology – Head and Neck Surgery*. 150(1_suppl):S1–S24.

Shulman S, Bisno A, Clegg A. Clinical practice guideline for the diagnosis and management of group A streptococcal pharyngitis: 2012 update by the Infectious Diseases Society of America. *Clinical Infectious Diseases*. 2012;55(10):1279–1282.

Svider P, Arianpour K, Mutchnick S. Management of epistaxis in children and adolescents: avoiding a chaotic approach. *Pediatric Clinics of North America*. 2018;65(3):607–621.

van den Aardweg MT, Rovers MM, de Ru JA, Albers FW, Schilder AG. A systematic review of diagnostic criteria for acute mastoiditis in children. *Otology & Neurotology*. 2008;29(6):751–757. https://doi.org/10.1097/MAO.0b013e31817f736b.

Wald E, Applegate K, Bordley C. Clinical practice guideline for the diagnosis and management of acute bacterial sinusitis in children aged 1–18 years. *Pediatrics*. 2013;132:262–280.

CHAPTER 23

NECK PAIN AND MASSES

Leah Kaye, MD, FAAP

TOP SECRETS

1. Refer patients with congenital muscular torticollis to PT as early as possible.
2. Ultrasound is the preferred imaging for a palpable neck mass

1. A 2-year-old boy presents to urgent care for a lump on his neck. He has been well besides upper respiratory infection (URI) symptoms 2 weeks ago, with no fever, weight loss, trouble breathing, or change in activity level or behavior. He has a 2-cm palpable lymph node in the anterior cervical chain. What characteristics suggest it is benign?
   Lymph node size <3 cm, no/mild erythema, no/mild tenderness, and no generalized lymphadenopathy. Children under 2 are also more likely to have reactive lymphadenopathy.

2. What node characteristics raise concern for malignancy?
   Location: supraclavicular nodes are malignant until proven otherwise. Nodes in the posterior triangle (behind or lateral to the sternocleidomastoid) are suspicious. Beware hard, irregular, firm, or rubbery nodes, or those that feel fixed to deep tissues. Fever, malaise, weight loss, or night sweats (B symptoms) raise concern for malignancy. Large nodes (initial size >3 cm) are more likely to be malignant, especially in the absence of signs of infection. Node persistence >6 weeks or increasing size during antibiotic therapy is concerning. Older children (5–18 years) are more likely to have malignant lateral neck masses than younger children. Patients may require a biopsy to evaluate for malignancy or other rare disorders such as Kikuchi disease (histolytic necrotizing lymphadenitis).

3. What imaging should I choose first for a palpable neck mass?
   Ultrasound. If you are concerned for deep mass, you cannot palpate. If the patient presents with difficulty breathing, difficulty swallowing, or significant limitation of range of motion, transfer for computed tomography (CT).

4. What are the most common organisms causing bacterial lymphadenitis?
   Staphylococcus aureus and group A streptococcus. Use cephalexin, amoxicillin-clavulanate, or clindamycin if you are starting empiric antibiotics. History should include pets (cat scratch fever), outdoor exposure (Lyme disease), and dental concerns (poor dentition or periodontal disease resulting in anaerobic infection). Fever is not always present. A small percentage will have return visits and require ED transfer for IV antibiotics, especially children under 1 year. Lymphadenitis not improving with IV antibiotics is concerning for atypical mycobacterium.

5. A 5-year-old presents with a neck lump x 7 days. He has had fatigue, poor appetite, and malaise for 10 days. The family adopted a kitten 4 weeks ago. He has a swollen, tender, indurated, warm right cervical lymph node. What diagnosis do you consider?
   Cat scratch disease (CSD; Bartonella henselae). CSD is transmitted via scratch or bite of an infected cat. Many patients do not recall an initial scratch. A papule or pustule on the skin often develops days after inoculation, followed by lymphadenopathy 1–2 weeks later. Approximately 25% of cases involve lymphadenopathy of the head or neck. Symptoms include fever, malaise, anorexia, headache, myalgia, arthralgia, arthritis, or vision changes. A third will have lymphadenopathy at other sites, and 15% will have splenomegaly.

6. What is the treatment for cat scratch disease?
   Most cases spontaneously resolve in 1–2 months; 10% of nodes will spontaneously suppurate. Use antibiotics (typically azithromycin) for acutely or severely ill immunocompetent patients, those with retinitis, hepatic, splenic involvement, or painful adenitis. Avoid incision and drainage (I&D) of the node to lessen the risk of fistula. All immunocompromised patients should be treated. You do not need to treat the cat with antibiotics, but cats should be treated for fleas, which carry the bacteria.

7. How can I tell a thyroglossal duct cyst from a dermoid cyst?
   Both are in the midline ventral neck. Thyroglossal duct cysts elevate when the tongue is protruded or the patient swallows. Dermoid cysts move with the movement of the overlying skin.

8. A 6-year-old female presents with a third episode of neck swelling and tenderness in one year. Infections resolve completely, then recur. What should you consider?
   Recurrent swelling or infection at the same location on the neck is suspicious for a branchial cleft cyst or thyroglossal duct cyst. Location is the key difference. Midline: thyroglossal duct cyst. Lateral neck: branchial cleft cyst. These may also present with recurrent swelling near the ear or recurrent parotid abscess.

9. **A 7-year-old febrile male is rushed in with stridor, respiratory distress, and drooling. He appears toxic and anxious and nods urgently when asked about a sore throat. He holds his neck hyperextended with his nose pointed up. He developed a sore throat 3 hours ago. What are you concerned for and what should you do?**
Acute onset of sore throat and fever with rapid progression to drooling, stridor, anxiety, and maintaining the "sniffing" position is concerning for epiglottitis. Other symptoms include dysphagia, "hot potato"/muffled voice, and tenderness to palpation over the hyoid bone. Transfer to the emergency department immediately for urgent ear, nose, and throat (ENT) and anesthesia consult to arrange emergent intubation in the operating room (OR). Defer diagnostics (labs, intravenous [IV] placement, imaging) to avoid worsening respiratory distress. The classic "thumb sign" on lateral neck x-ray (severe edema of the epiglottis) has poor sensitivity and specificity. Humidified oxygen or racemic epinephrine may be used while awaiting transport. Treat with a second- or third-generation cephalosporin. Etiologies include group A strep, S. aureus, Klebsiella pneumoniae, H. parainfluenzae, Moraxella, Neisseria, Pseudomonas, and beta-hemolytic strep. H. flu type b, while less common in the post-Hib vaccination era, is still a potential cause.

10. **A 3-year-old patient presents with new-onset torticollis, fever, and irritability. What should you rule out?**
Retropharyngeal abscess.

11. **What are the common symptoms of retropharyngeal abscess?**
Fever, restricted neck movements, neck pain, and cervical lymphadenopathy. Others include drooling, trismus, torticollis, neck swelling, and dysphagia. Respiratory distress is rare. Of all cases, 80% occur in children under 5. Risk factors include recent URI or recent oropharyngeal trauma. Complications include sepsis, mediastinitis, necrotizing fasciitis, airway obstruction, internal jugular vein thrombosis, and carotid artery aneurysms.

12. **What imaging should you order if concerned for retropharyngeal abscess?**
Is there any respiratory distress? If so, transfer to the emergency department for urgent CT and surgical consult. If not, obtain lateral neck x-rays with neck extension to look for widening of the soft tissues (prevertebral space).
   Are the x-rays normal and the airway intact? Consider other diagnoses.
   Are the x-rays concerning? Transfer for CT and/or ENT consult.

13. **A 15-year-old male presents with a sore throat x 5 days, new-onset neck swelling, fever, shortness of breath, and rigors. He is tender to palpation along his lateral left neck. Rapid strep is negative. What testing should you consider next?**
This presentation is concerning for Lemierre syndrome (septic thrombophlebitis or thrombosis of the internal jugular), commonly caused by fusobacterium. Although uncommon, it carries a high mortality rate. It occurs by the spread of a primary parapharyngeal infection (sore throat), which spreads internally to the jugular and can cause septic embolization. There is often pain out of proportion to the exam. Obtain a neck ultrasound to examine the jugular.

14. **A 15-year-old female presents with sore throat x 8 days, fever, and new left ear and neck pain. The past 2 days it "feels like swallowing glass," and her voice sounds strange. On exam, her uvula is deviated to the right, with left-sided tender cervical lymphadenopathy and foul breath. What do you suspect and what testing should you order?**
Peritonsillar abscess (PTA), which is a collection of pus behind the tonsil in the superior arch of the soft palate. PTA typically presents with a sore throat, fever, malaise, dysphagia, muffled/"hot potato" voice, or referred ear pain. It can be a complication of treated or untreated strep pharyngitis. It is most common in older children and adolescents. The most common etiology is group A strep, but it can be polymicrobial including aerobes and anaerobes. On exam, the uvula typically deviates away from the affected side. There can be lymphadenopathy on the affected side, drooling, foul-smelling breath, trismus, muffled voice, and fever. Transfer for imaging and ENT consult.

15. **An 18-month-old presents 2 days after completing a 10-day course of antibiotics for otitis media. He is still febrile, and his left ear is red. On exam, he has left ear proptosis, postauricular swelling, and a bulging left tympanic membrane. What should you do next?**
Send to the emergency department for CT with contrast to evaluate for mastoiditis. Treatment includes IV antibiotics, ENT consult, and sometimes surgical drainage. It is most common in children under 2 years.

16. **What are the presenting symptoms, causes, and treatment of acute infectious parotitis?**
Parotitis typically presents with swelling, pain, and erythema over the parotid gland (acute swelling of the cheek that extends to the angle of the mandible). Other symptoms include fever, trismus, and pain with mastication. It is typically unilateral, or if bilateral, one side is significantly worse. Causes can be divided into viral, bacterial, autoimmune, and idiopathic (Table 23.1). If suppurative, treat with oral antibiotics. In all cases, use hydration, warm massage, and sialagogues (such as sour candy or sour foods).

Table 23.1 Causes of Parotitis

Viral	Mumps (paramyxovirus), Epstein-Barr, parainfluenza, HIV, influenza A, Coxsackie, adenovirus, CMV, parvovirus B19
Bacterial	Most common: S. aureus, S. viridans, H. influenzae, Peptostreptococcus, S. pneumoniae, E. coli, bacteroides, actinomyces, Bartonella, mycobacterium
Autoimmune	Sjögren syndrome, juvenile idiopathic arthritis (JIA), IgA deficiency, rheumatoid arthritis, sarcoidosis
Idiopathic	Juvenile recurrent parotitis: 5% caused by recurrent stones; otherwise idiopathic. Salivary stones are rare in children.

17. A 3-week-old's parents feel a mass over the right side of their son's neck. His head is always tilted right. He is otherwise well appearing and afebrile with no history of trauma. On exam, you note a tight sternocleidomastoid on the right with a smooth, well-circumscribed mass in the inferior third of the muscle. The child's head is tilted to the right. His chin is pointed left. What is the most likely diagnosis?

    Congenital muscular torticollis (CMT). Torticollis is a twisting of the head and neck caused by shortening of the sternocleidomastoid. It can be divided into paroxysmal (episodic) and nonparoxysmal (static, unchanging) causes (Table 23.2).

Table 23.2 Causes of Torticollis

Nonparoxysmal Torticollis	
Congenital muscular torticollis	Fibrosed hematoma or developmental fibroma in the sternocleidomastoid starts to shrink, shortening the sternocleidomastoid and producing torticollis. Associated with craniofacial asymmetry.
Osseous torticollis	Congenital: Klippel-Feil syndrome, congenital atlantoaxial dislocation, ligamentous laxity (e.g., Marfan), achondroplasia, Morquio syndrome Traumatic: cervical spine trauma causing atlantoaxial subluxation, vertebral fractures Inflammatory: cervical adenitis, otitis media, Grisel syndrome* CNS: posterior fossa tumor, basal ganglia injury (HIE), spinal cord tumors Peripheral nerve: brachial plexus injury
Ocular torticollis	CN IV palsy; tilting head to minimize diplopia Spasmus nutans
Soft tissue infections	Cervical adenitis, retropharyngeal abscess, sternocleidomastoid myositis
Paroxysmal Torticollis	
Benign paroxysmal torticollis	Self-limited, rare, presents at 2 weeks to 4.5 months Recurrent torticollis, vomiting, pallor, irritability, ataxia, drowsiness. Torticollis can alternate sides with different attacks Starts to improve at 2 years; usually resolves by age 3 Family history of migraine is common No treatment; can consider antiemetics
Sandifer syndrome	Gastroesophageal reflux with abnormal posturing. Look for reflux symptoms such as regurgitation, anorexia, irritability, FTT, cough Treat with reflux therapy and reflux precautions
Acute dystonic reaction	Common causes: antiemetics, neuroleptics, antidepressants, antihistamines, anticonvulsants, cough suppressants, anticholinergics, drugs of abuse Treatment: removal of the drug, diphenhydramine
Increased ICP	Pseudotumor cerebri

CN, Cranial nerve; *CNS*, central nervous system; *FTT*, failure to thrive; *HIE*, hypoxic-ischemic encephalopathy; *ICP*, intracranial pressure.
*Nontraumatic atlantoaxial subluxation from inflammatory ligamentous laxity following an infectious process.

18. **What kind of imaging should I order for afebrile new-onset torticollis?**
Consider ultrasound to better delineate the mass and rule out tumor, and radiographs of the cervical spine to look for C1-C2 subluxation. MRI or CT should be used only for suspected intracranial pathology.

19. **What is the treatment for the patient with congenital muscular torticollis?**
Referral to physical therapy to learn positioning techniques and stretching exercises, starting as young as possible. The majority of children improve with physical therapy. If there is no improvement in 6 months, their provider may refer them to surgery.

20. **A child with trisomy 21 keeps his head tilted toward the left. On exam, he has a tight, tender sternocleidomastoid on the right. What are you concerned for?**
Atlantoaxial instability. The difference in tilt (head tilted away from the tight sternocleidomastoid, not toward) is a key clue to steer you away from congenital muscular torticollis. Another concerning factor is the patient's history of trisomy 21, which is associated with atlantoaxial dislocation. Look for tenderness of the spinous process of the axis as well.

21. **What should you order if you are concerned for atlantoaxial instability?**
Start with cervical spine radiographs. Head CT may be necessary for confirmation. Patients will need a spine consult.

KEY POINTS

1. Supraclavicular lymph nodes are concerning for malignancy.
2. Ear proptosis and fever are concerning for mastoiditis.
3. Absence of respiratory distress does not rule out retropharyngeal abscess.
4. Upper limb, gait, or cranial nerve abnormalities, or signs of increased intracranial pressure with torticollis are concerning for posterior fossa tumor.
5. Avoid I&D of the node in cat scratch disease, as it increases the risk of fistula.

BIBLIOGRAPHY

Abudinen-Vasquez S, Marin MN. Management of pediatric head and neck infections in the emergency department. *Pediatr Emerg Med Pract.* 2020;17(11):1–24. Epub 2020.

Aladag Ciftdemir N, Eren T, Ciftdemir M. A rare cause of torticollis: Grisel syndrome. *Journal of Tropical Pediatrics.* 2017;64(3):245–248. doi:10.1093/tropej/fmx050.

Akhavan M. Ear, Nose, Throat. *Emergency Medicine Clinics of North America.* Published online June 2021. doi:10.1016/j.emc.2021.04.012.

Chafin JB, Bayazid L. Pediatric salivary gland disease. *Pediatric Clinics of North America.* 2022;69(2):363–380. doi:10.1016/j.pcl.2022.01.004.

Dayasiri K, Rao S. Fifteen-minute consultation: evaluation of paediatric torticollis. Archives of Disease in Childhood—Education & Practice Edition. Published online November 19, 2021:edpract-2020-319668. doi:10.1136/archdischild-2020-319668.

Dowdy RAE, Cornelius BW. Medical management of epiglottitis. *Anesthesia Progress.* 2020;67(2):90–97. doi:10.2344/anpr-66-04-08.

Esposito S, De Guido C, Pappalardo M, et al. Retropharyngeal, parapharyngeal and peritonsillar abscesses. *Children (Basel).* 2022;9(5):618. doi:10.3390/children9050618.

Greene KA, Lu V, Luciano MS, et al. Benign paroxysmal torticollis: phenotype, natural history, and quality of life. *Pediatric Research.* 2021;90(5):1044–1051. doi:10.1038/s41390-020-01309-1.

Ho ML. Pediatric neck masses. *Radiologic Clinics of North America.* 2022;60(1):1–14. doi:10.1016/j.rcl.2021.08.001.

King SK. Lateral neck lumps: a systematic approach for the general paediatrician. *J Paediatr Child Health.* 2017;53(11):1091–1095. doi:10.1111/jpc.13755.

Long M, Reddy DN, Akiki S, Barrowman NJ, Zemek R. Paediatric acute lymphadenitis: emergency department management and clinical course. Paediatrics & Child Health. Published online September 21, 2019. doi:10.1093/pch/pxz125.

Masab M, Surmachevska N, Farooq H. Kikuchi disease 2022 Jun 27. StatPearls [Internet]. Treasure Island (FL): StatPearls Publishing; 2022.

Nelson CA, Moore AR, Perea AE, Mead PS. Cat scratch disease: US clinicians' experience and knowledge. *Zoonoses and Public Health.* 2017;56(1):67–73. doi:10.1111/zph.12368.

Okura Y, Shimomura M, Nawate M, Takahashi Y, Kobayashi I. Age-related clinical manifestation of suppurative cervical lymphadenitis in children. *Clinical Pediatrics.* 2022;61(8):530–534. doi:10.1177/00099228221095939.

Patel PN, Levi JR, Cohen MB. Lemierre's syndrome in the pediatric population: trends in disease presentation and management in literature. *International Journal of Pediatric Otorhinolaryngology.* 2020;136:110213. doi:10.1016/j.ijporl.2020.110213.

Sargent B, Kaplan SL, Coulter C, Baker C. Congenital muscular torticollis: bridging the gap between research and clinical practice. *Pediatrics.* 2019;144(2):e20190582. doi:10.1542/peds.2019-0582.

Zangwill KM. Cat scratch disease and Bartonellaceae. *Pediatric Infectious Disease Journal.* 2021;40(5S):S11–S15. doi:10.1097/inf.0000000000002776.

CHAPTER 24

COUGH

Saamia Masoom, MD, Sarah D. Meskill, MD, MS

TOP SECRETS

1. The differential diagnosis for pediatric cough is broad, and most etiologies are self-limited. Perform a detailed history and physical exam to differentiate mild symptoms from dangerous complications.
2. The mainstay for most cases of pediatric cough is supportive care: encourage hydration, monitor urine output, suction as needed, and treat fever with antipyretics. Additional treatments may be added based on clinical indication.

1. **A 5-year-old boy presents to your urgent care center with a 2-day history of persistent cough associated with fever, runny nose, and trouble breathing. What is your differential diagnosis?**
   Cough is one of the most common pediatric complaints with a myriad of causes (Table 24.1). Although the etiology of cough is usually self-limited, a detailed history and physical exam can exclude other potentially dangerous conditions.

2. **A 10-year-old girl with a history of asthma presents to your urgent care center with shortness of breath and difficulty speaking. She is tachypneic with intercostal retractions. What is the first-line treatment for an acute asthma exacerbation?**
   Acute exacerbations of asthma should be treated with systemic corticosteroids, high-dose beta-agonists, and anticholinergics. Timeliness of medication administration is a key principle in the management of acute asthma exacerbations, as studies have shown decreased length of stay, hospitalization, and symptom scores with early

Table 24.1 Differential Causes of Cough

AIRWAY NEOPLASM	CONGENITAL ANOMALIES	INFECTIOUS ETIOLOGY	INFLAMMATION/ IRRITATION	OTHERS
Hemangioma	Cleft palate	Bronchiolitis	Allergic rhinitis	Otic foreign body
Lymphoma	Laryngotracheomalacia	Bronchitis	Asthma	Medications (ACE inhibitors)
Mediastinal tumors	Laryngeal webs	Bronchiectasis	Cystic fibrosis	Psychogenic
Papilloma	Pulmonary sequestration	Croup	Congestive heart failure	Swallowing dysfunction
Polyps	Tracheoesophageal fistula	Laryngitis	Chemical fumes/ particulates	Vasculitis (granulomatosis with polyangiitis)
	Tracheal webs	Pleural effusion	Foreign body	Vocal cord dysfunction
	Vascular rings/slings	Pleuritis	Gastroesophageal reflux	
		Pulmonary abscess	Granulomatous disease	
		Tonsillitis	Smoking	
		Tuberculosis		
		Sinusitis		
		Upper respiratory infection		

ACE, Angiotensin-converting enzyme inhibitors.

Table 24.2 Acute Asthma Exacerbation Medication Dosing

	Short-Acting Beta$_2$ Agonists		
	Nebulizer		
WEIGHT (KG)	UNIT DOSE (0.5%)	CONTINUOUS	MDI PUFFS
<5	1.25 mg (0.25 mL)	5 mg/hr	2
5–10	2.5 mg (0.5 mL)	10 mg/hr	4
10–20	3.75 mg (0.75 mL)	15 mg/hr	6
>20	5 mg (1 mL)	20 mg/hr	8
	Ipratropium Bromide		
5–10	250 mcg	Up to 3 doses	
>10	500 mcg		
	Systemic Corticosteroids		
Prednisone (5-day course)	2 mg/kg	Max 60 mg	po
Dexamethasone (IM or PO, q24h x 2)	0.6 mg/kg	Max 8–16 mg	po, IM

Table 24.3 Differential Causes of Wheezing

INFECTIOUS/ INFLAMMATORY	INTRALUMINAL OBSTRUCTION	EXTRALUMINAL OBSTRUCTION
Bronchiolitis	Foreign body	Vascular ring/sling
Bronchopulmonary dysplasia	Congestive heart failure	Cystic malformation of lung
Cystic fibrosis	Alpha-antitrypsin deficiency	Congenital lobar emphysema
Pneumonia	Cholinergic poisoning	Masses (tumor, papilloma, hemangioma)
Aspiration (GERD, TEF)	Vocal cord dysfunction	

GERD, Gastroesophageal reflux disease; *TEF*, tracheoesophageal fistula.

administration of oral steroids, such as in triage. Combined treatment regimens take several hours to reach peak effect; thus, timeliness is key (Table 24.2).

3. **Is dexamethasone an effective alternative to oral prednisone in the treatment of pediatric asthma exacerbations?**
Yes. Providers should consider a two-dose regimen of dexamethasone as an alternative to a 5-day course of prednisone/prednisolone in the acute management of asthma exacerbations (see Table 24.2).

4. **Should I order a chest x-ray in a child with an acute asthma exacerbation?**
Chest x-rays (CXRs) are of limited use in the evaluation of a patient with asthma and rarely lead to a change in management. CXRs should be limited to cases where there is a clinical suspicion of a radiographic abnormality, such as persistent rales and asymmetry of breath sounds, high fever, crepitus in the neck, very poor response to therapy, or sudden deterioration. A CXR may be helpful in distinguishing from other causes of wheezing in early childhood (Table 24.3).

5. **What are historical risk factors for high-risk/fatal asthma that I should consider when dispositioning my patient?**
   - Prior intubation or intensive care unit (ICU) admission
   - Greater than two hospitalizations in past year
   - Greater than three emergency department visits in past year
   - Use of more than two beta-agonist canisters per month
   - Comorbid conditions
   - Emergency department visit or hospitalization in past month
   - Past history of severe sudden exacerbations
   - Current/recent withdrawal of systemic corticosteroids

6. **When do I need to send a child to an emergency department with an acute asthma exacerbation?**

   Children who are not responsive to conventional treatment of beta-2 agonists, anticholinergics, and systemic corticosteroids with persistent respiratory distress or oxygen requirement <90% should be transferred to a higher level of care. It should be noted that patients receiving beta-agonists may sometimes experience transient hypoxia (V/Q mismatch). As such, determination of persistent oxygen requirement should be made at least 30–60 minutes after the last treatment.

7. **A 10-month-old infant presents to your urgent care center in January with a 3-day history of fever, runny nose, cough, and decreased oral intake. On examination, the infant is smiling with a respiratory rate of 70 breaths per minute, appears well hydrated, and has wheezing throughout all lung fields on auscultation. What is your diagnosis?**

   This infant most likely has bronchiolitis, a common viral respiratory illness that significantly affects young children from birth to 2 years of age. Lower respiratory tract viruses cause significant edema and epithelial sloughing in the small bronchioles that then manifests as respiratory distress, including retractions and nasal flaring. The most common viral cause of bronchiolitis is respiratory syncytial virus (RSV); however, there are many different respiratory viruses that cause the same symptoms. Bronchiolitis is a completely clinical diagnosis. History will be notable for viral symptoms such as runny nose, congestion, and cough. Fever is sometimes present. Younger infants may present with apnea as their only symptom. A physical exam is notable for tachypnea and variable abnormal lung sounds; there can be wheezing, crackles, or even rhonchi throughout the lung fields. Distress is noted by nasal flaring, grunting, subcostal or intercostal retractions, and tachypnea.

8. **What can be done to treat bronchiolitis?**

   Unfortunately, not much. If patients have a fever, antipyretics can be given. Nasal suctioning with saline can relieve some distress, as patients are typically obligate nose breathers and congestion worsens the respiratory distress associated with bronchiolitis. There is no role for corticosteroids, inhaled steroids, beta-agonists, cough suppressants, nebulized hypertonic saline, or nebulized epinephrine, as there is little evidence that such treatments decrease the length or severity of illness. Antibiotics should only be given if a concomitant bacterial infection is diagnosed. If patients are dehydrated or their breathing makes them unable to adequately take in fluids, nasogastric (NG) or intravenous (IV) fluids can be given.

9. **Should I order a CXR or laboratory studies in an infant with bronchiolitis?**

   Not routinely. Many infants with bronchiolitis will have abnormal CXR findings; however, these findings have not been found to correlate with disease severity. Similarly, laboratory studies, including viral studies, are not routinely indicated.

10. **Are there certain factors that place some infants at increased risk when diagnosed with bronchiolitis?**

    • Age less than 12 weeks
    • Hemodynamically significant heart disease
    • Chronic lung disease
    • History of prematurity
    • Immunodeficiency

11. **When do I need to send a patient with bronchiolitis to the emergency department?**

    Patients with persistent respiratory distress that is not relieved by nasal suctioning, fever control, or positioning should be assessed by an emergency physician, as should those who are dehydrated or unable to adequately hydrate themselves secondary to respiratory distress, choking with feeds, or vomiting. Younger infants presenting with apnea should also be transferred for further evaluation.

12. **A 12-month-old infant presents to your urgent care with 2 days of fever, runny nose, and "barky" cough. This afternoon, he has been breathing harder than usual, making a high-pitched sound with each breath even while sitting quietly. What is your diagnosis?**

    Croup is a viral infection that causes inflammation of the larynx and trachea. Symptoms start with runny nose and congestion, then progress to include fever, "barky" cough (similar to a seal), and stridor, especially when agitated or crying. Patients with stridor at rest are considered to be more ill.

13. **What is the treatment for croup?**

    Current recommendations are to give dexamethasone 0.15–0.6 mg/kg with a maximum dose of 8–16 mg. The oral route is best as the IM route can cause more agitation; IM should be reserved for patients with vomiting or severe distress. Although rarely necessary, steroids can be redosed in 6–24 hours. Nebulized racemic epinephrine should only be used in those patients who have stridor at rest. Racemic epinephrine is administered as 0.05 mL/kg per dose (maximum of 0.5 mL) of a 2.25% solution diluted to 3 mL total volume with normal saline. It is given via nebulizer over 15 minutes. A child who receives racemic epinephrine for stridor at rest should be observed for at least 2 hours to monitor for rebound stridor.

14. **What other diagnoses should I consider in a patient with suspected croup?**
In a patient with sudden onset of stridor and difficulty breathing without any preceding viral illness, foreign body aspiration should be considered. In unvaccinated, ill-appearing children, acute epiglottitis can also present with distress, cough, and stridor. Ill-appearing children with drooling, fever, and tripoding can also have a posterior retropharyngeal abscess. These patients require emergent transfer to a higher level of care where difficult pediatric airways can be managed.

15. **Should I order a neck x-ray or any other studies in an infant with croup?**
Not routinely. X-rays do not aid in diagnosis or help with determining the severity of presentation. X-rays should be reserved for those patients with concern for foreign body aspiration or other diagnoses for which there is no response to treatments. If a neck x-ray is obtained, the most classic finding is subglottic narrowing with a normal epiglottis, known as the "steeple sign." This is in contrast to patients with epiglottitis who have swelling of the epiglottis, called the "thumb sign," or increased prevertebral edema seen with a retropharyngeal abscess. Viral studies are not helpful, as they will not change management or have any prognostic factors for the severity of illness.

16. **A 3-year-old unvaccinated girl presents with 1 week of persistent cough. During your exam, you hear her cough several times in succession, followed by a high-pitched "whoop" sound. What is your diagnosis?**
This patient's presentation is concerning for pertussis. The classic presentation of pertussis occurs in three stages. The first stage, or catarrhal phase, lasts 1–2 weeks and is similar to a viral upper respiratory infection with watery rhinorrhea, mild cough, and low-grade fever. The difference from a viral URI is that the cough worsens throughout the first stage. The second stage, or paroxysmal phase, is when the classic "whoop" of pertussis is heard. This stage is marked by increasing severity of episodes of coughing spells with long episodes of coughing with little respiratory effort. This is when the child struggles to breathe and could have cyanosis and gagging. This stage lasts from 2–8 weeks. The third stage, or convalescent phase, is when the patient is slowly improving from the illness over several weeks to months. The median duration of cough in untreated patients is 112 days.

17. **How do I diagnose pertussis?**
Pertussis should be diagnosed clinically. In children younger than 4 months, there might not be the "whooping" sound, so apnea, seizures, and cyanosis should be used as clues to the diagnosis of possible pertussis. Confirmatory testing by culture or polymerase chain reaction (PCR) is required to meet national reporting guidelines. Serology is not useful in patients younger than 4 months or if they have received the vaccine in the last year.

18. **What is the treatment for pertussis? Should I treat family members?**
Treatment for pertussis should be started as soon as possible while awaiting confirmatory testing. Azithromycin is recommended, though alternate regimens are available (Table 24.4). Azithromycin has the same efficacy and fewer side effects than other treatment options. Therapy is best when initiated within 7 days of symptoms. Close contacts and high-risk individuals (patients who are immunocompromised, pregnant, younger than 4 months of age, or have moderate to severe asthma) should be treated with postexposure prophylaxis with the same treatment as the infected patient. Infants less than 4 months of age are at high risk for severe or fatal pertussis. These infants should be considered for evaluation at an emergency department.

19. **A 15-year-old presents to your urgent care center with 5 days of fever, cough, chest pain, and difficulty breathing. How do I diagnose pneumonia?**
Pneumonia is a clinical diagnosis. Common historical components of pneumonia include cough, fever, chest pain, and difficulty breathing. On exam, there can be respiratory distress as noted by tachypnea, retractions, and hypoxia in addition to focal auscultatory findings such as crackles or decreased lung sounds. In cases of basilar pneumonia, abdominal pain may be the presenting sign. Only the absence of tachypnea has been linked to the absence of pneumonia. Routine CBC or cultures (either blood or sputum) are not necessary in children who will be treated as outpatients.

20. **When should I get a CXR in a child whom I suspect has pneumonia?**
CXRs should be saved for those patients with severe distress, persistent hypoxia, outpatient treatment failure, or any other indication that the patient would need admission for therapy. Outpatient CXRs have not been shown to affect outcomes.

21. **What is the best antibiotic choice for pneumonia in children?**
As the cause varies by age, so does the treatment (Table 24.5). Amoxicillin 90 mg/kg/day divided into two doses for 10 days should be given to all patients with suspected pneumonia except in cases of allergy. Azithromycin should be added for school-age children. When influenza is in season, patients with influenza-like illness in the first 48 hours of symptoms should also be covered empirically with antiviral therapy.

22. **When do I need to send a child with pneumonia to the emergency department?**
Patients who are persistently hypoxic (less than 90% on room air while awake) will require supplemental oxygen and therefore need to be admitted. Other reasons for admission are significant respiratory distress or inability to maintain hydration.

Table 24.4 Recommended Antimicrobial Therapy and Postexposure Prophylaxis for Pertussis in Infants, Children, Adolescents, and Adults[a]

	Recommended Drugs			ALTERNATIVE
AGE	AZITHROMYCIN	ERYTHROMYCIN	CLARITHROMYCIN	TMP-SMX
<1 month	10 mg/kg/day as a single dose daily for 5 days[b,c]	40 mg/kg/day in 4 divided doses for 14 days	Not recommended	Contraindicated at younger than 2 months of age
1–5 months	See above	See above	15 mg/kg/day in 2 divided doses for 7 days	2 months of age or older: TMP, 8 mg/kg/day; SMX, 40 mg/kg/day in 2 doses for 14 days
>6 months and children	10 mg/kg as a single dose on day 1 (max 500 mg), then 5 mg/kg/day as a single dose on days 2 through 5 (max 250 mg/day)[b,d]	40 mg/kg/day in 4 divided doses for 7–14 days (max 1–2 g/day)	15 mg/kg/day in 2 divided doses for 7 days (max 1 g/day)	See above
Adolescents and adults	500 mg as a single dose on day 1, then 250 mg as a single dose on days 2 through 5[b,d]	2 g/day in 4 divided doses for 7–14 days	1 g/day in 2 divided doses for 7 days	TMP, 320 mg/day; SMX, 1600 mg/day in 2 divided doses for 14 days

SMX, Sulfamethoxazole; TMP, trimethoprim.
[a]Centers for Disease Control and Prevention: Recommended antimicrobial agents for the treatment and postexposure prophylaxis of pertussis: 2005 CDC guidelines. MMWR Recomm Rep. 54(RR-14):1–16, 2005.
[b]Azithromycin should be used with caution in people with prolonged QT interval and certain proarrhythmic conditions.
[c]Preferred macrolide for this age because of risk of idiopathic hypertrophic pyloric stenosis associated with erythromycin.
[d]A 3-day course of azithromycin for PEP or treatment has not been validated and is not recommended.

Table 24.5 Antibiotic Choice by Age for Treatment of Pneumonia[a]

AGE	FIRST LINE	ALTERNATE OPTIONS FOR PENICILLIN-ALLERGIC PATIENTS
6 months–5 years	Amoxicillin: 90 mg/kg divided twice a day for 10 days (max 4 g/day)	Cefdinir: 14 mg/kg per day divided twice a day for 10 days (max 600 mg/day) OR Clindamycin: 30–40 mg/kg per day divided into 3 doses for 10 days (max 1.8 g/day)
>5 years	Amoxicillin: 90 mg/kg divided twice a day for 10 days (max 4 g/day) AND Azithromycin: 10 mg/kg on day 1 followed by 5 mg/kg daily for 4 more days	As above for amoxicillin AND Doxycycline: 4 mg/kg per day divided twice a day for 10 days (max 200 mg/day)

[a]Adapted from UpToDate.

23. A 4-year-old boy presents with 2 days of fever and cough. His parent reports that his at-home COVID-19 test was positive. How do you evaluate and counsel this patient?
Acute COVID-19 infection may present with a variety of respiratory symptoms that can mimic croup, asthma, and bronchiolitis. Perform a thorough history and physical exam to determine whether the child is in significant distress, hypoxic, unable to maintain hydration, and or exhibiting signs of a secondary bacterial infection. If not,

only supportive care is indicated as with any pediatric viral cough illness: encourage hydration, monitor urine output, perform nasal suctioning for infants and younger children, and treat fever with antipyretics. Refer to local guidelines for the most up-to-date guidance regarding isolation and treatment.

KEY POINTS

1. Acute exacerbations of asthma should be treated with a combination of timely systemic corticosteroids, short-acting beta$_2$ agonists, and anticholinergics.
2. In the routine treatment of bronchiolitis, there is no role for beta-agonists, systemic steroids, inhaled steroids, nebulized hypertonic saline, or nebulized epinephrine.
3. In patients with croup, if a patient has stridor at rest, racemic epinephrine should be given and then the patient will need to be monitored for at least 2 hours.
4. The presentation of pertussis, also known as whooping cough, may vary based on the patient's stage of illness: catarrhal (first 1–2 weeks), paroxysmal (next 2–8 weeks), or convalescent (weeks to months); treatment should be started while confirmatory testing is pending.
5. Chest x-rays are not indicated in patients with suspected pneumonia unless they are exhibiting severe distress, persistent hypoxia, outpatient treatment failure, or any other indication that the patient would need hospital admission for therapy.

Acknowledgments

The authors would like to thank Dr. Esther Maria Sampayo, MD, MPH, for her contributions to this chapter in the previous edition.

BIBLIOGRAPHY

Barson WJ. Pneumonia in children: epidemiology, pathogenesis, and etiology. UpToDate. Available at: http://www.uptodate.com/contents/pneumonia-in-children-epidemiology-pathogenesis-and-etiology?source=see_link&sectionName=Community-acquired+pneumonia&anchor=H15#H15. Published March 14, 2022. Accessed July 13, 2022.
Bradley JS, Byington CL, Shah SS, et al. The management of community-acquired pneumonia in infants and children older than 3 months of age: clinical practice guidelines by the Pediatric Infectious Diseases Society and the Infectious Diseases Society of America. *Clinical Infectious Diseases.* 2011;53(7):e25–e76.
Cloutier MM, Baptist AM, Blake KV, et al. 2020 Focused Updates to the Asthma Management Guidelines: a report from the National Asthma Education and Prevention Program Coordinating Committee Expert Panel Working Group. *Journal of Allergy and Clinical Immunology.* 2020;146(6):1217–1270.
Keeney GE, Gray P, Morrison AK, Levas MN, et al. Dexamethasone for acute asthma exacerbations in children: a meta-analysis. *Pediatrics.* 2014;133(3):493–499.
Kimberlin DW, Barnett ED, Lynfield R, et al. Pertussis (Whooping Cough). *Red Book: 2021-2024 Report of the Committee on Infectious Diseases.* 32nd ed. Itasca, IL: American Academy of Pediatrics; 2021.
McInerny TK, Adam HM, Campbell DE, et al. Bronchiolitis. *American Academy of Pediatrics Textbook of Pediatric Care.* 2nd ed. Itasca, IL: American Academy of Pediatrics; 2016.
Ralston SL, Lieberthal AS, Meissner HC, et al. Clinical practice guideline: the diagnosis, management, and prevention of bronchiolitis. *Pediatrics.* 2014;134:e1474.

CHAPTER 25

CHEST PAIN

Siraj Amanullah, MD, MPH, Jay Pershad, MD, MMM, CPE

A 14-year-old male presents to an urgent care facility for new-onset intermittent chest pain since he has started to play competitive basketball for the first time. Pain is exertional, retrosternal, with no radiation, pressure-like squeezing, with resolution after rest. On the day he presented, he had an episode of chest pain with dizziness and near syncope. On examination, he has a heart rate of 85 beats per minute, a respiratory rate of 25 breaths per minute, and blood pressure of 130/75 mm Hg. He has a normal respiratory and chest wall exam. He has a systolic ejection (crescendo–decrescendo) murmur between the apex of the heart and the left sternal border that becomes more prominent in a standing position.

1. **What are the concerning features of this patient's chest pain presented in the scenario?**
   Exertional chest pain with dizziness and/or syncope is concerning for cardiac pathology. The characteristic of his murmur suggests hypertrophic obstructive cardiomyopathy. His electrocardiogram (ECG) is shown in Fig. 25.1. He will be best managed by an urgent referral to a pediatric cardiologist and refraining from any exertional activity until evaluated.

2. **How common is chest pain in the pediatric population?**
   Chest pain is one of the common reasons to seek medical care and is reported to be 0.3–0.6% of emergency department visits.

3. **How serious is chest pain in children?**
   The majority of pediatric patients with chest pain have a benign etiology. Less than 5% of chest pain complaints have been reported to be due to urgent or serious conditions. With COVID-19-related multisystem inflammatory syndrome (MIS-C) and vaccination-associated myocarditis, a broader differential diagnosis needs to be considered when assessing patients with chest pain. In most cases, a careful history and physical examination are still sufficient to rule out a serious pathology, without the need for extensive workup.

4. **What are the components of a good history and physical examination in assessment of a pediatric patient with chest pain?**
   History of onset, duration, character, frequency, radiation, association with exertion, assessment of associated symptoms (fever, syncope, dyspnea, sweating), recent COVID-19 infection or vaccination, past medical history, and family history can help differentiate various etiologies of chest pain. Physical examination includes cardiac, respiratory, and abdominal exam especially assessing for hypoxia, tachypnea, tachycardia, fever, cardiac murmurs, gallop rhythm, and rubs; signs consistent with inflammatory syndromes (Kawasaki Disease, MIS-C) point toward a need for urgent diagnostic workup. Fig. 25.2 shows an algorithmic approach to a pediatric patient with chest pain and when cardiology referral is warranted.

5. **What are important past medical and family history in patients with chest pain?**
   Past medical history includes congenital heart disease, cystic fibrosis, Kawasaki disease, Marfan syndrome, Turner syndrome, Noonan syndrome, Ehlers-Danlos syndrome, ankylosing spondylitis, systemic lupus erythematosus, sickle cell disease, asthma, anxiety, and panic attacks. Family history of prolonged QT syndrome, sudden cardiac death, and cardiomyopathy warrant additional testing and/or consultation.

6. **What is the most common cause of chest pain in pediatric patients?**
   Chest wall pain due to muscular strain or costochondritis remains the most common etiology of chest pain in pediatric patients. Pain is reproducible with history of recent physical or sports activity, heavy backpacks, trauma, or cough.

7. **What are the characteristic historical or physical findings in patients with chest wall pain?**
   Costochondritis pain is usually worse with breathing or exercise, mostly unilateral, anterior, reproducible at the costochondral areas, involving two or more costochondral joints, and may persist for weeks. If there is localized inflammation, pain, swelling, and erythema of one costochondral joint (usually the second/third joint), the condition is called Tietze syndrome. Pleurodynia (Bornholm disease) features paroxysms of sharp chest pain associated with coxsackievirus infection.

8. **What are the other causes of benign chest pain?**
   Precordial catch (Texidor twinge) is usually left-sided, recurrent, lasting for a few seconds, with a point location in an intercostal space, worsening on deep breathing or bending down, and improving with shallow breathing. Unilateral burning or sharp pain in a dermatomal distribution is typical of herpes zoster. Various breast conditions can also present with chest pain. Esophageal spasms can lead to severe retrosternal chest pain, while

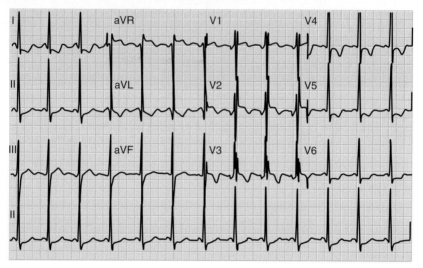

Fig. 25.1 Male teenager with severe HOCM with left atrial enlargement, left ventricular hypertrophy, and diffuse ST-T changes. (Courtesy Dr. James Ziegler, MD, Department of Pediatrics, Brown Medical School, Hasbro Children's Hospital, Providence, RI, USA.)

gastroesophageal reflux can lead to burning pain after meals or worsening with lying down. Noncardiac chest pain can be due to psychosocial stressors or conditions such as depression, anxiety, stress, conversion, or somatization. It is usually reported as frequent, recurrent, severe, lasting for varied durations, spanning over months to years, with no consistent relationship to activity, usually without any other associated symptoms, with or without hyperventilation or obvious anxiety, affecting daily life routine.

9. **Which medical conditions can present with sudden chest pain?**
   Serious conditions for an urgent care physician to consider with acute onset of atraumatic chest pain: acute asthma, spontaneous pneumothorax or pneumomediastinum, acute chest syndrome in patients with sickle cell disease, myocarditis, and, uncommonly, pulmonary embolism or aortic dissection. Sudden onset of chest pain in an otherwise healthy young child may also be due to foreign body ingestion. Sudden increase in intrathoracic pressure associated with trauma, asthma, pneumonia, vomiting, weightlifting, inhalation of recreational drugs, or hookah may lead to pneumomediastinum or pneumothorax (Fig. 25.3). Pain is unilateral with shortness of breath with pneumothorax. Pneumomediastinum pain is in the neck and retrosternal area with subcutaneous emphysema and Hamman sign (crunchy sound over precordium). If it is associated with profound vomiting, then esophageal perforation needs to be ruled out. Fever, cough, respiratory distress, and chest pain are presenting signs of acute chest crisis in patients with sickle cell disease. Cocaine abuse can present with angina with chest tightness, nausea, sweating, vomiting, or shortness of breath. Aortic dissection is rarely seen in pediatric patients and is associated with collagen vascular disorders. Unexplained tachycardia with chest pain preceded by viral prodrome is concerning for myocarditis. Chest pain in a patient with signs and symptoms consistent with MIS-C suggests myocardial inflammation and dysfunction (https://www.cdc.gov/mis/mis-c/hcp/index.html).

10. **How common is cardiac pathology in pediatric patients with chest pain?**
    Cardiac disease as an etiology of chest pain is very rare in pediatric patients, with a reported incidence of 0.6–1.2% of all etiologies. Almost all of these conditions can be suspected based on historical clues, physical exam findings, and judicious use of ECG.

11. **How common is myocardial ischemia in pediatric patients?**
    Acute myocardial ischemia is extremely rare in pediatric patients with male gender in the teenage years; substance abuse like cocaine and tobacco are identified as risk factors. Other at-risk etiologies of acute ischemia are cardiac structural abnormalities, hypertension, infection or inflammation, or sequelae of prior inflammatory conditions, like Kawasaki Disease.

12. **What are the characteristic historical and physical examination findings in patients with structural cardiac abnormalities and chest pain?**
    A cardiac cause of chest pain is very infrequent, but clinical implications can be serious. A thorough history and physical can be very helpful in ruling out a cardiac cause in pediatric patients presenting to an urgent care setting (Table 25.1). Hypertrophic cardiomyopathy (HOCM) is associated with exertional chest pain, occasionally syncope, and murmur with the Valsalva maneuver. Though by itself rare, it is one of the most common etiologies of sudden

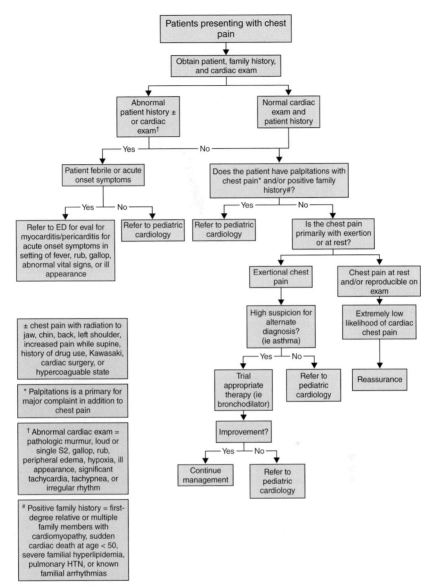

Fig. 25.2 Approach to assessment of a pediatric patient with chest pain. (From Friedman KG, Alexander ME. Chest pain and syncope in children: a practical approach to the diagnosis of cardiac disease. *J Pediatr.* 163(3):896–901, e1–e3, 2013 (Fig. 2, p. 10). Note: As mentioned in the algorithm, symptoms suggestive of unstable vital signs or cardiac exam concerning for failure should be urgently referred to an emergency department.)

cardiac deaths. HOCM is associated with atrial fibrillation and coronary artery anomalies. Dilated cardiomyopathy patients present with chest pain and shortness of breath. Very few structural heart defects present with chest pain, including mitral valve prolapse, coronary artery anomalies, and severe aortic and pulmonary outlet obstruction. Pain due to mitral valve prolapse is vague, could be nonexertional, is along the cardiac apex, and may have a midsystolic click that is pronounced when standing. Those with anomalous coronary artery and severe outflow tract obstruction have exertional angina pain with murmur along the upper sternum on physical exam.

13. **What other cardiac pathologies may present with chest pain?**
    Other diagnoses considered as potential causes of chest pain include cardiomyopathy, myocarditis, pericarditis, specific coronary anomalies, pulmonary hypertension, pulmonary embolism, and aortic dissection. Pericarditis

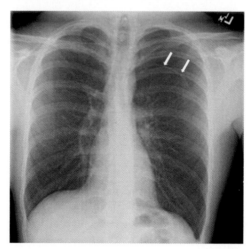

Fig. 25.3 Left-sided spontaneous pneumothorax in a teenager with acute chest pain. (Courtesy Jay Pershad, MD, MMM, Department of Pediatrics and Emergency Medicine, University of Tennessee Health Sciences Center, Le Bonheur Children's Hospital, Memphis, TN 38103.)

pain is sharp, positional, and stabbing and improves with leaning forward. Chest pain on exertion with syncope and or palpitation may be due to ventricular or supraventricular tachyarrhythmia (Fig. 25.4). Lyme carditis patients can present with fatigue, chest discomfort, or near syncope with severe first-degree heart block (Fig. 25.5) or third-degree atrioventricular block. Viral myocarditis presents with mild chest pain with tachycardia out of proportion to fever, muffled heart sounds, and a gallop rhythm.

14. **What is the association of chest pain and myocarditis with COVID-19 infection?**
Just like other viral etiologies, myocarditis has also been seen in patients with acute COVID-19 infections or due to its sequelae of MIS-C. Post-COVID-19 mRNA vaccine-associated myocarditis has been reported in adolescents. It has an extremely low incidence when compared with the number of vaccines administered. The presentation has been observed after the second dose, and usually within a week, in young males, with no residual impact on cardiac function (https://www.cdc.gov/vaccines/covid-19/clinical-considerations/myocarditis.html).

15. **How common is pulmonary embolism in pediatric patients?**
It is uncommon in otherwise healthy pediatric patients. It should be considered in patients with risk factors and chest pain or unexplained persistent tachypnea or tachycardia. High-risk conditions associated with pulmonary embolism in pediatrics include hypercoagulable states, use of birth control pills, recent abortion or surgery, cancer, prolonged immobilization, lower extremity trauma, central venous lines, prior history of DVT or embolism, and travel on long flights. Classic presentation includes acute dyspnea, pleuritic chest pain, cough, hemoptysis, and/or sinus tachycardia, with decreased breath sounds over the affected area and pleural rub. The incidence of pulmonary embolism in hospitalized patients with acute COVID-19 infection has been reported to be higher than in the general population. The overall numbers were still extremely low (<1%). There are screening criteria based on history and physical exam variables that are well described and validated in adults to rule out pulmonary embolism (e.g., PERC, Wells score, Geneva criteria). These have not been validated in pediatrics.

16. **What are the important ancillary tests as part of evaluation of chest pain?**
Pulse oximetry is one of the most important, in addition to other vital signs. Electrocardiogram and chest radiography are the most common and should be guided by careful history and physical examination.

17. **When is a chest x-ray warranted in the setting of chest pain?**
A chest radiograph is not indicated in every patient with acute asthma exacerbation but may be indicated in the presence of persistent chest pain or hypoxia despite appropriate treatments. A radiograph can exclude suspected pneumothorax, pneumomediastinum, cardiomegaly (myocarditis, pericarditis, cardiomyopathy), foreign body, and pneumonia.

18. **What are the abnormal ECG findings in a patient with chest pain?**
The following ECG abnormalities are considered abnormal in a pediatric patient with chest pain: evidence of ventricular hypertrophy, ST-T abnormalities, high-grade atrioventricular (AV) block, ventricular or atrial ectopy, QTc >470 msec, PR depression, low QRS voltages, and an S1Q3 inverted T3 pattern. Patients with HOCM usually have evidence of left ventricular hypertrophy with left atrial enlargement and may have diffuse ST-T wave changes (see Fig. 25.1). However, ECG may be normal in 5–10% of such patients.

Table 25.1 Cardiac Causes of Chest Pain and Red Flag History, Exam, and ECG Findings

CAUSE	HISTORY	PHYSICAL EXAM FINDINGS	ECG FINDINGS
HCM	Positive family history Exercise intolerance Exertional chest pain Syncope and/or arrhythmia	Dynamic systolic murmur	Left ventricular hypertrophy or left axis deviation ST-segment or T-wave changes Q waves Arrhythmias, ventricular premature beats Ventricular preexcitation (Wolff-Parkinson-White)
Dilated cardiomyopathy	Family history Decreased exercise tolerance, syncope Heart failure symptoms	Gallop Mitral regurgitation murmur	Intraventricular conduction delay High or low QRS voltages Arrhythmia, premature beats
Anomalous coronary artery origin	Exertional chest pain Exertional syncope	Usually normal	Usually normal
Coronary ischemia	• Predisposing conditions • History of Kawasaki disease • Cardiac surgery or heart transplant • Systemic arteriopathy (Williams syndrome) • Severe familial hypercholesterolemia • Drug use: cocaine, sympathomimetics • Anginal chest pain	Tachycardia Tachypnea New murmur or gallop	ST-segment depressions or elevation T-wave changes Q waves
Severe left ventricular outflow tract obstruction	Exertional symptoms Exertional syncope	Loud systolic murmur	Left ventricular hypertrophy Left ventricular strain pattern
Arrhythmia	Palpitations Syncope Positive family history	Irregular rhythm	Atrial arrhythmia Ventricular arrhythmia Premature contractions Ventricular preexcitation (Wolff-Parkinson-White)
Pericarditis	Positional chest pain Predisposing factors: • Rheumatologic conditions • Malignancy • Mediastinal radiation • Infection (HIV, tuberculosis, viral) • Renal failure • Recent cardiac surgery	Cardiac rub Tachycardia/tachypnea Distant heart sound, JVD	Diffuse ST-segment changes T-wave inversion
Myocarditis	Fever Viral prodrome Short duration of symptoms New onset heart failure symptoms	Tachycardia Tachypnea With or without gallop rhythm, ventricular ectopy Cardiovascular collapse	Diffuse ST-segment changes T-wave inversions PR depressions Ventricular ectopy Low QRS voltages

Continued on following page

Table 25.1 Cardiac Causes of Chest Pain and Red Flag History, Exam, and ECG Findings (*Continued*)

CAUSE	HISTORY	PHYSICAL EXAM FINDINGS	ECG FINDINGS
Aortic dissection	Personal or family history of bicuspid aortic valve or connective tissue disorders (e.g., Marfan, Loeys-Dietz, Ehlers-Danlos type IV) Acute onset, sharp or tearing type of pain	Marfanoid body habitus	See coronary ischemia above
Pulmonary embolus	Pain description: acute onset, pleuritic, associated dyspnea	Right ventricular heave (elevated right ventricular pressure)	Right ventricular hypertrophy
	Personal or family risk factors (inherited thrombophilia, hypercoagulable state, immobilization, medications)	Loud and/or unsplit S2 (if right ventricular pressure elevated)	Right ventricular stain pattern

JVD, Jugular venous distention.
From Friedman KG, Alexander ME. Chest pain and syncope in children: a practical approach to the diagnosis of cardiac disease. *J Pediatr.* 163(3):896–901, e1–e3, 2013 [Table IV, pages 15–16].

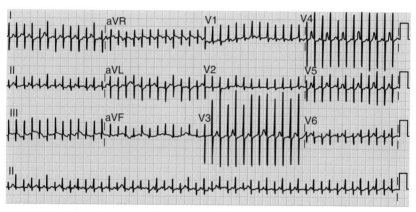

Fig. 25.4 Patient with sudden onset of pallor, chest discomfort, and palpitations associated with narrow complex tachycardia on ECG with absent P waves. (Courtesy Dr. Siraj Amanullah, MD, MPH, Department of Emergency Medicine and Pediatrics, Brown Medical School, Hasbro Children's Hospital, Providence, RI, USA.)

The best screening tool for myocarditis is ECG (sinus tachycardia, ST changes), with more than 90% of patients with ECG changes. Pericarditis patients may have diffuse ST-segment elevation (in up to 60% of patients) with PR depression in inferior leads and V2–V6. Pulmonary embolism patients are most likely to have sinus tachycardia alone with otherwise normal ECG. It is important to note that only a few patients with a large embolus may have a prominent S wave in lead 1, Q wave in lead 3, and inverted T wave in lead 3 or in V1–V3, right axis deviation, or right bundle branch block (RBBB), and these changes are not specific for pulmonary embolism. Patients with outflow tract obstruction usually have left ventricular hypertrophy. Patients with coronary artery disease or anomalies may show ST-segment elevation associated with cardiac ischemia.

19. **What is the role of laboratory workup in pediatric patients with chest pain?**
Laboratory tests are indicated when a cardiac etiology or pulmonary embolism is suspected. They should not be performed universally. A serum troponin level should be obtained in a workup for myocarditis, cardiac ischemia, or MIS-C. Natriuretic peptide tests are helpful in the evaluation of MIS-C. They are often elevated in patients with myocardial dysfunction but can be normal in patients with myocarditis. The role of D-dimers and effective cut-off values have not been reliably established in pediatric patients with suspected pulmonary embolism. Recent

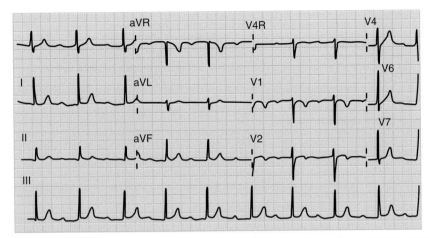

Fig. 25.5 Patient with fatigue, chest discomfort, and near syncope on exertion with prolonged PR interval associated with Lyme carditis. (Courtesy Dr. Siraj Amanullah, MD, MPH, Department of Emergency Medicine and Pediatrics, Brown Medical School, Hasbro Children's Hospital, Providence, RI, USA.)

studies have shown the values to be remarkably elevated in adolescent patients with PE when compared to those without, but the values can be still high in those patients without PE. It is for the patients with low risk of PE, that D-dimers value can be helpful to rule out PE.

20. **What are the steps in management of patients with benign chest pain?**
    If a patient has a benign cause for chest pain, reassurance, rest, and supportive care with use of acetaminophen or nonsteroidal antiinflammatory drugs is advised.

21. **When should a pediatric patient with chest pain be referred for urgent evaluation to an emergency department?**
    Ill appearance, fever, hypotension, respiratory distress, low oxygenation, significant unexplained tachycardia, tachypnea, irregular rhythm, peripheral edema, or other signs of congestive heart failure such as hepatomegaly, gallop or jugular venous distention, pathologic murmur, or rub. Exertional syncope and/or palpitations with acute chest pain with an abnormal EKG or chest radiograph may warrant urgent referral to a tertiary center.

22. **When can a patient with chest pain be referred for outpatient evaluation by a cardiologist?**
    Patients with exertional chest pain that resolves with rest without signs of life-threatening arrhythmia can be referred for urgent outpatient cardiac workup.

23. **When is it appropriate to abstain a child from physical activity with chest pain?**
    Patients with exertional chest pain should be refrained from sports until seen by a pediatric cardiologist. Those with a benign etiology of chest pain should not refrain from physical activities as this will create unnecessary anxiety for the patient and their family.

KEY POINTS

1. Chest pain associated with exertion and or syncope warrants careful evaluation for a cardiopulmonary etiology.
2. A cardiology referral is recommended for patients with chest pain and a positive family history of first-degree relatives with cardiomyopathy, prolonged QTc, sudden death <50 years, or severe hyperlipidemia.
3. Abnormal ECG findings in a patient with pediatric chest pain include evidence of ventricular hypertrophy, ST-T abnormalities, high-grade AV block, ventricular or atrial ectopy, QTc >470 msec, PR depression, low QRS voltages, and/or an S1Q3 inverted T3 pattern.
4. Chest pain with acute COVID-19 infection, after recent vaccination or when suspected MIS-C, requires further evaluation and may warrant emergency department referral.

BIBLIOGRAPHY

Barbut G, Needleman JP. Pediatric chest pain. *Pediatr Rev.* 2020;41(9):469–480. doi:10.1542/pir.2019-0058. PMID: 32873561.
Bergmann KR, Kharbanda A, Haveman L. Myocarditis and pericarditis in the pediatric patient: validated management strategies. *Pediatr Emerg Med Pract.* 2015;12(7):1–22. [quiz 23].
Bozkurt B, Kamat I, Hotez PJ. Myocarditis with COVID-19 mRNA vaccines. *Circulation.* 2021;144(6):471–484. doi: 10.1161/CIRCULATIONAHA.121.056135. Epub 2021 Jul 20. PMID: 34281357; PMCID: PMC8340726.

Chima M, Williams D, Thomas NJ, Krawiec C. COVID-19-associated pulmonary embolism in pediatric patients. *Hosp Pediatr.* 2021;11(6):e90–e94. doi:10.1542/hpeds.2021-005866. Epub 2021 Mar 30. PMID: 33785517.

Eslick GD. Epidemiology and risk factors of pediatric chest pain: a systematic review. *Pediatr Clin North Am.* 2010;57(6):1211–1219.

Friedman KG, Alexander ME. Chest pain and syncope in children: a practical approach to the diagnosis of cardiac disease. *J Pediatr.* 2013;163(3):896–901. e1–e3.

Johnson NN, Toledo A, Endom EE. Pneumothorax, pneumomediastinum, and pulmonary embolism. *Pediatr Clin North Am.* 2010;57(6):1357–1383.

Kane DA, et al. Needles in hay: chest pain as the presenting symptom in children with serious underlying cardiac pathology. *Congenit Heart Dis.* 2010;5(4):366–373.

Kane DA, et al. Needles in hay II: detecting cardiac pathology by the pediatric chest pain standardized clinical assessment and management plan. *Congenit Heart Dis.* 2016.

Law YM, Lal AK, Chen S, et al. American Heart Association Pediatric Heart Failure and Transplantation Committee of the Council on Lifelong Congenital Heart Disease and Heart Health in the Young and Stroke Council. Diagnosis and management of myocarditis in children: a scientific statement from the American Heart Association. *Circulation.* 2021;144(6):e123–e135. doi:10.1161/CIR.0000000000001001. Epub 2021 Jul 7. Erratum in: Circulation. 2021;144(6):e149. PMID: 34229446.

Mahle WT, Campbell RM, Favaloro-Sabatier J. Myocardial infarction in adolescents. *J Pediatr.* 2007;151(2):150–154.

McDonnell CJ, White KS, Grady RM. Noncardiac chest pain in children and adolescents: a biopsychosocial conceptualization. *Child Psychiatry Hum Dev.* 2012;43(1):1–26.

Park M. *Pediatric Cardiology for Practitioners.* 6th ed. Philadelphia: Saunders; 2014.

Patel T, Kelleman M, West Z, et al. Comparison of multisystem inflammatory syndrome in children-related myocarditis, classic viral myocarditis, and COVID-19 vaccine-related myocarditis in children. *J Am Heart Assoc.* 2022;11(9):e024393. doi:10.1161/JAHA.121.024393. Epub 2022 Apr 27. PMID: 35475362; PMCID: PMC9238597.

Patocka C, Nemeth J. Pulmonary embolism in pediatrics. *J Emerg Med.* 2012;42(1):105–116.

Ramiz S, Rajpurkar M. Pulmonary embolism in children. *Pediatr Clin North Am.* 2018;65(3):495–507. doi:10.1016/j.pcl.2018.02.002. PMID: 29803279.

Siripanthong B, Nazarian S, Muser D, et al. Recognizing COVID-19-related myocarditis: the possible pathophysiology and proposed guideline for diagnosis and management. *Heart Rhythm.* 2020;17(9):1463–1471. doi:10.1016/j.hrthm.2020.05.001. Epub 2020 May 5. PMID: 32387246; PMCID: PMC7199677.

Sharaf N, Sharaf VB, Mace SE, Nowacki AS, Stoller JK, Carl JC. D-dimer in adolescent pulmonary embolism. *Acad Emerg Med.* 2018;25(11):1235–1241. doi:10.1111/acem.13517. Epub 2018 Aug 10. PMID: 30010232.

CHAPTER 26

ABDOMINAL PAIN

Karen Y. Kwan, BS, MD

TOP SECRETS

1. Bilious emesis should prompt emergent workup for distal obstruction, including malrotation with volvulus.
2. Polyethylene glycol (Miralax) is first-line treatment for functional constipation in children.
3. Intussusception must be suspected in afebrile children ages 6 months to 2 years of age with episodic abdominal pain and vomiting.

ABDOMINAL PAIN

1. **How common is acute abdominal pain in childhood?**
   Abdominal pain is one of the most common complaints in childhood, accounting for approximately 9% of childhood outpatient visits and frequently requiring urgent evaluation. The cause is usually a benign self-limiting condition (see Table 26.1), with the challenge to identify potentially life-threatening conditions (see Table 26.2). Diagnosis can be differentiated by a child's age and clinical characteristics such as symptoms and physical exam findings.

COMMON CAUSES

2. **What is the most common medical cause of abdominal pain in children?**
   Gastroenteritis is the most common cause of abdominal pain in children. The most frequent viruses include rotavirus, Norwalk virus, adenovirus, and enterovirus. *Escherichia coli*, *Campylobacter*, *Salmonella*, *Shigella*, and *Yersinia* are the most common bacterial agents.
   - Pet birds and reptiles can be a source of salmonella infections.
   - Outbreaks of *E. coli* O157, which can cause hemolytic uremic syndrome, have been linked to petting zoos.

3. **Describe symptoms of gastroenteritis**
   Acute gastroenteritis may present with fever, generalized abdominal pain, and cramp-like pain followed by the onset of diarrhea. In the absence of diarrhea, gastroenteritis should be a diagnosis of exclusion.
   - Gastroenteritis is most likely with a sick contact or family member with similar symptoms.

Table 26.1 Acute Abdominal Pain Etiologies by Age

AGE	<1 YEAR	1–5 YEARS	5–12 YEARS	>12 YEARS

Common/Urgent	Colic
	GERD
	Constipation
	Gastroenteritis
	UTI
		Gastroenteritis
		Constipation
		UTI
		Pharyngitis
		Henoch-Schönlein
		  purpura (HSP)
		Mesenteric adenitis
		Group A Strep (>2yr)
			Gastroenteritis
			Constipation
			Gastritis
			Functional Pain
			UTI
			Pharyngitis
			Pneumonia
			HSP
			Mesenteric adenitis
			Group A strep
				Gastroenteritis
				Constipation
				Gastritis
				UTI
				Dysmenorrhea
				Mittelschmerz
				PID
				Threatened
				  abortion
				Group A strep

Emergent	Pyloric Stenosis
	Intussusception
	Volvulus
	Incarcerated hernia
	Hirschsprung
	Necrotizing
	  enterocolitis
	Meckel
	  Diverticulum
	Trauma/NAT
		Appendicitis
		Intussusception
		Volvulus
		Trauma
		Sickle cell crisis
			Appendicitis
			Trauma
			Sickle cell crisis
			DKA
				Appendicitis
				Testicular torsion
				Ovarian torsion
				Ectopic pregnancy
				Pancreatitis
				Cholecystitis
				DKA

DKA, diabetic ketoacidosis; *NAT*, nonaccidental trauma; *PID*, pelvic inflammatory disease; *UTI*, urinary tract infections.

Table 26.2 Emergent Abdominal Pain Evaluation

CATASTROPHIC PRESENTATION	SUSPECT INTESTINAL OBSTRUCTION	SUSPECT APPENDICITIS OR TORSION	SUSPECT HEPATOBILIARY
• Very sick appearing • Listless or septic • Severe pain • Unstable vitals	• Abdominal • distension/firmness • Bilious emesis	• Periumbilical/RLQ • Suprapubic/LLQ • Anorexia • Nausea/vomiting • Fever	• RUQ or epigastric pain • Hepatomegaly • Jaundice • Nausea/vomiting
↓	↓	↓	↓
• Perforated viscus • Intraabdominal bleed • Necrotizing • Enterocolitis • Volvulus • Bowel ischemia	Neonate • Volvulus • 2 mo–2 years • Intussusception • Hirschsprung • Incarcerated hernia	• CBC, UA • Imaging US/CT • Surgery Consult	• Acute pancreatitis • Acute cholecystitis • Choledocholithiasis • Cholangitis • Hepatitis

CBC, complete blood count; *CT*, computer tomography; *LLQ*, left lower quadrant; *RLQ*, right lower quadrant; *RUQ*, right upper quadrant; *UA*, urinalysis; *US*, ultrasound.

4. **A 10-year-old male patient presents to your urgent care center with 3 days of intermittent abdominal pain, associated with nonbilious vomiting and decreased appetite. He strains with bowel movements and his stool consists of small balls of fecal matter. He is afebrile and his vitals are stable. On exam, he has left lower quadrant abdominal tenderness. What is the most likely diagnosis?**
Constipation is one of the most common chronic disorders of childhood. It is responsible for 3% of all primary care visits for children and up to 25% of pediatric gastroenterology visits. Children may present with a chief complaint of colicky abdominal pain, hard pellet-like stools, difficulty or pain with defecation, abdominal distension, vomiting, and/or anorexia. On examination, there is often left-sided or suprapubic tenderness.

5. **What is considered constipation in children?**
Constipation is likely in children with at least two of the following characteristics: fecal incontinence/encopresis, painful defecation, less than three stools weekly, large stools palpable in rectum on abdominal exam, or retentive posturing.

6. **What is functional constipation?**
Constipation without any evidence of organic etiology. It is also known as fecal withholding, functional fecal retention, or nonorganic constipation. Functional constipation may occur with toilet training, changes in routine or diet, stressful events, illness, lack of accessible toilets (e.g., at school), or a busy child who defers defecation.

7. **How do you diagnose constipation?**
A history and physical examination are usually sufficient to distinguish functional constipation from constipation with an organic etiology. History should review type of diet; prior history with therapies; frequency, consistency, and size of stools (use Bristol stool chart); age of onset of symptoms; meconium passage after birth; recent stressors; withholding behaviors, pain, or bleeding with bowel movements; abdominal pain; and fecal incontinence. Physical exam should include an abdominal exam; external examination of the perineum, perianal areas, thyroid, and spine; and a neurologic evaluation for appropriate reflexes (cremasteric, anal wink, and patellar).

8. **Is abdominal radiography recommended for diagnosing constipation?**
Abdominal radiography is not recommended for initial evaluation due to a lack of interobserver reliability and accuracy, but it may be useful to determine the extent of fecal impaction and differentiate between encopresis and diarrhea. It can be used in clinical circumstances in which a rectal examination is unreasonable (child with a history of trauma) or the diagnosis is uncertain.

9. **How is constipation treated?**
Treatment consists of acute oral or rectal disimpaction, followed by maintenance therapy for at least 2 months, in order to empty the rectum and allow the rectum to contract to normal size. Polyethylene glycol (PEG) is first-line treatment for disimpaction followed by maintenance. Oral therapies include osmotics (polyethylene glycol, magnesium citrate), stimulants (senna bisacodyl), and lubricants (mineral oil). Rectal agents include enemas (mineral oil, phosphate, normal saline) and suppositories (bisacodyl, glycerin).

10. **What symptoms are red flags for an underlying organic cause of constipation?**
    - Delayed passage of meconium
    - Significant abdominal distension
    - Abnormal development

- Constipation since birth
- Bloody stools (absence of anal fissure)
- Weight loss and/or failure to thrive

11. **What diagnosis must be considered in a neonate or infant presenting with constipation, poor feeding, and a weak cry?**
Infant botulism needs to be considered. Infant botulism is characterized by constipation followed by neuromuscular paralysis or "floppiness." Symptoms include constipation, history of poor feeding, difficulty latching and suckling, lethargy, and a weak cry. Exposure to honey or a construction site may be the cause.

12. **In a child presenting with constipation since birth, what disorder must be considered?**
Hirschsprung disease must be considered in infants and children with a history of constipation since birth and/or delayed meconium passing (>48 hours). Children diagnosed later in childhood may have a history of poor growth, severe refractory constipation, and intermittent vomiting. History and physical exam findings may include signs of enterocolitis, abdominal distension and pain, poor feeding, and foul-smelling watery stools.

13. **What are the most common presenting symptoms of urinary tract infection (UTI) in children aged 2 to 5 years?**
Abdominal pain and fever are the most common presenting symptoms of UTI in children 2–5 years of age. Infants may have a fever, vomiting, or anorexia; children >5 years are more likely to have classic UTI symptoms including dysuria, polyuria, and/or flank discomfort. Consider screening for UTI in toilet-trained children with any of the following:
- Urinary frequency
- Dysuria
- Nausea/vomiting
- Urinary incontinence
- Abdominal/suprapubic/flank pain
- Hematuria
- Prior UTI history: Fever ≥2 days without source
- Fever ≥5 days without a source

14. **What is referred abdominal pain and what are the most common causes?**
Referred pain is felt in areas remote from the affected organ and may come from extraabdominal conditions including:
- Pneumonia
- Streptococcal pharyngitis
- Diabetic ketoacidosis (DKA)
- Pelvic/genitourinary etiologies
  - Dysmenorrhea
  - Endometriosis
  - Ovarian cyst or torsion
  - Pelvic inflammatory disease
  - Testicular torsion/epididymitis

15. **What are the clinical features of infantile colic?**
Infantile colic affects up to 10–20% of infants during the first 3–4 weeks of life. It typically presents with screaming/crying, knees drawn up to the abdomen, or the appearance of abdominal pain. Clinical features suggestive of the diagnosis of colic include:
- A daily pattern of paroxysmal crying lasting at least 3 weeks
- Crying usually in the afternoon or evening
- Crying relieved with flatus or bowel movement
- Normal feeding and appropriate weight gain
- Normal physical exam

EMERGENT CAUSES

16. **A 14-day-old full-term female infant is brought into your office with new onset of vomiting with every feed for the last 8 hours. The emesis was initially the color of breast milk, but the last two episodes are the color of "green grass." Her parents state she is also fussy and crying more than usual. On exam, you note the infant is afebrile and fussy, and her abdomen is distended with guarding. What is your next step in management?**
Bilious emesis should prompt emergent workup for distal obstruction, including malrotation with volvulus. Immediate referral to an emergency department is warranted. Volvulus is abnormal twisting of the gut resulting in bowel obstruction and/or bowel ischemia. Abdominal two-view x-rays can be obtained to assess for obstruction findings:
- Free air
- Linear pneumatosis indicating bowel perforation
- Air-fluid levels and paucity of gas in lower intestines indicating obstruction

- Midgut volvulus: "Double bubble" sign with distended duodenal bulb and stomach
- Cecal volvulus: "Coffee bean" shaped air-filled cecum (25% of patients)
- Sigmoid volvulus: "Bent inner tube" showing distended U-shaped sigmoid colon
  If you suspect peritonitis due to necrotic bowel, imaging studies should not delay emergent operative management.

17. A 6-week-old full-term male is brought in with nonbilious vomiting for the past 2 days. He spits up usually, but his vomiting is progressively worsening and now he is vomiting very forcefully, immediately after all his feeds. He appears to be hungry after vomiting. What surgical condition do you need to rule out?

Pyloric stenosis is the most common surgical condition in infants. Pyloric stenosis is hypertrophy of the pyloric smooth muscle, which results in narrowing of the pylorus lumen and progressive obstruction as the pylorus thickens and elongates. The onset can be sudden (over a few days) or gradual (over 1–2 weeks with signs of growth failure), and vomiting is often described as "projectile" forceful vomiting. Obstruction of the pylorus muscle leads to gastric outlet obstruction, which leads to vomiting every feed, severe dehydration, hypovolemic shock, and electrolyte imbalances such as hypochloremia, hypokalemia, and metabolic alkalosis. Suspected pyloric stenosis needs to be emergently worked up and evaluated.

18. How do you diagnose pyloric stenosis and what is the treatment?

US of the pylorus is the diagnostic imaging of choice (sensitivity and specificity near 100%) with pyloric canal length ≥1.4 cm and muscle thickness ≥0.3 cm. Treatment is immediate intravenous fluid resuscitation and correction of electrolyte derangements. Once initial rehydration is complete, the definitive curative treatment is surgical pyloromyotomy.

19. A 16-month-old female presents with 2 days of recurrent 5–10-minute bouts of inconsolable crying, legs drawing up to her chest, along with several episodes of nonbilious nonbloody vomiting. In between episodes, she acts normal. On exam, she is afebrile and may have some diffuse right-sided abdominal tenderness. What abdominal emergency diagnosis do you need to consider?

Intussusception is the most common abdominal emergency of early childhood and commonly occurs between 3 months and 3 years of age. Intussusception is telescoping or invagination of one portion of the intestine into a more distal portion, commonly occurring at the junction of the terminal ileum and cecum (90% of cases). The classic triad of paroxysmal abdominal pain, vomiting (usually afebrile), and bloody "currant jelly" stool is seen in one-third of patients. If intussusception is suspected, the patient should be referred immediately to an emergency department for definitive diagnosis.

20. How do you diagnose and treat an intussusception?

Definitive diagnosis is made by abdominal ultrasound (sensitivity 98–100%, specificity 88–100%). A "target" or "doughnut" sign is noted with a hypoechoic outer rim with a central hyperechoic core on transverse view. Treatment is reduction by barium or air contrast enema with pediatric surgeon consultation for definitive intervention if the enema fails or in the rare case of perforation from the enema.

21. A 2-year-old male is brought in by his mother after she witnessed him putting something into his mouth 2 hours ago, and noted to have some gagging that is now resolved. He has had no difficulty breathing and he was able to drink some water and eat part of a banana. He is now holding his stomach and complaining of pain. He has had no vomiting, diarrhea, or fever. On exam, he is mild to moderately tender in the midabdominal area. What is your next step?

A majority (80%) of foreign body (FB) ingestions are witnessed; initial imaging includes AP and lateral radiographs of the neck, chest, and abdomen.
- Identify and locate a radiopaque FB
- Identify air-fluid levels in case of perforation
- Lateral views to distinguish location in trachea vs. esophagus

22. What are symptoms associated with complications of FB ingestion?

Patients with these symptoms should be made NPO and referred to a higher level of care in anticipation of anesthesia for FB removal.
- Vomiting
- Abdominal pain or distension
- Gastrointestinal bleeding
- Airway compromise

23. What FB characteristics are high risk for impaction or complications with ingestion?

It is important to assess the location and type of FB to determine the obstruction, impaction, and risk for complications.
- Sharp objects represent 10–15% of ingestions and have a higher risk of perforation (15–35%), and long objects >2.5 cm have a higher risk of impaction.
- Button batteries (characterized by telltale "ring" or "halo" on x-rays) can cause erosion, tissue necrosis, and perforation within several hours, especially if retained in the stomach.

- Multiple magnets lead to impaction by attraction across loops of bowel, resulting in necrosis and perforation.
- Superabsorbent polymers (e.g., expanding water beads) cause exponential expansion, leading to obstruction.

24. **What is the most common surgical cause of abdominal pain in children?**
Appendicitis, with approximately 70,000 pediatric cases/year, is the most common nontraumatic surgical condition in children presenting with acute abdominal pain. Approximately 1 in 15 people develop appendicitis, with a peak incidence of 9–12 years of age. Lymphoid or fecalith obstructs the appendiceal lumen, and the appendix becomes distended, with ischemia and necrosis developing.

25. **What are the three most predictive clinical features of appendicitis?**
Right lower quadrant (RLQ) abdominal pain, guarding, and migration of periumbilical pain within 6–48 hours to localize in the right lower quadrant. Less than 50% of pediatric patients will present with the classic presentation. Younger children present with atypical symptoms that may delay diagnosis, resulting in increased risk of complications. Omentum in children under 5 years old is underdeveloped, and if the appendix perforates, this may result in diffuse peritonitis with a nonspecific presentation. The misdiagnosis rate in children less than 2 years old is nearly 100%, due to the difficulty in localizing abdominal pain in nonverbal children. Many cases present similar to other common pediatric diagnoses such as constipation and gastroenteritis.

26. **What are some methods to reproduce RLQ pain in children with suspected appendicitis?**
When children are found to have RLQ pain, it is often reproduced with hopping, coughing, or rebound pain on examination.

27. **Describe the two physical exam signs that are indicative of appendicitis in children.**
The two physical exam findings are the obturator sign and the Rovsing sign.
    The obturator sign is pain elicited with passive internal rotation of the flexed right thigh.
    The Rovsing sign is obtained by pushing on the abdomen in the left lower quadrant, which elicits pain in the right lower quadrant.

28. **What is the psoas sign?**
Pain on passive extension of the right thigh with the patient lying on the left side.

29. **What laboratories should be sent for suspected appendicitis?**
White blood cell (WBC) count, C-reactive protein (CRP), urinalysis, and urine pregnancy; also consider serum chemistry. Combining the use of WBC and CRP increases sensitivity of laboratory evaluation for possible appendicitis.

30. **What is the radiographic diagnostic study of choice for diagnosing pediatric appendicitis?**
Ultrasound (US) is now the diagnostic modality of choice in pediatrics. To reduce the risk of radiation and long-term sequelae with abdominal computed tomography (CT), US and clinical decision rules (CDRs) can be used to make the diagnosis of appendicitis. The Pediatric Appendicitis Score (PAS) is frequently used with US, which increases diagnostic reliability (sensitivity 98.6%). Watchful waiting and serial abdominal examinations have a significant role in diagnosing pediatric appendicitis. CT scans provide better diagnostic information for perforated appendicitis or suspected intraabdominal abscesses.

31. **In a male patient presenting with localized abdominal pain, why should the genital area always be examined?**
The male scrotum and testes should always be examined to rule out testicular torsion/pathology and inguinal hernias. Referred abdominal pain may occur due to the stomach and small intestine having shared innervation with the testicle and epididymis.

TESTICULAR

32. **What surgical emergency needs to be considered when an adolescent male presents with vomiting, abdominal pain, and a swollen, painful testicle?**
Testicular torsion, a surgical emergency, presents with excruciating pain, scrotal swelling, nausea, and/or vomiting. Rapid diagnosis and detorsion are necessary to maximize testicle survival. Torsion is caused by the twisting of the spermatic cord, resulting in compression of the testicular artery and reduced or absent blood flow to the testicle. Torsion is the most common cause of testicular demise in adolescent males.

33. **What are the risk factors for testicular torsion?**
Presents in adolescence with 90% of cases due to congenital malformation, lack of proper fixation of the testis and epididymis to the scrotum, or the "bell-clapper deformity." Trauma is responsible in 4–8% of cases.

34. **What is the physical exam of a patient with testicular torsion?**
A torsed testicle is typically tender, with scrotal swelling, erythema, or discoloration. The testicle may have a horizontal lie and may be elevated. The probability of testicular torsion is high with an absent ipsilateral cremasteric reflex.

35. When is the onset of irreversible ischemia in testicular torsion?
Irreversible ischemia begins around 6 hours after onset of symptoms. Diagnosis and treatment within the 6-hour time period are optimal to minimize the risk of testicular necrosis and loss.

36. What diagnostic imaging is used to diagnose testicular torsion?
Scrotal ultrasound with Doppler is used to detect blood flow to the testicle. In children, flow is harder to detect, leading to false-positive results. However testicular torsion is a clinical diagnosis, and surgical exploration should be done emergently when suspicion is high despite imaging studies. Scrotal ultrasound can also differentiate an incarcerated inguinal hernia from testicular torsion.

37. Can manual detorsion be attempted at the patient's bedside?
Bedside manual detorsion may be attempted as long as definitive treatment is not delayed. This is done by rotating the testicle 180–360 degrees from medial to lateral.

OVARIAN

38. What are the signs and symptoms of ovarian torsion?
The most common symptom is sudden onset of sharp pelvic or lower abdominal pain (80–100%). The pain may be intermittent (15%), leading to a delayed diagnosis. In a younger child, the pain could be nonspecific and difficult to localize or describe. Nausea and vomiting are common and present in approximately 75% of the cases. Severe symptoms, such as acute abdominal pain or tenderness, fever, vomiting, and pallor, can mimic an acute surgical abdomen.

39. How common is ovarian torsion in premenarchal girls?
Ovarian torsion is rare in premenarchal girls. In one case series of 22 children, the mean age at presentation was 10 years. The majority of patients (70–75%) are younger than 30 years.

40. What are the risk factors for ovarian torsion?
Risk factors include ovarian cysts or masses, pregnancy, and history of pelvic inflammatory disease. Ovarian masses or cysts >4–6 cm are implicated in 50–60% of cases of ovarian torsion.

41. What is the study of choice to differentiate ovarian torsion versus other ovarian processes?
Ultrasound with Doppler is the study of choice. Findings for ovarian torsion may include an enlarged unilateral ovary, a heterogeneous mass, absent arterial flow, or fluid in the cul-de-sac. Ultrasound assists in the detection and diagnosis of other etiologies such as ovarian cyst, tubo-ovarian abscess, ectopic pregnancy, or appendicitis.

42. What is the definitive treatment for ovarian torsion?
Surgical or gynecologic urgent referral or transfer should be initiated immediately. Definitive treatment is surgical with laparoscopic or open detorsion with ovariopexy of the viable ovary. Ovariopexy for the contralateral ovary is typically performed.

43. What diagnosis must be considered in postmenarchal girls with acute abdominal pain?
Pregnancy, ectopic pregnancy, and threatened abortion must be considered in the diagnosis of abdominal pain in postmenarchal girls. Some adolescents have irregular menses and may not realize they are pregnant. Classic symptoms of threatened abortion and ectopic pregnancy are amenorrhea, abdominal pain, and vaginal bleeding. Ectopic pregnancy needs to be ruled out emergently in an emergency department, with subsequent rupture associated with life-threatening hemorrhage.

GALLSTONES

44. What are the signs and symptoms of gallstones in children?
No single symptom is highly sensitive or specific for cholelithiasis in children. Biliary colic may be present with persistent or episodic pain in the right upper quadrant (RUQ) and/or epigastrium. Pain may radiate to the right shoulder, back, or flank with nausea and vomiting after eating fatty foods. Pain lasting longer than 4–6 hours suggests biliary obstruction.

45. How common is cholelithiasis in children?
Gallstones are rare in children, but recently the incidence of pediatric gallbladder disease has been increasing, paralleling the rise of obesity in children. A large number (40%) of children with gallstones are asymptomatic, and complications arise when stones obstruct the cystic duct (cholecystitis) or common bile duct (choledocholithiasis) or cause an infection of the common bile duct (cholangitis).

46. What is the imaging modality of choice for diagnosis of choledocholithiasis?
Ultrasound is the modality of choice with excellent sensitivity and specificity. It is noninvasive and does not involve radiation exposure. Gallbladder distension, wall thickening, pericholecystic fluid suggesting choledocholithiasis, and stones as small as 2 mm can be visualized.

47. **What is a Murphy sign?**

A Murphy sign is worsening pain or inspiration arrest when the RUQ is palpated. It is highly sensitive in adults with cholecystitis.

48. **How do you treat uncomplicated cholelithiasis?**

Treatment for uncomplicated cholelithiasis is symptomatic with pain control and a low-fat diet. Routine ultrasound surveillance is appropriate for asymptomatic cases. Removal of the gallbladder in asymptomatic children with cholelithiasis is not standard practice, with the exception of those with sickle cell anemia.

49. **How do you treat symptomatic cholelithiasis?**

Laparoscopic cholecystectomy is the standard in the treatment of symptomatic cholelithiasis. It has been proven to be safe and effective in children, with a low rate of postoperative complications.

50. **How do you treat patients with biliary stone complications?**

Ill-appearing patients likely suffering from biliary stone complications should be stabilized with analgesics, antiemetics, and antibiotics and transferred/admitted. Patients with unresolved biliary colic or any suspicion of cholecystitis, cholelithiasis, cholangitis, or pancreatitis should be referred and admitted.

51. **What laboratory tests should be done to evaluate causes of diffuse or RUQ abdominal pain?**

The following are reasonable tests to evaluate causes of abdominal pain.
- Chemistries including aspartate transaminase (AST), alanine transaminase (ALT), direct and indirect bilirubin, and γ-glutamyltransferase (GGT; liver disease, cholangitis)
- Amylase and lipase (pancreatitis)
- CBC with differential (anemia and leukocytosis)
- C-reactive protein (elevated in choledocholithiasis and appendicitis)
- Urinalysis and urine pregnancy (urinary tract infections, pregnancy, diabetes screen)

PANCREATITIS

52. **What are the signs and symptoms of acute pancreatitis in children?**
- Abdominal pain (87%)
- Sharp, constant pain in the epigastric area
- Pain may radiate to the back or sides
- Pain and vomiting worsen after eating
- Nausea, vomiting, and anorexia (64%)
- Abdominal tenderness (77%)
- Abdominal distension (18%)

53. **What is the most common cause of acute pancreatitis in children?**

Blunt trauma to the pancreas is the most common cause of acute pancreatitis in children. Traumatic pancreatitis can result from motor vehicle accidents, bicycle/scooter handlebar injuries, and inflicted injury from child abuse. Pseudocysts may develop 2–3 weeks after the traumatic pancreatitis episode. In 25% of childhood cases, the etiology of pediatric pancreatitis is unknown.

54. **How do you diagnose pancreatitis?**

The diagnosis is clinical and can be made if two or more of these criteria are fulfilled: symptoms consistent with acute pancreatitis (abdominal pain, nausea, vomiting, and abdominal tenderness), elevated lipase and/or amylase, and imaging consistent with pancreatitis.

55. **What imaging is useful for diagnosing acute pancreatitis?**

Ultrasound is the imaging of choice for acute pancreatitis, as it can assess the pancreatic size, inflammation, and texture. It can also assess biliary stone obstruction and the presence of pseudocysts or abscesses.

56. **How do you treat acute pancreatitis in children?**

The treatment of pancreatitis is supportive inpatient care with pancreatic rest, no oral intake or adhering to a low-fat elemental diet, fluid resuscitation, pain medication, and parenteral nutrition if unable to eat. Meperidine (Demerol) is preferred to morphine for pain control because it is less likely to cause spasm of the sphincter of Oddi, which can worsen the pancreatitis. Acute uncomplicated cases of childhood pancreatitis have an excellent prognosis.

HEPATITIS

57. **What causes hepatitis in children?**

Hepatitis may result from both infectious (viral, bacterial, fungal, and parasitic organisms) and noninfectious (medications, toxins, and autoimmune) causes. Possible viral exposures include blood transfusions, intravenous or intranasal drug use, sexual or sexual abuse history, and travel history. It is important to consider exposure to medications, such as acetaminophen commonly found in children's cold medications, or toxins such as poisonous wild mushrooms.

58. **What are some viruses that can cause acute hepatitis?**
Following is a list of some viruses associated with acute hepatitis.
- Hepatitis viruses: five main types, including hepatitis A, B, C, D, and E
- Cytomegalovirus (CMV), part of the herpesvirus family
- Epstein-Barr virus (EBV), commonly associated with infectious mononucleosis
- Herpes simplex virus (HSV), varicella zoster virus (VZV), enteroviruses, rubella, parvovirus, and adenovirus (adenovirus type 41 has been linked to acute liver failure)

59. **What are the symptoms and treatment of acute hepatitis in children?**
The most common symptoms of acute hepatitis include flu-like symptoms, fever, abdominal pain, nausea, vomiting, fatigue, anorexia, jaundice, myalgias, dark urine, and clay-colored stools. Medications are not routinely given for treatment of uncomplicated acute viral hepatitis. All patients with suspected or confirmed HBV or HCV infection should be referred to a gastroenterologist or hepatologist for further evaluation and treatment.

Patients with evidence of fulminant hepatitis, hepatic encephalopathy, significant vomiting, dehydration, or electrolyte abnormalities require hospital admission.

60. **What laboratory tests should be sent for suspected acute hepatitis?**
- ALT, AST, and lactate to evaluate hepatocellular injury
- Prothrombin time (PT), partial thromboplastin time (PTT), albumin, and ammonia to evaluate the liver's functional capacity
- Alkaline phosphatase, GGT, and total/direct bilirubin to detect biliary obstruction
- Serum electrolytes, blood urea nitrogen (BUN), creatinine, and glucose
- Acetaminophen levels if suspect acetaminophen toxicity
- Hepatitis A antibody (IgM, anti-HAV), hepatitis B core antibody (IgM anti-HBc), and surface antigen (HbsAg)
- Anti-HCV antibody testing and qualitative polymerase chain reaction (PCR) for HCV

61. **Is radiographic imaging necessary to diagnose acute hepatitis?**
Abdominal ultrasound or CT scan may be necessary to rule out other abdominal pathology such as abdominal masses, gallbladder disease, or biliary tract obstruction.

KEY POINTS

1. Age is a key factor in evaluating abdominal pain in order to make a rapid diagnosis and initiate treatment to minimize morbidity.
2. Constipation is one of the most common causes of childhood abdominal pain and is a diagnosis of exclusion.
3. Children presenting with constipation since birth need to have Hirschsprung disease ruled out.
4. Testicular torsion is a time-sensitive emergency, requiring immediate diagnosis and a 6-hour time window for treatment to minimize testicle necrosis and loss.
5. Ovarian torsion in premenarchal girls is rare, but abdominal pain in adolescent females warrants a pregnancy test and a diagnostic ultrasound study to evaluate ovaries for torsion or other ovarian pathology.
6. Consider referred abdominal pain from extraabdominal sources, such as pneumonia, Streptococcal pharyngitis, or DKA, if a patient has a history or concurrent symptoms of a URI, sore throat, or viral illness.

BIBLIOGRAPHY

Barcega BR, Piroutek MJ. Constipation. In: Hoffman RJ, et al., ed. *Fleisher & Ludwig's 5-Minute Pediatric Emergency Medicine Consult.* 2nd ed. Wolters Kluwer Health; 2019:148–149. VitalSource Bookshelf.

Cavallaro SC. Ovarian Torsion. In: Hoffman RJ, et al., ed. *Fleisher & Ludwig's 5-Minute Pediatric Emergency Medicine Consult.* 2nd ed. Wolters Kluwer Health; 2019:622–623. VitalSource Bookshelf.

Centers for Disease Control and Prevention. Acute Hepatitis and Adenovirus Infection Among Children — Alabama, October 2021–February 2022. Available at: https://www.cdc.gov/mmwr/volumes/71/wr/mm7118e1.htm. Published April 29, 2022. Accessed October 1, 2022.

Costello MC, Garcia Pena BM. Pain, Abdominal. In: Hoffman RJ, et al., ed. *Fleisher & Ludwig's 5-Minute Pediatric Emergency Medicine Consult.* 2nd ed. Wolters Kluwer Health; 2019:624–625. VitalSource Bookshelf.

Ellison AM. Hepatitis, Acute. In: Hoffman RJ, et al., ed. *Fleisher & Ludwig's 5-Minute Pediatric Emergency Medicine Consult.* 2nd ed. Wolters Kluwer Health; 2019:422–423. VitalSource Bookshelf.

Graham KN, Bachur RG, eds. *Fleisher and Ludwig's Textbook of Pediatric Emergency Medicine.* 7th ed. Wolters Kluwer; 2016:109–114.

Kim JS. Acute abdominal pain in children. *Pediatr Gastroenterol Hepatol Nutr.* 2013;16(4):219–224.

Leung AK, Sigalet DL. Acute abdominal pain in children. *Am Fam Physician.* 2003;67(11):2321–2326.

Loening-Baucke V, Swidsinski A. Constipation as cause of acute abdominal pain in children. *J Pediatr.* 2007;151:666–669.

Loiselle J. Pancreatitis. In: Hoffman RJ, et al., ed. *Fleisher & Ludwig's 5-Minute Pediatric Emergency Medicine Consult.* 2nd ed. Wolters Kluwer Health; 2019:646–647. Available from: VitalSource Bookshelf.

Mehta S, Lopez ME, Chumpitazi BP, Mazziotti MV, Brandt ML, Fishman DS. Clinical characteristics and risk factors for symptomatic pediatric gallbladder disease. *Pediatrics.* 2012;129(1):e82–e88.

Raymond M, Marsicovetere P, DeShaney K. Diagnosing and managing acute abdominal pain in children. *JAAPA.* 2022;35:16–20.

Reust CE, Williams A. Acute abdominal pain in children. *Am Fam Physician*. 2016;93(10):830–836.

Seiden JA. Intussusception. In: Hoffman RJ, et al., ed. *Fleisher & Ludwig's 5-Minute Pediatric Emergency Medicine Consult*. 2nd ed. Wolters Kluwer Health; 2019:488–489. VitalSource Bookshelf.

Seiden JA. Foreign Body Ingestion. In: Hoffman RJ, et al., ed. *Fleisher & Ludwig's 5-Minute Pediatric Emergency Medicine Consult*. 2nd ed. Wolters Kluwer Health; 2019:308–309. VitalSource Bookshelf.

Seiden JA. Pyloric Stenosis. In: Hoffman RJ, et al., ed. *Fleisher & Ludwig's 5-Minute Pediatric Emergency Medicine Consult*. 2nd ed. Wolters Kluwer Health; 2019:774–775. VitalSource Bookshelf.

Shah SR, Sinclair KA, Theut SB, et al. Computed tomography utilization for the diagnosis of acute appendicitis in children decreases with a diagnostic algorithm. *Ann Surg*. 2016;264(3):474–481.

Sharma A, Chauhan N, Alexander A, et al. The risks and the identification of ingested button batteries in the esophagus. *Pediatr Emerg Care*. 2009;25(3):196–199.

Sharp VJ, Kieran K, Arlen AM. Testicular torsion: diagnosis, evaluation, and management. *Am Fam Physician*. 2013;88(12):835–840.

Snyder MJ, Guthrie M, Cagle S. Acute appendicitis: efficient diagnosis and management. *Am Fam Physician*. 2018;98(1):25–33.

Subramaniam S, Chao JH. Ovarian Cyst/Mass. In: Hoffman RJ, et al., ed. *Fleisher & Ludwig's 5-Minute Pediatric Emergency Medicine Consult*. 2nd ed. Wolters Kluwer Health; 2019:620–621. VitalSource Bookshelf.

Tabbers MM, DiLorenzo C, Merger MY, et al. Evaluation and treatment of functional constipation in infants and children: evidence-based recommendations from ESPGHAN and NASPGHAN. *J Pediatr Gastroenterol Nutr*. 2014;58:258–274.

UpToDate. Causes of acute abdominal pain in children and adolescents. Available at: https://www.uptodate.com/contents/causes-of-acute-abdominal-pain-in-children-and-adolescents#H84421646. Published 2022. Accessed October 1, 2022.

CHAPTER 27

NAUSEA, VOMITING, DIARRHEA, AND DEHYDRATION

Christopher M. Pruitt, MD

TOP SECRETS

While there are no clinical tools superior to clinician gestalt in the assessment of dehydration in children, oliguria is not usually associated with significant dehydration.

In the young child (approximately 6–36 months of age) with isolated vomiting, always consider the diagnosis of ileocolic intussusception.

1. **What are the common reasons for vomiting in pediatric patients?**
   Children vomit with almost any kind of illness, so the list of causes is extensive. However, gastroenteritis is by far the most common cause of vomiting in children of any age.

2. **What are the usual culprits for gastroenteritis?**
   The answer depends on your practice setting. While bacterial and parasitic causes are more commonly encountered in resource-poor settings, in developed countries, viruses are much more prevalent.

3. **If vomiting is so common, how can I know if a dangerous condition might be present (Table 27.1)?**
   - Appearance of the vomit: bright green or yellow (bilious)
   - Pain: especially severe or constant
   - Exam: marked tenderness or distension
   - Signs or symptoms of elevated intracranial pressure

4. **Why is bilious emesis worrisome? Is it always?**
   Vomiting of bile can herald an intestinal obstruction distal to the sphincter of Oddi. More frequently, however, bilious emesis simply follows vomiting of nonbilious contents and does not indicate an emergency.

5. **A 13-day-old female patient presents with two episodes of vomiting in the past few hours. The parents show you a blanket with a small bright yellow stain from her emesis. What should you do?**
   Bilious emesis in young infants should be considered an emergency until proven otherwise. This is a classic presentation (even if the infant is well appearing) for neonatal obstruction, the most common cause being intestinal malrotation entraining volvulus. This child should have an urgent upper gastrointestinal (GI) study.

6. **How do I know if the baby I'm seeing simply has reflux?**
   Physiologic reflux ("spitting up") is the most common cause of vomiting in infants. Clues to this diagnosis are well appearance, normal growth, and nonacute presentation. Reflux typically peaks in the second month of life and usually does not require pharmacologic intervention.

7. **A 7-week-old infant has had worsening vomiting for 5 days. There is no bile. The caregiver thinks that the emesis is becoming more forceful. What diagnosis should you consider?**
   Hypertrophic pyloric stenosis usually presents in the second month of life, and it is more common in males. Given the anatomic location of the obstruction, the vomitus is nonbilious. Babies are often well appearing, and unless they present later in the course of illness, the "classic" electrolyte pattern of a hypochloremic, hypokalemic metabolic alkalosis will be absent. They have progressive "projectile" vomiting and lack satiety. The diagnosis is made by ultrasound.

8. **List some common causes for a presenting complaint of "blood in the stool" for infants and young children.**
   - Lack of true blood (red dyes, cefdinir)
   - Anal fissures
   - Infectious diarrhea
   - Swallowed maternal blood
   - Milk protein intolerance (infants)
   - Ileocolic intussusception (late finding)

Table 27.1 Worrisome Causes of Vomiting by Age Group

INFANCY	EARLY CHILDHOOD	ADOLESCENCE
Volvulus from malrotation	Intussusception	Appendicitis
Pyloric stenosis	Toxic ingestion	Toxic ingestion
Increased intracranial pressure	Increased intracranial pressure	Increased intracranial pressure
Inborn errors of metabolism	Diabetic ketoacidosis	Diabetic ketoacidosis
Other causes of obstruction	Appendicitis	Torsion of ovary/testis

9. **My patient has had fever and diarrhea but now has blood in the stool. Guaiac testing is positive. The child looks well. Given the presence of blood, is there anything different that should be done?**
   While routine stool cultures are not recommended for children with acute diarrhea, up to 20% of cultures will grow a bacterial pathogen when gross blood is present. Therefore, it is advisable to obtain a stool culture in this setting. Nevertheless, antibiotic treatment is not recommended for healthy children in most cases of bacterial enteritis.

10. **What diagnosis should always be considered in older infants and young children with isolated vomiting?**
    Ileocolic intussusception is the most common gastrointestinal emergency in young children. The usual age range is 6–36 months of age, but all the "classic" findings (vomiting, pain, lethargy, abdominal mass, "currant jelly" stools) are not usually present. Kids can appear well, especially if the obstruction is intermittent. The preferred diagnostic modality is ultrasound, and hydrostatic air enema is usually successful in reducing intussusception.

11. **Does a complaint of vomiting blood in a child often portend a worrisome cause?**
    No. Though serious causes should be explored via history and physical, the most common causes for hematemesis are swallowed blood from the upper airways (e.g., colds, epistaxis) or small Mallory-Weiss tears that usually heal on their own.

12. **Why does constipation often present with "diarrhea"?**
    Kids with constipation often have watery feces that move past the impacted distal stool. A detailed history will help you arrive at the right diagnosis.

13. **What is the most common reason for hyponatremic dehydration in infants?**
    While most children have isotonic dehydration, infants whose caregivers improperly prepare or dilute formula can cause hypotonic dehydration in these young children. Left unrecognized and untreated, these infants can progress to seizures and even death.

14. **In an ill-appearing child with dehydration, what lab value is the most important to check initially?**
    In younger children, hypoglycemia should be suspected and rapidly corrected. Up to 10% of young children with dehydration have hypoglycemia. For well-appearing patients, mild hypoglycemia can be administered enterally; for ill-appearing children, or for significantly low glucose levels, correct intravenously with 0.5 g/kg dextrose.

15. **My patient's caregiver says that he hasn't urinated in 18 hours. This means he has significant dehydration, right?**
    Perhaps, but not usually. Less than one of every five parents who report oliguria will have a child with considerable dehydration (Table 27.2). Unfortunately, though parents are often told to watch for this at home, this is an unreliable means for a caregiver to accurately gauge dehydration. You should still ask about urine output; other conditions can cause dehydration that may be associated with an *increase* in urine output (most notably diabetes mellitus, but also diabetes insipidus or other conditions that impair renal concentration). Oliguria may also indicate kidney injury (e.g., hemolytic-uremic syndrome).

16. **How helpful is urine specific gravity in detection of dehydration?**
    Excluding conditions that alter urine osmolarity, highly concentrated urine does not always indicate significant dehydration, and a low specific gravity doesn't mean the patient isn't dehydrated. It simply is not a very helpful measure of hydration in children.

17. **At the patient's bedside, how am I supposed to know whether they are dehydrated?**
    Clinician "gestalt" may be just as good as scoring instruments for dehydration. However, the best clinical tools for assessing dehydration combine features of the physical exam, most notably general appearance, dry mucous membranes, and absence of tears.

Table 27.2 Reliability of Clinical Findings in Dehydration

CLINICAL FINDING	SENSITIVITY	SPECIFICITY	POSITIVE PREDICTIVE VALUE	NEGATIVE PREDICTIVE VALUE
Decreased skin elasticity	0.35	0.97	0.57	0.93
Capillary refill >2 sec	0.48	0.96	0.57	0.94
General appearance	0.59	0.91	0.42	0.95
Absent tears	0.67	0.89	0.40	0.96
Abnormal respirations	0.43	0.86	0.37	0.94
Dry mucous membranes	0.80	0.78	0.29	0.99
Sunken eyes	0.60	0.84	0.29	0.95
Abnormal radial pulse	0.43	0.86	0.25	0.93
Tachycardia (HR >150)	0.46	0.79	0.20	0.93
Decreased urine output	0.85	0.53	0.17	0.97

Data from Gorelick MH, Shaw KN, Murphy KO. Validity and Reliability of Clinical Signs in the Diagnosis of Dehydration in Children. *Pediatrics.* 99(5):E6.

18. **What medications should be used in children with vomiting and/or diarrhea?**
A single dose of ondansetron (best to use orally disintegrating form) is likely to reduce vomiting and facilitate oral rehydration for infants and children and has been shown to reduce hospitalization and the need for parenteral fluids. Conversely, well-designed clinical trials have failed to demonstrate any benefit of probiotics for infectious diarrhea in children.

19. **You are seeing a 3-year-old male with 4 days of profuse diarrhea and some vomiting. You believe he is moderately dehydrated. How should you rehydrate this child?**
Extensive research has demonstrated great success with enteral rehydration in children with mild to moderate dehydration. Oral rehydration solutions (ORS) with balanced sodium and glucose enable the intestinal cotransport mechanisms for passive water absorption. One trial demonstrated that initial rehydration with half-diluted apple juice followed by the child's preferred oral fluids did better than those with ORS. The fluid deficit is replaced over 4 hours, usually in 5-minute increments. Mild dehydration equates to roughly 50 mL/kg body water loss, and moderate dehydration to 100 mL/kg; this means the mildly dehydrated child gets approximately 1 mL/kg per aliquot, and 2 mL/kg if moderately dehydrated.

20. **When would you not advise a rehydration solution for a child with diarrhea?**
The sodium and glucose in rehydration solutions render them highly osmolar. If the child is not dehydrated, ingestion of such liquids can exacerbate diarrhea. Infants without dehydration should continue to drink breastmilk or formula; consider dilution of high-sugar beverages for older children. If intravenous fluids are needed, order isotonic (0.9% saline or lactated Ringer) fluid in volumes of 20 mL/kg (up to 1 liter), usually over 20–30 minutes. Never bolus hypotonic fluids or dextrose-containing fluids (unless the latter is needed for rapid correction of hypoglycemia).

KEY POINTS

1. Complaints of blood in vomit or stool are usually associated with nonemergencies in healthy children.
2. Ileocolic intussusception should always be considered in the young child (about 6–36 months of age) with isolated vomiting.
3. Parental report of oliguria is the least predictive sign of pediatric dehydration.
4. While ondansetron is helpful in children with vomiting, probiotics have not been consistently proven effective for children with infectious diarrhea.
5. If dehydration is not severe, most children can be successfully treated with appropriate oral rehydration solutions or diluted apple juice followed by their preferred fluids.

BIBLIOGRAPHY

Falszewska A, Szajewska H, Dziechciarz P. Diagnostic accuracy of three clinical dehydration scales: a systematic review. *Arch Dis Child.* 2018;103(4):383–388.
Freedman SB, Willan AR, Boutis K, et al. Effect of dilute apple juice and preferred fluids vs electrolyte maintenance solution on treatment failure among children with mild gastroenteritis: a randomized clinical trial. *JAMA.* 2016;315(18):1966–1974.

Gorelick MH, Shaw KN, Murphy KO. Validity and reliability of clinical signs in the diagnosis of dehydration in children. *Pediatrics.* 1997;99(5):E6.

Niño-Serna LF, Acosta-Reyes J, Veroniki AA, et al. Antiemetics in children with acute gastroenteritis: a meta-analysis. *Pediatrics.* 2020;145(4):e20193260.

Reid SR, Losek JD. Hypoglycemia complicating dehydration in children with acute gastroenteritis. *J Emerg Med.* 2005;29(2):141–145.

Schnadower D, Tarr PI, Casper TC, et al. Lactobacillus rhamnosus GG versus placebo for acute gastroenteritis in children. *N Engl J Med.* 2018;379(21):2002–2014.

Spandorfer PR. Dehydration. In: Shaw KN, Bachur RG, eds. *Textbook of Pediatric Emergency Medicine.* Lippincott Williams & Wilkins; 2015:128–134.

Steiner MJ, Nager AL, Wang VJ. Urine specific gravity and other urinary indices: inaccurate tests for dehydration. *Pediatr Emerg Care.* 2007;23(5):298–303.

Whittington LA, Stevens DC, Jones SA, et al. Visual diagnosis: an 11-month-old with nausea, vomiting, and an abdominal mass. *Pediatr Rev.* 2013;34(12):e47–e50.

CHAPTER 28

URINARY AND UROLOGIC COMPLAINTS

Jennifer F. Anders, MD, Jennifer N. Fishe, MD

1. **The classic symptoms of urinary tract infection include dysuria, urgency, and frequency. What are the most common signs of urinary tract infection in preverbal and nonverbal children?**

   Urinary tract infection (UTI) may present with a myriad of signs and symptoms. In the neonate, UTI may present as fever or sepsis without an obvious source. Fever may be the only symptom in infants as well. Other manifestations of UTIs can be nonspecific. Systemic symptoms may include irritability, fatigue, fussiness, decreased oral intake, decreased urine output, or failure to thrive. Gastrointestinal (GI) symptoms are common and may include vomiting, diarrhea, and abdominal pain (especially suprapubic) or back pain. This may lead caregivers to conclude the patient has gastroenteritis or a food allergy.

   Beyond 2–3 years of age, symptoms more often point to the urinary tract; these include frequency, urgency, retention or incontinence, dysuria, and occasionally hematuria. This can present as a previously toilet-trained child beginning to have "accidents."

   Foul-smelling urine is often mentioned by caregivers but has little diagnostic meaning.

   In children who lack bladder sensation (e.g., spina bifida) and who receive regular straight catheterization, a change in the quality of the urine (cloudier, change in odor) may be the only sign. Such children may also present with fever, change in level of alertness, or vomiting.

2. **When should a urinalysis be obtained in a child with suspected UTI?**

   For an infant less than 2 months of age, urinalysis should always be obtained as part of the complete evaluation of fever without a source. For children over 2 months of age, the decision to obtain urinalysis is guided by the child's clinical status. Once antimicrobial therapy is initiated, the opportunity to make a definitive diagnosis is lost; therefore, urinalysis and culture should be obtained prior to antibiotic therapy.

   If a child with an unexplained fever does not need immediate antibiotic treatment, the clinician can use clinical history and exam findings to assess the likelihood of UTI. Laboratory investigation for UTI should be reserved for those children with concerning symptoms including dysuria, urgency, frequency, suprapubic pain, fever with no obvious source, fever with emesis (and absence of diarrhea), costovertebral angle tenderness, other unexplained abdominal pain, or irritability without an alternate explanation.

   Since specific UTI symptoms of dysuria, urgency, or frequency are not available for most diapered or preverbal children, alternative risk stratification tools have been created. The approximate rate of UTI in febrile children 2–24 months of age is 5%; the risk is significantly lower for circumcised boys. Higher risk of UTI can be predicted for children with prior history of UTI, those of non-black race, and those with higher temperatures (>39°C), longer duration of fever (>24 hours), or signs of systemic toxicity. For children 2–24 months with one or more risk factors, urinalysis is recommended, and if pyuria is present, a culture should be obtained to confirm UTI. An online version of this tool is freely available at UTICalc.pitt.edu.

3. **When and how should urine be obtained for culture in a child with suspected UTI?**

   If antimicrobial therapy is to be initiated, then a urine specimen suitable for culture should be obtained before antimicrobial agents are given. Urine specimens suitable for culture include those obtained by clean catch midstream collection, urethral catheterization, or suprapubic aspiration. Adhesive bag urine collection is often used for children who are not toilet trained. Such bag specimens may be used for urinalysis (UA) but should be assumed to be contaminated with perineal flora and not be used for culture.

   One option is to obtain a urinalysis with a bag specimen, and if the UA is normal and the patient is otherwise not at high risk for UTI, the evaluation can be considered complete. If the UA is abnormal, a second urine sample should be obtained by a clean method (clean catch, urethral catheterization, or suprapubic aspiration) and sent for culture to confirm the diagnosis and provide bacterial identification and sensitivities.

4. **What are the alternative methods for urine to be obtained for culture from children of various ages?**

   In children who are not able to cooperate with a clean catch urine collection, culture samples should only be obtained via catheterization or suprapubic aspiration. Cultures of urine specimens collected in a bag applied to the perineum have an unacceptably high false-positive rate and are valid only when they yield negative results.

   Ideal handling of a bagged urine specimen includes (a) the perineal skin is well cleansed before bag application, (b) the bag is removed promptly after voiding, and (c) the specimen is refrigerated or processed immediately. Despite claims that this collection technique has a low contamination rate with ideal handling, there is an unavoidable but significant contamination in the two groups at the highest risk for UTI: the vagina in girls and the prepuce in uncircumcised boys.

5. **How can you differentiate pyelonephritis from cystitis in pediatric patients?**
Distinguishing pyelonephritis from cystitis is difficult in young patients because they may have clinical overlap and younger patients often have only nonspecific symptoms. Hence, pyelonephritis and cystitis are often discussed together as one clinical entity, generically covered by the term "urinary tract infection."

While strict differentiation between upper and lower tract disease in children is often not feasible, there are some features more suggestive of pyelonephritis: high fever (>40°C), ill or toxic appearance, flank pain, or costovertebral angle tenderness and emesis.

Features suggestive of limited cystitis include well appearance, suprapubic pain, and normothermia or low-grade fever.

6. **What are some widely accepted empiric antibiotic strategies for pediatric UTI?**
Oral or parenteral treatment is equally efficacious for most pediatric UTIs (cystitis or pyelonephritis). Antibiotic choice should be based on local antimicrobial sensitivity patterns (if available) and should be individually adjusted to sensitivity testing from the patient's urine culture.

There is no single preferred duration of therapy, but most recent guidelines suggest at least 3–5 days for simple cystitis without fever and 7–14 days for febrile UTI. Shorter courses of 1–3 days of antibiotic treatment currently do not have a robust evidence base.

Intravenous (IV; parenteral) antibiotic therapy should be initiated if the patient is less than 2 months of age, has a toxic appearance or other signs of systemic illness, cannot tolerate oral intake, has other adverse anatomic factors (e.g., obstruction to urinary flow), or has a known positive culture for a pathogen not susceptible to oral agents (Boxes 28.1 and 28.2).

It is essential to know local susceptibility patterns because there is substantial geographic variability. Up to 60% of *Escherichia coli* strains demonstrate resistance to ampicillin and amoxicillin/clavulanate; therefore, these drugs should not be used as monotherapy unless local patterns of susceptibility are known to be favorable.

7. **How does antibiotic therapy for children with pyelonephritis differ from therapy for cystitis?**
Historically, treatment of pyelonephritis has been initiated with IV antibiotics until the patient becomes afebrile. This may still be warranted in ill-appearing children or those with complicating factors. However, ample evidence supports the outpatient treatment of uncomplicated pediatric pyelonephritis when the child can tolerate oral fluids and antibiotics, has normal renal function, and is not septic. The widely recommended treatment course is 7–14 days of oral cephalosporin (e.g., cephalexin, cefdinir, cefixime, or cefpodoxime). It is important to note that nitrofurantoin should not be used for suspected pyelonephritis because it does not achieve therapeutic concentrations in the bloodstream.

8. **What follow-up should be planned for a child with diagnosis of urinary tract infection?**
Ideally, the child should have a follow-up within 48 hours to ensure that the current infection is being adequately treated, including ability to tolerate the prescribed antibiotic and verification that any symptoms are resolving. The follow-up should include review of urine culture results and sensitivities and allow for changes in antibiotic treatment if needed to match the sensitivity results. Children should seek care earlier if their condition worsens.

9. **When is hospitalization necessary for a child with urinary tract infection?**
Many UTIs may be treated with oral antibiotics in the outpatient setting. However, children who cannot tolerate oral antibiotics or fluids, children with signs of sepsis (e.g., persistent tachycardia, hypotension, delayed capillary

---

Box 28.1 Oral Antibiotic Options for Pediatric UTI

Cephalexin 100 mg/kg/day ÷ qid
Cefixime 8 mg/kg/day given once daily
Cefpodoxime 10 mg/kg/day ÷ bid
Cefdinir 14 mg/kg/day given once daily
Nitrofurantoin 7 mg/kg/day ÷ qid or (as macrocrystal/monohydrate) 100 mg bid
Trimethoprim/sulfamethoxazole 8–10 mg/kg/day of trimethoprim component ÷ bid

---

Box 28.2 Parenteral (IV) Antibiotic Options for Pediatric UTI

Ampicillin 200 mg/kg/day ÷ qid PLUS gentamicin 5–7.5 mg/kg/day in a single dose
Cefazolin 75 mg/kg/day ÷ tid
Ceftriaxone 75 mg/kg/day (IV or IM) in a single dose or ÷ bid
Cefepime 200 mg/kg/day ÷ bid

refill) or renal dysfunction (decreased urine output, urinary retention/obstruction), and infants less than 2 months of age should be hospitalized and receive IV antibiotics. In addition, children require IV antibiotics for cultures positive for pathogens for which there is no susceptible oral antibiotic. Hospitalization should also be considered for children with genitourinary anatomic abnormalities (e.g., ureteropelvic junction obstruction, posterior urethral valves, bladder extrophy) or children with indwelling urinary catheters.

10. **What is the definition of true hematuria? What is the differential diagnosis of false hematuria?**
True hematuria is confirmed by microscopy with greater than five red blood cells (RBCs) present in the urinalysis. False hematuria, presenting with red urine or apparent gross hematuria, or a positive dipstick for hemoglobin without RBC on microscopy, may be caused by myoglobinuria, hemolysis, crystal urates, or ingestion of foods including beets and blackberries, aniline dyes, or medications including Pyridium and rifampin.

11. **What is the differential diagnosis for true hematuria in a child?**
There are numerous causes of hematuria in children. Tables 28.1 and 28.2 list a variety of common causes, with the most common highlighted in bold.

12. **When should a child with hematuria be referred to an emergency department for immediate evaluation?**
A child with hematuria should be referred for emergent evaluation if there is concern for nephritis or if the hematuria is accompanied by proteinuria; such children require further laboratory evaluation for evidence of renal dysfunction. Hematuria with hypertension (>90th percentile for height) should also have prompt emergent

Table 28.1 Common Causes of Gross Hematuria in Children

BENIGN CAUSES	PATHOLOGIC CAUSES
Exercise	**UTI (urethritis, cystitis, pyelonephritis)** Trauma (kidney, bladder, urethra)
Idiopathic hypercalciuria without nephrolithiasis	**Acute poststreptococcal glomerulonephritis (APSGN)**
	Nephrolithiasis
	Sickle cell trait or disease
	Obstruction (ureteropelvic junction obstruction)
	Foreign body
	Wilms tumor
	Renal vein thrombosis (ex-premature infants)
	Polycystic kidney disease
	Genitourinary tract arteriovenous malformation (rare)
	Tuberculosis

Table 28.2 Common Causes of Microscopic Hematuria in Children

BENIGN	PATHOLOGIC
Asymptomatic isolated hematuria	**Trauma**
Benign familial hematuria	Nephritic syndrome (e.g., lupus, membranoproliferative glomerulonephritis)
	Alport syndrome
	IgA nephropathy
	Vasculitis (Wegener)
	Henoch-Schönlein purpura
	Hemolytic-uremic syndrome

Box 28.3 Most Frequent Etiologies of Kidney Stones in Children

Dehydration
Diet (high sodium, low calcium intake)
Infection
Metabolic abnormalities (most frequently hypercalciuria)

Box 28.4 Causes of Acute Urinary Retention in Children

Mechanical obstruction (anatomic abnormality, blood clot, stone, stricture from catheterization, neoplasm)
Infection (UTI, vaginitis)
Fecal impaction
Neurologic disorder (dysfunctional voiding, acute myelitis)
Behavioral
Drug effect (opioids)
Idiopathic

referral. Children with suspected trauma to the kidneys, bladder, pelvis, or urethra also need emergent evaluation. Any patient with decreased urine output, no urine output, signs of volume overload on physical exam (such as periorbital or scrotal edema), or signs of urinary tract obstruction (from blood clots) should be referred to an emergency department.

13. What are the most frequent causes of renal stones in children?
See Box 28.3. The incidence of renal stones in pediatric patients is increasing. Children with renal stones should be referred to a urologist or nephrologist for a metabolic workup (studies estimate at least 30% of children with renal stones will have an underlying metabolic disorder). Calcium oxalate stones are the most frequent type (40%–60%).

14. What can cause acute urinary retention in a child?
Acute urinary retention is a urologic emergency and may progress to bladder injury if not relieved promptly. Emergent treatment may include urethral catheterization to drain the bladder. Additional treatments would be guided by the underlying cause (Box 28.4).

15. An 8-year-old boy presents with complaints of penile pain, swelling, and dysuria. His parents report that they are no longer able to retract the child's foreskin after a traumatic retraction the week prior. What is the diagnosis and how is this condition treated?
Phimosis is the inability to retract the foreskin over the glans of the penis in an uncircumcised male. It can be physiologic or pathologic, which is caused by adhesions or scar tissue from inflammation or infection. A urinalysis and culture should be obtained in symptomatic patients.
Physiologic phimosis can be managed safely with topical steroids such as 1%–2.5% hydrocortisone ointment. A treatment course of up to 3–6 weeks of therapy is generally sufficient. This should be combined with gentle manual retraction of the foreskin. When performing gentle retractions, careful replacement of the foreskin to its original position is imperative. Patients with symptomatic or pathologic phimosis should be referred to a urologist for evaluation. A portion of patients may require circumcision to correct the phimosis.

16. Your 8-year-old patient seen last week with phimosis returns today complaining of worsening penile pain and swelling. You examine his penis and find the glans appears extremely red and swollen relative to the penile shaft. His foreskin appears tight, like a constricting band around the glans. What is the next step?
He has paraphimosis, a urologic emergency where the retracted foreskin cannot be returned to the normal resting position due to swelling. Distal edema and swelling worsen, which results in ischemic changes and the development of gangrene and tissue necrosis if left untreated. Paraphimosis can be precipitated by the caregiver retracting the foreskin behind the glans for cleaning. It occurs in uncircumcised or partially circumcised males.
Treatment involves returning the glans to its position within the foreskin. Numerous techniques have been described, with manual reduction being the least invasive. First hold steady pressure on the head of the penis, squeezing distally to proximally in order to reduce swelling. Ice packs may be a helpful adjunct as well. Then place both thumbs on the glans, and index and middle fingers proximal to the phimotic ring. Apply steady pressure on the glans and attempt to move the phimotic ring distally over the glans, thus reducing the paraphimosis. Adequate analgesia should be provided. Pain control can also be achieved by local lidocaine infiltration to achieve penile

block. Second-line therapies include needle decompression. If conservative measures fail, an emergency dorsal slit procedure should be performed by a urologist.

17. **A 15-month-old circumcised boy presents with swelling of the penis. You examine his diaper area to find a grossly swollen, boggy area on the shaft of the penis just proximal to the glans. The glans appears slightly swollen and red. You astutely diagnose him with balanoposthitis. How is this condition treated?**
Balanitis is defined as inflammation of the glans penis. When the foreskin is also involved, it is termed "balanoposthitis." It is usually the result of irritation from prolonged exposure to a wet diaper or similar hygiene issues in uncircumcised males. It can also be seen with trauma due to forceful foreskin retraction or excessive washing with exposure to soap or other irritants. The most important aspect of treatment is good local and topical hygiene. Sitting the baby in a shallow tub of lukewarm water for 5–10 minutes twice a day is the most efficient way to rinse and soothe the inflamed area. (Note: Infants and toddlers must ALWAYS be attended in a bath, no matter how shallow the water!) Additional analgesia should be provided to patients with severe pain.

In addition for boys nearly toilet trained, allowing them to go without a diaper for certain periods of time will allow air circulation to the area and promote resolution. A diaper rash ointment (zinc oxide, petroleum jelly) applied to the area will protect the skin from further irritation by urine or diaper contents. If candida diaper rash is suspected, an antifungal cream can also be applied to the area. If the area is particularly red, painful, or has tense (rather than boggy) swelling, oral antibiotic therapy for possible cellulitis may be considered.

18. **A 5-year-old African American girl is brought in by her mother, who saw streaks of blood in her underpants. On physical exam, you find a circle of bright red and friable mucosa between her clitoral hood and vaginal introitus. What is the diagnosis and how will you manage it?**
This is the typical presentation of urethral prolapse, which is a protrusion of distal urethral mucosa through the external urethral meatus. Urethral prolapse can be seen in prepubertal and postmenopausal women. For unknown reasons, in prepubertal girls, it occurs most often in African Americans. The finding of genital bleeding in a prepubertal girl often causes anxiety for caregivers and may provoke questions about sexual abuse. In the absence of specific allegations of sexual abuse, the diagnosis of urethral prolapse can be provided with reassurance.

Most cases of urethral prolapse can be managed conservatively, with sitz baths and good hygiene. Topical estrogen cream can be used to temporarily estrogenize the vaginal mucosa and promote resolution. Most patients can be appropriately discharged from urgent care with primary care or urologic follow-up. Send a urinalysis and culture if the patient complains of urinary symptoms. Do not attempt to manually reduce the urethral prolapse. In rare cases, a very edematous prolapsed segment might obstruct urination. In the event of acute bladder outlet obstruction, excessive pain, or excessive bleeding, immediate evaluation by a urologist is warranted. A small portion of patients may require surgical intervention to resect the prolapsed urethral segment. Surgery is usually reserved for chronic prolapse that fails the conservative approach outlined above but may be indicated acutely in severe cases.

19. **What is the difference between primary enuresis and secondary enuresis, and what initial management of primary enuresis can be initiated in urgent care?**
It is important to differentiate between primary and secondary enuresis when evaluating a child older than 5 years. Children who have never achieved nighttime dryness and wet the bed during sleep have primary enuresis. Children who develop enuresis after a dry period of at least 6 months have secondary enuresis. First-line therapies for children with primary enuresis include restriction of fluids before bedtime, bed alarm therapy, or desmopressin therapy.

20. **What urgent evaluation should be done for a child with secondary enuresis?**
Initial evaluation should include a history, exam, and urinalysis. Several conditions such as diabetes mellitus, diabetes insipidus, constipation, obstructive sleep apnea, chronic kidney disease, and urinary tract infection may be associated with secondary enuresis.

Patients with secondary enuresis should be evaluated for recent psychosocial stressors, poor voiding habits, and caffeine intake or stool retention. Routine urinalysis can screen for many items on this differential including glucosuria (diabetes mellitus), low specific gravity (diabetes insipidus), and white blood cells (WBCs) or nitrites to suggest UTI.

KEY POINTS

1. Urinary tract infections can present with subtlety in young children. Unexplained fever or vomiting in a preverbal or diapered child is ample reason to consider UTI.
2. Bag-collected urine specimens are not appropriate for urine culture due to a high rate of contamination.
3. It is vital to know local antibiotic susceptibility patterns when choosing empiric therapy for UTI.

BIBLIOGRAPHY

Hernandez JD, Ellison JS, Lendvay TS. Current trends, evaluation, and management of pediatric nephrolithiasis. *JAMA Pediatr.* 2015;169(10):964–970.

Kaplan BS, Pradham M. Urinalysis interpretation for pediatricians. *Pediatric Annals.* 2013;42(3):45–51.

Nevo A, Mano R, Livne PM, Sivan B, Ben-Meir D. Urinary retention in children. *Urology.* 2014;84:1475–1479.

Pohlman GD, Phillips JM, Wilcox DT. Simple method of paraphimosis reduction revisited: point of technique and review of literature. *J Pediatric Urology.* 2013;9:104–107.

Ramakrishnan K. Evaluation and treatment of enuresis. *Am Fam Physician.* 2000;78:489–496.

Sas DJ. An update on the changing epidemiology and metabolic risk factors in pediatric kidney stone disease. *Clin J Am Soc Nephrol.* 2011;6(8):2062–2068.

Shaw K, Blackstone MM, Lopez P, Rober C. UTI, febrile. In: Shaw KN, Bachur RG, eds. *Fleisher & Ludwig's Textbook of Pediatric Emergency Medicine.* 7th ed. Philadelphia: Lippincott Williams & Wilkins; 2016.

Subcommittee on Urinary Tract Infection and Steering Committee on Quality Improvement and Management Urinary Tract Infection. Clinical practice guideline for the diagnosis and management of the initial UTI in febrile infants and children 2–24 months. *Pediatrics.* 2011;128:595–610.

Vunda A, Vanderuin L, Gervaix A. Urethral prolapse: an overlooked diagnosis of urogenital bleeding in pre-menarchal girls. *J Pediatrics.* 2011;158:682–683.

CHAPTER 29

VAGINAL COMPLAINTS

Atsuko Koyama, MD, MPH, Kathryn S. Brigham, MD

1. **What is the best position to perform a genital exam on a prepubertal child?**
   Children approximately 2 years and older are best examined in the supine frog-leg or prone knee-chest position (see Figs. 29.1 and 29.2). Children may be more comfortable lying with their parent (if in a supine frog-leg position) and/or keeping the underwear on (can be pulled to the side) during the exam. The United States has high rates of child sexual abuse (1 in 4 girls); therefore, it is paramount to practice trauma-informed care. Physicians should use appropriate terms for genital anatomy, limit the number of people in the exam room, always explain the procedure prior to examination, and allow the child to stop the exam at any time. Some children may need an exam under sedation.

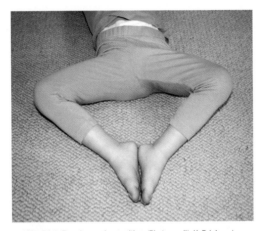

Fig. 29.1 Frog-leg supine position. (Photo credit: K. Brigham.)

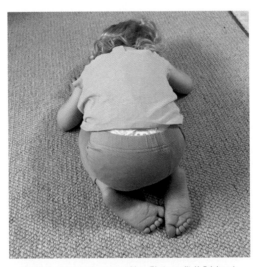

Fig. 29.2 Knee-chest prone position. (Photo credit: K. Brigham.)

2. What is the best way to examine a prepubertal child?
   1) Provide gentle lateral traction or gently grip the labia and pull anteriorly.
   2) The hymen often gapes open if you ask the child to cough or take a deep breath.
   3) Use an angiocath and flush a small amount of warm water or saline to expose the vaginal canal. Use a small swab if needed to separate the labia and/or identify anatomy.
   4) If vaginal culture is not needed, a small amount of lido jelly can be used for anesthesia.

3. What are the differences between prepubertal and pubertal genital exams?
   1) In the preterm infant, the labia minora and clitoris are prominent.
   2) In the full-term infant, the labia majora is full and may cover other structures due to maternal estrogen effects. The labia minora is thickened.
   3) The normal prepubertal clitoral glans is 3 mm x 3 mm.
   4) The appearance of the hymen changes with age. In newborns, the hymen is thick, pale pink, and redundant due to maternal estrogen, but then develops into the prepubertal hymen, which is relatively thin and smooth-edged. With puberty, the hymen becomes thicker and more redundant, and may assume a fimbriated or crescentic appearance and increase in elasticity.

4. What are important considerations in genital exams for transgender patients?
   Only examine relevant anatomy. Use general terms for anatomy (genital vs. vaginal or penile) and/or ask patients what terminology they use. **Transgender females** who have undergone vaginoplasty retain the prostate and have a blind ending pouch without a cervix or fornices. An anoscope is recommended if an exam is indicated. Testing and treatment for prostatitis should be considered. **Transgender males** may have vaginal atrophy from testosterone therapy, making lubricant important if a bimanual or speculum exam is indicated. Genital samples should have clear labeling as vaginal or cervical source if the patient's sex is noted as male. Strongly consider patient self-collection of genital samples for patient comfort.

5. What are important considerations in genital exams for those at risk for or who have undergone female genital mutilation/cutting (FGC)?
   Although there are estimates that more than 500,000 girls and women in the U.S. have had or are at risk of FGC, exact numbers are unavailable given the lack of recognition and reporting. First and foremost, providers need to be aware of the possibility of FGC when examining patients and know when to refer to specialists, as indicated. See references below for terminology, counseling, management, and legal/ethical considerations.

6. How should you approach vaginitis in prepubertal girls?
   The most common signs and symptoms of vaginitis include vulvar erythema, vulvar edema, vaginal bleeding, vaginal discharge, pruritis, vaginal irritation, and/or dysuria.

7. What should discharge instructions be for outpatient management of nonspecific vaginitis?
   If there is no identifiable treatable cause for vaginitis AND symptoms are acute onset and mild without vaginal bleeding or discharge, consider conservative management. Recommend loose-fitting clothing, cotton underwear, limit bubble baths and soap to the genital area, avoid long periods in wet swimwear, and advise wiping front to back. Also recommend soaking in a sitz bath or voiding in the bathtub if dysuria, and cool compresses if vulvar/vaginal pain/swelling. If the patient has progressively worsening symptoms or develops purulent discharge, obtain culture and treat appropriately.

8. How do you evaluate prepubertal girls for vaginal foreign bodies?
   The knee-chest position for children over 2 years of age generally allows clinicians to visualize the vagina and cervix. Vaginal irrigation using a Foley catheter with a syringe filled with normal saline after a topical anesthetic can be performed if direct visualization and removal with a Calgi swab fails. Rarely, examination under sedation and/or pelvic ultrasound is required.

9. How do you distinguish between labial adhesions and lichen sclerosis? How are they treated?
   Labial adhesions are much more common than lichen sclerosis, but both may cause vaginal irritation and bleeding. **Labial adhesions** present in infancy and in early childhood, likely due to the lack of estrogen, and usually resolve with estrogenization at puberty. They are thin, pale, semitranslucent adhesions between the posterior labia minora and can progress anteriorly, occasionally leaving only a pinpoint opening. In asymptomatic patients, conservative management with a bland ointment, such as A and D ointment, and observation is appropriate. First-line therapy for symptomatic and/or large labial adhesions is estrogen cream applied twice daily to the point of fusion; if no improvement after 2–3 weeks of therapy, low-dose steroid creams can be trialed. Classic skin findings of **lichen sclerosis** include a symmetric hourglass pattern of the vulvar and perianal area with atrophic, white-colored plaques. First-line therapy is high-dose topical steroids; if that fails, topical calcineurin inhibitors are a second-line therapy.

10. What is the differential diagnosis for urethral prolapse?
    Urethral prolapse presents as a friable, annular mass anterior and separate from the vaginal introitus and can present with bleeding or dysuria. The peak age of presentation is 5–8 years of age. A urine catheterization can be

performed to confirm that the mass is part of the urethra and connected to the bladder. If not necrotic, it usually improves with estrogen cream and sitz baths. Masses that are less annular and more "grape-like" are concerning for **sarcoma botryoides**. A pelvic ultrasound to assess for pelvic masses and a tissue biopsy would be indicated. If the mass were adjacent to the urethra, white in color, and found in a neonate, it would be more consistent with a **paraurethral cyst**. In these cases, a renal ultrasound evaluating for renal pathology would be warranted to evaluate for other anomalies such as urethral diverticula and ectopic ureteroceles.

11. What is the best management of perineal trauma?

Superficial lacerations in the perineal area that are not bleeding can be treated conservatively with only symptomatic care, such as ice packs and nonsteroidal antiinflammatory drugs (NSAIDs) for small hematomas. Sitz baths can provide pain relief, and voiding in the bathtub or shower can be helpful for dysuria. Significant/active bleeding or complicated lacerations involving the anus, urethra, vagina, cervix, and/or large hematomas will likely need further examination under sedation and management/repair by a surgical specialist. An indwelling urinary catheter should be inserted if there is concern for enlarging hematomas, placing the patient at risk for urinary obstruction and distortion of genital anatomy.

12. How do you diagnose and manage Bartholin gland abscesses?

Bartholin glands secrete mucus and are found in the posterior labia majora at 4 and 8 o'clock. These glands can develop an abscess, presenting as painful, fluctuant, and with a large labial mass. They generally require incision and drainage and placement of a Word catheter to prevent recurrence. Marsupialization is also an option but requires an experienced clinician to perform. Antibiotics are only necessary with concomitant cellulitis, recurrent abscess, or culture-positive methicillin-resistant *Staphylococcal aureus,* or for patients with high risk of complications.

13. What is the differential diagnosis for vaginal ulcers?

Diagnosis should be based on history of sexual activity, travel, systemic signs/symptoms, and similar past episodes. Lesions may be single versus multiple, painful versus painless, and with or without lymphadenopathy. Noninfectious causes include fixed drug reactions, Behçet syndrome, and trauma. Behçet syndrome is uncommon and typically affects young adults, but it can be seen in children. The hallmark of Behçet is the recurrent and usually painful intraoral, urogenital, and cutaneous ulcers, but it has many systemic manifestations. Infectious causes include sexually transmitted infections and, rarely, non–sexually transmitted infections such as acute genital ulcerations (Lipschütz ulcer). Herpes and chancroid cause painful ulcers; syphilis, lymphogranuloma venereum, and granuloma inguinale are generally painless. Lipschütz ulcers may be due to primary Epstein-Barr virus (EBV) infection and are painful. Lipschütz ulcers have also been reported after COVID-19 infections and vaccinations.

14. Which infections are most concerning for sexual abuse?

Cases of gonorrhea, chlamydia, syphilis, trichomonas, anogenital human papillomavirus (HPV), genital herpes, and non-transfusion-acquired human immunodeficiency virus (HIV) in children make sexual abuse/assault likely but not definite. In the neonatal period, there may be cases of vertical transmission of these infections.

15. When should you be concerned about commercial sexual exploitation (CSE)?

Most children enter into CSE at approximately 12–16 years of age. Risk factors include a history of running away from home, truancy, child maltreatment, involvement with child protective services or the juvenile justice system, multiple sexually transmitted infections (STIs), and/or repeat pregnancies. Specific questions targeting this include: "Has anyone ever asked you to have sex in exchange for something you needed or wanted (money, food, shelter, or other items)?" "Has anyone ever asked you to have sex with another person?" "Has anyone ever taken sexual pictures of you or posted such pictures on the internet?" Familiarize yourself with local resources and your closest child protection services team. The National Human Trafficking Resource Center Hotline is 1-888-373-7888.

16. What are the signs of pelvic inflammatory disease (PID)?

The minimum requirement for the diagnosis of PID is pelvic or lower abdominal pain and either (1) uterine tenderness, (2) cervical motion tenderness, or (3) adnexal tenderness. Other signs and symptoms are quite variable. There should be a low threshold for treating empirically given complications of untreated PID including increased rates of ectopic pregnancy, chronic pelvic pain, and infertility. Outpatient treatment is ceftriaxone 500 mg intramuscular once plus doxycycline 100 mg BID for 14 days with metronidazole 500 mg BID for 14 days, OR cefoxitin 2 g IM once and probenecid 1 g PO administered concurrently once plus doxycycline 100 mg PO BID x 14 days with metronidazole 500 mg PO BID for 14 days. Alternative regimens are available at https://www.cdc.gov/std/treatment-guidelines/pid.htm. Close follow-up within 72 hours to ensure improvement of symptoms is required; if the patient fails to improve within that time period, additional parenteral treatment is indicated.

17. Which STIs should I test for?

HPV, chlamydia, trichomoniasis, herpes simplex virus (HSV), and gonorrhea are the five most common STIs among sexually active adolescents. Highly sensitive nucleic acid amplification tests (NAAT) for chlamydia, gonorrhea, and trichomoniasis should be sent using self-collected vaginal swabs (most sensitive), urine, or cervical swabs for sexually active patients with vaginal discharge, dysuria, genital pain, lower abdominal pain, or symptoms of PID. In some cases (sexual assault evaluation, failed treatment), cultures requiring a special medium may be indicated. Polymerase chain reaction (PCR) testing for HSV should also be sent if vaginal ulcers are present. Empiric treatment for gonorrhea, chlamydia, trichomoniasis, and HSV is indicated if the history and physical exam findings are consistent with these infections. Nontreponemal serologic testing for rapid plasma reagin (RPR), Venereal Disease Research Laboratories (VDRL), or toluidine red unheated serum test (TRUST) can be used to screen for syphilis with treponemal tests for confirmation in patients who have signs/symptoms concerning for syphilis: diffuse maculopapular rash on trunk, extremities, or palms and soles or a painless genital ulcer. HPV testing is only performed as part of cervical cancer screening.

18. **What are important considerations when evaluating a female for sexual assault?**
    - Pubertal state and sex assigned at birth: STI testing varies based on pubertal status and sex assigned at birth, including specimen source (urine vs. anatomic sites) and type of test (NAAT vs. culture).
    - Time since incident: evidence collection and postexposure prophylaxis, empiric STI testing, and emergency contraception all depend on time since incident. Consider referring to providers with specialized training in sexual abuse/assault evaluation if no emergent needs.
    - Availability of a trained sexual assault nurse examiner (SANE) for evidence collection.
    - Safety concerns: involve a child protection team (if available), police, and a social worker. Consider if other children are at risk in the home.
    - STI testing: serum and genital/rectal/oral specimen collection.
    - Medications: postexposure HIV prophylaxis, hepatitis B vaccination and/or immunoglobulin, emergency contraception, gonorrhea/chlamydia/trichomoniasis treatment, and antinausea medication.

19. **A 17-year-old female requests emergency contraception. What are her options?**
    Emergency contraception (EC) is most effective within 72 hours after unprotected sex but can be administered up to 120 hours after unprotected sex. The copper intrauterine device (Cu-IUD) and levonorgestrel IUDs are the most effective forms of emergency contraception; however, both are off-label as EC in the United States. The Cu-IUD also provides up to 10 years of contraception and does not wane in efficacy from 72–120 hours or with increased body mass index (BMI). Ulipristal acetate (UPA), a progesterone receptor modulator, and levonorgestrel (LNG), a progestin-only pill, prevent or delay ovulation and are more easily accessible as forms of EC. UPA is more effective in patients with BMIs over 30 and for patients who are over 72 hours after unprotected sex when compared to LNG; both should be given as a one-time dose as soon as possible after unprotected sex. The dose for LNG is 1.5 mg and UPA is 30 mg.

20. **What is the differential diagnosis for abnormal uterine bleeding in adolescents?**
    Anovulatory cycles are the most common cause of abnormal uterine bleeding (AUB) in adolescents. For sexually active patients, STIs are also a common cause. Patients with bleeding disorders such as von Willebrand disease, platelet dysfunction, and thrombocytopenia can present at initiation of menses with menorrhagia. Testing for von Willebrand should be considered prior to administration of hormonal contraception, as estrogen increases von Willebrand levels, leading to false-negative results. Polycystic ovarian syndrome (PCOS) and changes in the hypothalamic-pituitary axis can also lead to AUB. Testosterone, follicle-stimulating hormone (FSH), and luteinizing hormone (LH) can be ordered, especially if hormonal contraception is started to control bleeding, as these medications affect these tests. Thyroid dysfunction should be screened for with a thyroid-stimulating hormone (TSH). Prolactin levels with or without brain computerized tomography (CT) should be considered in patients with AUB and neurologic findings, galactorrhea, or vision deficits to evaluate for prolactinoma. 17-hydroxyprogesterone can be sent for rare cases of late-onset congenital adrenal hyperplasia (CAH).

21. **A 14-year-old girl presents with 14 days of heavy vaginal bleeding, 2 days of dizziness, and an episode of syncope. A pregnancy test is negative. How do you decide between inpatient and outpatient management?**
    The workup for mild AUB can be pending and/or deferred to a primary care provider, but for patients with moderate to severe AUB, inpatient management should be considered. A complete blood count (CBC) and reticulocyte count should be obtained to evaluate the degree of anemia and necessity of hormonal and iron therapy along with assessment of hemodynamic status.

    Mild: hemoglobin (Hgb) >12 mg/dL
    Moderate: Hgb 10–12 mg/dL
    Severe: Hgb <10 mg/dL

    Patients with tachycardia, headaches, dizziness, syncopal episodes, and moderate to severe anemia should be considered for inpatient management. Unless estrogen is contraindicated, treatment should include monophasic combined oral contraceptive pills (OCPs). Exogenous estrogen promotes endometrial proliferation and heals bleeding sites, and progestin stabilizes the uterine lining. Specific medication and dosing schedules vary, but recommendations are generally for monophasic combined OCPs, one tab one to four times a day until bleeding stops, and then tapered down to either typical use of daily OCPs or continuous cycling of daily OCPs, depending on the degree of anemia, bleeding, and symptoms. Antinausea medications are generally indicated given the high doses of estrogen. If estrogen is contraindicated, progestin-only pills can be used, though generally less effective.

IV estrogen is only considered in patients with severe acute hemorrhage who are unable to tolerate oral medications, are unstable, and are critically ill. Iron should also be given to all patients.

22. **When should primary amenorrhea (absence of menses prior to 15 years of age in a girl with normal breast and pubic/axillary hair development) be further evaluated urgently?**
Once pregnancy is ruled out, other causes of primary amenorrhea can generally be evaluated by a primary care provider. Other diagnoses to consider are disorders of the hypothalamic-pituitary-ovarian axis, eating disorders/female athlete triad, thyroid disorders, primary ovarian insufficiency, hyperprolactinemia, PCOS, and anatomic abnormalities (imperforate hymen, hematocolpos, Müllerian agenesis). A thorough history and physical exam should enable directed evaluation.

23. **What is the first-line treatment for primary dysmenorrhea?**
Primary dysmenorrhea is thought to be prostaglandin-mediated, making NSAIDs the first-line treatment. Evidence is lacking to support the use of any one particular NSAID. If NSAIDs are not sufficient, combined hormonal contraceptives should be considered, which can also be given in a continuous manner to prevent the patient from having any withdrawal bleeds. If dysmenorrhea continues despite these interventions, a gynecologic consult would be appropriate.

24. **Your 17-year-old patient had an intrauterine device (IUD) placed 2 weeks prior and now presents with moderate to severe lower abdominal pain that started after IUD insertion. She reports no fever, vomiting, diarrhea, constipation, back pain, or UTI symptoms. How should you approach her evaluation?**
Rule out ectopic pregnancy. If the patient is pregnant, refer to gynecology for possible removal of the IUD. Send urinalysis and STI testing. Treat empirically for STIs and/or UTIs as indicated. In cases of PID, females should be treated without removal of the IUD. Regardless of the results of STI tests, evaluate IUD location by ultrasound. The proper location of the copper IUDs is at the fundus; progestin-releasing IUDs can be anywhere within the uterus. Consider immediate removal if not in the proper location, at the lower uterine segment, or in the cervix. Discharge with contraception, if so desired. If the IUD is not located in the uterine cavity, consider abdominal radiography to evaluate for IUD migration or uterine perforation. If an IUD is intraperitoneal or embedded in the myometrium, refer to gynecology.

25. **A 16-year-old patient is changing 1–2 pads per hour for the past 5 hours and passing blood clots the size of a dime. She has had some abdominal cramping, which has been tolerable with ibuprofen. She reports ordering medication abortion pills online and taking the second set of pills yesterday. How should you manage this patient?**
Patients may disclose that they have obtained medication abortion pills from a variety of sources. Self-managed abortions (SMA) are defined as abortions obtained outside formal health care settings, which most commonly include self-sourced medications (mifepristone and/or misoprostol, often obtained online), but the term can also include the use of herbs, blunt abdominal trauma, or the introduction of instruments into the intrauterine cavity. Research has shown that SMA with mifepristone and misoprostol is generally safe and effective. People who have SMAs are able to date their pregnancy and use these medications appropriately without the need to seek care at a medical facility. Approximately 7% of pregnant people in the U.S. have attempted SMA at some point in their lifetime, although SMA rates tend to be higher in states with greater abortion restrictions.

This patient is experiencing normal symptoms after a medication abortion. A pelvic ultrasound is not needed unless the patient (1) is bleeding through more than two pads per hour for 2 consecutive hours, (2) has blood clots larger than a lemon, (3) has severe pain not controlled with nonsteroidal antiinflammatories, or (4) exhibits persistent pregnancy symptoms (breast tenderness/pain, nausea/vomiting/morning sickness). Providers should be aware of state laws around abortion provision, to ensure both providers and patients are protected against criminalization.

KEY POINTS

1. Most adolescents will have regular menstrual cycles within 2 years of their menarche.
2. Pregnancy should be ruled out regardless of the patient's sexual history or absence of menarche if other signs of puberty are present.
3. Hormonal contraceptive pills have a variety of indications other than just contraception, as they can be useful in treating abnormal uterine bleeding and dysmenorrhea.

BIBLIOGRAPHY

Abdulcadir J, Sachs Guedi N, Yaron M, eds. Female genital mutilation/cutting in children and adolescents: Illustrated guide to diagnose, assess, inform, and report. Switzerland; 2022. https://link.springer.com/book/10.1007/978-3-030-81736-7.

Bacon JL, Romero ME, Quint EH. Clinical recommendations: labial adhesions. *J Pediatr Adol Gyn.* 2015;28(5).

Conti J, Cahill EP. Self-managed abortion. *Curr Opin Obstet Gynecol.* 2019;31(6):435–440.

Deutsch MB, Wesp L, eds. *Guidelines for the primary and gender-affirming care of transgender and gender nonbinary people.* 2nd ed. Center of Excellence for Transgender Health; 2016. https://transcare.ucsf.edu/guidelines/physical-examination.

Emergency Contraception. Centers for Disease Control and Prevention, 2 November 2018. https://www.cdc.gov/reproductivehealth/contraception/mmwr/spr/emergency.html. Accessed 27 September 2022.

Fast Facts: Preventing Child Sexual Abuse. Centers for Disease Control and Prevention, 6 April 2022. https://www.cdc.gov/violenceprevention/childsexualabuse/fastfact.html. Accessed 27 September 2022.

Gala PK, Akers AY, Wolff M. Gynecology emergencies. In: Shaw KN, Bachur RG, eds. *Fleisher & Ludwig's Textbook of Pediatric Emergency Medicine*. 8th ed. Wolters Kluwer; 2021. *EBSCOhost*. https://eds-p-ebscohost-com.treadwell.idm.oclc.org/eds/ebookviewer/ebook/ZTY4MHN3d19fMzA1MTk1NF9fQU41?sid=acb0ab45-87d8-473d-9b34-36d42be60ddf@redis&vid=0&format=EK&rid=1.

Gray SH, et al. Abnormal vaginal bleeding in the adolescent. In: Emans SJ, Laufer MR, DiVasta AD, eds. *Emans, Laufer. Goldstein's Pediatric & Adolescent Gynecology*. 7th ed. Philadelphia: Wolters Kluwer; 2020.

Identifying victims of human trafficking: What to look for in a healthcare setting. National Human Trafficking Resource Setting. https://humantraffickinghotline.org/sites/default/files/What%20to%20Look%20for%20during%20a%20Medical%20Exam%20-%20FINAL%20-%202-16-16_0.pdf.

Marjoribanks J, Ayeleke RO, Farquhar C, et al. Nonsteroidal anti-inflammatory drugs for dysmenorrhea. *Cochrane Database of Syst Rev*. 2015;7:CD001751.

Molnar J, O'Connell MS, Mollen C, et al. Sexual assault: child and adolescent. In: Shaw KN, Bachur RG, eds. *Fleisher and Ludwig's Textbook of Pediatric Emergency Medicine*. 8th ed. Philadelphia: Wolters Kluwer; 2021. *EBSCOhost*. https://web-p-ebscohost-com.treadwell.idm.oclc.org/ehost/ebookviewer/ebook/ZTY4MHN3d19fMzA1MTk1NF9fQU41?sid=13daab1c-c339-4de2-9a2f-8136b998949f@redis&vid=0&format=EK&rid=1.

Popatio S, Chiu YE. Vulvar aphthous ulcer after COVID-19 vaccination. *Pediatr Dermatol*. 2022;39(10):153–154.

Roett MA. Genital ulcers: differential diagnosis and management. *Am Fam Physician*. 2020;101(5):355.361.

Turok DK, et al. Levonorgestrel vs. copper intrauterine devices for emergency contraception. *N Engl J Med*. 2021;384:335–344.

Upadhya KK. AAP Committee on Adolescence. *Emergency contraception. Pediatrics*. 2019;144(6):e20193149.

Workowski KA, Bachmann LH, Chan PH et al. Sexually transmitted infections treatment guidelines, 2021. *MMWR Recomm Rep*. 2021;70(No. 4):1–187.

Young J, Nour NM, et al. Diagnosis, management, and treatment of female genital mutilation or cutting in girls. *Pediatrics*. 2020;146(2).

CHAPTER 30

SKIN RASHES AND INFECTIONS

Jennifer E. Sanders, MD, Sylvia E. Garcia, MD, Michelle N. Marin, MD

1. **True or false:** *Ixodes scapularis* is the vector causing all cases of Lyme disease in the United States.
   False. *Ixodes scapularis* is the tick vector transmitting the spirochete *Borrelia burgdorferi*, the cause of Lyme disease in the East, including New England and the eastern mid-Atlantic states as far south as Virginia (≥90% of all cases), as well as the upper Midwest. *Borrelia mayonii* causes Lyme disease in the northern midwestern states. *Ixodes pacificus* is the tick vector in the west. Most cases occur between April and October, but cases can occur year-round. In addition to outdoor activities, cases in urban areas and backyards have been reported. Most bites are from nymphs, which are small and hard to identify. The highest incidence of infection in the United States is in children between 5–9 years of age and adults between 55–69 years of age. The incubation period from tick bite to appearance of erythema migrans (EM) ranges from 3–32 days.

2. **What are the clinical manifestations associated with the three stages of Lyme disease?**
   Early localized disease occurs within 3–30 days postexposure to a tick bite. The characteristic lesion is erythema migrans, which occurs in up to 89% of cases. Early disseminated disease can have multiple EM lesions or no associated dermatologic findings. Other manifestations include cranial nerve palsies, especially cranial nerve VII (Bell palsy), lymphocytic meningitis, polyradiculitis, ophthalmic changes, and nonspecific systemic symptoms. Carditis and heart block can occur but are less common in children. Late disease (months to years postexposure) is rare in previously treated patients. In children, late disease presents as pauciarticular arthritis affecting the large joints, especially the knees. Neurologic complications, including encephalitis, are rare.

3. **Is the rash of erythema migrans alone sufficient for initiating treatment of Lyme disease?**
   Yes. EM is the most common clinical manifestation of early localized Lyme disease and the most common manifestation in children. Appearing 7–14 days after tick detachment, and initially as a painless red macule or papule, it expands into a nonpruritic erythematous annular lesion, occasionally with central clearing and a diameter ≥5 cm (Fig. 30.1). The center may appear necrotic or vesicular. It may be confused with hypersensitivity reactions, which

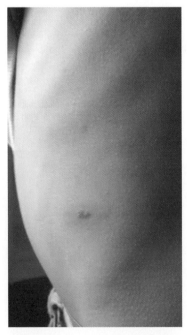

Fig. 30.1 Erythema migrans. Erythematous annular lesions with central clearing. (Image courtesy of Sylvia E. Garcia, MD.)

occur while the tick is attached or within 48 hours of detachment, are ≤5 cm in diameter, and disappear in 1–2 days. Associated symptoms may be present, including fever, headache, malaise, myalgias, and arthralgias. Treatment prevents progression to the early disseminated and late stages of Lyme disease.

4. **What is southern tick-associated rash illness?**
Southern tick-associated rash illness (STARI) is an illness with an EM-like rash and mild flu-like symptoms. It is caused by the bite of the tick *Ambylomma americanum*, also known as the Lone Star Tick, but does not transmit *B. burgdorferi*. Despite its name, STARI is known to occur in the South as well as the Midwest, mid-Atlantic, and some New England states. This illness has not been associated with any of the disseminated complications of Lyme disease. Its etiology and treatment are unknown.

5. **What diagnostic serologic testing is available for Lyme disease?**
Recognition of Lyme disease rests primarily on recognition of clinical illness in patients who have been in an endemic area; testing for nonspecific symptoms is discouraged. Early localized disease is rarely seropositive. Standard testing is done by two-tiered assay: a sensitive, but not specific, enzyme-linked immunosorbent assay (ELISA or EIA) or immunofluorescent antibody (IFA), and the Western immunoblot, or alternatively, a second EIA. Positive or equivocal results for ELISA, EIA, or IFA necessitate further testing, as false-positive results can occur from cross-reactivity with spirochetal, viral, and autoimmune diseases. The presence of two IgM bands or five IgG bands on the Western immunoblot is a positive result.

6. **What is the first-line antibiotic therapy for erythema migrans in pediatric patients with early localized disease?**
First-line therapy for the treatment of EM in all pediatric patients includes doxycycline, amoxicillin, or cefuroxime. The use of doxycycline has not been well studied in pregnant or lactating patients, but other recommended antibiotic therapy remains the same. Macrolides are not recommended as first-line therapy but may be used if the patient is unable to take the approved drug regimens.

7. **True or false: Successful tick removal involves complete removal of the mouthparts.**
True. Ticks should be promptly removed in order to decrease the transmission of disease. Removal should be attempted with the use of fine-tipped tweezers, grasping the tick where the mouth parts attach to the skin. Steady outward pressure should be applied, with care not to twist, crush, or squeeze the tick's body. If the mouthparts become detached and stay embedded in the skin and cannot be easily removed, only topical disinfection is required. Attempted removal of embedded mouthparts can cause local tissue damage and have no effect on the risk of contracting Lyme disease.

8. **Can tick bites be prevented?**
In addition to avoiding tick-infested areas, use of protective clothing, tick and insect repellants, showering after being outdoors, and close inspection for ticks on both humans and pets are recommended. Permethrin-treated clothing is approved for all ages and for pregnant women; it may be sprayed on clothes but not directly onto the skin. DEET is approved for use in children over 2 months of age, but only formulations containing no more than a 30% concentration. It should not be sprayed on objects that young children might chew or suck.

9. **Should chemoprophylaxis be provided to patients after sustaining a tick bite?**
Because the risk of contracting Lyme disease after a tick bite is ≤3% in highly endemic areas, routine use of chemoprophylaxis or serologic testing is not recommended. The risk increases after engorgement, especially if attachment is beyond 36 hours. A single dose of doxycycline in older children and adults may be used if all the following requirements are met: the tick has been attached for more than 36 hours and can be identified as *I. scapularis*, prophylaxis can be started within 72 hours of tick removal, high local rate of infection, and the use of doxycycline is not contraindicated. Amoxicillin prophylaxis has not been well studied. Prophylaxis is recommended in children of all ages. If unable to take doxycycline, no alternative therapy should be given, with initiation of therapy only if symptoms develop.

10. **Is follow-up necessary after tick removal and/or administration of antibiotic prophylaxis?**
Yes. Close monitoring for signs or symptoms of Lyme disease for up to 30 days is recommended. Medical attention should be sought if a skin lesion or viral-like illness occurs within 1 month of tick removal.

11. **What is the most common cause of the pictured skin lesion (Fig. 30.2)?**
The pictured lesion (Fig. 30.2) is the superficial bacterial infection, impetigo. The nonbullous type is primarily caused by *S. aureus* and *Streptococcus pyogenes*. *S. aureus* accounts for roughly 80% of cases, GAS 10%, and other bacteria 10%. The bullous type is caused by *S. aureus*. Impetigo is highly contagious and is the most common bacterial skin infection in children.

12. **How does impetigo usually present clinically?**
It is most commonly seen in children ages 2–5 years. Nonbullous impetigo begins as erythematous papules, which evolve into vesicles and pustules. These vesicles and pustules rupture to produce a "honey crust" on an erythematous base, primarily on the face or areas of irritation. Bullous-type impetigo is most commonly seen in neonates and infants. Lesions usually occur on intact skin in the intertriginous areas, though they can be seen

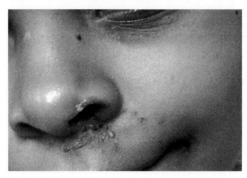

Fig. 30.2 Nonbullous impetigo. Vesicles and pustules with overlying honey-colored crust. (Image courtesy of Sylvia E. Garcia, MD.)

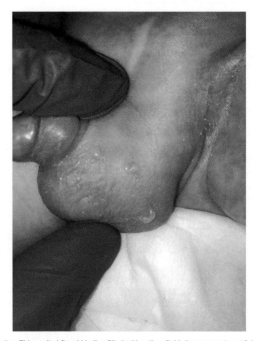

Fig. 30.3 Bullous impetigo. Thin-walled flaccid bullae filled with yellow fluid. (Image courtesy of Jennifer E. Sanders, MD.)

anywhere on the body. The bullae are small (<3 cm), thin-walled, flaccid lesions containing a clear-to-yellowish fluid (Fig. 30.3.). The lesions tend to rupture easily, usually within 1–3 days, leaving behind a collarette scale on an erythematous base or multiple concentric rings, resembling onion slices.

13. **How is impetigo diagnosed?**
    Diagnosis can be made on clinical presentation. Honey-colored crusting should raise clinical suspicion for impetigo. Superficial wound cultures may be helpful to identify the causative organism but should not delay treatment.

14. **What is the initial treatment of impetigo?**
    Impetiginous lesions will usually resolve on their own; however, treatment is recommended to decrease transmission, improve cosmetic appearance, and relieve discomfort. Topical treatment with mupirocin is the preferred method for patients with limited disease for both bullous and nonbullous impetigo. Patients with more extensive disease or who are immunocompromised should also be treated with oral antibiotics, such as dicloxacillin and cephalexin.

15. **How do the skin lesions in tinea corporis (body)?**
Tinea corporis, more commonly known as "ringworm," usually begins as pruritic, round (ovoid or circular), erythematous, scaling patches. These lesions spread centrifugally with central clearing and a raised scaling border. There may be clusters of lesions that coalesce. Pustules may be present around the edge of the lesion.

16. **Describe the various scalp lesions seen in tinea capitis.**
Tinea capitis can present with scaling scalp lesions with overlying alopecia that enlarge centrifugally over time. Alopecia with black dots may also be seen without scaling lesions. The black dots represent the distal ends of the hair follicles that have broken off. Patients may also present with diffuse scaling with minimal hair loss. Finally, some patients may develop a kerion due to an intense inflammatory response. A kerion is a thick, boggy plaque with pustules, crusting, and/or drainage. Kerions should not be confused with an abscess and should not be lanced.

17. **How are tinea infections diagnosed?**
Classic lesions do not require a confirmatory diagnosis, but skin scraping can be useful when the diagnosis is uncertain. Scrapings of skin lesions are treated with potassium hydroxide (KOH) on a slide and examined under a microscope. Positive scrapings will demonstrate segmented hyphae.

18. **What is the difference in treatment for tinea corporis and tinea capitis?**
First-line treatment for tinea corporis infections is topical antifungals, such as azoles, allylamines, butenafine, ciclopirox, and tolnaftate. For tinea capitis or onychomycosis (fungal infection of the nail), first-line treatment is with oral medication. Tinea capitis is treated with oral griseofulvin or terbinafine, while onychomycosis is treated with oral terbinafine or itraconazole. Oral treatment is also indicated for patients with extensive skin involvement or who fail topical treatment.

19. **Describe the appearance of an urticarial lesion.**
Urticarial lesions are raised, circumscribed, erythematous plaques. Lesions are usually intensely pruritic, often with central pallor. The plaques may develop over minutes to hours. Urticarial lesions do not typically leave residual markings. Urticaria is considered acute when it has been present for less than 6 weeks.

20. **What is the pathophysiology of urticarial lesion development?**
Urticarial lesions develop from the degranulation of mast cells, causing the release of histamine, in the superficial dermis due to some triggering factor.

21. **What are the most common causes of urticaria in children?**
- Infections: viral, bacterial, and parasitic
- Allergic reaction to food, medication, and insect stings/bites
- Medications causing direct, non-IgE-mediated mast cell activation (such as narcotics, muscle relaxants, vancomycin, and contrast media)
- Nonsteroidal anti-inflammatory drugs (NSAIDs), due to abnormality in arachidonic acid metabolism
- Less common: serum sickness, physical stimuli, or hormone-associated disorders

22. **How is acute urticaria treated?**
Almost two-thirds of cases of acute urticaria are self-limited. Treatment focuses on identifying the underlying cause and relieving symptoms of pruritus and associated angioedema. First-line treatment is with H_1 blockers. Second-generation antihistamines are preferred over first-generation due to increased sedation and anticholinergic effects seen with first-generation antihistamines. Short courses of steroids can be used in addition to antihistamines for severe or refractory cases.

23. **What causes the dermatitis of poison ivy, poison oak, and poison sumac?**
Poison ivy, poison oak, and poison sumac are plants that belong to the plant genus *Toxicodendron*. All plants within this genus contain the allergenic compound urushiol, which causes plant-associated contact dermatitis.

24. **Who is at risk for a reaction from exposure to poison ivy, poison oak, or poison sumac?**
Different *Toxicodendron* plants can be found throughout the United States, and 50% of people exposed to plants of the *Toxicodendron* genus will have a cutaneous reaction regardless of their ethnicity or skin type.

25. **What does a contact dermatitis rash post-*Toxicodendron* plant exposure look like?**
The rash is extremely pruritic and will appear as plaques, papules, vesicles, and/or bullae in a streak-like or linear pattern on the area of the skin exposed to the plant. If contact dermatitis is found on the face or genitals, significant edema may be present.

26. **Is the *Toxicodendron* contact dermatitis contagious?**
No, postexposure the rash will erupt in different parts of the body at different time intervals. Therefore, it is not a contagious dermatitis. However, individuals may inadvertently spread the resin containing urushiol to other parts of the body, or to other people due to scratching.

27. **What are the treatment options for *Toxicodendron* contact dermatitis?**
Patients only require symptomatic treatment with topical corticosteroids, cold compresses, and calamine lotion. If a patient has a known exposure, they should wash the body with mild soap or dish soap and hot water. The sooner the patient can wash, the more urushiol can be removed. One study demonstrated that washing 10 minutes after exposure can remove 50% of the urushiol, but that number falls to 10% after 30 minutes and 0% after 1 hour. Severe dermatitis may benefit from a 2-week tapering course of oral corticosteroids such as prednisone.

28. **Which virus causes cutaneous warts?**
Cutaneous warts are caused by human papillomavirus (HPV) infecting the epithelial tissues and mucous membranes of the host.

29. **Which age groups within the pediatric population primarily are affected by cutaneous warts?**
The school-age and adolescent populations are mainly affected by cutaneous warts. It is estimated that 10–20% of children will have a cutaneous wart at some point in their childhood.

30. **What are the common appearances of common cutaneous warts?**
Verrucae vulgaris, also known as common warts, are rough, hard, raised, dome-shaped lesions commonly found on the hands and usually asymptomatic.
  Plantar warts, or verrucae plantaris, affect the soles of the feet and appear as hyperkeratotic papules that obscure skin lines, occasionally with tiny red or black dots from thrombosed capillaries. They are usually symptomatic.
  Flat or juvenile warts are smooth, flesh-colored papules usually on the face and neck that vary in size and are more common in young children than in adolescents.

31. **Without therapeutic intervention, can a wart regress?**
About two-thirds of cutaneous warts will disappear without therapeutic intervention, especially in younger children and for nonplantar warts. It can take up to 2 years for a wart to self-resolve.

32. **What are some prescription methods for wart removal?**
First-line treatments include topical salicylic acid and cryotherapy with liquid nitrogen. Topical salicylic acid is superior to placebo and may be a gentler treatment option, thus better tolerated by younger children. Parents should be warned that this treatment may cause burning and irritation to local unaffected skin. Higher concentrations effectively treat plantar warts. Filing the wart down can enhance success. Salicylic acid can often be combined with other treatments to improve response. The treatment course should not extend beyond 12 weeks.
  Cryotherapy with liquid nitrogen is a more aggressive treatment option, used primarily in older children and adolescents secondary to pain and blistering associated with treatment. Healing and resolution will usually occur after one treatment session and 7 days following cryotherapy. Patients with darker skin tones should be made aware of the risk of hypopigmentation after healing.

33. **How can I distinguish herpetic gingivostomatitis from herpangina?**
Gingivostomatitis presents with ulcerations and grouped vesicles on the gums, hard palate, and tongue (Fig. 30.4). The vesicles rupture and become yellow with a surrounding red halo. Over time the vesicles coalesce to form larger ulcers. The gingiva tends to be friable and bleeds easily. Herpangina, on the other hand, presents with well-circumscribed erosions and ulcerations on the tonsillar pillars and soft palate.

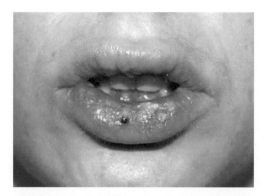

Fig. 30.4 Herpetic gingivostomatitis. Shallow ulcerations with overlying crusting noted on the lip. (Image courtesy of Ee T. Tay, MD.)

34. **Should I treat herpetic gingivostomatitis?**

Supportive care is focused on maintaining hydration and pain control. Gingivostomatitis is painful, and patients should be provided pain medications such as NSAIDs. Magic mouthwash, which consists of diphenhydramine, or Maalox with or without viscous lidocaine may also help the patient's pain, though clinical trials have not shown benefit in the use of this or other topical therapies. Oral antivirals are not routinely recommended for the treatment of herpetic gingivostomatitis but have been shown to benefit a limited group of patients with primary gingivostomatitis. They are recommended if there is severe dehydration or pain within 96 hours of presentation.

35. **How do I treat a first-time outbreak of genital herpes?**

There are several treatment options for a primary outbreak of genital herpes:
- Acyclovir (400 mg po tid for 7–10 days)
- Valacyclovir (1 g po bid for 7–10 days)
- Famciclovir (250 mg po tid for 7–10 days)
  Sitz baths and topical anesthetics may also provide some relief.

36. **When do I need to be worried about genital herpes?**

Genital herpes in a non–sexually active child should raise suspicion for child abuse. A thorough history and physical should be performed, and a report should be made to child protective services if an alternative diagnosis or explanation cannot be uncovered.

In patients with genital herpes who are having urinary retention secondary to pain, hospitalization should be considered for a urinary catheter and intravenous (IV) pain medications.

37. **How do I treat scabies?**

Permethrin 5% cream applied from the neck to the soles of the feet and washed off 8–14 hours later is the treatment of choice for pediatric patients 2 months of age and older. Sulfur ointments have been used successfully in adults and children, including those younger than 2 months of age, but may cause skin irritation and have an unpleasant odor. Lindane 1% lotion is equally as effective as permethrin, but it has higher rates of neurotoxicity and therefore should not be used in pediatric patients. Oral ivermectin can be used in children greater than 15 kilograms but not in smaller children and infants, as there is not much safety data to authorize use in this population.

38. **What is crusted scabies?**

Crusted scabies, or Norwegian scabies, tend to occur only in immunocompromised patients. It may initially present with erythematous patches, but then a thick scaly crust appears that can also fissure. These fissures allow ports of entry for bacteria, which can lead to sepsis. Concomitant treatment with permethrin 5% cream and oral ivermectin is recommended.

39. **What are the treatment options for contact dermatitis?**

Contact dermatitis is typically treated with topical corticosteroids. Low- to moderate-potency steroids, such as hydrocortisone 1–2%, triamcinolone 0.1%, and hydrocortisone valerate, are usually potent enough to clear contact dermatitis. Patients may also benefit from antihistamines to help control itching.

40. **What about a rash can help me distinguish contact dermatitis from other causes of dermatitis?**

Contact dermatitis is broadly divided into two main categories: irritant and allergic. Irritant contact dermatitis occurs immediately after exposure while allergic contact dermatitis causes a delayed inflammatory response. The skin tends to be erythematous and edematous, and fluid-filled vesicles may form. Contact dermatitis tends to be well demarcated and is often more itchy than painful, which helps differentiate it from cellulitis.

41. **How does pityriasis rosea present?**

Pityriasis rosea often starts with a herald patch, which is an annular, sharply demarcated pink lesion that becomes scaly with some central clearing (Fig. 30.5). It usually occurs on the chest, back, or neck. Days or weeks later, lesions that appear similar to the herald patch occur on the trunk and proximal extremities. Classically, a "Christmas tree" pattern may be seen on the back.

The rash may last 2–3 months. Follow-up is unnecessary if the rash resolves during that time.

42. **What can I do to treat pityriasis rosea?**

Treatment of pityriasis generally involves supportive care with antihistamines to help control itching. Limited use of medium potency topical steroids such as hydrocortisone valerate and mometasone furoate may also be helpful for itching but should be monitored by a healthcare professional for skin atrophy.

43. **What are some mimickers of pityriasis rosea?**

See Table 30.1.

44. **What are the high-yield tests in the diagnosis of cellulitis?**

There are no definitive tests for the diagnosis of cellulitis. It is a clinical diagnosis. This infection involves the dermal and subcutaneous layers of the skin. The lesion will be warm, erythematous, and tender. Occasionally

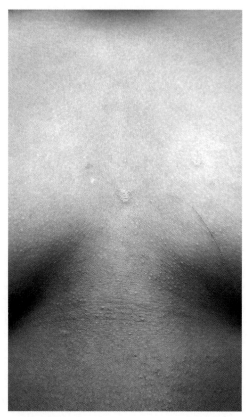

Fig. 30.5 Herald patch in pityriasis rosea. A single annular pink patch noted on the chest with a fine overlying scale. (Image courtesy of Sylvia E. Garcia, MD.)

Table 30.1 Mimickers of Pityriasis Rosea (PR)

CONDITION	HOW IT DIFFERS FROM PR
Secondary syphilis	Involves palms and soles
Guttate psoriasis	Thicker overlying scale
Nummular eczema	Involves the extremities more than the trunk
Tinea corporis	Usually a single lesion

the lesion may be indurated and can be difficult to differentiate from an abscess. In these cases, point-of-care ultrasound may be used to locate a subcutaneous fluid collection consistent with an abscess. There is no need to obtain a complete blood count or blood culture for the diagnosis of cellulitis. A white count will not change the initial management of cellulitis. The rate of bacteremia in children with cellulitis is low, and therefore a blood culture is not indicated in the evaluation of cellulitis.

45. **What are the optimal antibiotic choices for the treatment of cellulitis?**
Group A streptococcus is the bacteria that accounts for over 70% of cellulitis infections. With the emergence of MRSA, however, there is a growing concern for it to be the offending agent of skin infections. When deciding on antibiotics, a clinician should take into account if the patient has had a previous MRSA skin infection or if there is a family history of MRSA infections. If the patient has no previous personal or family history of MRSA infection, then treatment should focus on Group A streptococcus coverage with cephalexin for 5 days. If there is a concern for a possible MRSA cellulitis, treatment with clindamycin alone or trimethoprim-sulfamethoxazole should be concomitantly given with cephalexin for 5 days.

Table 30.2 Kawasaki Mnemonic: CRASH and Burn

KAWASAKI MNEMONIC: CRASH AND BURN
Conjunctivitis (limbic sparing)
Rash (nonpruritic)
Adenopathy (unilateral side or single node)
Strawberry tongue
Hands & feet (swelling & peeling later in illness course)
Burn Fever of 103–104°F for ≥5 days

46. **I just saw a child with 5 days of high-grade fever and rash, should Kawasaki be on my differential?**

   Yes. Typical Kawasaki is a medium-sized vasculitis that can be diagnosed clinically as fever for 5 or more days plus four of the five signs: bilateral, nonexudative bulbar conjunctivitis; rash; erythema of the lips and oral mucosa; extremity changes; and cervical lymphadenopathy (often a single enlarged node). Extremity changes include erythema of palms and soles or swelling of the dorsum of the hands and feet. Desquamation of the fingers is a late finding. The rash in Kawasaki disease can be variable but often is maculopapular, morbilliform, scarlatiniform, or urticarial. Vesicular and bullous lesions are not usually associated with Kawasaki. A useful mnemonic to remember clinical symptoms is "CRASH and burn" (Table 30.2).

47. **What workup and treatment are recommended for Kawasaki disease?**

   Typical Kawasaki can be diagnosed clinically. Laboratory testing can be useful in patients with incomplete or atypical Kawasaki disease. Lab findings include elevated C-reactive protein (CRP)/erythrocyte sedimentation rate (ESR), leukocytosis >15,000, thrombocytosis >450,000 after 1 week of illness, normocytic normochromic anemia for age, elevated alanine transaminase (ALT), low albumin (<3), and sterile pyuria. An echocardiogram is performed to evaluate for coronary artery dilation or ectasias, the most significant complication of Kawasaki disease. Patients with Kawasaki disease should be admitted and treated with intravenous immunoglobulin (IVIG) and high-dose aspirin. Treatment should be initiated within 10 days of the start of illness to decrease the risk of cardiac sequelae.

48. **Is there any treatment for erythema multiforme?**

   Erythema multiforme is a self-limited process. Treatment consists of stopping any inciting agents, as well as pain control and anti-itch medications. Topical corticosteroids and oral diphenhydramine may be useful for itching.

49. **Do all patients with Stevens-Johnson syndrome need to be admitted?**

   Patients with Stevens-Johnson syndrome (SJS) require intensive care and should be referred to the local emergency department or admitted to the hospital. Patients with SJS are managed similarly to burn patients with special attention to hydration, wound care, pain control, nutritional support, and monitoring for infections.

50. **Are all children with fever and petechial rash seriously ill?**

   Not necessarily. In a study of 190 children with fever and petechial rash, 8% (15) had an invasive bacterial illness. Of that 8%, half had meningitis. The remainder of those patients had otitis media, Group A streptococcal infections, and likely viral syndrome. All of those children had petechiae below the nipple line and appeared ill on presentation.

51. **Do all children with a petechial rash need labs drawn?**

   Petechiae should raise concerns to practitioners; however, the presence of petechiae does not always indicate serious illness. For example, children with forceful coughing or vomiting may present with petechiae on the face. In those children with diffuse or widespread petechiae, it is prudent to do some bloodwork, including complete blood count and coagulation factors to evaluate for idiopathic thrombocytopenic purpura, neoplastic disorders, hemolytic uremic syndrome, vasculitis syndrome, and autoimmune disorders.

52. **Do I need to treat my 6-year-old patient who has varicella?**

   Probably not. Varicella is a self-limited process in healthy children less than 12 years of age. Oral antiviral therapy with acyclovir, or its analogs, is recommended for immunocompetent children and adolescents who are at risk of complications from varicella. This includes unvaccinated adolescents, secondary cases in household contacts, patients with chronic disease, and those taking chronic steroids or salicylates. The dose of acyclovir is 20 mg/kg per dose four times daily for 5 days.

53. **My 12-month-old patient had several days of high fever and now has a rash. Should I check labs?**

   Probably not. Roseola classically presents with 3–5 days of fever that abruptly resolves followed by the eruption of a blanching maculopapular rash that tends to start on the trunk and spread to the face and extremities. The rash is usually present for 1–2 days and then resolves. Complications of roseola include seizures, encephalitis, and aseptic meningitis. Children with complications or those who are ill-appearing would require laboratory evaluation.

KEY POINTS

1. The appearance of erythema migrans alone is sufficient to start antibiotic therapy in endemic areas, preventing the progression of Lyme disease.
2. Blood cultures, cutaneous aspirates, and biopsies are not routinely recommended in immunocompetent patients with cellulitis.
3. Herpetic gingivostomatitis is self-limited and typically does not require oral antivirals.
4. Genital herpes in a child should raise suspicion for child abuse.
5. Petechiae below the nipple should raise concerns for serious bacterial infection in infants with fever.

Acknowledgments
The authors would like to thank Dr. Bellis for her contributions to this chapter in the previous edition.

BIBLIOGRAPHY

Albrecht M. Treatment of varicella (chickenpox) infection. http://www.uptodate.com/; 2012.
Asero R. New-onset urticaria. http://www.uptodate.com/; 2022.
Baddour LM. Impetigo. http://www.uptodate.com/; 2022.
CDC Guidelines: Crusted Scabies. https://www.cdc.gov/parasites/scabies/health_professionals/meds.html; 2019.
Goldstein BG, Goldstein AO. Pityriasis rosea. http://www.uptodate.com/; 2022.
Goldstein BG, Goldstein AO. Scabies: Management. http://www.uptodate.com/; 2021.
Goldstein BG, Goldstein AO, Morris-Jones R. Cutaneous warts (common, plantar, and flat warts). http://www.uptodate.com/: 2022.
Hepburn MJ, Dooley DP, Skidmore PJ, Ellis MW, Starnes WF, Hasewinkle WC. Comparison of short-course (5 days) and standard (10 days) treatment for uncomplicated cellulitis. *Arch Intern Med.* 2004;164(15):1669–1674.
High WN, Roujeau JC. Stevens-Johnson syndrome and toxic epidermal necrolysis: management, prognosis and long-term sequelae. http://www.uptodate.com/; 2016.
Keel MA, Clements DA. Herpetic gingivostomatitis in young children. http://www.uptodate.com/; 2022.
Kimberlin DW, Barnett ED, Lynfield R, Sawyer MH, eds. Herpes Simplex, *Red Book: 2021–2024 Report of the Committee on Infectious Diseases.* 32nd ed. American Academy of Pediatrics; 2021.
Lantos PM, Rumbaugh J, Bockenstedt LK, et al. Clinical practice guidelines by the Infectious Disease Society of America (IDSA), American Academy of Neurology (AAN), and American College of Rheumatology (ACR): 2020 Guidelines for prevention, diagnosis and treatment of Lyme disease. *Clin Infect Dis.* Published online November 30, 2020. DOI: https://doi.org/10.1093/cid/ciaa1215. The full guideline is available at: www.idsociety.org/practice-guideline/lyme-disease/.
Lee HY. Stevens-Johnson syndrome and toxic epidermal necrolysis: management, prognosis and long-term sequelae. http://www.uptodate.com/; 2022.
Levy ML. Contact dermatitis in children. http://www.uptodate.com/; 2020.
McCrindle BW, Rowley AH, Newburger JW, et al. American Heart Association Rheumatic Fever, Endocarditis, and Kawasaki Disease Committee of the Council on Cardiovascular Disease in the Young; Council on Cardiovascular and Stroke Nursing; Council on Cardiovascular Surgery and Anesthesia; and Council on Epidemiology and Prevention. Diagnosis, Treatment, and Long-Term Management of Kawasaki Disease: A Scientific Statement for Health Professionals From the American Heart Association. *Circulation.* 2017;135(17):e927–e999. Erratum in: Circulation. 2019 Jul 30;140(5):e181–e184. PMID: 28356445.
Mead P, Peterson J, Hinckley A. Updated CDC recommendation for serologic diagnosis of Lyme disease. *MMWR Morb Mortal Wkly Rep.* 2019;68:703. http://dx.doi.org/10.15585/mmwr.mm6832a4.
Mukkada S, Buckingham SC. Recognition of and prompt treatment for tick-borne infections in children. *Infect Dis Clin North Am.* 2015;29(3):539–555.
Pope M, Kyriakides K, Hoffman C. Treatment of warts in pediatrics: a review. *J Fam Med Dis Prev.* 2020;6:132.
Prok L, McGovern, T. Poison ivy (Toxidendron) dermatitis. http://www.uptodate.com/; 2022.
Sexton DJ, McClain MT. Southern Tick-Associated Rash Illness (STARI). http://www.uptodate.com/; 2021.
Tremblay C, Brady MT. Roseola infantum (exanthem subtium). http://www.uptodate.com; 2022.
Wetter DA. Erythema multiforme: pathogenesis, clinical features and diagnosis. http://www.uptodate.com/; 2021.

CHAPTER 31

LIMP

Robert D. Wilkinson, DO, Bryan Upham, MD, MSCE

TOP SECRETS

Most causes of limp in children can be treated in the urgent care setting, but if there are high-risk features such as fever, young age, abnormal neurological or abdominal exams, or others, referral to the pediatric ED is needed. See Table 31.1.

Having the caregiver range the patient's joints and palpate the legs, back, and abdomen while you observe from a distance is particularly helpful with infants and toddlers.

1. An 18-month-old female presents with a 2-day history of limp. She has no chronic medical conditions, and they deny trauma and fever. The patient cries when you enter the room, making the exam difficult. Your next best step is to:
   A) Use distraction.
   B) Sit across the room.
   C) Have the parent palpate the child's legs, abdomen, and back.
   D) Inform the caregiver they will have to return when the child is better behaved.
   E) A, B, and C.
      E. Getting a meaningful exam from a toddler can be challenging. Distraction with a toy, book, or cell phone and sitting at the child's level across the room may help. ***Having the caregiver range the patient's joints and palpate the legs, back, and abdomen while you observe from a distance for signs of discomfort can be particularly helpful.***

QUESTIONS 2–5

A 16-month-old male is brought in for limp. He twisted his leg while walking last night and has been limping since. He has no chronic diseases, no history of fevers, and is well appearing. You have his mother range his joints and palpate his legs, back, and abdomen, starting with the unaffected limb and finishing with the suspected area. He grimaces with palpation of the right tibia. Neurologic examination and pulses are normal. He will walk with an antalgic gait, placing most weight on the left leg.

2. What is the most likely diagnosis?
   Due to his age and lack of other symptoms, toddler's fracture is the most likely diagnosis. The differential diagnosis for an antalgic gait is large but can be divided by trauma and systemic symptoms (Fig. 31.1).

3. What is the most appropriate initial workup for this patient?
   A) Anterior/posterior (A/P) and lateral x-rays of the right tibia
   B) X-rays of the entire right lower extremity
   C) X-rays of the right tibia, inflammatory markers, blood cultures, and Lyme titers
   D) Referral to the ED
      A. A/P and lateral x-rays of the most affected area (right tibia only) are appropriate. Oblique views can be helpful if A/P and lateral x-rays are not revealing. Answer B is reasonable if the location of the pain can't be pinpointed. Answer C is incorrect because without fever, in a well-appearing child with focal tibia tenderness,

---

Table 31.1 Risk Factors Requiring Transfer to the Emergency Department

- Inability to bear weight
- Young age (<2 years) or ill appearance
- Infection (fever, joint tenderness)
- History of hematologic disorder
- Acute abnormal neurologic examination
- Long bone fracture or nonaccidental trauma
- Open or displaced fractures or dislocations
- Concern for compartment syndrome
- Pelvic causes, such as appendicitis and testicular or ovarian torsion
- Concern for neoplasia
- SCFE

Diagnosis of a Child with an Antalgic Gait

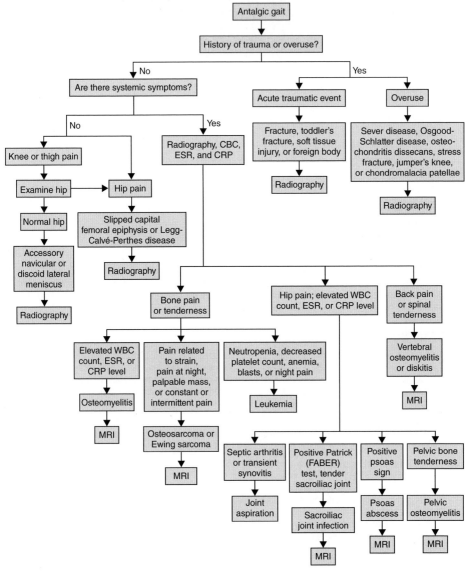

Fig. 31.1 Diagnostic approach to a limping child with an antalgic gait. (*CBC,* Complete blood count; *CRP,* C-reactive protein; *ESR,* erythrocyte sedimentation rate; *MRI,* magnetic resonance imaging; *WBC,* white blood cell.) (Adapted with permission from Sawyer JR, Kapoor M. The limping child: a systematic approach to diagnosis. *Am Fam Physician.* 2009;79(3):215–224.)

lab work isn't necessary. Answer D isn't correct because, while there is the risk factor (see Table 31.1) of age less than 2 years old, the H&P are consistent with a toddler's fracture.

4. **X-rays for the patient above show a nondisplaced spiral right distal tibia fracture. You give ibuprofen. What's your next best step?**
   A) Splint the leg, call child protective services (CPS), and arrange for medical transportation to the ED.
   B) Discuss mom's preference for a splint, short-leg controlled ankle motion (CAM) boot, or no immobilization. Apply immobilization if requested and discharge to home.
   C) Consult orthopedic surgery.

Diagnosis of a Child with a Nonantalgic Gait

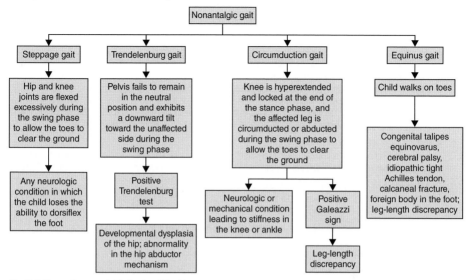

Fig. 31.2 Diagnostic approach to a limping child with a nonantalgic gait. (Adapted with permission from Sawyer JR, Kapoor M. The limping child: a systematic approach to diagnosis. *Am Fam Physician.* 2009;79(3):216.)

B. Toddler's fractures occur in children 9 months to 3 years who twist on a planted foot. These fractures are stable, resolve within 3–4 weeks, and treatment has evolved to include the options of a short leg splint, short pediatric CAM boot, or even no immobilization. Shared decision-making with the care provider is a reasonable approach. Answer A is incorrect because a nondisplaced distal tibia spiral fracture is consistent with a toddler's fracture and contacting CPS isn't appropriate. Answer C is incorrect because it is unnecessary. The child can follow up with their primary care provider, but local practice varies.

5. **What if the x-rays are negative for a suspected toddler's fracture?**
   Many toddler's fractures are not apparent on initial x-rays. If there are no other high-risk features (see Table 31.1), these x-ray-negative toddler's fractures are generally treated the same way as x-ray-positive fractures, but closer follow-up may be warranted to exclude other causes.

6. **How is "limp" defined, anyway? And what about an antalgic gait?**
   Limp is a derivation from age-appropriate gait pattern. For this chapter, we'll also include not using the limb. Abnormal gaits are most commonly antalgic (shortening of stance phase due to pain) but may be steppage (flexion of the hip and knee to allow toes to clear the ground), Trendelenburg (pelvis tilts down to the unaffected side), circumduction, and equinus (toe stepping). The differential diagnosis differs for nonantalgic gaits (Fig. 31.2).

7. **A 3-year-old male presents with 1 day of fever, left leg pain, and refusal to walk. He is otherwise healthy and has no history of trauma. He is febrile to 38.9°C and ill but awake, alert, and interactive. His blood pressure is normal. He is given ibuprofen in triage, and 90 minutes later he is improved but still unable to bear weight. The abdomen is soft and nontender, but any internal or external rotation of his left hip causes extreme pain. Your next best step is:**
   A) Transfer immediately to the closest general ED.
   B) Transfer immediately to the closest pediatric ED.
   C) Perform A/P and frog-leg views of the pelvis.
   D) Start an IV, check inflammatory markers, blood culture, Lyme titers, and a hip ultrasound.
   E) Discharge to home with close follow-up.
   B. This child has a fever, an inability to bear weight, and a hip exam concerning for septic arthritis (SA). See Table 31.1. While closer, a general ED won't have access to the pediatric orthopedic surgeons needed. Answer C is incorrect because while A/P and frog-leg views of the pelvis are appropriate for ruling out slipped capital femoral epiphysis (SCFE) and Legg-Calvé-Perthes (LCP), they are not helpful in SA. Answer D is an appropriate workup in a pediatric ED in a Lyme endemic area, but not in an urgent care or general ED, because the workup may include hip aspiration, and the treatment requires a pediatric orthopedic surgeon. Answer E is incorrect (see Table 31.1).

8. A 5-year-old male presents with a 2-day history of limp. Last week the child had a cough and fever, but it has since resolved. There is no history of trauma. The child is afebrile, and his joints all appear normal except that he has pain with internal and external rotation of the left hip. Sensation and pulses are intact. He can ambulate and is improved with ibuprofen. What's your next best step?
   A) Transfer immediately to the closest ED.
   B) Transfer immediately to the closest pediatric ED.
   C) Perform A/P and frog-leg views of the pelvis.
   D) Start an IV, check inflammatory markers, blood culture, Lyme titers, and a hip ultrasound.
   E) Discharge to home with close follow-up.
        E. Transient synovitis (TS), aka toxic synovitis, is most likely given this history and exam. Answers A, B, and D are not indicated given the history, age, ability to bear weight, and improvement with ibuprofen.

9. What causes TS?
   The cause of TS is not clear but is often seen in children 3–8 years old after an upper respiratory infection. It is one of the most common reasons for evaluation for atraumatic limp in children and is managed as an outpatient with NSAIDs.

10. For the patient in question 7, what about LCP or SCFE?
   The patient is in the right age group (3–12 years) for LCP, but the history of LCP is usually more chronic and not associated with recent illness. SCFE is common in early adolescence.

11. How can you differentiate septic arthritis (SA) from transient synovitis (TS)?
   A) By history
   B) By laboratory values
   C) By Kocher criteria
   D) By A, B, C, ultrasound, and hip joint aspiration
       D. The only true way to differentiate the two is by aspiration of synovial fluid from the hip under fluoroscopic guidance. However, this is invasive and usually requires procedural sedation. The Kocher and Caird criteria can be helpful.

12. What are the "Kocher and Caird criteria" for septic arthritis?
   Kocher developed less invasive criteria (inability to bear weight, erythrocyte sedimentation rate (ESR) ≥40 mm/hr, serum white blood cell count (WBC) >12,000 cells/μL, fever >38.5°C) with the likelihood of septic arthritis increasing for each factor (1 = 3%, 2 = 40%, 3 = 93%, 4 = 99%). Caird added C-reactive protein (CRP) with a CRP of >2.0 mg/dL (20 mg/L) as a fifth factor concerning for septic arthritis.

13. What about procalcitonin for septic arthritis?
   Procalcitonin >2.5 ng/L is specific but not sensitive, so it is NOT a good screening test.

14. Is MRI helpful for septic arthritis?
   MRI can be helpful but usually requires procedural sedation, and availability is limited.

15. A 15-year-old male presents with limp and left leg pain for 1 month. You obtain a plain radiograph (Fig. 31.3). Which passage would best describe the findings and diagnosis?
   A) The lesion is in the distal femur, which is one of the most common locations for Ewing sarcoma.
   B) The classic sunburst appearance is caused by calcified blood vessels radiating out from the lesion often found in osteosarcoma.
   C) The lesion shows onion skinning often found in Ewing sarcoma.
   D) The lesion is most likely a benign bone cyst and requires nonurgent follow-up with an orthopedic surgeon.
       B. The patient's bone pain is being caused by an osteosarcoma. The most common sites for development of osteosarcoma are the metaphysis of the most rapidly growing bones (distal femur, proximal humerus, and proximal tibia). Ewing sarcoma is most often found in either the pelvis or diaphysis of the femur. Furthermore, Ewing sarcoma classically has layers of periosteal reaction called "onion skinning," while osteosarcoma is composed of calcified blood vessels radiating out from the lesion, causing a "sunburst" pattern.

16. What are the two most common malignant bone tumors?
   Osteosarcoma and Ewing sarcoma comprise the most frequently encountered malignant bone tumors in children and adolescents.

17. You obtain an x-ray of a 17-year-old female softball player who developed ankle pain after twisting her ankle rounding third base. She is pointing to her lateral malleolus and has pain with ambulation. The radiology report reads as follows: "Soft tissue swelling around the ankle without signs of a fracture. A lesion in the superior aspect of the visible tibia with sharp edges without extension into the surrounding bone. The cortex appears normal." Which of the following is the best next step?
   A) Place the patient in an ankle stirrup and have them follow up with their primary care provider if the pain continues longer than 3 days.
   B) Place a short leg posterior splint and send her to the closest emergency department for further imaging.

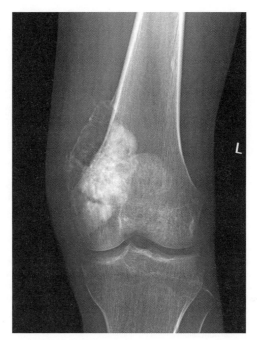

Fig. 31.3 Anterior/posterior (AP) plain film of a 15-year-old male presenting with limp and left leg pain for 1 month. (From: Czerniak MD. Dorfman and Czerniak's Bone Tumors. 2nd ed. Elsevier; 2016, Fig. 5.6.)

C) Tell her mother the x-ray shows some swelling of the ankle but is otherwise normal.

D) Explain that it looks like she has an ankle sprain. Recommend rest, ice, compression, and elevation over the next 3 days and close follow-up if there is no improvement. Also mention that there was an incidental finding of a benign bone cyst for which she should have nonurgent follow-up with an orthopedic surgeon.

     D. There may be nothing to do; however, patients should be told about the findings and given appropriate follow-up. An obvious division between the normal bone and the lesion along with a lack of destruction of the cortex and no extension into surrounding tissues help make benign bone mass more likely.

18. A 12-year-old male presents with a limp and left knee pain off and on for weeks. It worsened after spending the day at the trampoline park for a friend's birthday yesterday. On exam, he has pain with flexion and rotation of the hip. You order a plain film radiograph (Fig. 31.4). What is the diagnosis?

The diagnosis of slipped capital femoral epiphysis (SCFE) is made on plain film radiographs. As seen in Fig. 31.4, there is classic posterior displacement of the femoral epiphysis. The use of both AP and frog-leg views can help confirm the diagnosis. If clinical suspicion is high despite normal radiographs, clinicians can order an MRI, which can demonstrate widening of the physis with surrounding edema. LCP or a late diagnosis of developmental dysplasia of the hip (DDH) can mimic SCFE. However, the use of plain films usually allows the clinician to differentiate the three diagnoses. In LCP, plain film will classically show a flattened, and later fragmented, femoral head. Plain film in DDH will be positive for a dysplastic femoral head and an increased center edge angle.

19. A 6-year-old male presents with his father to the urgent care. The mother sent them because the child has been limping for the last 2 days causing him to miss school. Which of the following pieces of information would require immediate referral to the pediatric emergency department?

A) Family history of lupus

B) History of a URI 1 week ago

C) Patient's temperature is 101.3°F at triage

D) A bruise on the anterior tibia during exam

     C. Luckily, for atraumatic causes of limp, transient synovitis (TS) is the most common, and it can be managed in the urgent care setting. Fever, however, places children at high risk for an infection, and they should therefore be referred to a pediatric center. See Table 31.1 for other reasons to transfer a patient to the ED.

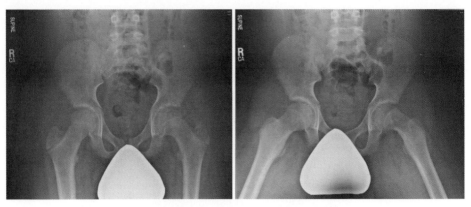

Fig. 31.4 Anterior/posterior (AP) and frog-leg plain film radiographs of a 12-year-old male complaining of left knee pain. (From: Berry: *Surgery of the Hip.* 1st ed. Elsevier; 2013. Fig. 42.5.)

20. Mom brings in a 4-month-old baby for crying since his diaper change this morning. He cries every time she picks him up or changes his diaper. The baby was fine when mom left for work last night. Vitals are normal when he is not crying, and there is no report of fevers. On examination, his left thigh is swollen, deformed, and painful to the touch and with movement. Which of the following would be most appropriate?
    A) Transfer via private vehicle to the closest pediatric emergency center
    B) Septic workup and hospital admission
    C) X-ray of the left leg, pain control, and splinting if fractured
    D) Contact law enforcement and child protective services and transfer to a pediatric center via ambulance if there is a femur fracture
    E) Computed tomography of the head, skeletal survey, and contact the local child abuse team if there is a femur fracture
    C, D, and E in combination are correct. Femur fractures require a high level of force, and without an appropriate mechanism, nonaccidental trauma (NAT) is the correct diagnosis. Answer A is not correct because while pain control and splinting are appropriate, sending the child with an NAT alone with the potential offenders is not. Answer B is not correct unless the patient is ill appearing and has had a fever.

21. A 4-year-old presents with 1 month of intermittent diffuse back pain, limp, tactile fevers, and no history of trauma. There is no focal back tenderness and full range of motion of all joints, but you do feel a spleen. The most appropriate next step is:
    A) Tell the family to get a new mattress for the child as her pain is likely musculoskeletal in nature.
    B) NSAIDs and outpatient pediatric orthopedist referral.
    C) Obtain standing and sitting x-rays of the lumbar spine.
    D) Explain to the family that you are worried because despite a normal exam, back pain in children can be a sign of a serious problem and you are sending them to the local pediatric emergency department where they will likely need blood work.
    D. Back pain in pediatric patients is concerning for infection or neoplasm in the absence of trauma. Blood work should be obtained, as abnormalities in two blood cell lines would be concerning for leukemia.

22. A 15-year-old female presents with severe right hip pain, vomiting, and limp with no history of trauma or overuse. She is afebrile and has tenderness to palpation of the right lower quadrant and right hip. Internal and external rotation of the hip worsens the pain. Ultrasound reveals no hip effusion and a normal appendix. X-rays are normal. CBC, CRP, ESR, UA, and urine pregnancy are unremarkable.
    What radiology study may help clarify the diagnosis?
    This presentation is most concerning for ovarian torsion. Ultrasound of the ovaries (either transabdominal for patients who are not yet sexually active or transvaginal for those who are) is the best next study.

KEY POINTS

1. Transient synovitis is the most common cause of atraumatic limp in children. Developmental dysplasia of the hip (DDH) in infants, Legg-Calvé-Perthes (LCP) in young school-aged children, and slipped capital femoral epiphysis (SCFE) in preteens and teens can cause limp.
2. Reassuring laboratory values can help distinguish septic arthritis from transient synovitis.
3. Pain can be referred from the back or pelvis to the hip (as in ovarian torsion) or hip to the knee (as in SCFE).
4. Back pain without trauma in children is abnormal and should be considered infectious or neoplastic until proven otherwise.
5. If the story does not fit, you must admit; that is, beware of nonaccidental trauma.

BIBLIOGRAPHY

Boutin A, Misir A, Boutis K. Management of toddler's fracture: a systematic review with meta-analysis. *Pediatr Emerg Care.* 2022;38(2):49–57.

Caird MS, Flynn JM, Leung YL, Millman JE, D'Italia JG, Dormans JP. Factors distinguishing septic arthritis from transient synovitis of the hip in children: a prospective study. *J Bone Joint Surg Am.* 2006;88(6):1251–1257.

Heinrich SD, Mooney JF. Fractures of the shaft of the tibia and fibula. In: Shaw KN, Wilkins KE, Barchur RG, eds. *Fleischer & Ludwig's Textbook of Pediatric Emergency Medicine.* 7th ed. Wolters Kluwer Publishers; 2016:280.

Kocher MS, Zurakowski D, Kasser JR. Differentiating between septic arthritis and transient synovitis of the hip in children: an evidence-based clinical prediction algorithm. *J Bone Joint Surg Am.* 1999;81(12):1662–1670.

Kost S, Thompson AD. Limp. In: Rockwood CA, Wilkins KE, Beaty JH, eds. *Rockwood and Wilkins' Fractures in Children.* 4th ed. Lippincott-Raven Publishers; 2006:1033.

Naranje S, Kelly DM, Sawyer JR. A systematic approach to the evaluation of a limping child. *Am Fam Physician.* 2015;92:10.

Nickel A, Bretscher B, Truong W, Laine J, Kharbanda A. Novel uses of traditional algorithms for septic arthritis. *J Pediatr Orthop.* 2022;42(2):e212–e217.

Payares-Lizano M. The limping child. *Pediatr Clin North Am.* 2020;67(1):119–138.

Schuh AM, Whitlock KB, Klein EJ. Management of toddler's fractures in the pediatric emergency department. *Pediatr Emerg Care.* 2016;32:7.

CHAPTER 32

HEAD AND NECK TRAUMA

Kara K. Seaton, MD, FAAP

HEAD INJURIES

A 3-year-old female is brought in by her mother for evaluation of a head injury after a fall off a bed. She had no loss of consciousness, crying immediately on impact. She had one episode of vomiting but is now calm and acting normally according to her mother. The child denies having a headache currently.

1. **How common are head injuries in children?**
   Pediatric head injuries account for approximately 800,000 emergency department visits per year in the United States. Head injuries are the most common cause of death and acquired disability for children in developed countries. The estimated prevalence for lifetime concussions or head injuries ranges from 3.6–7.0% for children (classified as ages 3–17) to 6.5–18.3% for adolescents (classified as ages 13–17) on US national surveys.

2. **What are some of the most common mechanisms leading to pediatric head injury?**
   Falls are the most common cause of head injury in children. Other common mechanisms include motor vehicle collisions, pedestrian or bike accidents, and sports and recreational activities. It is also important to consider nonaccidental trauma, as this is a potentially life-threatening cause of head injury in infants and younger children and should not be missed.

3. **How do we define clinically important traumatic brain injury?**
   Many children sustain head injuries, but only a few will have injuries that fall into the category of clinically important traumatic brain injury (ciTBI). These injuries cause significant immediate or long-term impact on the child or result in the child's death. Generally, these injuries include depressed or basilar skull fractures, bleeding requiring neurosurgical intervention, injury requiring the child to be intubated for more than 24 hours, or injury severe enough to warrant hospital admission longer than 48 hours.

4. **What types of injuries are considered ciTBIs?**
   Head injuries are frequently characterized by diffuse and focal injury patterns. Diffuse injuries include diffuse axonal injury (DAI), cerebral edema, hypoxic ischemic encephalopathy, and diffuse vascular injury. Concussions are also classified as diffuse injuries. Focal injuries include cerebral contusions and hemorrhage in the subdural, subarachnoid, or epidural spaces.

5. **How do diffuse injuries usually occur?**
   Diffuse injuries occur from shearing forces, often with a rapid acceleration-deceleration event or rotational force. Infants may suffer these types of injuries when shaken vigorously back and forth. Cerebral edema frequently occurs in severe trauma. It can occur as a result of hypoxia or changes in cerebral blood flow and from inflammatory mediators and vascular leak postinjury.

6. **What are the different types of focal injuries?**
   A *cerebral contusion* occurs from a direct impact of the brain against the intracranial bony surfaces and may lead to focal neurologic deficits. *Subdural hematomas* result from bleeding between the dura and the arachnoid membranes, typically from tearing of the bridging veins. This can occur from direct trauma or shaking. This type of injury is more common in children two years of age and younger. It may occur as a result of nonaccidental trauma. *Subarachnoid hemorrhage* occurs from bleeding of the vessels that supply the pia mater. Accumulation of blood occurs in layers along the bony surface, and bleeding can be quite extensive. *Epidural hemorrhage* is the collection of blood between the skull and the dura and may be from an arterial or venous source. Temporal epidural hemorrhage classically results from injury to the middle meningeal artery.

7. **What are important age-related considerations when evaluating a child with a head injury?**
   Younger children (<2 years) should be considered separately from older children. Clinical assessment is decidedly more difficult in infants, who are unable to report symptoms or may have subtle or nonspecific signs of injury. It is important to consider the risk of inflicted or abusive injury in children. Traumatic brain injury is a leading cause of death from abuse in children. Clinicians need to consider the possibility of inflicted trauma in infants who present with a head injury, especially if the reported mechanism of injury does not seem to match the severity of the injury.

8. **I need to evaluate a child who just sustained a head injury at my urgent care facility. Are there specific things I should consider when determining a plan of care?**
   The primary goal of evaluating a child with a head injury is to determine the severity of the injury and recognize injuries that require further management. Children with potentially serious injuries need to be rapidly identified

Table 32.1 Criteria for Children at Low Risk of ciTBI by Age (A child must meet all of these criteria to be considered low-risk)

CHILDREN <2 YEARS	CHILDREN ≥2 YEARS
Acting normally per parents	Normal mental status (GCS ≥14)
Known, low-risk mechanism	Known, low-risk mechanism
No loss of consciousness	No loss of consciousness
No nonfrontal scalp hematoma	No vomiting
No signs of basilar skull fracture	No signs of basilar skull fracture
No concern for abuse	No complaints of severe headache

and transferred to an appropriate facility for definitive care. Ideally, this would be a pediatric certified trauma center that includes access to pediatric neurosurgeons. The secondary goal of evaluation includes minimizing unnecessary radiation exposure.

9. **Why should minimizing radiation be a priority?**
   Computed tomography (CT) is considered the standard of care for assessing traumatic head injuries. However, this form of imaging exposes children to ionizing radiation. Young children are more sensitive to radiation, and thus there is an increased risk of cancer mortality associated with head CTs in children. It is important to balance the risk of the child having a significant injury with the potential future risk of malignancy.

10. **Are there established guidelines that can help me determine a child's risk of clinically important TBI and make an educated decision about imaging?**
    Yes! In the US, the Pediatric Emergency Care Applied Research Network (PECARN) has developed and validated clinical decision rules for children with a low risk of serious head injuries. The rules are derived from a large, multicenter, prospective trial that included over 43,000 patients. These guidelines help standardize patient evaluations, rapidly identify children with potentially serious intracranial injury, and minimize the use of CT scans in low-risk patients. Such rules are useful when evaluating healthy children who present to the emergency department within 24 hours of injury, and in whom there is no suspicion for nonaccidental trauma. For children in the younger age group, the low-risk rule had a sensitivity of 100% and a negative predictive value of 100%. In the older age group, the sensitivity of the low-risk rule was 96.8% with a negative predictive value of 99.95%.

11. **Can I use the PECARN criteria for all children with head injuries?**
    Not all children will be eligible for the PECARN pathway. The PECARN rules are intended to identify *low-risk* children not requiring further assessment. Children who are at moderate or high risk for significant intracranial injury, including those with Glasgow Coma Scale (GCS) <14, require transfer to a pediatric trauma center. Children with underlying neuropathology, such as brain tumors or preexisting neurologic disorders, warrant separate consideration. Finally, children with ventriculoperitoneal (VP) shunts or bleeding disorders may have a higher risk of serious injury than otherwise healthy children or may have intracranial bleeding with a less severe mechanism of injury.

12. **What are the PECARN criteria by which children qualify as low risk for serious injury?**
    Table 32.1 describes the criteria for children who qualify as low risk based on the PECARN guidelines.

13. **How do I know what counts as a severe mechanism?**
    The PECARN criteria use well-defined descriptions to classify mild and severe mechanisms. If the mechanism fails to meet the criteria for one or the other, it is generally considered to fall within the moderate risk category. Mild mechanisms include ground-level falls or injuries resulting from a child running into a stationary object. Severe mechanisms include motor vehicle accidents with ejection, death of another passenger, rollover accidents, and pedestrians or bicyclists struck by a motor vehicle. Falls greater than 3 feet for children less than 2 years, falls greater than 5 feet for children older than 2 years, and head strikes by a high-impact object are also considered severe mechanisms.

14. **Are there certain symptoms that suggest a child might be at higher risk for ciTBI and therefore need urgent imaging?**
    Symptoms suggestive of serious injury include altered mental status, loss of consciousness, focal neurologic findings, posttraumatic seizure, persistent vomiting, or evidence of a depressed or basilar skull fracture. Consider that infants with bulging fontanel, nonfrontal scalp hematoma, irritability, poor feeding, or lethargy may also be at risk of serious TBI. Older children with significant TBI may complain of worsening or severe headaches.

15. **What if I am concerned for ciTBI in my patient?**
    Children with suspected or proven ciTBI need to be transported to a qualified pediatric trauma center as rapidly and safely as possible. Be aware that such patients have a risk of worsening neurologic status and herniation.

Table 32.2 PECARN Recommendations[*] for Determining the Use of CT Scan to Evaluate Children With Head Injuries and GCS 14–15

AGE	CLINICAL FEATURES	RISK OF CITBI	RECOMMENDATIONS
<2 years	GCS = 14 or Altered mental status or Palpable skull fracture	4.4%	• CT recommended • Transfer to a trauma center
	Nonfrontal scalp hematoma or Loss of consciousness ≥5 seconds or Severe mechanism or Not acting normally per parents	0.9%	• Observation versus CT[**] • Consider transfer if worsening signs/symptoms
	Acting normally per parents and None of the features listed above	<0.02%	• CT not recommended • Discharge with home care instructions
≥2 years	GCS = 14 or Altered mental status or Signs of basilar skull fracture	4.3%	• CT recommended • Transfer to a trauma center
	Loss of consciousness or History of vomiting or Severe mechanism or Severe headache	0.8%	• Observation versus CT[**] • Consider transfer if worsening signs/symptoms
	Appropriate mental status and None of the features listed above	<0.05%	• CT not recommended • Discharge with home care instructions

[*]Data adapted from Kupperman N, Holes JF, Dayan PS, et al. Identification of children at very low risk of clinically-important brain injuries after head trauma: a prospective cohort study. *Lancet.* 2009;374:1160–1170 [Fig. 3, p 1168].

[**]CT scan may be obtained based on physician experience, if the patient exhibits worsening signs or symptoms during the observation period, if the patient is under 3 months of age, or if the parental preference is for CT.

These children will frequently have altered mental status (GCS <14). Other concerning signs include pupillary changes, bradycardia, hypertension, and respiratory depression. Such children may need airway protection with intubation prior to transfer.

16. **How can I use the PECARN criteria to help me make an informed decision about management?**
Table 32.2, adapted from the original study, summarizes the PECARN recommendations for children who present with head injuries and have a GCS of 14 or 15.

17. **What about children with skull fractures?**
Simple, linear, unilateral, and nondepressed skull fractures are common in children and account for 75% of all pediatric skull fractures. Most of these are uncomplicated, with only 15–30% having an underlying intracranial injury. The goal of evaluation of skull fractures is to separate children with uncomplicated fractures from those with more complex injuries.

18. **What counts as a complicated skull fracture?**
Complicated skull fractures are more likely to be associated with underlying injury. There is also a correlation between complex skull fractures and nonaccidental trauma. Complicated fractures include:
- Fractures that are large or cross suture lines
- Complex or burst fracture pattern
- Bilateral or multiple fractures
- Depressed fractures
- Basilar skull fractures
- Open skull fractures

19. **Are there physical exam findings that might suggest skull fracture?**
Infants may have a scalp hematoma or significant soft tissue swelling in the area of the fracture. Crepitus or palpable skull defects are occasionally found. Patients with basilar skull fractures may present with nystagmus, hearing loss, hemotympanum, periorbital ecchymosis, Battle sign, CSF otorrhea or rhinorrhea, or facial nerve palsies. Patients with such findings need imaging, with CT scan as the preferred mechanism.

20. **Do all pediatric patients with skull fractures need to be admitted?**
    Not necessarily. Children may be discharged without admission if they meet **all** of the following criteria:
    - Have a simple, unilateral, nondisplaced skull fracture.
    - There is no underlying intracranial injury.
    - No other distracting traumatic injury is present.
    - Complete neurologic exam is normal.
        Admission is necessary for children with complicated injuries, including complex or basilar skull fractures, or when there is a suspicion of nonaccidental trauma.

21. **When do I have to worry about nonaccidental trauma in children with head injuries?**
    Traumatic brain injury is the leading cause of death from abuse in children. Thus, clinicians always need to consider abusive head injury when evaluating children with head injuries, especially infants. Up to 30% of infants with other abuse-related injuries may have occult head injuries, even if they are asymptomatic from a neurologic standpoint.

22. **How will children with abusive head injuries present to care?**
    Detecting abuse-related head injuries is often difficult. The history may be incomplete or lack a clear history of trauma. During evaluation, consider whether the mechanism and developmental abilities of the child are consistent with the injury. Remember that abusive head trauma can occur at any age but is most common in children less than 1 year of age, with a peak at 8–12 weeks. Infants may present with nonspecific symptoms, such as fussiness, poor feeding, or vomiting. In severe cases, infants may present with apnea, seizures, and coma. Additionally, abusive head trauma should be considered in children of any age with developmental disabilities.

NECK INJURIES

An 8-year-old male is brought in by his parents complaining of neck pain after being struck in the neck with a hockey stick during practice. He fell to the ice initially but was able to ambulate afterward. He complains of posterior neck pain but denies numbness or tingling in the extremities.

23. **What should I consider when evaluating a child with a neck injury?**
    Both penetrating and blunt neck trauma in children are uncommon but potentially life-threatening. Children have large heads, short necks, and mobile laryngotracheal structures, making them less susceptible to penetrating trauma and airway fractures than adults. However pediatric neck injuries are often severe given the small area of the neck and the large number of vital structures that pass through it. Significant neck trauma is often associated with extracervical injuries, including injuries to the head, face, airway, chest, or upper digestive systems.

24. **What are common complications of neck injuries in children?**
    Penetrating neck injuries are unusual injuries in children but may lead to vascular injuries and complications such as aneurysms, dissections, occlusions, or fistulas. Blunt neck trauma often results from motor vehicle accidents, clothesline or handlebar injuries, sports, strangulation or hanging injuries, or nonaccidental trauma. Blunt trauma may lead to laryngeal or airway injuries, esophageal injuries, or cervical spine injuries. Vascular injuries are less common in blunt trauma.

25. **What should I do if a child presents with penetrating neck trauma?**
    Although penetrating injuries are uncommon, clinicians should have a high suspicion for serious injury in these children. Primary management for such patients includes ensuring a patent and stable airway, control of hemorrhage, and prevention of injury progression. Early, safe transfer to an appropriate pediatric trauma center should be prioritized. Injuries should be imaged with CT angiography to assess for vascular injury. For injuries that penetrate the outer layer of musculature, surgical evaluation is recommended.

26. **Are there special considerations for cervical spine injuries in children?**
    Cervical spine injuries (CSI) are rare in children, but when such injuries occur, there is a higher risk of upper cervical injuries (C1–C4). This occurs because the fulcrum of the spine is at higher cervical levels in younger patients, with infants having the fulcrum at C2–C3 level, and the fulcrum lowering to C3–C4 by age 5–6 years. Children also have relatively weak neck muscles compared to adults. Certain preexisting conditions make children more susceptible to neck injuries, including trisomy 21 and achondroplasia. Sports and recreational activities associated with a higher risk of cervical spine injuries include diving, football, hockey, gymnastics or cheer, trampoline, or nonmotorized vehicle crashes or falls.

27. **I know that there are adult criteria for the detection of cervical spine injury. Can the same criteria be used for pediatric patients?**
    The NEXUS criteria are often used in adults to detect cervical spine injury and have been shown to have greater than 99% sensitivity for detecting spinal injuries in adults. However, when applied to children less than 18, the NEXUS criteria were 57–100% sensitive and only 20–54% specific. The PECARN group has investigated cervical

spine injuries in children. The group found good sensitivity in identifying C-spine injuries if one or more of the following eight factors are present:
- Altered mental status
- Neurologic deficits
- Neck pain
- Torticollis
- Significant torso trauma
- High-risk motor vehicle accident
- Diving injury
- Preexisting condition that increases the risk of cervical spine injury

28. **What do I do if a child with neck pain and a concerning mechanism of injury presents to my urgent care for evaluation?**
If there is concern for cervical spine injury, the child should be placed in an appropriately sized cervical collar. Avoid hyperextension of the spine. Cervical spine films may be used in initial evaluation, but CT or MRI should be considered if x-rays are abnormal or if there are neurologic deficits. If there is concern for significant injury, the child should be transferred to an appropriate pediatric trauma center. When in doubt, assume all children with multiple traumatic injuries or concerning mechanisms have a significant head or neck injury; it is important not to miss an unstable spine. Obtunded patients cannot be clinically cleared with regard to the cervical spine and should remain in a cervical collar.

KEY POINTS

Head Injuries
1. Children with clinically important head injuries, including intracranial bleeding and complicated skull fractures, should be rapidly identified and transferred to an appropriate pediatric trauma center.
2. Identifying infants with significant head injuries is often difficult, as they may be asymptomatic or have nonspecific symptoms.
3. Pediatric head trauma guidelines can be helpful to minimize the use of CT scans in children at low risk for significant injury.

Neck Injuries
1. Neck injuries are uncommon in children but may be severe due to the large number of vital structures and the high cervical fulcrum of the spine.
2. Children with neck injuries should be appropriately immobilized in a cervical collar and transferred to a qualified pediatric trauma center.
3. Consider cervical spine injuries in children presenting with a concerning mechanism (especially diving or axial loading) who complain of neck pain, have focal neurologic findings, or torticollis.

BIBLIOGRAPHY

Babcock L, Olsen CS, Jaffe DM, Leonard JC. Cervical spine injuries in children associated with sports and recreational activities. *Pediatr Emer Care.* 2018;34:677–686.
Kupperman N, Holes JF, Dayan PS, et al. Identification of children at very low risk of clinically-important brain injuries after head trauma: a prospective cohort study. *Lancet.* 2009;374:1160–1170.
Leonard JC, Kupperman N, Olsen C, et al. Factors associated with cervical spine injury in children after blunt trauma. *Ann Emerg Med.* 2011;52(2):145–155.
Lumba-Brown A, Yeates K, Sarmiento K, et al. Centers for Disease Control and Prevention guideline on diagnosis and management of mild traumatic brain injury among children. *JAMA Pediatr.* 2018;172(11):e182853.
McManemy JK, Jea A, Ducis K. Neurotrauma. In: Shaw KN, Bacher RG, eds. *Fleisher & Ludwig's Textbook of Pediatric Emergency Medicine.* 8th ed. Wolters Kluwer; 2021:1254–1262.
Nigrovic LE, Kupperman N. Children with minor blunt head injury presenting to the emergency department. *Pediatrics.* 2019;144(6):e20191495.
Schutzman S, Mannix R. Injury: Head. In: Shaw KN, Bacher RG, eds. *Fleisher & Ludwig's Textbook of Pediatric Emergency Medicine.* 8th ed. Wolters Kluwer; 2021:268–274.
Woodward GA, Keilman A. Neck trauma. In: Shaw KN, Bacher RG, eds. *Fleisher & Ludwig's Textbook of Pediatric Emergency Medicine.* 8th ed. Wolters Kluwer; 2021:1214–1253.

CHAPTER 33

CHEST AND ABDOMINAL TRAUMA

Peggy Tseng, MD, Emily Rose, MD

TOP SECRETS

1. An abdominal seat belt sign on physical exam is associated with a high risk of intraabdominal injuries.
2. Abnormal mental status, abnormal vital signs, respiratory symptoms, penetrating trauma, or multiple traumatic injuries should prompt emergent transfer to an emergency department for evaluation and treatment.

1. **What is the most common mechanism of chest or abdominal trauma in children?**
   Blunt trauma in pediatric patients accounts for approximately 90% of injuries, usually sustained from falls, motor vehicle collisions (MVC), or other vehicle-related accidents (e.g., auto vs. pedestrian or bicycle), and nonaccidental trauma.
   Penetrating trauma less commonly occurs from gunshot wounds (GSW), stabbing, or impalement.

2. **How do injury patterns differ in children compared to adults who sustain thoracic trauma?**
   The chest wall of a child is more compliant than that of an adult, so serious intrathoracic injuries may occur without rib fractures or even obvious physical signs on the chest wall. Due to their compliant musculoskeletal structures, rib fractures require more significant force than the same fractures in adults and are therefore a red flag for severe injury or nonaccidental injury.

3. **Why are children more vulnerable to blunt intraabdominal trauma compared to adult patients?**
   Infants and toddlers have relatively compact torsos with larger viscera, especially the liver and spleen, which extend below the costal margin, so they are more exposed to direct injury. They also have small anterior-posterior diameters, which provide a smaller area over which the force of injury is dissipated. This, in combination with less overlying fat and weaker abdominal musculature to cushion intraabdominal structures, places pediatric patients at higher risk for intraabdominal injuries following blunt trauma.

4. **A 3-year-old girl is brought to your urgent care after a 5-foot fall at the playground. What are assessment and management priorities in examination of a pediatric patient with traumatic injuries to the chest and abdomen?**
   The initial management should be to identify and stabilize any life-threatening injuries. Airway, breathing, and circulation are essential and part of any traumatic primary exam. If any component of the trauma primary exam is absent or severely compromised, emergent intervention is needed; immediately transfer to a higher level of care. Any hemodynamically unstable child with suspected intrathoracic or intraabdominal injury needs to be stabilized emergently and should be transferred to an emergency department with trauma capabilities for resuscitation and possible operative intervention.

5. **What additional information should be gathered after a traumatic event?**
   Gather information regarding the mechanism from witnesses if available. Obtain a history from the patient or the patient's family and perform a thorough secondary physical exam. Key elements of the patient include the mechanism of injury, time since the injury, and the patient's presentation at the scene of the injury. Was there any loss of consciousness? Were there any witnesses to the injury?
   Does the patient complain of any chest pain or abdominal pain? Any difficulty breathing? Nausea or vomiting? Has the patient been able to tolerate food?

6. **What are major considerations in motor vehicle accidents?**
   Was the patient restrained? Was the patient in a car seat, facing forward or backward? Where in the car was the patient seated? Where was the impact on the vehicle? Were any other people in the accident severely injured? How fast was the vehicle traveling and were airbags deployed?

7. **What is important history to obtain in penetrating trauma?**
   If the penetrating trauma was due to a gunshot, how many shots were fired? If the wounds were due to impalement, how long was the object that penetrated the patient? Was the whole object removed and witnessed to be intact? Are the injuries present consistent with the given mechanism?

8. **When should you consider nonaccidental trauma?**
   Any serious injury such as intracranial hemorrhage, a long bone fracture (except a spiral tibial fracture), or hollow viscous injury should have a significant mechanism of injury on history. Any discrepancy between the history and the physical or diagnostic findings or signs of significant force (such as a rib fracture) should prompt you to consider inflicted injury. Consider if a mechanism of injury is inconsistent with a patient's developmental abilities

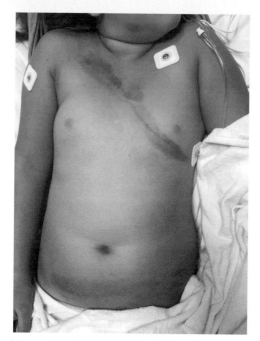

Fig. 33.1 Seat belt sign in a pediatric patient.

(e.g., bruising in a nonmobile infant). Any pattern injury is concerning for inflicted injury (bruising/burns/marks that correspond to infliction with instruments or do not occur through natural play environmental interactions). Also, note frequent visits for injuries. Children with inflicted injuries may present with multiple visits for injuries that may not individually raise concern.

9. **A 1-year-old boy comes to your urgent care after a fall from a bed. Your primary exam is normal. Describe key components of the secondary exam of the chest in a pediatric trauma patient**
Evaluate respiratory status including breath sounds, respiratory rate, and signs of distress such as nasal flaring or retractions. Assess the chest wall for focal tenderness, crepitus, abrasions, ecchymosis, or lacerations. Remember that open wounds may be the track of a penetrating wound. Paradoxical chest wall movement is important to note because a flail segment bulges during expiration. Decreased or absent breath sounds may indicate pneumothorax, hemothorax, or pulmonary contusion. Distant or muffled heart tones may suggest hemopericardium. Injury to the great vessels may result in hypotension, peripheral pulse abnormality, or neurologic deficit.

10. **What are the red flag physical exam findings after chest and abdominal trauma?**
Respiratory distress in a child after trauma is a red flag for serious injury and potential for decompensation. Chest pain with neck discomfort is concerning for mediastinal free air, and distended neck veins are associated with pericardial tamponade. Children should be transferred to the emergency department for further evaluation with any abnormalities of lung auscultation, respiratory rate, chest rise pattern, and oxygen saturation.
     In abdominal trauma, focal tenderness, distension, vomiting, and bruising are red flags for injury. Any sign of rigidity or rebound tenderness is a late finding and concerning for severe abdominal injury.

11. **A 7-year-old girl comes to your urgent care after she was a passenger in a motor vehicle accident. On physical exam you find what is shown in Fig. 33.1. What is the name of this physical finding and what is its significance?**
This is a seat belt sign. It is ecchymosis due to the acceleration and deceleration of the body against a seat belt in an MVC.
     Children with seat belt signs over the abdomen from MVCs are almost 3 times more likely to suffer an intraabdominal injury (IAI) and are over 10 times more likely to suffer gastrointestinal injuries such as hollow viscous or mesentery. There is a lower association of injury if the seat belt sign is localized to only the chest.
     A child with a seat belt sign over the abdomen should be transferred to the emergency department with trauma capabilities, as there is a significant associated risk of IAI. Further investigation is required, including serial abdominal exams, laboratory studies, and frequently CT scans.

12. **Which laboratory studies are indicated after chest trauma?**
    There are no specific laboratory studies indicated for pediatric chest trauma. In general, with all trauma, if significant injury is suspected, hemoglobin and hematocrit are important to evaluate for hemorrhage. Serial hemoglobin and hematocrit levels are more useful as a marker of ongoing blood loss, because a single value may not reflect the current degree of hemorrhage. Type and screen or cross-match blood is needed, especially for any patients in whom you suspect serious injury and who may have the potential to decompensate and need blood transfusion.

13. **Are there any specific laboratory studies helpful in evaluating pediatric abdominal trauma?**
    Serial hemoglobin/hematocrit levels evaluate for blood loss and are more clinically useful if significant intraabdominal injury is suspected. Elevated aspartate transaminase (AST) (>60–200 IU/L) or elevated alanine transaminase (ALT) (>25–125 IU/L) is sensitive in detecting hepatic injuries if imaging is not obtained.
    Other tests such as amylase and lipase have poor discriminatory ability to diagnose or exclude injuries and are typically not indicated.
    Gross hematuria (which is typically ≥50 RBCs per high-power field) often indicates kidney injury. Microscopic hematuria is typically not clinically significant in asymptomatic patients without other associated injuries.

14. **Which imaging is indicated in thoracic trauma?**
    Chest x-ray (CXR) is the imaging of choice for most pediatric thoracic trauma, as it is widely available, inexpensive, and can identify life-threatening injuries like large hemothorax or pneumothorax. Bedside ultrasonography may be more sensitive than CXR for experienced providers. Chest computed tomography (CT) should not routinely occur in pediatric thoracic trauma because of the low incidence of cardiac and great vessel injury and high radiation exposure.

15. **What is the role of the extended focused assessment with sonography for trauma (eFAST) in pediatric trauma?**
    The eFAST is a standardized point-of-care ultrasound that does not expose children to radiation and is used to rapidly identify hemoperitoneum, pneumothorax, hemothorax, and pericardial effusion. The eFAST includes views of the right upper quadrant, left upper quadrant, bladder, lungs, and heart, and can be quickly repeated during reassessment. It can be used to rule in pneumothorax, pericardial effusion, and intraabdominal free fluid in the trauma setting.
    eFAST has more limited utility in the stable pediatric trauma patient due to suboptimal sensitivity for detecting injury. Patients with severe injury may have a normal scan, and prepubertal patients without injury may have a small amount of physiologic pelvic fluid on exam. However, when used in an unstable child with concern for IAI, a positive eFAST finding can be useful for expediting acute interventions without delay.

16. **When is CT scan indicated in children with chest trauma?**
    Consider further diagnostic investigation in cases of severe thoracic injury with an abnormal CXR. Aortic injuries are rare but highly lethal, and when red flags for injury are present in mechanism, physical exam, or diagnostic imaging, it is imperative to consider transfer to a trauma center for an emergent chest CT scan and trauma surgeon evaluation.
    Mechanism red flags for aortic injuries are usually high-velocity acceleration/deceleration injuries (most commonly high-speed MVCs or falls from height). Abnormal CXR red flags for aortic injuries consist of an obscured aortic knob, left apical cap, or wide mediastinum, and physical exam red flags for aortic injuries include asymmetric, diminished, or absent peripheral pulses.
    A large pneumothorax or hemothorax seen on CXR requires immediate intervention. Crepitus in the chest should raise suspicion for tracheobronchial injury. Both abnormalities require ED transfer and CT imaging.
    Imaging for penetrating trauma depends on the mechanism. High-velocity injuries (e.g., gunshot wounds) frequently require CT imaging even if the initial CXR is normal. Stab wounds may only require a CXR and ultrasound (often serially performed). Transfer to the ED is typically recommended in penetrating trauma.

17. **Who can be classified as low risk for intraabdominal injury?**
    Though significant intraabdominal injury can occur with seemingly trivial trauma, those with low risk for injury include: (adapted from the PECARN prediction rule by Holmes et al. 2013)
    - Glasgow Coma Scale ≥14
    - No evidence of abdominal wall trauma or seat belt sign
    - No abdominal tenderness on exam
    - No complaints of abdominal pain
    - No vomiting
    - No thoracic wall trauma
    - No decreased breath sounds
    - No concern for physical abuse
    - No serious associated injuries

18. Your patient with the seat belt sign is complaining of abdominal pain. When should you consider CT scan for abdominal trauma in children?

Indications for abdominal CT scan to evaluate for IAI in the hemodynamically stable patient include the following: (adapted from the PECARN prediction rule by Holmes et al. 2013)

- Inability to tolerate oral intake
- Persistent abdominal tenderness (outside of superficial minor bruises or abrasions not associated with a seat belt)
- Gross hematuria
- Hematemesis or blood in the stool
- Seat belt sign with abdominal pain
- Positive eFAST with chest pain, abdominal pain, or other symptoms concerning for IAI
- Elevated AST (>200 IU/L) or elevated ALT (>125 IU/L)
- Hemodynamic instability or decreased hemoglobin or hematocrit

19. You evaluate a 10-year-old boy who is complaining of abdominal pain after he fell off his bicycle. He sustained a direct blow from the handlebars into his abdomen. Does a negative CT scan of the abdomen rule out IAI?

No. CT is insensitive for hollow viscous injury, and these injuries should be suspected in patients with persistent/progressive tenderness. Hollow viscous injuries include mesenteric injuries, duodenal hematomas, and bowel perforation. The mechanism involves a direct blow and discrete point of energy transfer to the abdomen from bicycle handlebars, seat belts during MVCs, and child abuse. Significant abdominal tenderness even after a prior normal CT scan should prompt urgent ED referral. Symptoms may also be delayed up to 24 hours after injury, so suspicion of injury should be maintained even with a subacute presentation.

20. Describe the most common traumatic chest wall injuries in a pediatric patient.

A tension pneumothorax is the most common immediate life-threatening thoracic injury in pediatric trauma and needs emergent intervention and transfer to a higher level of care. More common and stable blunt injuries include pulmonary contusion, non-tension pneumothorax, and rib fractures.

Less commonly, penetrating trauma may result in hemothorax or pneumothorax, followed by pulmonary contusion, pulmonary laceration, and blood vessel injury.

21. Does the location of rib fracture in a chest trauma patient correlate with injury?

Yes. The upper ribs (1–3) are usually protected by the scapula, humerus, and clavicle, and a significant amount of force is required to fracture them. Further investigation to evaluate for associated organ injuries such as pulmonary contusion and intrathoracic vessels is often required in patients with upper rib fractures.

Lower rib fractures may be associated with injury to the abdominal organs such as liver and spleen injuries.

22. What physical exam findings are concerning for cardiac contusion?

Consider blunt cardiac injuries in pediatric patients with physical findings of anterior chest wall trauma, sternal fracture, new murmurs or muffled heart tones, or any arrhythmia including sinus tachycardia in the absence of hemorrhage.

23. What testing is indicated to screen for cardiac contusion?

Obtain a chest radiograph to evaluate for noncardiac injuries and an electrocardiogram (ECG). Cardiac contusions may manifest as tachycardia or various arrhythmias. Cardiac contusion is unlikely with a normal ECG.

Cardiac troponin test in pediatric trauma is controversial. An abnormal ECG (including sinus tachycardia) in chest trauma warrants an ED referral for further investigation.

24. Does every pediatric patient with chest trauma mandate a CXR?

No, there are some children with isolated minor trauma that may not require any imaging if paired with low physician concern for underlying injury based on mechanism and exam.

A CXR is likely to be normal in patients with a normal GCS of 15, normal vital signs (especially respiratory rate, pulse oximetry, and blood pressure), no femur fracture, and no localized findings on chest auscultation and examination (including signs of trauma).

25. What types of patients who sustain abdominal trauma can we care for in the urgent care setting?

If a patient has no evidence of abdominal wall or chest wall trauma, no seat belt sign, normal GCS of 15, no abdominal pain or tenderness, no absent or decreased breath sounds, and no vomiting, then some researchers have found that this can make a child very low risk (<0.1%) of having clinically important blunt abdominal injuries. However, clinical judgment is still necessary, as this does not account for the mechanism of injury, vital signs, laboratory results, and clinician gestalt. Additionally, a positive screen does not mandate a CT scan but should strongly still consider transfer to an emergency department for serial exams, assessment with ultrasound, and/or laboratory evaluation. When in doubt, a patient should be transferred to the emergency department for evaluation.

26. When should transfer to a higher level of care be considered?

Abdominal pain or tenderness and/or a seat belt sign on exam should prompt further diagnostic investigation in the emergency department (Fig. 33.2).

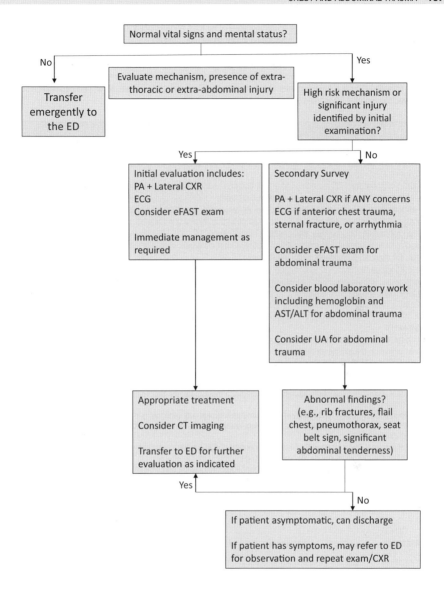

Fig. 33.2 Pediatric algorithm for blunt chest and abdominal trauma. (Adapted from Initial Evaluation and Stabilization of Children with Thoracic Trauma. https://www-uptodate-com; Accessed July 19, 2016.)

Severe pain, abnormal findings on radiography other than nondisplaced rib fractures in an older child, or a high-impact mechanism such as a penetrating injury should be referred.

Any abnormal vital signs including tachypnea, hypoxia, tachycardia, or hypotension; any altered mental status; or multiple traumatic injuries indicate life-threatening injury. Obviously, immediately life-threatening injuries such as airway obstruction, tension pneumothorax, massive hemothorax, and cardiac tamponade require emergent paramedic transportation to a trauma center. In any hemodynamically unstable patient, testing and evaluation in urgent care would only delay ED evaluation and treatment.

KEY POINTS

1. Consider nonaccidental trauma in children younger than 2 years of age with rib fractures, abdominal pain/bruising, associated serious injury such as long bone fractures or intracranial injury, and no history of significant accidental mechanism of injury.
2. Children with normal GCS, normal vital signs, and no focal findings or tenderness on chest or back examination are at low risk for having findings on chest radiography.
3. An abdominal seat belt sign on physical exam is associated with high risk of intraabdominal injuries. This finding, with or without symptoms, should prompt further evaluation and consideration of a transfer to a hospital setting for testing, observation, and possible intervention.
4. Abnormal mental status, vital signs, or multiple traumatic injuries should prompt emergent transfer to a trauma center for evaluation and treatment.
5. Penetrating trauma occurs less commonly in children and is associated with higher injury risk. The urgent care provider should have a low threshold to transfer to the emergency department for further evaluation and management.

BIBLIOGRAPHY

Chan KK, Joo DA, McRae AD, et al. Chest ultrasonography versus supine chest radiography for diagnosis of pneumothorax in trauma patients in the emergency department. *Cochrane Database Syst Rev.* 2020;7(7):CD013031. Published 2020 Jul 23. doi:10.1002/14651858.CD013031.pub2.

Hannon MM, Middelberg LK, Lee LK. The initial approach to the multisystem pediatric trauma patient. *Pediatr Emerg Care.* 2022;38(6):290–298. doi:10.1097/PEC.0000000000002722.

Holmes JF, et al. A clinical decision rule for identifying children with thoracic injuries after blunt torso trauma. *Ann Emerg Med.* 2002;39(5):492–499.

Liang T, Roseman E, Gao M, Sinert R. The utility of the focused assessment with sonography in trauma examination in pediatric blunt abdominal trauma: a systematic review and meta-analysis. *Pediatr Emerg Care.* 2021;37(2):108–118. doi:10.1097/PEC.0000000000001755.

Netherton S, Milenkovic V, Taylor M, Davis PJ. Diagnostic accuracy of eFAST in the trauma patient: a systematic review and meta-analysis. *CJEM.* 2019;21(6):727–738. doi:10.1017/cem.2019.381.

Ozcan A, Ahn T, Akay B, Menoch M. Imaging for pediatric blunt abdominal trauma with different prediction rules: is the outcome the same? *Pediatr Emerg Care.* 2022;38(2):e654–e658. doi:10.1097/PEC.0000000000002346.

Springer E, Frazier SB, Arnold DH, Vukovic AA. External validation of a clinical prediction rule for very low risk pediatric blunt abdominal trauma. *Am J Emerg Med.* 2019;37(9):1643–1648. doi:10.1016/j.ajem.2018.11.031.

CHAPTER 34

EXTREMITY TRAUMA

Joel M. Clingenpeel, MD, MPH, MS.MEdL, Michelle Georgia, DO, Kristin Herbert, DO, MPH

TOP SECRETS

- The pliability of the pediatric skeleton results in unique fracture patterns including "plastic" fractures (torus, greenstick, and bowing) and fractures involving the growth plate, which are described using the Salter-Harris classification.
- If the fracture and the history/mechanism are discordant (mechanism not plausible based on child's developmental age), keep nonaccidental trauma high in your differential diagnosis for young children.

1. **What is the Salter-Harris fracture classification?**
   The Salter-Harris classification system is used when describing fractures and their relation to the growth plate (physis). The system classifies fractures according to the level of involvement of the physis, metaphysis, and epiphysis. As physeal fractures account for 15–30% of bony injuries in children, this classification system is extremely important in pediatrics. Before the fusion of growth plates, the physis is predisposed to fracture, as it is weak compared to the surrounding bone. The classification system has five types (I–V) and will be further described in upcoming questions, but for now, remember that the higher the Roman numeral, the more serious the injury and greater the potential for growth disturbance.

2. **Sort the fractures in Fig. 34.1 through Fig. 34.5 according to the Salter-Harris classification (I–V) (Fig. 34.6).**
   Answer: fractures are type III, IV, I, II, and V, respectively, as seen in Figs. 34.1–34.5.
   You can remember types I–V with the mnemonic SALTR (Slipped, Above, Lower, Through/Transverse, Rammed/Ruined). Salter I (Slipped): fracture is confined within the physis, often not visible on radiographs. Look for widening of the physis or evidence of epiphyseal displacement (Fig. 34.3 shows displacement). Salter II (Above): the fracture involves the physis and up into the metaphysis. Salter III (Lower): fracture involves the physis and extends down through the epiphysis. This is the lowest classification of an intraarticular fracture. Salter IV (Through/Transverse): this is also an intraarticular fracture but involves the metaphysis, physis, and epiphysis; therefore, it goes through all three. Salter V (Rammed/Ruining): also known as a crush or compression fracture that damages the physis. Often not seen on initial radiographs and retrospectively diagnosed once growth arrest has occurred. Fig. 34.5 shows a follow-up x-ray of a child with an axial load mechanism to the ankle.

3. **Describe clinical and historical clues that suggest a child has a nursemaid's elbow needing reduction rather than an elbow fracture necessitating radiographs.**
   A nursemaid's elbow, an anatomic entrapment of the annular ligament between the radial head and capitellum, results from axial traction on the distal aspect of the child's extremity. Most elbow fractures, in contrast, involve

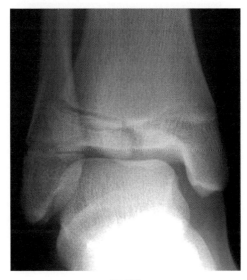

Fig. 34.1

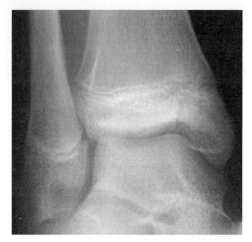

Fig. 34.2

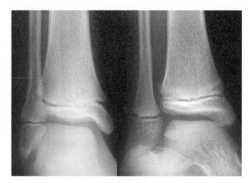

Fig. 34.3

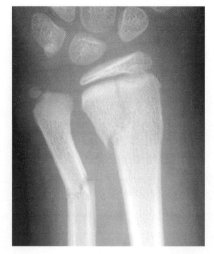

Fig. 34.4

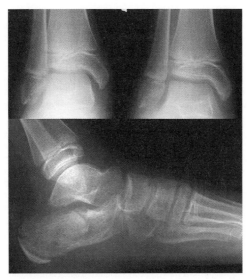

Fig. 34.5 Descriptions for Figs. 34.1–34.5 are embedded in the answer to question 2. (From Yamamoto LG, Chung SMK, Inaba AS. Salter-Harris. Radiology Cases in Pediatric Emergency Medicine 1 [case 18], University of Hawaii John A. Burns School of Medicine.)

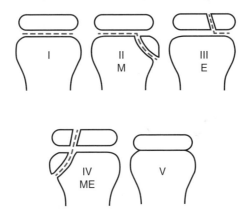

Fig. 34.6 Diagram of the Salter-Harris classification. (M, metaphyseal involvement; E, epiphyseal involvement.) (From Yamamoto LG, Chung SMK, Inaba AS. Salter-Harris. Radiology Cases in Pediatric Emergency Medicine 1 [case 18]. University of Hawaii John A. Burns School of Medicine.)

blunt trauma to the elbow or a fall on an outstretched hand. Children with nursemaid's deformity usually present with the arm held closely to the side, pronated, and partially flexed. While these children refuse to move the elbow, in contrast to children with a fracture, there is usually no swelling or ecchymosis and no pinpoint bony tenderness to the distal humerus or proximal radius and ulna.

4. **What pediatric extremity fractures are suspicious for nonaccidental trauma?**
   Any extremity fracture may be the result of abuse, particularly if associated with other injuries concerning for abuse, or if the fracture and the history/mechanism are discordant (mechanism not plausible based on the child's developmental age). The following extremity fracture patterns have the greatest specificity for abuse and should always arouse a high index of suspicion: femur or spiral extremity fractures in preambulatory children, multiple fractures in various stages of healing, and metaphyseal corner/chip fractures (which result from forced axial traction to an extremity).

5. **Explain compartment syndrome and describe injury mechanisms or fractures that place a patient at risk for its development.**
   Compartment syndrome occurs when there is elevated pressure within an extremity's fascial compartment resulting in decreased perfusion. This is a surgical emergency; without treatment, resultant ischemia to the muscles, nerves, and vessels can ensue. Common orthopedic injuries associated with compartment syndrome include crush

extremity injuries, proximal tibiofibular fractures, displaced supracondylar fractures, midshaft radius and ulna fractures, and elbow dislocation. Additionally, constrictive dressings and casts placed soon after injury that are not "bivalved" to allow space for the ongoing swelling have been associated with compartment syndrome.

6. **What signs and symptoms are concerning for possible compartment syndrome?**
Swollen and taut soft tissue in the traumatized region as well as pain out of proportion to the injury are usually the first (and sometimes only) clues to the diagnosis. Pain out of proportion should never be ignored, especially if the pain is made worse with passive extension of the muscles in the compartment. There are five signs/symptoms commonly affiliated with compartment syndrome, which one can remember as the five Ps: pain, paresthesia, pallor, paralysis, and pulselessness.

7. **What are "plastic fractures?"**
Torus, greenstick, and bowing fractures are commonly referred to as "plastic fractures" and are unique to children because of the pliability of pediatric bones. Torus (aka "buckle") fractures are common and result from the cortex of a long bone bulging without a visible fracture. Generally, these heal well with simple immobilization. Greenstick fractures occur when a bone bends and breaks on just one side, looking like a young, malleable green tree stick when bent. These are treated with a removable splint/cast immobilization and sometimes closed reduction, depending on the fracture. Bowing fractures are uncommon and, when seen, are usually in the forearm in children between the ages of 2 and 5. These injuries will often require reduction to prevent permanent bone angulation.

8. **Describe the location of injury and treatment of a "toddler's fracture."**
These fractures involve the distal third of the tibia, and as the fracture line is often spiral or oblique, it can be difficult to see on radiographic series without an oblique view. As the fractures are nondisplaced, there is no need for reduction. Management involves supportive care for 3–4 weeks. While no immobilization is absolutely necessary, most children will dislike bearing weight, so a walking boot or a long leg splint is commonly placed.

9. **What are humeral fat pads and when is their presence concerning for fracture?**
Anterior and posterior fat pads (Fig. 34.7 shows a small anterior fat pad on lateral, and Fig. 34.8 shows a large posterior fat pad on lateral) are seen as radiographic silhouettes around the distal humerus and are radiographic signs of an elbow effusion. In the setting of trauma and distal humeral pain, a poster fat pad should be considered evidence of an occult supracondylar fracture. Anterior fat pads can also be seen with occult supracondylar fractures, but they are far less specific and are visible in some children after blunt trauma without osseous injuries. Large ballooning anterior fat pads (aka "sail signs") are more specific than small anterior fat pads for osseous injuries in children.

10. **Name two lines you should draw on every pediatric lateral elbow film to screen for subtle fractures/dislocations (Figs. 34.7 and 34.8).**
The anterior humeral line and radiocapitellar line. A line drawn anterior to the humerus that does not pass through the middle or posterior third of the capitellum is concerning for an occult supracondylar fracture (with posterior displacement of the capitellum). A line drawn from the middle of the radius should point to the capitellum in every view. A misaligned radiocapitellar line is concerning for either a radial head dislocation or a Monteggia injury pattern.

11. **What is a Tillaux fracture and in what age group does it usually occur?**
Tillaux fracture (Fig. 34.9) is a traumatic Salter III fracture of the anterolateral distal tibia. Forced external rotation of the foot is the usual mechanism of the injury as the anterior inferior tibiofibular ligament avulses the anterolateral corner of the distal tibial epiphysis. Distal tibial physeal closure commences in a medial to lateral direction with full fusion usually occurring between 12–15 years of age. This fracture occurs in older children and adolescents whose medial tibial growth plate is fused but in whom the lateral tibial physis is still open.

12. **Explain the Gartland classification for supracondylar fractures (Fig. 34.10).**
Gartland type I supracondylar fractures are nondisplaced and have an anterior humeral line that usually intersects a portion of the capitellum. Gartland type II fractures have extension of the fractures and are partially displaced with an abnormal humeral line. A differentiating feature of the type II fracture is that the posterior aspect of the humerus remains intact. Type III Gartland fractures have a circumferential break in the cortex with complete displacement of the fracture fragments.

13. **What is the appropriate treatment and disposition for the three types of supracondylar fractures?**
Type I fractures can usually be splinted and followed up with orthopedics in 48 hours. Type III fractures require operative repair and sometimes emergent reduction if the neurovascular status of the upper extremity is compromised. The disposition of the type II fracture without neurovascular compromise is made in consultation with orthopedics. Some of these fractures are appropriate for short-term splinting, and others will require admission for neurovascular checks and definitive repair.

14. **How are clavicle fractures treated in children?**
In most cases, a medial or distal clavicle fracture can be treated with immobilization with a sling alone or a sling and swathe combination. The use of a figure-eight brace for clavicle fractures has not been shown to be more effective than a sling. A midshaft fracture with greater than 2 cm of displacement, fractures with greater than 1.5 cm of clavicle shortening, or grossly unstable distal injuries may need closed or open reduction with fixation. Other clavicle fractures needing evaluation

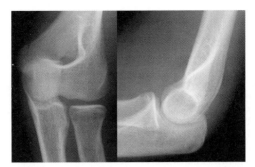

Fig. 34.7 Normal AP and lateral radiograph of the elbow. Note that the anterior humeral line passes through the middle of the capitellum. The radiocapitellar line also points directly at the capitellum. (From Yamamoto LG. Test Your Skill in Reading Pediatric Elbows. Radiology Cases in Pediatric Emergency Medicine 2 [case 18]. University of Hawaii John A. Burns School of Medicine.)

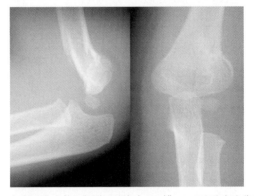

Fig. 34.8 AP and lateral radiograph of the elbow. Note that the anterior humeral line passes anterior to the capitellum, representing a supracondylar fracture. The radiocapitellar line is normal and not consistent with a Monteggia injury pattern. (From Yamamoto LG. Test Your Skill in Reading Pediatric Elbows. Radiology Cases in Pediatric Emergency Medicine 2 [case 18]. University of Hawaii John A. Burns School of Medicine.)

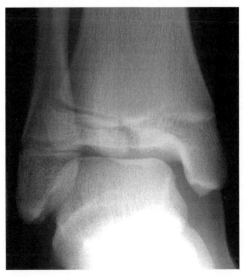

Fig. 34.9 AP radiograph of the distal tibia revealing a Tillaux fracture. (From Yamamoto LG, Chung SMK, Inaba AS. Salter-Harris. Radiology Cases in Pediatric Emergency Medicine 1 [case 18]. University of Hawaii John A. Burns School of Medicine.)

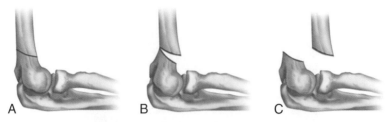

Fig. 34.10 (A) Gartland classification type I, (B), type II, and (C), type III for supracondylar fractures. (From Alton TB, Werner SE, Gee AO. Classifications in brief: the gartland classification of supracondylar humerus fractures. *Clin Orthop Relat Res.* 2015;473(2):738–741. http://dx.doi.org/10.1007/s11999-014-4033-8 [Fig. 3A-C].)

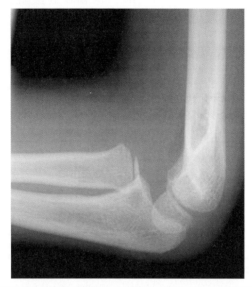

Fig. 34.11 Lateral radiograph of the elbow revealing a Monteggia dislocation. Note that the radiocapitellar line does not point to the capitellum. (From Young LL. Monteggia's Injury. Radiology Cases in Pediatric Emergency Medicine 1 [case 15]. University of Hawaii John A. Burns School of Medicine.)

by an orthopedic surgeon include any open fracture, fractures that are posteriorly displaced, any fracture causing neurovascular compromise, or fractures that cause tenting of the skin that can lead to skin necrosis and an eventual open fracture.

15. **What is the management of a displaced proximal humerus fracture?**
Proximal humerus fractures can remodel even with large amounts of angulation. In children, angulation up to 50° is often acceptable. In adolescence, there is more variability regarding the acceptable degree of angulation, but most authors advocate accepting up to 20°–50°. Management of proximal humerus fractures is typically a sling or shoulder immobilization device for 3–4 weeks. Splints to this area often cause more pain than stabilization and are generally not recommended. Operative indications include fractures of the articular surface, comminuted fractures, neurovascular compromise, or pathological fractures through a bone cyst.

16. **What is the usual mechanism of injury of supracondylar fractures and what nerve is sometimes compromised as a complication?**
The mechanism of injury for this common pediatric fracture is usually a fall on an outstretched arm with hyperextension of the elbow. The anterior interosseous branch of the median nerve (which has no sensory innervation) is most commonly injured. Injury of this nerve causes mild weakness of the flexor digitorum profundus to the index finger and of the flexor pollicis longus. Assessment of the anterior interosseous nerve function is performed by having the patient make an "OK" sign and then testing the index finger and thumb for strength in this position.

17. **Describe the Monteggia and Galeazzi fracture dislocation patterns that are associated with forearm trauma.**
Monteggia fracture (Fig. 34.11) is when there is a fracture of the proximal ulnar shaft in addition to a radial head dislocation (proximal radioulnar joint subluxation or dislocation). Suspicion for this type of fracture should be

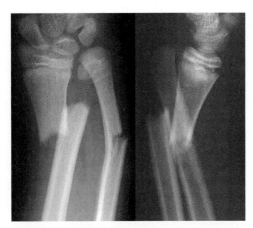

Fig. 34.12 AP and lateral radiograph of the wrist revealing a distal radial fracture and dislocated distal ulna consistent with a Galeazzi fracture. (From Yamamoto LG, Chung SMK. Galeazzi's Injury. Radiology Cases in Pediatric Emergency Medicine 1 [case 16]. University of Hawaii John A. Burns School of Medicine.)

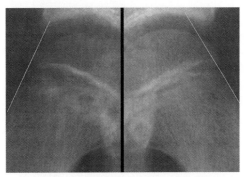

Fig. 34.13 The image on the left (right hip) reveals a Klein line that does not intersect the proximal femoral epiphysis, which is consistent with a slipped capital femoral epiphysis. The image on the right (left hip) is normal. (From Yamamoto LG. Thigh and Knee Pain in an Obese 10-Year-Old. Radiology Cases in Pediatric Emergency Medicine 2 [case 10]. University of Hawaii John A. Burns School of Medicine.)

heightened if there is swelling or pain over the elbow in the setting of an ulnar fracture. A lateral radiograph of the elbow will demonstrate misalignment of the radiocapitellar line. A Galeazzi fracture (Fig. 34.12) is a radial shaft fracture with a distal radioulnar joint dislocation. Both injuries require immediate orthopedic consultation, since failure to promptly reduce the dislocations in these fracture/dislocation injuries could lead to deformity and poor arm function.

18. **What is a Klein line?**
    A Klein line is drawn on an anteroposterior femoral radiograph to screen a child for a subtle slipped capital femoral epiphysis (SCFE). A SCFE is a Salter-Harris type I fracture of the proximal femoral physis with epiphyseal displacement. On the radiographs, the proximal femoral epiphysis will have an abnormal position in relation to the metaphysis. In a moderate or severe slip, the appearance resembles ice cream sliding off a cone. A Klein line is drawn along the superior border of a femoral epiphysis. If the Klein line does not intersect the epiphysis at all, it supports the diagnosis of a subtle SCFE (Fig. 34.13).

19. **How do you tell an avulsion fracture of the proximal fifth metatarsal from a normal apophysis?**
    An avulsion fracture at the most proximal portion of the fifth metatarsal occurs when there is avulsion of the bony tuberosity at the attachment site of the peroneus brevis and the lateral band of plantar fascia. The mechanism of injury for this type of fracture is plantar flexion with forced inversion of the foot/ankle. On a physical exam, the patient will have tenderness and potentially swelling/bruising over the fifth metatarsal. A radiograph of an avulsion fracture (Fig. 34.14) usually shows a fracture perpendicular to the long axis of the fifth metatarsal. The normal apophysis of the fifth metatarsal (Fig. 34.15) becomes visible on radiographs between ages 9–14 and appears as

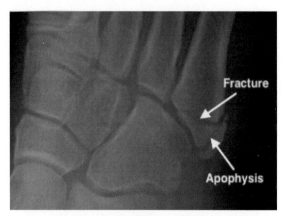

Fig. 34.14 Fifth metatarsal tuberosity avulsion fracture with radiolucency perpendicular to the long axis of the metatarsal. Also shown is the fifth metatarsal apophysis with an oblique orientation of the radiolucency that runs parallel to the metatarsal. Case courtesy of Dr. Alexandra Stanislavsky, Radiopaedia.org, rID: 10842. (Copyright 2023 Dr Alexandra Stanislavsky and Radiopaedia.org).

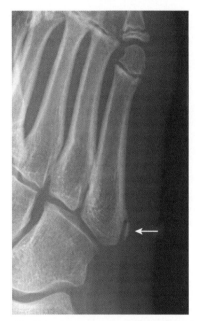

Fig. 34.15 Apophysis (*arrow*) of the base of the fifth metatarsal. Note the oblique orientation with the radiolucency aligned in parallel to the fifth metatarsal diaphysis. (From Keats, Theodore E, Strouse, Peter J. Anatomic Variants. Caffey's Pediatric Diagnostic Imaging. Elsevier; 2008.)

a small fleck of calcification lying parallel to the shaft of the fifth metatarsal. A comparison view of the normal foot may be helpful for obliquely oriented lucencies.

20. **What are the Ottawa ankle rules and how are they applicable to children?**
    The Ottawa ankle rules are physical exam findings that help predict the likelihood of an osseous ankle injury. Ankle radiographs are suggested if there is pain in the malleolar region accompanied by any of the following: (1) bone tenderness at the posterior edge or the tip of lateral malleolus; (2) bony tenderness at the posterior edge of the tip of the medial malleolus; and/or (3) inability to bear weight for a least four steps, both immediately after the injury and at the time of evaluation. Pooled data from several small trials suggest the rules are likely useful in children, but some studies have shown diminished sensitivity in comparison to adult cohorts.

KEY POINTS

1. The Salter-Harris classification describes growth plate fractures and has five levels that guide acute management as well as overall prognosis.
2. Fractures concerning for NAT include femur and spiral extremity fractures in preambulatory children, multiple fractures in various stages of healing, and corner/chip fractures of the metaphysis.
3. Torus, greenstick, and bowing fractures are often collectively referred to as "plastic fractures" and are unique to children because of the pliability of the pediatric skeleton.
4. Toddler's fractures are subtle radiographic fractures and involve the distal third of the tibia in ambulatory preschool children.
5. The Ottawa ankle rules recommend ankle radiographs if there is bony pain at the medial or lateral malleolus along with an inability to bear weight after an ankle injury.

BIBLIOGRAPHY

Almeida SI, Rios J, Costa Lima S, Oom P. Applying the Ottawa ankle rules in a pediatric emergency department. *Pediatr Emerg Care.* 2022;38(3):e1123–e1126. doi:10.1097/PEC.0000000000002528.
Egol KA, Koval KJ, Zuckerman JD. *Handbook of Fractures.* 6th ed. Wolters Kluwer Health; 2019.
Lien J. Pediatric orthopedic injuries: evidence-based management in the emergency department. *Pediatr Emerg Med Pract.* 2017;14(9).
Manske RC. *Fundamental Orthopedic Management for the Physical Therapist Assistant - E-Book.* Elsevier Health Sciences; 2021:167–172, 287.
Paul AR, Adamo MA. Non-accidental trauma in pediatric patients: a review of epidemiology, pathophysiology, diagnosis and treatment. *Transl Pediatr.* 2014;3(3):195–207.
Shah AS, Samora JB. Monteggia fracture dislocation in children. In: Waters PM, Skaggs DL, Flynn JM, eds. *Rockwood and Wilkins' Fractures in Children.* 9th ed. Wolters Kluwer; 2020:658–664.
Sheffer BW, Villarreal ED, Ochsner MG, Sawyer JR, Spence DD, Kelly DM. Concurrent ipsilateral tibial shaft and distal tibial fractures in pediatric patients: risk factors, frequency, and risk of missed diagnosis. *J Pediatr Orthop.* 2020 Jan;40(1):e1–e5.
Skaggs DL, Flynn JM. Supracondylar fractures of the distal humerus. In: Flynn JM, Skaggs DL, Waters PM, eds. *Rockwood and Wilkins' fractures in children.* 8th ed. Wolters Kluwer Health; 2015:582–627.

CHAPTER 35

COMMON NEWBORN COMPLAINTS

Nadine Aprahamian, MD, FAAP, Toni Clare Hogencamp, MD

CENTRAL CYANOSIS VERSUS ACROCYANOSIS IN INFANTS

1. **What is the difference between central cyanosis and acrocyanosis?**

   Cyanosis is a common clinical finding in newborn infants. Central cyanosis is caused by reduced arterial oxygen saturation. Central cyanosis can be associated with life-threatening illnesses such as cardiac, metabolic, neurologic, infectious, and parenchymal and nonparenchymal pulmonary disorders. Healthy newborns have central cyanosis up to 5–10 minutes after birth as the oxygen saturation rises to 85–95%. Persistent cyanosis is always abnormal and should be evaluated and treated promptly. By contrast, acrocyanosis is seen in healthy newborns and refers to intense peripheral vasoconstriction and variable perfusion in the extremities. As opposed to central cyanosis, in acrocyanosis the mucous membranes of the neonate remain pink. This may persist for 24–48 hours, and it is usually not pathologic. Acrocyanosis can also be seen in infants when crying, regurgitating, vomiting, coughing, or breath-holding.

2. **In a cyanotic newborn, how could pulmonary disease be distinguished from cyanotic congenital heart disease?**

   Historically the hyperoxia test was used to differentiate cyanosis secondary to pulmonary versus congenital heart disease. However, the routine pulse oximetry screening for critical congenital heart disease has replaced the hyperoxia test. If the screening test is positive, then an echocardiogram must be obtained. Additional tests include blood gas, complete blood count, and blood culture.

3. **Which congenital heart lesions present with cyanosis on day 1 of life?**
   - Transposition of great arteries with an intact ventricular septum
   - Tricuspid valve atresia
   - Pulmonary valve atresia with intact ventricular septum
   - Tetralogy of Fallot
   - Ebstein anomaly of the tricuspid valve
   - Total anomalous pulmonary venous return
   - Hypoplastic left heart syndrome
   - Truncus arteriosus

ORAL CANDIDIASIS

4. **How do newborns acquire oropharyngeal candidiasis?**

   Transmission of fungi from maternal vaginal candidal colonization is the primary means of infection in newborns. It can also be transmitted during breastfeeding. It affects up to 3–5% of healthy newborns. Median age of onset is reported to be 9–10 days of life. On examination, the thrush presents as white plaques with or without an erythematous base on the buccal or lingual mucosal surface of the mouth. Infants are usually asymptomatic; however, it may interfere with feeding due to discomfort. Mild punctate areas of bleeding confirm the diagnosis during scraping. Nystatin 100,000 U/mL as a dose of 0.5 mL to each side of the mouth given four times daily is the treatment of choice for oral candidiasis.

NEWBORN RASHES

A 4-week-old baby girl presents with a rash limited to the cheeks and forehead. She is otherwise feeding and growing well. She is afebrile.

5. **Is there a difference between neonatal cephalic pustulosis (neonatal acne) and infantile acne?**

   Neonatal cephalic pustulosis is a variant of acne vulgaris that presents at birth or in the first weeks of life (Fig. 35.1). This occurs in about 20% of newborns. It is due to androgenic hormones, both maternally derived and endogenous. The lesions appear pustular and erupt on the neck and head of the newborn around 3 weeks of age. The lesions self-resolve within 1–3 months as the androgenic levels drop. Occasionally, neonatal acne can be treated with topical azole antifungal preparations or topical steroids to speed up clearance.

   Infantile acne is uncommon and typically presents at 3–4 months of life. It is due to hyperplasia of sebaceous glands secondary to androgen stimulants and is more common in boys. It can self-resolve by the first year of life but can persist until 3 years of age. Treatment may be required because of concern for scarring. If increased inflammation is noted, benzoyl peroxide 2.5% may be applied.

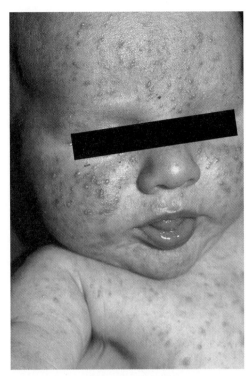

Fig. 35.1 Neonatal acne. (From Paller AS, Mancini AJ. *Hurwitz Clinical Pediatric Dermatology*. Saunders; 2011:167–183. Fig. 8.17.)

6. **How is seborrheic dermatitis (cradle cap) treated at home?**
   Seborrheic dermatitis presents as a yellow scaly rash on the scalp and may involve the head, eyes, ears, eyebrows, nose, and back of the head. It occurs in areas rich in sebaceous glands. The pathogenesis is not clear, but it may be due to maternal androgens. It may resolve spontaneously in weeks to several months. Seborrheic dermatitis is treated with emollients such as white petroleum, vegetable oil, mineral oil, or baby oil followed by shampooing with a mild anti-dandruff shampoo containing selenium 25% for 2–4 weeks. A soft brush can be used to remove the loosened scales. This treatment can be done once daily for 1 week. If the seborrheic dermatitis is extensive or persistent, low-potency topical steroids may be used. Ketoconazole 2% shampoo twice a week for 2 weeks may also be applied. If lesions are inflamed or there is a facial involvement, then a low-potency topical steroid may be applied.

7. **What are the differences between erythema toxicum neonatorum (ETN) and transient neonatal pustular melanosis?**
   Erythema toxicum neonatorum (ETN) is noted in 20% of neonates in the first 72 hours of life. Etiology is unknown. It presents as multiple erythematous macules and papules that rapidly progress to pustules on an erythematous base. The rash presents over the trunk and proximal extremities, sparing palms and soles. They may be present at birth but can be seen at 24–48 hours of life and usually resolve within 7 days. Peripheral eosinophilia may be present in 7–18% of patients. Transient neonatal pustular melanosis (Fig. 35.2) is less common than ETN. Small pustules are seen on a nonerythematous base, and they are usually present at birth. As the pustules rupture, erythematous macules with surrounding scale may develop and can persist for weeks to months. These pustules contain neutrophils.

8. **What is the difference between milia and miliaria?**
   Milia are white papules caused by retention of keratin. They are firm and, unlike pustules, not easily denuded by pressure. Milia consist of epithelial lined cysts arising from hair follicles. On examination, the rash is found on the nose and cheeks, and it resolves within the first weeks of life. Miliaria is rarely present at birth; it is caused by an accumulation of sweat beneath the eccrine sweat ducts at the level of the stratum corneum resulting in the formation of 2- to 3-mm sweat retention vesicles. In infants, the lesions are noted over the head, neck, and upper trunk. Miliaria can develop in the first week of life due to warming of the infant such as incubation, occlusion dressings or clothing, or fever.

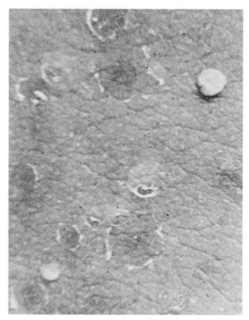

Fig. 35.2 Transient neonatal melanosis. (From Diseases of the Neonate. *Nelson Textbook of Pediatrics*, 2004. Fig. 637.2.)

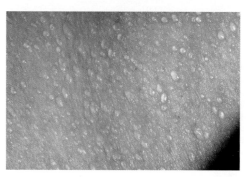

Fig. 35.3 Miliaria crystallina. (From Dermatoses Resulting from Physical Factors. *Andrews' Diseases of the Skin*. Saunders; 2011:18–44. Fig. 3.3.)

9. What are the different types of miliaria?
   - Miliaria crystallina (Fig. 35.3) presents as small thin-walled vesicles without inflammation.
   - Miliaria rubra (Fig. 35.4) occurs when the obstructed sweat leaks into the dermis and causes an inflammatory response that results in erythematous papules and pustules.
   - Miliaria pustulosa results from localized inflammation consisting of pustules over an erythematous base.
   - Miliaria profunda is papular or papulopustular and skin colored.

10. What is the differential diagnosis of sucking blisters?
    Herpes simplex virus infection, bullous impetigo, congenital syphilis or candidiasis, neonatal lupus erythematous, and hereditary bullous diseases. Other clinical signs and symptoms along with positive maternal history usually accompany these disorders.

11. What is the difference between cutis marmorata and harlequin color change?
    Cutis marmorata (Fig. 35.5) is asymmetric reticular mottling of the skin noted on the extremities and trunk. It is a vascular response to cold and usually resolves with warming, and no treatment is required. Harlequin color change is noted when an infant is lying on one side of the body. There is an intense reddening of the dependent side and blanching of the nondependent side with a demarcated line at the midline. It can range from a few

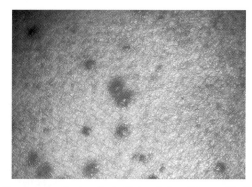

Fig. 35.4 Miliaria rubra. (From Dermatoses Resulting from Physical Factors. *Andrews' Diseases of the Skin.* Saunders; 2011:18–44. Fig. 3.4.)

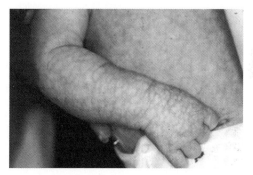

Fig. 35.5 Cutis marmorata. (From Neonatal skin disorders. Selbst: *Pediatric Emergency Medicine.* 2008. Fig. 39.4.)

seconds to 20 minutes. It is benign and self-limited, and it can be seen up to 3 weeks after birth. This is more common in preterm infants than in term infants. The etiology is unclear. It may be due to immaturity of the autonomic regulation of cutaneous blood vessels.

HYPERBILIRUBINEMIA

A 4-day-old, 38-week-gestation male presents to urgent care for a bilirubin check. The mother notes worsening jaundice. He was discharged home on day 2 of life after successfully breastfeeding for a 24-hour period. At the time of discharge, his physical examination was noted for mild jaundice and a cephalohematoma. Currently, he has 5% weight loss from birth, and his parents report slightly decreased urine output. He has stooled once today. On physical examination, he has jaundice to the abdomen and has a resolving cephalohematoma. Otherwise, he has a normal examination including normal neurologic examination. The total bilirubin is 20 mg/dL. The mother's blood type is O+; the baby's blood type is to be determined.

12. What are the patient risk factors for development of hyperbilirubinemia?
    - Gestational age <35 weeks
    - Jaundice less than 24 hours or before discharge
    - Predischarge total serum bilirubin (TSB) >75th percentile
    - Hemolysis from any cause
    - Cephalohematoma or other bruising
    - Exclusive breastfeeding with suboptimal intake
    - Macrosomia
    - Down syndrome
    - Genetic ancestry suggestive of red blood cell disorders such as glucose-6-phosphate dehydrogenase deficiency (G6PD)
    - Sibling previously requiring phototherapy

13. **What are the hyperbilirubinemia neurotoxicity risk factors?**
    - Gestational age <38 weeks
    - Hemolytic disease
    - Sepsis
    - Significant clinical instability in the last 24 hours
    - Albumin <3.0 g/dL

14. **Which newborns require evaluation for hyperbilirubinemia?**
    All newborns should be visually screened for jaundice in the first 8–12 hours of life. Infants who develop jaundice <24 hours of life are at increased risk for severe hyperbilirubinemia often due to isoimmune hemolytic disease.
    At least one measurement of total bilirubin prior to discharge is indicated to identify hyperbilirubinemia in all newborns. Measurements of total serum bilirubin (TSB) or transcutaneous bilirubin (TcB) are acceptable.

15. **What are the physiologic causes of hyperbilirubinemia in newborns?**
    - Neonatal jaundice is caused mainly by changes in bilirubin metabolism that result in increased bilirubin production.
    - The newborn infant produces two to three times more bilirubin than adults. This is due to increased numbers of red blood cells in newborns, which also have a shorter life span.
    - There is a decreased bilirubin clearance mainly due to the deficiency of the enzyme uridine diphosphogluconurate glucuronosyltransferase.
    - There is also an increase in the enterohepatic circulation, further increasing the bilirubin load.

16. **What are the clinical manifestations of neurotoxicity due to hyperbilirubinemia?**
    Hypertonia or hypotonia, arching, torticollis, opisthotonos, fever, and a high-pitched cry are some of the signs and symptoms seen in patients presenting with bilirubin toxicity.

17. **When should a patient be referred to the emergency room (ER) and what are the guidelines for phototherapy?**
    The American Academy of Pediatrics (AAP) released updated clinical guidelines in 2022. Identification and treatment of hyperbilirubinemia are aimed at preventing neurotoxicity. Phototherapy thresholds are stratified by risk of neurotoxicity but have been simplified to no risk vs. risk. Gestational age, days of life of the newborn, and neurotoxicity risk combine to determine the level of total serum bilirubin (TSB) requiring treatment.

18. **When is an additional evaluation for hyperbilirubinemia indicated?**
    If a newborn presents with total bilirubin values greater than the 95th percentile or hemolytic disease is suspected, further evaluation for jaundice etiology is required.
    Initial testing includes blood type and direct Coombs test. If the patient is receiving phototherapy or has a rapid rise in total serum bilirubin, especially crossing percentiles, additional tests should be obtained including complete blood count and smear along with direct bilirubin. It is an option to perform reticulocyte count and G6PD. Rising reticulocyte count during the first 72 hours of life is consistent with red cell destruction. A G6PD measurement should be done if the patient is of Mediterranean, Nigerian, or East Asian descent and has a total bilirubin concentration >18 mg/dL.
    Additional testing should also be done if jaundice is present at or beyond 3 weeks of life. These laboratory tests include newborn thyroid and galactosemia screen; there is also a need to evaluate the infant for signs and symptoms of hypothyroidism.

19. **At which total serum bilirubin levels should phototherapy be initiated?**
    Phototherapy thresholds vary by gestational age of the newborn and their current age in hours as well as the risk factors for neurotoxicity. These values can be found in the most recent update to the AAP Clinical Practice Guideline: Management of Hyperbilirubinemia in the Newborn Infant 35 or More Weeks of Gestation, published in 2022.

20. **How soon should a newborn be followed up in clinic after discharge from the hospital?**
    Newborn follow-up to assess hyperbilirubinemia after hospital discharge considers the age of the newborn, their phototherapy threshold, and TSB. The difference between the phototherapy threshold value and the TSB helps guide the timing of follow-up.

21. **Should a baby with hyperbilirubinemia continue breastfeeding?**
    There is no contraindication to continue breastfeeding. This can reduce bilirubin levels and increase the efficacy of phototherapy. Supplementation with expressed breast milk or formula is also adequate, especially if there is excessive weight loss (>12th percentile of birth weight) or the infant appears to be dehydrated. Intravenous fluids should be considered in these patients as well.

BRUE (BRIEF RESOLVED UNEXPLAINED EVENTS)

A 2-month-old female infant presents to urgent care due to cessation of breathing noted by her mother after feeding while at home. This episode lasted about 10 seconds, and the patient appeared to turn blue around the mouth. The infant has been well since the episode, but due to parental concerns, she was brought to your urgent care for further evaluation. Examination: vital signs T 37°C, pulse 130, respirations 24, BP 80/50, O_2 saturation 100% on room air. Her examination was unremarkable.

22. **What defines BRUE (brief resolved unexplained events)?**
   Brief resolved unexplained events (BRUE) are unexpected episodes that are frightening to the caregiver and include color change, altered breathing (absent, decreased, or irregular), marked change in muscle tone, and changes in the level of responsiveness.

23. **Which patients could be classified as low risk presenting with BRUE?**
   If there is no concern on history and physical examination, patients who are identified as low risk include infants with all of the following:
   - Age >60 days
   - Born >32 weeks' gestation and corrected gestational age >45 weeks
   - No CPR by trained medical provider
   - Events lasted <1 minute
   - No prior events preceding the current one
   - No concerning history or exam features (see warning signs below)

24. **What are some of the warning signs that would increase the likelihood of BRUE being medically significant, thus necessitating referral to a local ER?**
   - Signs of systemic illness: toxic appearance, lethargy, unexplained recurrent vomiting, or respiratory distress
   - Signs of nonaccidental trauma, suggested by:
     - Evidence of trauma or bruising
     - Event inconsistent with child's developmental stage
   - Significance of event:
     - Significant physiologic compromise during the event, such as significant generalized cyanosis or loss of consciousness
     - Resuscitation (CPR) required by a caregiver
   - History of prior BRUE, especially within the past 24 hours
   - History of clinically significant event or unexpected death in a sibling
   - Dysmorphic features, congenital anomalies, or any known syndromes

25. **When is a workup indicated for BRUE?**
   Most infants at low risk require no further evaluation.
   Provide: education about BRUE and discuss next steps and appropriate follow-up as well as resources for CPR training.
   Consider: serial observation and continuous pulse oximetry and/or 12-lead EKG.
   Unnecessary: laboratory studies, home cardiorespiratory monitoring, and initiation of acid suppression therapy. Admission is solely for cardiorespiratory monitoring.

26. **Is sudden infant death syndrome (SIDS) related to brief resolved unexplained events (BRUE)?**
   Studies have not shown a causal relationship between preexisting apnea and SIDS. The vast majority of SIDS patients do not experience BRUE or apnea prior to death. Also, the risk factors for SIDS differ from those of BRUE. The risk factors for SIDS include male sex, prematurity, low birth weight, maternal smoking, low socioeconomic status, poor prenatal care, young maternal age, multiple gestation, and unsafe sleeping conditions. The risk factors for BRUE are a prior history of apneas, pallor, cyanosis, difficulty feeding, recent upper viral respiratory symptoms, and age younger than 10 weeks.

VOMITING

A 3-week-old girl with frequent spit-up after feeding is now spitting up with every feed. The last episode was projectile in nature. She has gained weight well since birth. There is no fever and no other sick contacts.

27. **What differentiates spitting up versus vomiting?**
   Of infants, 50% will have daily episodes of spitting up due to esophageal sphincter immaturity; overfeeding may also play a role. Spitting up will generally result in small amounts of breast milk or formula coming from the mouth, usually shortly after feeding. This may be more forceful with burping.
   In contrast, vomiting is a coordinated expulsion of gastric content that may be associated with anatomic abnormality, obstruction, infection, or other nongastrointestinal causes. In infants, it is important to differentiate true vomiting from spitting up.

28. **What are the causes of vomiting in infants (Table 35.1)?**

29. **How do I know if an infant has reflux?**
   It is important to differentiate physiologic gastroesophageal regurgitation (GER) from pathologic gastroesophageal reflux disease (GERD). GERD may manifest as fussiness, persistent regurgitation, vomiting, or failure to gain weight. Diagnostic testing with pH probe or direct endoscopy is ideal but impractical in small infants.

Table 35.1 Causes of Vomiting in Infants	
GASTROINTESTINAL Obstruction	*Neurologic*
• Pyloric stenosis	• Hydrocephalus
• Malrotation with intermittent volvulus	• Subdural hematoma
• Intestinal duplication	• Intracranial hemorrhage
• Hirschsprung disease	• Intracranial mass
• Antral/duodenal web	*Infectious*
• Incarcerated hernia	• Sepsis
• Other gastrointestinal disorders	• Meningitis
◦ Achalasia	• Urinary tract infection
◦ Gastroparesis	• Pneumonia
◦ Gastroenteritis	• Otitis media
◦ Eosinophilic esophagitis/gastroenteritis	• Hepatitis
◦ Food allergy	*Cardiac*
Metabolic/endocrine	• Congestive heart failure
• Galactosemia	• Vascular ring
• Hereditary fructose intolerance	*Toxic*
• Urea cycle defects	• Lead
◦ Amino and organic acidemias	• Iron
◦ Congenital adrenal hyperplasia	• Vitamins A and D
◦ Renal obstructive uropathy	• Medications (e.g., ipecac, digoxin, theophylline)
• Renal insufficiency	
Others	
• Pediatric falsification disorder (Munchausen syndrome by proxy)	
• Child neglect or abuse	
• Autonomic dysfunction	

Modified from Pediatric Gastroesophageal Reflux Clinical Practice Guidelines: Joint Recommendations of the North American Society for Pediatric Gastroenterology, Hepatology, and Nutrition (NASPGHAN) and the European Society for Pediatric Gastroenterology, Hepatology, and Nutrition (ESPGHAN). *J Pediatr Gastroenterol Nutr.* 49:498–547.

30. **What can I do to treat reflux?**

Guidelines exist for initial management of suspected reflux. Physiologic reflux can be treated with upright positioning during and after feeding. One may also try hydrolyzed formula or thickened formula, as cow's milk protein allergy may play a role in reflux.

In infants with suspected GERD who are symptomatic, a trial of ranitidine may be done for 2–4 weeks.

31. **How fast should infants gain weight?**

All newborns will lose some weight after birth due to fluid shifts and limited caloric intake in the first few days of life. Infants may lose up to 10% of body weight but should regain this by 2 weeks of age. After this initial period of weight loss, newborns are expected to gain ½ ounce to 1 ounce (15–30 g) per day. Generally, infants will double their birth weight by age 6 months and triple it by 1 year.

32. **What is failure to thrive?**

Failure to thrive (FTT) is the failure to gain weight and/or length as expected over a course of time. Use of standardized growth charts from the Centers for Disease Control and Prevention (CDC) or the World Health Organization (WHO) helps track growth. Infants who are losing weight or are "falling off their curve" (dropping down 2 percentile curves over the course of time) are considered FTT and should undergo an evaluation.

Table 35.2 Diagnosis of Crying Infants

MORE BENIGN	MORE SERIOUS/LIFE-THREATENING
Anal fissure	Abusive head trauma/child abuse
Colic	Congestive heart failure
Corneal abrasion	Congenital heart disease/SVT
Feeding difficulties	Drugs or drug withdrawal
Gas	Incarcerated hernia
Hair tourniquet	Infection
Hernia (unincarcerated)	Sepsis
Milk protein allergy	Meningitis
Nasal congestion	Respiratory distress
Otitis media	Urinary tract infection
Oral thrush (severe)	Injury
Reflux	Intussusception
	Metabolic disturbances
	Testicular/ovarian torsion

From Hogencamp TC. An urgent care approach to excessively crying infants. *J Urgent Care Med.* 2012;6(12):9–18.

It is important to note that growth charts for certain conditions (e.g., Down syndrome or Turner syndrome) also exist, as growth patterns are different for this population.

33. **What are the signs and symptoms of pyloric stenosis?**
Pyloric stenosis occurs in approximately 0.2% of infants and typically presents between the ages of 3 and 4 weeks (1–12 weeks). Infants will have acute onset of persistent vomiting, which may become projectile due to the obstruction caused by the enlarged pylorus. It is generally nonbilious. Ultrasound will reveal an enlarged pylorus. Intravenous (IV) hydration is required until a pyloromyotomy can be performed.

34. **What is the evaluation of an infant with bilious emesis?**
Bilious vomiting is concerning for obstruction and, in infants, may be related to malrotation with midgut volvulus. In addition to vomiting, infants will often have irritability and may present in extremis due to gut necrosis. Malrotation is a congenital anomaly where the gut is malrotated. This increases the risk of volvulus, where the small intestine compresses the superior mesentery artery, causing gut necrosis. Volvulus is a surgical emergency requiring immediate transfer to a pediatric facility.

35. **How do I approach the evaluation of a crying infant? There must be something I am missing.**
All infants cry! Crying is a primitive form of communication. Crying infants can cause significant stress for parents and seasoned providers. Crying increases during the first few weeks of life and peaks at approximately 2 months. A systematic approach to the crying infant will ensure you evaluate all potential causes (Table 35.2).

A complete head-to-toe examination, including removing the diaper, will help determine any physical causes of the crying. A serious underlying cause will be found in approximately 5% of infants who present with crying. Two-thirds of the time, history of the physical examination will lead to the diagnosis, although most infants presenting with crying will have a normal examination and no definitive diagnosis. One of the most common diagnoses of infants presenting with crying is urinary tract infection.

36. **How do I rule out colic as a cause for crying?**
Colic is a distinct syndrome of excessive crying. The exact cause of colic is unknown, and treatment is aimed at consoling the infant and supporting the family. There are no tests to rule out colic, but it is certainly important to rule out other serious causes of crying.

Colic is a clinical diagnosis defined as episodes of intense, often inconsolable crying with no identifiable physiologic cause. To diagnose colic, think about the rule of 3s:
- Lasting 3 hours per day
- More than 3 days per week
- Occurring in the last ⅓ of the day (evening)
- Colic begins after 3 weeks and disappears by 3–4 months of age

37. **A 1-month-old has had no bowel movement in 3 days. He is feeding well without vomiting. He has normal urine output. He has been crying all day. Is he constipated?**
Newborns will have their first meconium stool within the first 24 hours of life. Stool will then transition to a mustard yellow seedy stool. In the first week of life, infants will often stool after each feeding. Over the course of the first several weeks, stool may decrease in frequency and take on a firmer consistency. Most infants will stool daily, but stooling every 2–3 days can also be normal, especially when transitioning from breastfeeding to formula or solid foods. Breastfed infants will often continue to have soft, seedy stool several times per day but may also go several days between stools.

Grunting, drawing up the legs, and straining are normal for infants while they are stooling because it is challenging to stool while lying flat on your back. To relieve some of this distress, parents may try rectal stimulation with a thermometer or a glycerin suppository, but reassuring parents about this normal stooling behavior is most helpful.

38. **When should I be concerned about constipation?**
For infants who have always had infrequent stools or who had delayed passage of meconium, consider evaluation for Hirschsprung disease. In Hirschsprung disease, there is aganglionosis of the rectal sphincter and distal colon, making it challenging to pass stool. Barium enema is diagnostic, as you can see the transition zone between the aganglionic and normal colon.

39. **What are the physical examination findings for nonaccidental trauma?**
The most common form of injury due to nonaccidental trauma in infants will be from brain injury due to vigorous shaking. This type of injury may present with irritability, vomiting, or poor feeding. There may not be other physical signs of abuse.

Fractures of the extremities or the skull may present with swelling at the fracture site and history of irritability.

Because infants are not mobile, maintain a high index of suspicion if physical findings (bruising or swelling) are not consistent with the history and examination.

40. **Are there other disorders that can mimic nonaccidental trauma?**
In infants, consider genetic disorders of bone formation that may contribute to pathologic fractures. Bleeding disorders or metabolic disorders may contribute to easy bruising. Consultation with a child abuse pediatrician at a local children's hospital is recommended.

Any concern for nonaccidental trauma in an infant should be referred to a pediatric center for further evaluation.

KEY POINTS

1. Acrocyanosis is seen in healthy newborns; it refers to the peripheral cyanosis around the mouth and the extremities including hands and feet.
2. The 97th percentile for bilirubin in a healthy full-term infant is 12.4 mg/dL for bottle-fed infants and 14.8 mg/dL for breastfed infants.
3. Brief resolved unexplained events (BRUE), formerly known as apparent life-threatening events (ALTE), unexpected episodes that are frightening to the caregiver, include apnea, color change, marked change in muscle tone, and choking or gagging.
4. Diagnostic testing for excessive crying should be guided by the history and physical examination.
5. Any concern for nonaccidental trauma in an infant should be referred to a pediatric center for further evaluation.

BIBLIOGRAPHY

Cohen BA, Davis HW. Dermatology. In: Zitelli BJ, Davis HW (Eds). *Atlas of Pediatric Physical Diagnosis.* 4th ed. Mosby: 257–314.
Freedman S, Al-Harthy N, Freedman J. The crying infant: diagnostic testing and frequency of serious underlying disease. *Pediatrics.* 2009;123:841–848. www.pediatrics.org/cgi/doi/10.1542/peds.2008-0113.
Hogencamp T. An urgent care approach to excessively crying infants. *JUCM.* 2012:9–18.
Kemper AR, Newman TB, Slaughter JL. Clinical practice guideline revision: management of hyperbilirubinemia in the newborn infant 35 or more weeks of gestation. *Pediatrics.* 2022;150(3):e2022058859. https://doi.org/10.1542/peds.2022-058859.
Maisels MJ, Clune S, Coleman K, et al. The natural history of jaundice in predominantly breastfed infants. *Pediatrics.* 2014;134(2):e340–e345. http://doi.org/10.1542/peds.2013-4299.
O'Connor NR, McLaughlin MR, Ham P. Newborn skin: Part I. Common rashes. *Am Fam Physician.* 2008;77(1):47–52.
Tieder JS, Bonkowsky JL, Etzel RA. Brief unexplained events (formerly apparent life-threatening events) and evaluation of lower risk infants: executive summary. *Pediatrics.* 2016;137(5):e20160591. https://doi.org/10.1542/peds.2016-0591.
Treadwell PA. Dermatoses in newborns. *Am Fam Physician.* 1997;56(2):443–450.
Vandenplas Y, Rudolph CD, Di Lorenzo C, et al. Pediatric gastroesophageal reflux clinical practice guidelines: joint recommendations of the North American Society for Pediatric Gastroenterology, Hepatology, and Nutrition (NASPGHAN) and the European Society for Pediatric Gastroenterology, Hepatology, and Nutrition (ESPGHAN). *J Pediatr Gastroenterol Nutr.* 2009;49(4):498–547. doi:10.1097/MPG.0b013e3181b7f563.

CONCUSSION

Jessica Knapp, CAQSM, Thomas Trojian, MD, MMB, CAQSM, FACSM, FAMSSM, RMSK

During a soccer game, a 14-year-old collides head-to-head with an opponent while jumping for the ball. After the collision she complains to the athletic trainer of a headache, nausea, and some dizziness. The sports medicine team evaluates her, diagnoses a concussion, and removes her from play. Her family asks, "What is a concussion?"

1. A concussion, sometimes called a mild traumatic brain injury (mTBI), occurs after a direct blow to the head or the face/neck/elsewhere on the body with an impulsive force transmitted to the head, with resultant neurologic or cognitive symptoms.

2. The patient's mother indicates she has seen several players collide with each other who were not removed from the game for a concussion and is curious about how common concussions are
   Approximately 3.8 million sports- and recreation-related concussions are seen annually.

3. What are some of the risk factors for a concussion?
   Athletes playing high-risk sports such as American football are at greater risk, but athletes in any sport can get concussions. A significant determinant of sustaining sports-related concussions is a prior concussion history; females have more concussions for comparable sports than males. Attention-deficit disorder, psychiatric disorders, or history of headaches/migraines can lengthen concussion recovery time. Sports such as wrestling, ice hockey, field hockey, lacrosse, football, rugby, soccer, basketball, baseball, and softball are examples of sports with high concussion rates.

4. What are the symptoms and signs of a concussion?
   a. The symptoms and signs of a concussion are divided into physical, cognitive, emotional, and sleep.
   b. Physical manifestations of concussion include nausea, dizziness, imbalance, visual problems, and sensitivity to light and sound.
   c. Cognitive impairments include mental fogginess, memory difficulties, difficulty with concentration, and confusion about recent events.
   d. Emotional symptoms of concussion include sadness, irritability, personality changes, depression, and nervousness.
   e. Sleep disturbances include difficulty initiating sleep, decreased sleep, and increased drowsiness.

5. Our patient's mother wants to know what to watch for and when to consider going to the emergency department. As the team doctor, you suggest watching for red-flag symptoms.
   These red-flag symptoms and signs include prolonged loss of consciousness (>1 minute), amnesia, neck pain over spinous process, deteriorating conscious state, increasing confusion or irritability, severe or increasing headache, repeated vomiting, unusual behavioral changes, seizure or convulsion, double vision, and weakness or tingling/burning in arms or legs.

6. Is imaging an appropriate next step in care?
   a. Regular imaging with computed tomography (CT) or magnetic resonance imaging (MRI) is not recommended, as imaging is usually normal with a concussion. Standard guidance has been created for imaging decision-making: Pediatric Emergency Care Applied Research Network (PECARN) head CT rules.
   b. PCARN Rules: Pediatric Head Trauma CT Guide
      i. Glasgow Coma Scale <15
      ii. Signs of basilar skull fracture
      iii. Altered mental status (agitation, somnolence, slow response, repetitive questions)
      iv. Vomiting
      v. Loss of consciousness
      vi. Severe headache
      vii. Severe mechanism of injury
         1. Fall >5 ft
         2. Motor vehicle accident with ejection, rollover, or fatality
         3. Bike/pedestrian vs. vehicle without a helmet
         4. Struck by high-impact object

7. How quickly do concussion symptoms appear?
Concussion symptoms are generally apparent after an injury but can often be delayed by 5–10 minutes; presentations up to 24 hours after impact have been reported.

8. You are at a college football game, and a receiver is hit while running with the ball. After the play they report feeling "slow" and having difficulty remembering the events leading up to the hit and after the impact. What are the three basic steps you should take to evaluate the injury?
   a. Remove the athlete from the game or practice and to a quiet location.
   b. Take away a piece of essential equipment (i.e., a helmet).
   c. Ask questions about symptoms and perform a complete cognitive and neurologic examination.

9. What should be included in the sideline neurologic exam?
Assess for amnesia, evaluate cranial nerves, peripheral sensation, extremity strength, and coordination, and perform a neurological screen.

10. What are some of the tools available for the evaluation of concussion?
   a. Balance Error Scoring System (BESS): consists of three tests lasting 20 seconds each, performed on a firm surface, with the eyes closed, and scored based on the number of errors in each trial.
   b. Sport Assessment Concussion Tool 5 (SCAT5): combines three tests: the Standard Assessment of Concussion (SAC), Maddock's questions, and the BESS. Orientation, immediate memory, concentration, and delayed recall are tested. SCAT5 is for ages 13 and above, and the Child Sport Assessment Concussion Tool 5 (Child SCAT5) is for ages 5–12.
      i. Sensitivity and specificity are best during the first 3 days after injury.
   c. King-Devick (KD) test: measures how fast an athlete can read aloud single-digit numbers from three test cards. Captures attention, language, and eye movement impairments. It has good sensitivity and specificity and can be done quickly.
   d. Vestibular-Ocular Motor Screening (VOMS): seven VOMS items include smooth pursuits, horizontal and vertical saccades, near point convergence (NPC), horizontal vestibular-ocular reflex (H-VOR), vertical vestibular-ocular reflex (V-VOR), and visual motion sensitivity. VOMS is the sum of headache, dizziness, nausea, and fogginess for each item.
   e. Tandem gait: heel-toe gait for three meters with a 180-degree turn around and return with heel-toe gait. Successful completion is in less than 14 seconds.
   f. Since these tests measure different areas of brain function, best to combine a test with a thorough history and complete neurological examination to rule out injuries like a bleed or spinal cord contusion.

11. What is the role of the Buffalo concussion treadmill test and treatment?
The Buffalo concussion treadmill test is a supplementary test based on the modified Balke treadmill test. The speed is constant, and the treadmill slope increases 1 degree every minute. It is useful for determining the heart rate threshold at which symptoms occur to help guide safe exercise levels in athletes below symptom provocation.

12. What is the role of neuropsychological testing in concussions?
Neuropsychological testing has become commonplace in concussion diagnosis but cannot be independently used to determine if a concussion has occurred. It measures neurologic deficit and can be helpful in patients with other neurologic illnesses. Concerns regarding reliability and positive predictive value are the focus of ongoing research.

13. Which specialty should evaluate and coordinate care for concussions?
The primary care team physician is best positioned to evaluate and treat concussions on the sideline and in the clinic. Primary care, emergency, and urgent care physicians are likely the first to evaluate if the concussion did not occur on the field of play. Between 80% and 90% of concussed older adolescents and adults return to preinjury levels of clinical function within 2 weeks. Younger athletes may take longer to recover with a return to preinjury level of function in the majority of athletes by 4 weeks. Providers with concussion expertise are most beneficial for patients whose symptoms persist beyond the expected time for recovery.

14. What is the primary treatment for concussion?
Twenty-four to 48 hours of physical and cognitive rest with activity as guided by the Buffalo concussion treadmill test after the initial rest period. Encouraging nonvigorous walking the next day has been shown to reduce symptoms in female athletes.

15. What is the role of medication in the management of concussions?
Symptomatic management of concussion is widely practiced with different medications depending on the patient's symptoms. There is no evidence that any particular medicine is effective in treating or altering the course of sports-related concussions.

Table 36.1 Some Accepted Treatments for Common Symptoms of Concussions

SYMPTOM	TREATMENT	COMMENTS
Headache	NSAIDs and acetaminophen Ice, massage, manual therapy for concomitant neck pain in acute setting Dim, quiet environment Amitriptyline	NSAIDs should be avoided acutely if concern for bleed, as they can theoretically increase bleeding risk Rebound headaches have been reported with frequent NSAID use
Sleep disturbances	Amitriptyline Melatonin	Good sleep hygiene should be encouraged
Balance, vertigo, and ocular dysfunction	Vestibular rehabilitation	Focus on vestibular-ocular exercises, smooth pursuit, gaze stabilization, and balance training

16. **What are the treatments for some of the common symptoms of a concussion?**
See Table 36.1.

17. **When is the appropriate time to return to school or work?**
There is no universal recommendation for when one can return to work or school because of the heterogeneity of concussion symptoms. The goal should be to disrupt life as little as possible and return to school or work as soon as possible.

18. **What are some reasonable accommodations that concussion patients may need?**
Reduced academic load at school or duties at the workplace, which may include shortened or altered schedules, should be considered. In the student athlete, adjustments may include excused school absences or lighter homework load, scheduled rest breaks during the day, extended time to complete homework assignments and projects, and extended time on tests.

19. **When is the appropriate return to play for athletes after sustaining a concussion?**
    a. Athletes should never return to play on the same day as diagnosis.
    b. Return to play should be considered when the concussed patient is asymptomatic, with a normal exam for 24 hours.
    c. Return to play should follow a stepwise progression for a minimum of 5 days.

20. **What is the recommended stepwise progression for return to play?**
    a. Return to play should begin with light aerobic activity followed by a sport-specific activity, noncontact training drills, full-contact practice, and ultimately complete return to play. If symptomatic or worsening during the process, the stepwise progression starts again.
    b. For noncontact sports, the BCTT can be used to determine readiness to return with no symptoms at 80% of the maximum expected heart rate.

21. **What is CTE, and will I get it if I get a concussion?**
CTE was initially described in the literature in boxers as dementia pugilistica. We now understand that having a TBI from any sport can increase neurodegenerative disease risk. The risk of CTE is considered to be quite low but is an area of active research.

22. **Can concussions be prevented?**
Prevention of concussion in contact sports is limited. The health claims of many products (specialized football helmets, headgear in soccer, custom-designed mouth guards) have limited scientific support and remain an active area of study not without significant debate in the medical community. Rule changes, enforcement of existing rules, technique changes, and neck strengthening have shown promise in reducing the number and severity of sports-related concussions.

KEY POINTS

- The Buffalo treadmill test helps guide early activity in concussion, and the return-to-play protocol is a stepwise plan that takes 24 hours for each stage.
- There is no evidence for a specific medication for concussion treatment.
- Advanced imaging is generally normal for a concussion.

Acknowledgments

The authors would like to thank Dr. Adae Amoeko for their contributions to this chapter in the previous edition.

BIBLIOGRAPHY

Echemendia RJ, Meeuwisse W, McCrory P, et al. The Sport Concussion Assessment Tool 5th edition (SCAT5): background and rationale. *Br J Sports Med.* 2017;51(11):848–850. doi:10.1136/bjsports-2017-097506. Epub 2017 Apr 26.

Kontos AP, Eagle SR, Marchetti G, et al. Discriminative validity of vestibular ocular motor screening in identifying concussion among collegiate athletes: a National Collegiate Athletic Association–Department of Defense Concussion Assessment, Research, and Education Consortium Study. *Am J Sports Med.* 2021;49(8):2211–2217. doi:10.1177/03635465211012359. Epub 2021 May 12.

Kelshaw PM, Cook NE, Terry DP, Iverson GL, Caswell SV. Child Sport Concussion Assessment Tool 5th edition: normative reference values in demographically diverse youth. *Clin J Sport Med.* 2022;32(2):e126–e133. doi:10.1097/JSM.0000000000000921.

Oldham JR, Difabio MS, Kaminski TW, Dewolf RM, Howell DR, Buckley TA. Efficacy of tandem gait to identify impaired postural control after concussion. *Med Sci Sports Exerc.* 2018;50(6):1162–1168. doi:10.1249/MSS.0000000000001540.

Sert ET, Mutlu H, Kokulu K. The use of PECARN and CATCH rules in children with minor head trauma presenting to emergency department 24 hours after injury. *Pediatr Emerg Care.* 2022;38(2):e524–e528. doi:10.1097/PEC.0000000000002011. PMID: 31929390. https://cdn-links.lww.com/permalink/jsm/a/jsm_2020_01_28_haider_19-313_sdc1.pdf.

CHAPTER 37

ACUTE NECK PAIN

Douglas Comeau, DO, CAQSM, FAAFP, FAMSSM, Deanna L. Corey, MD, CAQSM

TOP SECRET

Patients complaining of neck pain that meets all NEXUS criteria do not require imaging. (See question 3.)

1. **In what environment do spinal cord injuries occur most often and what percentage of those injuries involve the cervical spine?**
   The majority of spinal cord injuries are a direct result of motor vehicle accidents (MVA) (38%), falls from heights (23%), gunshot wounds/violence (15%), and sports-related activities (10%). Of these acquired spinal injuries, the cervical spine accounts for 65% of MVAs, 53% of falls from heights, 37% of gunshot/violence, and 97% of diving injuries (diving is a subset of sports-related activities).

2. **When approaching a patient with a suspected acute cervical spine injury, what should the primary survey consist of?**
   First, check ABCDEs and determine if lifesaving maneuvers are needed. If the patient is in stable condition, maintain inline immobilization until the cervical spine is cleared.

   A – Airway: Establish and/or maintain an open airway via the jaw thrust maneuver (jaw thrust generates less cervical spine motion than the head tilt/chin lift).
   B – Breathing: Ensure the patient is breathing (look, listen, and feel for signs of breathing). If absent, rescue breathing may be needed.
   C – Circulation: Locate a palpable pulse. If absent, CPR may be needed.
   D – Disability: Identify level of consciousness by utilizing the Glasgow Coma Scale.
   E – Exposure: Remove clothing when necessary.

3. **What findings indicate cervical spine immobilization?**
   Based on the Canadian C-Spine Rule, if the patient is >65 years old, if the patient had a dangerous mechanism of injury (fall >3 feet, axial load to head, MVA >100 km/hr or 62 mph, motorcycle/bicycle collision), or if there is paresthesia in the extremities, then immobilization is indicated. Patients are considered low risk if they meet all the following criteria: involved in a simple rear-end MVA, sitting or standing independently at any time, delayed onset of neck pain, and no midline C-spine tenderness. Range of motion can be safely assessed in low-risk patients. If the patient is unable to actively rotate the neck 45 degrees left and right, then immobilization is indicated. Once immobilized, the patient should be transported for imaging (100% sensitivity, 42.5% specificity).
   The National Emergency X-Radiography Utilization Study (NEXUS) can be used to determine low-risk patients who do not require immobilization and imaging. If there is no midline tenderness, no focal neurologic deficit, normal alertness, no intoxication, and no painful distracting injuries, then the patient does not require immobilization and imaging (99.6% sensitivity, 12.9% specificity).

4. **What is the optimal method of immobilization for clinically significant acute cervical spine injuries?**
   The most stable form of biomechanical immobilization is obtained through the use of a rigid cervical collar, rigid spine board, and head immobilization once on the board. The inclusion of strapping furthers the biomechanical immobilization of the thoracolumbar spine.

5. **Which imaging modality should be utilized when assessing acute cervical spine injuries?**
   In adults and adolescents, computed tomography (CT) scans should be utilized as the initial imaging modality of choice due to superior sensitivity and specificity. If unavailable, radiographs can be utilized (anterior-posterior, lateral, atlantoaxial views). Radiographs should be used for children to limit radiation exposure.

6. **What are some commonly seen upper cervical spine (C1–C2) injuries?**
   See Table 37.1.

7. **What are some commonly seen lower cervical spine (C3–C7) injuries?**
   See Table 37.2.

8. **Can there be isolated soft tissue injuries in the cervical spine?**
   Yes, these types of injuries are referred to as whiplash injuries and typically occur from hyperflexion/hyperextension acceleration mechanisms. They result in muscular spasms and muscle strains and can also cause ligamentous sprains and instability. They should be managed with active physical therapy and not be immobilized if stability is not compromised.

Table 37.1 Common Upper Cervical Spine (C1–C2) Injuries

MECHANISM OF SPINAL INJURY	STABILITY
Flexion	
Flexion teardrop fracture	Extremely unstable
Bilateral facet dislocation	Always unstable
Atlantooccipital dislocation	Unstable
Anterior atlantoaxial dislocation with/without fracture	Unstable
Odontoid fracture with lateral displacement fracture	Unstable
Subluxation	Potentially unstable
Wedge fracture	Stable
Transverse process fracture	Stable
Clay shoveler's fracture	Stable
Flexion-Rotation	
Rotary atlantoaxial dislocation	Unstable
Unilateral facet dislocation	Stable
Extension	
Posterior neural arch fracture (C1)	Unstable
Hangman fracture (C2)	Unstable
Posterior atlantoaxial dislocation with/without fracture	Unstable
Extension teardrop fracture	Usually stable in extension
Compression	
Jefferson fracture (C1)	Extremely unstable
Burst fracture of vertebral body	Stable
Isolated fracture of articular pillar and vertebral body	Stable

Kanwar R, et al. Emergency department evaluation and treatment of cervical spine injuries. *Emerg Med Clin N Am.* 2015;33:241–282.

9. What are stingers/burners?

    Stingers/burners are traction or compression injuries to the nerve roots or the brachial plexus, which result in neuropraxia. They present with shooting pain from the neck/shoulder to the hand with associated paresthesia, numbness, burning, or weakness.

10. Are these injuries an emergency?

    No, typically symptoms related to stingers/burners will resolve after a few minutes. As long as there are no additional injuries present (to the spine, brain, or spinal cord), it is safe to return the patient to sports participation once symptoms resolve and motor/sensory function is completely restored.

11. Can the spinal cord be injured without damaging bony structures?

    Yes, this type of injury is referred to as spinal cord injury without radiographic abnormality (SCIWORA). This is predominately an injury found in children due to their hypermobile joints/lax ligaments, and there is transient vertebral displacement and subsequent realignment that results in a damaged spinal cord. Normal alignment will be appreciated on radiographs, but evidence of spinal cord injury can be found on magnetic resonance imaging (MRI).

12. When should there be concern for a vascular injury?

    Although blunt cerebrovascular injury is uncommon, it carries a high risk of permanent neurologic deficits. Indications for screening for vascular injury are:
    - Unexplained neurologic deficits in patients with hyperextension/hyperflexion injuries
    - Severe blunt trauma to the neck or a seat belt injury
    - Cervical spine or skull base fractures adjacent to or involving vascular foramina
    - Le Fort II or Le Fort III facial fractures
        Digital subtraction angiography is considered the gold standard for diagnosing cerebrovascular injuries.

Table 37.2 Common Lower Cervical Spine (C3–C7) Injuries

MECHANISM OF INJURY	STABILITY
Flexion	
Bilateral facet dislocation	Extremely unstable
Flexion teardrop fracture	Unstable
Posterior ligamentous injury	Severe = unstable; mild = stable
Wedge fracture	Stable
Compression fracture	Stable
Clay shoveler's fracture	Stable
Flexion-Rotation	
Unilateral facet dislocation with/without fracture	Stable
Extension	
Extension teardrop fracture	Usually stable in extension
Compression	
Burst fracture	Stable

Kanwar R, et al. Emergency department evaluation and treatment of cervical spine injuries. *Emerg Med Clin N Am.* 2015;33:241–282.

KEY POINTS

1. Sports with the highest rate of acute cervical spine injuries include American football, wrestling, diving, ice hockey, skiing/snowboarding, and gymnastics.
2. Initial cervical spine injury management should be to establish ABCDE (airway, breathing, circulation, disability, and exposure) and then to maintain inline immobilization until any serious injury can be cleared.
3. The NEXUS (National Emergency X-Radiography Utilization Study) criteria and the Canadian C-Spine Rule are highly sensitive decision-making tools that provide guidelines as to when to immobilize and obtain imaging following acute injury.
4. CT scans are the preferred imaging modalities for acute injury diagnostics of adolescents and adults. Radiographs remain the gold standard for children.

Acknowledgments

The authors would like to thank Nicholas Pfeifer, EdM, ATC for his contributions to this chapter's first edition.

BIBLIOGRAPHY

Ahn H, et al. Pre-hospital care management of a potential spinal cord injury patient: a systematic review of the literature and evidence-based guidelines. *J Neurotrauma.* 2011;28(8):1341–1361.

Banerjee R, et al. Catastrophic cervical spine injuries in the collision sport athlete, part 1. *Amer J Sports Med.* 2004;32(4):1077–1087.

Casa D, et al. National Athletic Trainers' Association position statement: preventing sudden death in sports. *J Athl Train.* 2012;47(1):96–118.

Christensen SWM, Rasmussen MB, Jespersen CL, Sterling M, Skou ST. Soft-collar use in rehabilitation of whiplash-associated disorders: a systematic review and meta-analysis. *Musculoskelet Sci Pract.* 2021;55(102426):102426.

De Jonge M, Kramer J. Spine and sport. *Semin Musculoskelet Radiol.* 2014;18:246–264.

DeVivo M. Epidemiology of traumatic spinal cord injury: trends and future implications. *Spinal Cord.* 2012;50:365–372.

Grossheim L, et al. Cervical spine injury: an evidence-based evaluation of the patient with blunt cervical trauma. *Emer Med Prac.* 2009;11(4):1–25.

Kanwar R, et al. Emergency department evaluation and treatment of cervical spine injuries. *Emerg Med Clin N Am.* 2015;33:241–282.

Pimentel L, et al. Evaluation and management of acute cervical spine trauma. *Emerg Med Clin North Am.* 2010;28(4):719–738.

Standaert C, Herring S. Expert opinion and controversies in musculoskeletal and sports medicine: stingers. *Arch Phys Med Rehabil.* 2009;90(3):402–406.

Stiell I, et al. The Canadian C-spine rule versus the NEXUS low-risk criteria in patients with trauma. *N Engl J Med.* 2003;349:2510–2518.

Walton D, et al. Risk factors for persistent problems following acute whiplash injury: update of a systematic review and meta-analysis. *JOSPT.* 2013;43(2):31–43.

CHAPTER 38

ACUTE LOW BACK PAIN

Brian A. Gottwalt, DO, Christopher M. Miles, MD

INTRODUCTION

Acute low back pain (ALBP) is defined as less than 6 weeks of pain between the costal angles and gluteal folds. This may be accompanied by radicular pain, which radiates down one or both legs and may indicate irritation of a nerve root.

Low back pain (LBP) consistently ranks among the five most common reasons for office visits in the US. Only 1% of patients with ALBP in the primary care setting have a serious underlying cause.

1. **What is the differential diagnosis of ALBP?**
   The differential diagnosis is broad and may be categorized into mechanical, nonmechanical, and visceral (Table 38.1). Most patients who present with ALBP are diagnosed with nonspecific, mechanical-type pain.

2. **What are emergent causes of ALBP that should prompt referral to the emergency department (ED)?**
   - Cauda equina syndrome (CES); occurs when there is compression on the lower spinal nerve roots that results in urinary retention or incontinence, bilateral lower extremity weakness, and/or saddle anesthesia
   - Spinal fracture
   - Infection (e.g., epidural abscess, vertebral osteomyelitis)
   - Cancer (CA)

3. **What symptoms/historical details are red flags that should prompt referral to the ED?**
   - Severe or progressive neurologic deficits (e.g., those seen in CES).
   - Trauma. Suspect fracture when there has been a significant mechanism of injury, including motor vehicle collision >35 mph, fall >15 feet, or automobile versus pedestrian.
   - The patient has a history of or risk factors for CA or osteoporosis and presents with sudden onset of LBP after a minor fall or heavy lifting. Suspect pathologic or compression fracture.
   - Fever, constitutional symptoms, or risk factors for infection. Risk factors for infection include immune compromise or immunosuppression (human immunodeficiency virus [HIV]/acquired immunodeficiency syndrome [AIDS], alcoholism, diabetes, chronic steroid use), intravenous drug use, recent spinal surgery or injection, or recent bacterial infection.
   - Known CA history or worsening LBP >4 weeks that is worse at night, not responsive to analgesics, and associated with unintentional weight loss and/or night sweats.

4. **What additional historical features, symptoms, or signs that may not be as concerning in adults are unique red flags for children? (Note: The above red flags are ALSO red flags for children.)**
   - Age <4 years
   - Pain that interferes with daily activity
   - Limp or altered gait
   - Back pain despite no clear mechanism of injury
   - Acute or repetitive trauma

5. **List key exam findings that are red flags and might suggest a concerning etiology**
   - Fever.
   - Midline tenderness: Sensitive but not specific for spinal infection, cancer, and compression fracture.
   - Sensory or motor deficit: Abnormal neurologic exam of the lower extremities (strength, sensation, reflexes, gait) or loss of anal sphincter tone.
   - Straight leg raise (SLR): With the patient supine, knee extended, and ankle dorsiflexed, passive hip flexion of the affected leg to 30–60 degrees reproduces radicular pain. This suggests nerve root irritation, most commonly at L5 or S1, often caused by a herniated disc.
   - Crossed SLR: SLR of the unaffected leg reproduces radicular pain in the affected leg and suggests nerve root irritation.
   - Slump test: While seated, the patient slumps forward, flexing the cervical, thoracic, and lumbar spine. The patient then extends the knee and dorsiflexes the ankle on the affected side. This reproduces radicular pain in the affected leg. Pain should then decrease with cervical spine extension. May better detect irritation to upper lumbar nerve roots.

Table 38.1 Differential Diagnosis of Acute Low Back Pain

MECHANICAL	NONMECHANICAL	VISCERAL
• Muscle strain	• Cancer	• Pelvic organ disease
• Sacroiliac joint dysfunction	• Infection	• Renal disease
• Degenerative disease	• Inflammatory arthritis	• Abdominal aortic aneurysm
• Disc herniation	• Scheuermann kyphosis	• Gastrointestinal disease
• Spinal stenosis	• Paget disease	
• Spondylolysis/spondylolisthesis		
• Fracture		
• Apophyseal injury		
• Congenital disease		

6. When is imaging indicated in the evaluation of ALBP?

For both adults and children, consider imaging when patients present with red flags on history or exam that raise suspicion for a serious underlying condition (cauda equina syndrome, fracture, infection, or CA). For adults, in the absence of red flag symptoms, imaging of the spine for nonspecific ALBP is not recommended before 6 weeks.

7. Which imaging modality is appropriate? Which views? (Fig. 38.1)

• X-ray of the lumbar spine to assess for lytic lesions or fracture in patients with ALBP and red flags for CA or fracture. Standing anteroposterior (AP) and lateral views are typically sufficient. Bilateral oblique views can be considered if there is concern for a pars interarticularis fracture (spondylolysis), but they increase radiation

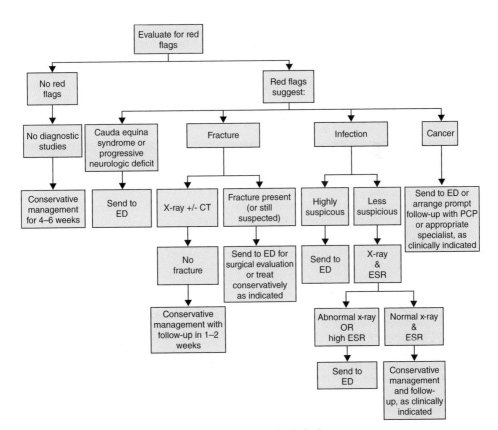

Fig. 38.1 Evaluation of acute low back pain.

exposure and likely offer little in the way of increasing diagnostic accuracy. Lateral flexion and extension views may be helpful if there is concern for instability (e.g., spondylolisthesis).
- MRI in patients with ALBP and red flags for spinal infection, cauda equina syndrome, or spinal cord compression/injury.
- CT without contrast for blunt trauma from a significant mechanism of injury (defined in question 3) with any of the following: back pain or midline tenderness, local signs of thoracolumbar injury, abnormal neurologic exam, cervical spine fracture, altered level of consciousness, major distracting injury, or alcohol or drug intoxication.

8. Are labs indicated in the evaluation of ALBP?
   If history or exam reveals red flags concerning for infection or malignancy, obtain a complete blood count (CBC) and erythrocyte sedimentation rate (ESR) or C-reactive protein (CRP). See Fig. 38.1.

9. How should patients with nonspecific, mechanical ALBP pain be treated in the outpatient setting?
   - Education: Discuss the expected course and establish goals of treatment. ALBP is often self-limited. With self-care, 75% of cases resolve within 4 weeks and 90% within 6 weeks. Treatment should focus on improving pain and function as well as reducing time away from work. Patients should stay active and avoid bed rest.
   - Nonpharmacologic: This is the preferred first-line therapy. Superficial heat is helpful in reducing pain and improving function. Massage, acupuncture, and spinal manipulation are reasonable if the patient is willing to try and the benefits outweigh the risks (including cost). Physical therapy may reduce pain recurrence but is typically reserved for those at risk of developing chronic low back pain. Exercise may improve pain and function if having radicular symptoms. Collectively nonpharmacologic interventions are preferred over pharmacologic for their side effect profile.
   - Pharmacologic: Nonsteroidal antiinflammatory drugs (NSAIDs) or acetaminophen are a second choice of first-line agents. After discussing potential adverse effects, consider the addition of a muscle relaxant. For patients with severe pain who are not responding to or are unlikely to respond to these options, the short-term use of opioids may be appropriate, after carefully weighing the risks and benefits. Current evidence does not support the use of systemic steroids.
   - Follow-up: Educate the patient on red flags (discussed above), which should prompt their return. Otherwise, the patient should follow up with a primary doctor in 4–6 weeks if the pain is not improving.

10. In the absence of red flags, what should you recommend regarding return to play (RTP)? Return to work?
    - The athlete may RTP when the pain has resolved at rest and with activity. Consider sports medicine consultation for guidance on RTP.
    - The patient should continue to work as pain permits, with possible job modifications. Refer to local regulations for workers' compensation cases.

KEY POINTS

1. Know the red flags that should prompt urgent/emergent evaluation.
2. Most patients do not need imaging.
3. For medical management:
   - Nonpharmacologic therapy is recommended as first line in most cases and includes heat, massage, acupuncture, spinal manipulation, exercise, and physical therapy.
   - Pharmacologic treatment if preferred or clinically indicated, starts with acetaminophen, NSAIDs, or short-term muscle relaxants.
4. Encourage patients to stay active. Bed rest is NOT helpful for acute low back pain (ALBP).
5. Follow-up should occur in 4–6 weeks if symptoms are not improving.

BIBLIOGRAPHY

2021 American College of Radiology ACR Appropriateness Criteria Low Back Pain guideline. Accessed September 2022.
AAFP Clinical Recommendations on Imaging for Low Back Pain - Choosing Wisely. Accessed September 2022.
Atlas SJ, Deyo RA. Evaluating and managing acute low back pain the primary care setting. *J Gen Intern Med.* 2001;16(2):120–131. doi:10.1111/j.1525-1497.2001.91141.x.
Bernstein RM, Cozen H. Evaluation of back pain in children and adolescents. *Am Fam Physician.* 2007;76(11):1669–1676.
Chou R. Low back pain. *Ann Intern Med.* 2021;174(8):ITC113–ITC128. doi:10.7326/AITC202108170.
Chou R. Nonpharmacologic therapies for low back pain. *Ann Intern Med.* 2017;167(8):606–607. doi:10.7326/L17-0395.
Duffy RL. Low back pain: an approach to diagnosis and management. *Prim Care. Prim Care.* 2010;37(4):729-iv. doi:10.1016/j.pop.2010.07.003.
Expert Panel on Neurological Imaging, Hutchins TA, Peckham M, et al. ACR Appropriateness Criteria Low Back Pain: 2021 Update. *J Am Coll Radiol.* 2021;18(11S):S361–S379. doi:10.1016/j.jacr.2021.08.002.
Expert Panel on Neurological Imaging and Musculoskeletal Imaging, Beckmann NM, West OC, et al. ACR Appropriateness Criteria® Suspected Spine Trauma. *J Am Coll Radiol.* 2019;16(5S):S264–S285. doi:10.1016/j.jacr.2019.02.002.

Henschke N, Maher CG, Refshauge KM, et al. Prevalence of and screening for serious spinal pathology in patients presenting to primary care settings with acute low back pain. *Arthritis Rheum.* 2009;60(10):3072–3080. doi:10.1002/art.24853.

Hollingworth P. Back pain in children. *Br J Rheumatol.* 1996;35(10):1022–1028. doi:10.1093/rheumatology/35.10.1022.

Jackson DW, Wiltse LL, Dingeman RD, Hayes M. Stress reactions involving the pars interarticularis in young athletes. *Am J Sports Med.* 1981;9(5):304–312. doi:10.1177/036354658100900504.

Majlesi J, Togay H, Unalan H, Toprak S. The sensitivity and specificity of the Slump and the Straight Leg Raising tests in patients with lumbar disc herniation. *J Clin Rheumatol.* 2008;14(2):87–91. doi:10.1097/RHU.0b013e31816b2f99.

Masci L, Pike J, Malara F, Phillips B, Bennell K, Brukner P. Use of the one-legged hyperextension test and magnetic resonance imaging in the diagnosis of active spondylolysis. *Br J Sports Med.* 2006;40(11):940–946. doi:10.1136/bjsm.2006.030023.

Qaseem A, Wilt TJ, McLean RM, et al. Noninvasive treatments for acute, subacute, and chronic low back pain: a clinical practice guideline from the American College of Physicians. *Ann Intern Med.* 2017;166(7):514–530. doi:10.7326/M16-2367.

CHAPTER 39

EVALUATION AND MANAGEMENT OF ACUTE SPRAINS AND STRAINS

Travis Bryan, DO, Laura J. Lintner, DO

TOP SECRETS

1. Beginning an active eccentric loading rehabilitation program early in the course of Achilles tendonitis has been shown to have long-term benefits.
2. Localized tenderness to palpation over lateral epicondyle and pain with resisted wrist and third finger extension can help diagnose lateral epicondylitis.

ACHILLES TENDON STRAIN (ACHILLES TENDINITIS)

A 65-year-old who is training for a half marathon presents with right posterior ankle pain. Pain is localized to just above the heel. There is no specific injury. Pain worsens with more activity, and there is intermittent swelling. Exam reveals mild fullness of the posterior right ankle and tenderness to palpation at the calcaneal insertion of the Achilles tendon. The patient has 5/5 strength in plantar and dorsiflexion of the right ankle. A Thompson test is negative, and x-rays show no bony abnormality. What is the best first step in management?
   A) Relative rest, protection, and initiation of an eccentric strengthening program
   B) Casting in the resting equinus position
   C) Obtain an MRI to rule out Achilles tendon rupture
   D) A cortisone injection to the Achilles tendon
      Answer: A. Casting in the resting equinus position is the initial treatment for an Achilles tendon rupture. MRI is not necessary to rule out a rupture, since this patient has a negative Thompson test. Cortisone injections to the Achilles tendon are not recommended and have been associated with Achilles tendon rupture.

1. **Describe the anatomy and function of the Achilles tendon.**
   The Achilles tendon is the largest and strongest tendon in the body. It originates from the combination of the medial and lateral heads of the gastrocnemius muscle and the deeper soleus muscle. It inserts distally on the posterior aspect of the calcaneus. Its primary function is plantar flexion, but it also helps with tibiotalar joint stabilization. There are two bursae related to the Achilles tendon: the retrocalcaneal bursa, which lies anterior to the tendon; and the superficial calcaneal bursa, which lies between the tendon and the overlying skin.

2. **How does Achilles tendonitis typically present?**
   Patients have pain, swelling, and impaired function of the ankle joint. Pain is worse in the morning or at the beginning of exercise. There are two types of Achilles tendonitis based on the location of pathology: midportion and insertional. Special tests include a painful arch sign (the thickened portion of the tendon moves in relation to the malleoli during active plantar flexion) and the Royal London test (the tender spot on the Achilles is improved in passive dorsiflexion compared to plantarflexion). While often a clinical diagnosis, musculoskeletal ultrasound or MRI can also be utilized to confirm the diagnosis.

3. **Once Achilles tendonitis has been diagnosed, what are some specific treatment options?**
   Rest, ice, protection, and activity modification are all appropriate initial forms of treatment. Active treatment with eccentric strengthening exercises has been shown to have long-term benefits. The mainstay of treatment is physical therapy (PT) to restore the tendon's strength and function. A 12-week eccentric loading protocol, Alfredson protocol, is the most common program for midportion tendinopathy. The modified Alfredson protocol (keeping the ankle out of active dorsiflexion) is often utilized for insertional tendinopathy.

4. **What are some medications and procedures that can be used?**
   Adjuvant use of oral or topical NSAIDs as well as the use of localized glyceryl trinitrate patches (used to increase blood flow through vasodilation) have shown benefits for pain and tendon healing. Nonsurgical procedures such as platelet-rich plasma (PRP) injections, extracorporeal shockwave therapy (ESWT), prolotherapy, and high-volume injectate (HVI) have all been documented in the literature and may be valid treatments for recalcitrant cases of Achilles tendinopathy. Postprocedural Achilles tendon rupture has been reported after corticosteroid injection.

5. **When does an Achilles tendon injury need to be referred to an orthopedic surgeon?**
   The patient should be referred when there is a concern for an Achilles tendon rupture. Typical presentation includes a history of a sudden "pop" at the back of the heel with subsequent pain. Thompson test supports disruption of the musculotendinous junction by squeezing the calf muscle. When torn, the foot does not plantar flex

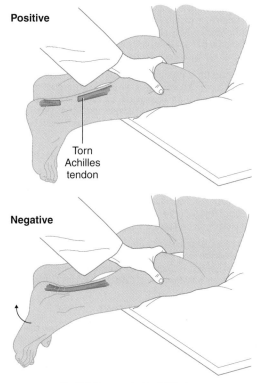

Positive

Torn
Achilles
tendon

Negative

Fig. 39.1 Thompson test for Achilles tear.

(or plantar flexes weaker than the contralateral side). While not all Achilles tendon ruptures require surgical repair, surgical consultation is critical to decision making.

See Fig. 39.1.

6. **What is the most appropriate management when concerned for an Achilles tendon rupture?**
The patient should be placed in a functional brace or cast in resting equinus (slight plantar flexion). X-rays should be obtained if there is concern for other associated bony injuries such as avulsion fractures. Musculoskeletal ultrasound can be an effective diagnostic tool to differentiate between complete and partial tears. MRI is recommended in cases of chronic rupture and equivocal exam findings.

QUADRICEPS TENDON STRAIN

A 17-year-old soccer player presents with anterior thigh pain. Initial symptoms occurred 2 weeks ago after playing in a tournament. She has now developed more pain, swelling, tenderness, and decreased range of motion with knee flexion. No other symptoms. What is the most likely complication of her initial injury?
A) A complete rectus femoris tear
B) Myositis ossificans
C) Quadriceps tendinopathy
D) Rectus femoris abscess
    Answer: B. A complete rectus femoris tear would result in difficulty with knee extension. Quadriceps tendon strain was likely the initial injury. A rectus femoris abscess would likely result in other infectious symptoms.

7. **What is the most common mechanism for a quadriceps strain?**
Acute strains commonly occur from a sudden, forceful, eccentric contraction of the quadriceps. They are typically seen after kicking or starting a sprint from a standing position. Excessive passive stretching of a maximally stretched muscle can also lead to this injury. Acute injuries typically occur distally while chronic injuries typically occur more proximally.

8. **What is the most common quadriceps muscle to be strained?**
Rectus femoris. This muscle crosses both the hip and knee joint as it originates at the ilium (anterior inferior iliac spine, AIIS) and inserts at the quadriceps tendon onto the patella. It functions to flex the hip and extend the knee.

9. **What is the typical presentation of a quadriceps strain?**

Patients complain of pain localized to the quadriceps muscle, often at the distal aspect, and have an appropriate mechanism of injury. Physical exam may demonstrate a muscle defect or bulge, ecchymosis, and tenderness. Pain occurs with resisted hip flexion and knee extension. If there is tenderness of the AIIS, an avulsion fracture should be considered. If the patient cannot passively fully extend their knee, then a tear or rupture should be considered.

10. **When is imaging indicated for a quadriceps strain?**

Imaging is not necessary to diagnose a quadriceps strain but should be utilized when there is concern for associated injuries or when diagnosis is uncertain. Radiographs are normal in a quadriceps strain but should be obtained when there is concern for an AIIS injury, especially in adolescents. Ultrasound may show hematoma formation and muscle fiber disruption. MRI can provide detailed information on muscle injury but is typically not necessary to diagnose a quadriceps strain.

11. **When someone sustains a quadriceps strain, what is the most appropriate initial management?**

The rehabilitation process for a quadriceps strain can be broken down into three phases. Phase one, acute management, includes POLICE (protection, optimal loading, ice, compression, elevation). Starting a physical rehab program in the acute phase has been shown to improve outcomes, including isometric and isotonic contractions, stabilizing exercises, and blood flow restriction (BFR). BFR has been shown to enhance muscle protein synthesis. Phases two and three are progressive increases in strengthening exercises and the addition of sport-specific drills.

12. **Name a complication of a quadriceps strain.**

Myositis ossificans. This is a reactive bone-forming process that occurs following a traumatic soft tissue injury. Presents as pain, limited ROM, and swelling. Radiographs are diagnostic. If athletes do not have recovery with conservative management (physical therapy with avoidance of passive stretching), then surgical excision may be necessary.

LATERAL EPICONDYLITIS (TENNIS ELBOW)

A 48-year-old carpenter presents to urgent care with worsening right lateral elbow pain over the past 2 months. The pain worsens during and after finishing work, and the patient has difficulty completing certain movements. The patient denies numbness or tingling in the arms or hands and has tried acetaminophen and naproxen with minimal relief. What physical exam tests should be performed to help diagnose this suspected condition?

A) Neer test, Hawkins/Kennedy test, Yocum test
B) Tinel test, Phalen test, Durkan test
C) Cozen test, Mill test, Maudsley test
D) Speed test, Yergason test, Ludington test

   The correct answer is C. The patient likely has lateral epicondylitis, or tennis elbow, related to the patient's occupation and the repetitive motions involved. Cozen, Mill, and Maudsley tests are useful for diagnosing lateral epicondylitis. A, B, and D are incorrect, as they are performed for other conditions (shoulder impingement, carpal tunnel syndrome, and biceps injury, respectively).

13. **Which muscles and tendons are involved in lateral epicondylitis?**

The common extensor tendon originates from the lateral epicondyle of the elbow and is directly involved. Within the common extensor tendon, the extensor carpi radialis brevis is almost always the primary tendon involved.

14. **Is lateral epicondylitis caused by inflammation of the tendons?**

No. Epicondylitis is a chronic tendinosis rather than an acute inflammatory process. Histologic studies of affected tendons show degenerative changes with fibroblastic proliferation leading to disorganized collagen and neovascularization.

15. **What are the risk factors for developing tennis elbow?**

Repetitive motions of the wrist including extension, forceful grasping and gripping movements, and rotary movements of the arm (e.g., using a screwdriver or wrench) are commonly implicated, especially if they are completed for more than 2 hours per day for several days. Other risk factors include smoking, obesity, and age (those 30–50 years of age have the highest risk). Lateral epicondylitis is common in racquet sport athletes and those who perform manual labor. It is estimated that 50% of tennis players above 30 years old will develop lateral epicondylitis.

16. **What physical examination tests aid in the diagnosis?**

Localized tenderness to palpation over the lateral epicondyle and distally along the common extensor origin. The Cozen test is performed by having the patient resist wrist extension with the elbow straightened while the wrist is pronated and radially deviated, and is considered positive with pain directly over the lateral epicondyle. The Maudsley test is performed by having the patient hold the middle finger against resistance in full extension, with a positive test reproducing pain over the lateral epicondyle. This movement directly tests the ECRB. The Mill test is positive when pain occurs over the lateral epicondyle while the patient is positioned in forearm pronation and wrist flexion and actively extending the elbow.

17. **What other diagnoses should be considered?**
    - Posterior interosseous nerve compression
    - Radiocapitellar arthritis
    - Cervical radiculopathy
    - Thoracic outlet syndrome
    - Inflammatory arthritis
    - Myofascial pain

18. **What are common treatments?**
    Rest and activity modification are the mainstays of treatment. Counterforce bracing, NSAIDs, icing, and soft tissue mobilization can also be helpful. A local injection of corticosteroid and anesthetic often provides short-term relief. PT and acupuncture may be beneficial. For patients with persistent lateral epicondylitis despite the treatments listed above, newer modalities including platelet-rich plasma injections, prolotherapy, and percutaneous needle tenotomy are becoming more readily utilized and researched. Operative treatment is reserved for those who have failed conservative management and only after other causes of lateral elbow pain have been excluded. Surgical management often includes a release of the common extensor tendon origin.

PATELLAR TENDINOPATHY

A 19-year-old collegiate basketball player presents to urgent care due to 6 weeks of progressive anterior right knee pain overlying the patella tendon. She believes the pain is related to increased conditioning. She has been using ice and acetaminophen with minimal relief. What is the most appropriate next step in initial management of the suspected condition?

A) Imaging, specifically x-ray
B) Rest, activity modification, strengthening exercises
C) Cortisone or PRP injection
D) Bracing and NSAIDs

The correct answer is B. The initial management for patellar tendinopathy is most often conservative including either rest from the inciting activity, strengthening exercises for the surrounding musculature, or activity modification. Bracing and NSAIDs can be utilized in the management of patellar tendinopathy but are often viewed as second-line treatment. Radiography is generally not indicated for the diagnosis of patellar tendinopathy. Cortisone injections are not utilized in the treatment of patellar tendinopathy. PRP injections are utilized in the treatment of persistent tendinopathy that has failed conservative measures.

19. **What is another name for patellar tendinopathy?**
    Jumper's knee (diagnosed frequently in jumping sports); sometimes referred to as patellar tendonitis. However, patellar tendinopathy can occur in any active person, not just those who jump or change direction. The term *patellar tendonitis* is also misleading, much like lateral epicondylitis, as the underlying pathology is noninflammatory and more associated with degeneration.

20. **How do patients typically present?**
    The most common presentation is anterior knee pain that is often worsened by jumping, decelerating, and changing direction. Pain is generally gradual and insidious in onset, occurring over a period of weeks to months. The Blazina classification system is utilized to help further evaluate the pain related to patellar tendinopathy. Phase 1: pain related to activity only. Phase 2: pain during and after activity. Phase 3: persistent pain with or without activities with notable deterioration of performance. There is often tenderness to palpation of the inferior pole of the patella, occasionally extending into the body of the tendon. Pain is associated with loading the knee extensors and applying increased stress to the patellar tendon. Applying pressure to the superior pole of the patella tilts the inferior pole, which gives the examiner the ability to better palpate the tendon origin. Pain with squatting and hopping can help diagnose and monitor recovery. Special testing used for diagnosis of patellar tendinopathy includes Basset sign, which reveals tenderness to palpation over the inferior pole of the patella in full extension but no tenderness in full flexion.

21. **What is the most common part of the tendon affected?**
    Tendon attachment to the inferior pole of the patella is most commonly involved. The distal tendon near the tibial insertion is less commonly involved, and midsubstance issues are rarely documented.

22. **What is the differential diagnosis?**
    - Patellar tendon rupture
    - Patellofemoral syndrome
    - Osgood-Schlatter disease (in adolescents)
    - Sinding-Larsen-Johansson Syndrome (in adolescents)

23. **How does tendinopathy appear on imaging?**

Increased signal is often seen on MRI, and areas of hypoechogenicity and thickening of the tendon are commonly seen on ultrasound. Ultrasound with Doppler can assess vascularity in the tendon and is more sensitive than MRI. MRI is generally limited to use in patients with chronic patellar tendon pain without improvement despite conservative measures or surgical planning.

24. **What is the typical management of patellar tendinopathy?**

Recovery can take weeks to months. Conservative management includes PT to strengthen the surrounding musculature, load reduction, and correction of biomechanical errors. Other treatment modalities utilized include ice, taping or strapping, or NSAIDs. Injections of autologous blood and PRP are being utilized more frequently for persistent patellar tendinopathy as promising research continues to be released. Notably, cortisone injections are contraindicated in patellar tendinopathy due to the increased rick of patellar tendon rupture. Surgery is generally reserved for patients with chronic patellar tendon pain that does not respond appropriately to conservative measures, patients with Blazina phase 3 classification, or those with imaging findings consistent with partial patellar tendon tears.

Acknowledgments

The authors would like to thank Lauren Borowski, MD, for her contributions in the first edition of this chapter.

BIBLIOGRAPHY

Hammond K, Kneer L, Cicinelli P. Rehabilitation of soft tissue injuries of the hip and pelvis. *Clin Sports Med*. 2021;40(2):409–428.

Jayanthi N. Elbow Tendinopathy (Tennis and Golf Elbow). UpToDate.com. https://www.uptodate.com/contents/elbow-tendinopathy-tennis-and-golf-elbow?search=lateral%20epicondylitis&source=search_result&selectedTitle=1~18&usage_type=default&display_rank=1. Updated October 24, 2022. Accessed September 30, 2022.

Jones T. Rectus Femoris Strain. Orthobullets.com. https://www.orthobullets.com/knee-and-sports/3104/rectus-femoris-strain. Updated June 1, 2021. Accessed September 29, 2022.

Karadsheh M. Achilles Tendon Rupture. Orthobullets.com. https://www.orthobullets.com/foot-and-ankle/7021/achilles-tendon-rupture. Updated on April 6, 2022. Accessed September 29, 2022.

Karadsheh M. Patellar Tendinitis. Orthobullets.com. https://www.orthobullets.com/knee-and-sports/3015/patellar-tendinitis. Updated August 13, 2021. Accessed September 30, 2022.

Moore D. Myositis Ossificans. Orthobullets.com. https://www.orthobullets.com/pathology/8042/myositis-ossificans. Updated October 27, 2021. Accessed September 30, 2022.

Praet S, Zwerver J. Patellar Tendinopathy. UpToDate.com. https://www.uptodate.com/contents/patellar-tendinopathy?search=patellar%20tendonitis&source=search_result&selectedTitle=1~24&usage_type=default&display_rank=1. Updated June 30, 2022. Accessed September 30, 2022.

von Rickenbach K, Borgstrom H, Tenforde A, Borg-Stein J, McInnis K. Achilles tendinopathy: evaluation, rehabilitation, and prevention. *Curr Sports Med Rep*. 2021;20(6):327–334.

Yoon R. Lateral Epicondylitis (Tennis Elbow). Orthobullets.com. https://www.orthobullets.com/shoulder-and-elbow/3082/lateral-epicondylitis-tennis-elbow. Published July 31, 2021. Accessed September 29, 2022.

CHAPTER 40

OVERUSE APOPHYSEAL INJURIES

Sahel Uddin, DO, Cayce Onks, DO, MS, ATC

TOP SECRETS

1. Apophysitis is an overuse injury in skeletally immature athletes that warrants rest and activity modification until pain is no longer present to prevent further irreversible injury.

1. **What is apophysitis?**
The apophysis is a protrusion of the bone that acts as an attachment point for ligaments and tendons. It is a secondary ossification center that will fuse with the main bone with maturation. In apophysitis, mechanical stress from the structures that are attached to the apophysis causes chronic tension and bony disruption. This phenomenon is often witnessed in young, skeletally immature athletes. As this area continues to grow, ossify, and enlarge, it may result in fibrous nonunion or union with bony enlargement. While many cases resolve with time, more recent research demonstrates that a large portion of cases can have lasting impacts with a decrease in function and chronic pain.

   The aim of this chapter is to educate on the presentation of various apophysitides, offer guidance that can be provided to patients, and provide some structure and ideas for treatment. The following chapter is limited to overuse apophyseal injuries.

2. **In patients with Osgood-Schlatter disease, will continued play result in long-term knee problems?**
Background: Osgood-Schlatter disease (OSD), sometimes referred to as Osgood-Schlatter syndrome, is one cause of anterior knee pain in young athletes. OSD was first described by Robert Osgood and Carl Schlatter in 1903. Due to chronic tension from the quadriceps muscle and patellar tendon, the apophyseal cartilage of the tibial tuberosity becomes separated from the anterior aspect of the tibia.

   The age of presentation is typically 12–15 years in boys and 8–13 years in girls. Boys have historically been attributed to having higher prevalence, but newer studies demonstrate a lack of difference partly due to the increasing number of female athletes. The pain is generally over the tibial tubercle and distal patellar tendon. It is aggravated by activities that load the quadriceps tendon in eccentric contraction and subsides with rest from activity. OSD has the highest incidence in sport-practicing adolescent populations, especially those participating in soccer. Other factors that are associated include increased quadriceps tightness and muscle imbalance.

   Physical examination: Patients will have tenderness to palpation over the tibial tuberosity, and a bony enlargement may be visualized. Pain with resisted knee extension may also be noted. The diagnosis of OSD is best made clinically.

   Imaging: Radiographic imaging can be used for unilateral cases to rule out diagnoses such as fractures, infections, or tumors, and a plain radiograph is usually recommended for this reason. Radiographs may demonstrate separation of the apophysis from the tibial tuberosity; however, this will not alter management. Magnetic resonance imaging (MRI) or computed tomography (CT) offer little in terms of establishing the diagnosis or treatment and should be reserved for refractory cases that do not respond to conservative management. Ultrasound is an inexpensive and safe option to assess the tibial tuberosity and may distinguish stages of disease; however, more research is needed.

   Treatment: OSD is generally a self-limiting condition and will resolve after the patient has completed growth. Approximately 90% will improve with conservative treatment. Patients may be treated with ice, nonsteroidal antiinflammatory drugs (NSAIDs), and knee padding. Physical therapy (PT) may be beneficial for strengthening and improving flexibility of the quadriceps, hamstring, and gastrocnemius muscles and iliotibial band. High-intensity quadriceps strengthening should be avoided in early rehabilitation. If an athlete complains of mild pain and no weakness, activity may continue as tolerated. The patient may initially require modification of activity to continue pain-free participation. If the athlete continues to have pain despite modifying activities, then complete rest is necessary, which can be guided by individual pain levels. The importance of rest should not be underestimated, as nonadherence may increase the risk of pain continuing into adulthood. Time of rest is variable and may require anywhere from 2 to 10 months. Surgical intervention is the last line of treatment and should be reserved for only those who are skeletally mature and continue to have symptoms despite appropriate conservative therapy. Corticosteroid use for this condition should be avoided due to risk of subcutaneous atrophy and tendon damage.

3. **Are radiographic images necessary to diagnose Sever disease?**
Background: Another location of pain seen in young athletes from apophysitis is in the posterior heel. This was first described by Sever in 1912. This condition is believed to result from traction of the Achilles tendon on the secondary ossification center of the calcaneus.

Presentation: The average age of onset is 11–15 years in boys and 8–13 years in girls. Boys are more commonly affected. Risk factors include high levels of athletic activity, obesity, increased height, and decreased ankle dorsiflexion. Pain is routinely described as "nonspecific" and aggravated by activity.

Physical examination: The diagnosis of Sever disease is best made clinically. Edema, erythema, and warmth are usually absent. There will be tenderness at the posteroplantar aspect of the calcaneus, and patients often have limited ankle dorsiflexion. Research demonstrates the most reliable physical examination findings are a positive squeeze test (lateral compression over the calcaneal tubercle) and barefoot one-leg heel standing. These have the highest sensitivity (97% and 100%, respectively) and specificity (each 100%) for making the diagnosis.

Imaging: Imaging for suspected Sever disease is low yield. Abnormalities over the calcaneus in a young athlete are neither sensitive nor specific. No radiographic sign has been found to be pathognomonic, and changes can be seen in asymptomatic, healthy individuals. For these reasons, radiographs should be reserved for ruling out pathologic abnormalities in recalcitrant cases. A lateral view provides the highest benefit. Ultrasound has also been investigated with some promise; however, further studies are needed.

Treatment: Calcaneal apophysitis is self-limited. Treatment options include rest, orthotics, PT, ice, and NSAIDs. Although several treatment options are available, it does not appear they have a large impact on time to resolution, as pain improves within 3 months. Heel lifts may be recommended, as those patients admitted to improved satisfaction with treatment; however, this comes with financial implications. Over-the-counter heel lifts would be desirable due to cost and availability over custom orthotics.

4. Do athletes with pelvic apophysitis face any risks should they continue to play in spite of pain?

Iliac crest apophysitis: There are many growth plates that can be affected in the pelvis; the most common is the iliac crest. Ossification of the iliac crest occurs from anterior lateral to posterior and typically takes 1 year to complete. This process begins in females around age 13 and males around age 15. Apophysitis of the iliac crest occurs anteriorly and is more commonly affected than posteriorly due to repeat traction from the external oblique, transversus abdominis, and tensor fascia lata muscle attachments. High-risk activities include running and gymnastics. Patients may report pain with coughing or sneezing. Physical examination reveals tenderness to palpation along the iliac crest, as well as tightness of the iliotibial band, hip flexors, and rectus femoris. The patient may have pain with resisted hip abduction. Radiographs may demonstrate a slight widening of the iliac apophysis. Treatment consists of weight-bearing modification and slow return to activity over about 6–12 weeks. When pain-free, the athlete can begin a hip abductor rehabilitation program. There is a risk of complete avulsion if the patient returns to intense activity too early. Fig. 40.1 demonstrates an iliac crest avulsion fracture.

Ischial apophysitis: Another affected growth center in the pelvis is the ischial apophysis, the site of hamstring insertion. Repetitive contraction of the hamstrings can cause the apophysis to become inflamed. It occurs between the ages of 13 and 25. Athletes complain of vague pain, with or without injury. Examination will show tenderness over the ischium and pain with straight leg raising. Progression to avulsion is a relatively common occurrence. Discussion of treatment in the literature is limited. A period of rest and refraining from sports is currently accepted. Conservative treatment should include partial weight bearing with use of crutches until pain-free and then therapy aimed at hamstring rehabilitation. Further treatment is controversial,

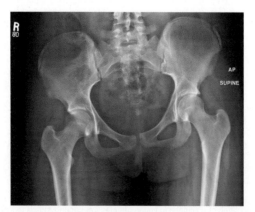

Fig. 40.1 Iliac crest avulsion fracture. There is a displaced ossification center of the left ilium. In apophysitis, the patient will complain of similar pain; however, the growth plate will remain unchanged. Comparison can be made to the right side. (From Duryea D, Penn State radiology archive.)

but surgical referral should be considered if bony displacement is greater than 1–2 cm or no symptom improvement occurs with 2 months of rest.

Other key areas of apophysitis: Other areas of the pelvis that are subject to apophyseal injury are the anterior superior iliac spine (ASIS), anterior inferior iliac spine (AIIS), and the lesser trochanter. The origin of the sartorius muscle is the ASIS, and injury can be due to sprinting. The rectus femoris, which is attached to the AIIS, is commonly injured by kicking in soccer. The lesser trochanter, which is attached to the iliopsoas tendon, can be injured from active hip extension and knee flexion. Due to the complexity of the hip anatomy, plain radiographs are important in confirming the diagnosis and ruling out avulsion. More advanced imaging, such as CT or MRI, is commonly unnecessary. Treatment is generally conservative, including non-weight bearing, then transitioning to routine activities with therapy progression focusing on the strength and flexibility of the offended muscle. Apophysitis in these areas can progress to acute avulsion fractures. For this reason, a suggested timeline for treatment includes 1 week of non-weight bearing followed by 2–3 weeks of limited activity and partial weight bearing, before initiating a therapy progression.

5. **In a young athlete with lateral foot pain, does a radiolucency parallel to the shaft and across the tubercle at the base of the fifth metatarsal raise concern for fracture?**
   Background: Apophysitis of the fifth metatarsal head, commonly referred to as Iselin disease, was first described in 1912 by Dr. H. Iselin. The apophysis is present at the attachment of the peroneus brevis, on the plantar aspect of the base of the fifth metatarsal.

   Presentation: The timing of occurrence for this injury is generally between ages 10–12 for girls and 12–14 in boys. This apophysitis occurs secondary to repeat tension from the peroneus brevis or by inversion injuries.

   Physical examination: Physical examination will reveal tenderness to palpation at the attachment site of the peroneus brevis and pain with resisted eversion or passive extreme plantar and dorsiflexion. An enlarged tuberosity, with edema or erythema, compared to the uninvolved side, may also be appreciated.

   Imaging: Radiographs are not necessary to make the diagnosis; however, oblique films may visualize the ossification center and reveal a small bone piece at the plantar-lateral edge of the tuberosity or enlargement of the apophysis. The apophysis crosses the tubercle parallel to the shaft, whereas fractures occur more transverse. This distinction may help prevent misdiagnosis on radiographs **(see Fig. 40.2 for example).** With a history of an acute inversion injury, radiographs should be obtained to make this differentiation.

   Treatment: Treatment is conservative with a period of rest, non-weight bearing, NSAIDs, bracing, and PT. A walking boot for 1 month before progressing to physical therapy, rather than the use of crutches, could also be considered.

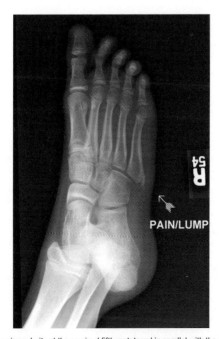

Fig. 40.2 Iselin apophysitis. The bony irregularity at the proximal fifth metatarsal is parallel with the shaft. This differs from a fracture to this area, as the fracture will occur more transverse, across the shaft. (From Duryea D, Penn State radiology archive.)

6. In patients with medial epicondyle apophysitis, are there any shoulder mechanics that make them more susceptible to this injury that could be addressed and improved through PT?

Background: Apophysitides of the upper extremity are rare due to a general lack of weight-bearing. For this reason, sports such as gymnastics increase the risk of injury. Overhead throwers also put enough stress on their elbow to cause injury. Throwers are more likely to injure their medial epicondylar apophysis (little league elbow), as the greatest amount of stress is transferred through this side of the joint. This is due to valgus extension overload and can also occur from tennis or swimming.

Presentation: Patients complain of medial-sided elbow pain and decreased throwing distance. History of overuse is quite common. For pitchers, the numbers and types of pitches thrown are important components of the history. Breaking pitches are thought to be exceptionally dangerous and should generally be avoided in the skeletally immature pitcher.

Physical examination: Physical examination demonstrates tenderness to palpation over the medial epicondyle and possible bony enlargement.

Imaging: Ossification center enlargement or detachment may be seen on radiograph.

Treatment: Treatment is rest from throwing for 4–6 weeks. After athletes are pain-free, they may slowly progress their throwing activities as tolerated. It is also important to address concomitant skeletal abnormalities, such as scapular dyskinesis, weak core strength, and spinal posture. These abnormalities can increase the force being transmitted through the elbow, increasing risk of injury. If the athlete is not compliant with a progression, decreasing pitch counts, and avoiding aggravating pitch mechanics, bony avulsion can occur. Surgery may be required in these circumstances.

Olecranon apophysitis: A similar apophyseal injury can occur at the location of the olecranon from repeated triceps contraction. Patients will elicit tenderness to palpation over the olecranon and pain with resisted elbow extension. A period of 4–6 weeks' rest is advised, and activity can gradually resume when the patient is pain-free. Radiographs may take 10 months to demonstrate bone consolidation. Return to play is determined clinically.

KEY POINTS

1. Individuals with Osgood-Schlatter disease may continue to play sports in spite of pain; however, they should use pain as their guide. An athlete should discontinue activities and rest if modification of activities does not alleviate pain.
2. Sever disease can be expected to improve within 3 months of diagnosis, regardless of therapeutic treatment.
3. Contrary to most other areas of apophysitis, concern around the pelvis should be evaluated with radiographs to rule out avulsion fracture.
4. Use caution when viewing radiographs in Iselin disease, as fractures can look similar to apophysitis.
5. If rest is not performed for little league elbow, the injury may progress to an avulsion fracture and could require surgical intervention.

Acknowledgments

The authors would like to thank Dr. Jayson Loeffert for contributions to this chapter in the previous edition.

BIBLIOGRAPHY

Canale S, Williams K. Iselin's disease. *J Pediatr Ortho.* 1992;12(1):90–93.

Corbi F, Matas S, Álvarez-Herms J, Sitko S, Baiget E, Reverter-Masia J, López-Laval I. Osgood-Schlatter disease: appearance, diagnosis and treatment: a narrative review. *Healthcare.* 2022;10(6):1011. https://doi.org/10.3390/healthcare10061011.

Circi E, Atalay Y, Beyzadeoglu T. Treatment of Osgood–Schlatter disease: review of the literature. In: *Musculoskeletal Surgery,* Vol. 101, Issue 3. Springer-Verlag Italia s.r.l; 2017:195–200. https://doi.org/10.1007/s12306-017-0479-7.

de Schepper E, Bindels P, Bierma-Zeinstra S, van Middelkoop M, Rathleff M, van Leeuwen GJ. Incidence and management of Osgood–Schlatter disease in general practice: retrospective cohort study. *Br J Gen Pract.* 2022;72(717):E301–E306. https://doi.org/10.3399/BJGP.2021.0386.

Frush T, Lindenfeld T. Peri-epiphyseal and overuse injuries in adolescent athletes. *Sports Health.* 2009;1:3.

Gholve PA, Scher DM, Khakharia S, Widmann RF, Green DW (n.d.). *Osgood Schlatter syndrome.*

Hasgoren B, Koktener A, Dilmen G. Ultrasonography of the calcaneus in Sever's disease. *Indian J Pediatr.* 2005;42(8):801–803.

James A, Williams C, Luscombe M, et al. Factors associated with pain severity in children with calcaneal apophysitis (Sever disease). *J Pediatr.* 2015;2:167.

Kujala U, Dvist M, Heinonen O. Osgood-Schlatter's disease in adolescent athletes; retrospective study of incidence and duration. *Am J Sports Med.* 1985;4:13.

Ladenhauf HN, Seitlinger G, Green DW. Osgood-Schlatter disease: a 2020 update of a common knee condition in children. *Curr Opin Pediatr.* 2020;32(1):107–112. doi.org/10.1097/MOP.0000000000000842.

Launay F. Sports-related overuse injuries in children. *Orthop Traumatol Surg Res.* 2015;1:101.

Leahy I, Schorpion M, Ganley T. Common medial elbow injuries in the adolescent athlete. *J Hand Ther.* 2015;28(2):201–210.

Nakase J, Goshima K, Numata H, et al. Precise risk factors for Osgood-Schlatter disease. *Arch Orthop Trauma Surg.* 2015;135(9):1277–1281.

Kose O. Do we really need radiographic assessment for the diagnosis of nonspecific heel pain (calcaneal apophysitis) in children? *Skeletal Radiol.* 2010;39(4):359–361.

Perhamre S, Lazowska D, Papageorgiou S, et al. Severs injury: a clinical diagnosis. *J Am Podiatr Med Assoc.* 2013;5:103.

Perhamre S, Lazowska D, Papageorgiou S, et al. Severs injury: a clinical diagnosis. *J Am Podiatr Med Assoc.* 2013;5:103.

Pointinger H, Munk P, Poeschl G. Avulsion fracture of the anterior superior iliac spine following apophysitis. *Br J Sports Med.* 2003;37(4):361–362.

Rachel J, Williams J, Sawyer J, et al. A novel approach to treatment for chronic avulsion fracture of the ischial tuberosity in three adolescent athletes: a case series. *J Pediatr Orthop.* 2011;31(5):548–550.

Ramponi DR, Baker C. Sever's disease (calcaneal apophysitis). *Adv Emerg Nurs J.* 2019;41(1):10–14. https://doi.org/10.1097/TME.0000000000000219.

Schoensee S, Nilsson K. Is radiographic evaluation necessary in children with a clinical diagnosis of calcaneal apophysitis (Sever disease). *Int J Sports Phys Ther.* 2014;7:9.

Villa FD, Renato A, Artur PC, Neves MC. Apophysitis. In: Espregueira-Mendes J, et al., eds. *Injuries and Health Problems in Football.* Springer; 2017:473–479.

Wiegerinck J, Zwiers R, Sierevelt I, et al. Treatment of calcaneal apophysitis: wait and see versus orthotic device versus physical therapy: a pragmatic therapeutic randomized clinical trial. *J Pediatr Orthop.* 2015;36(2):162–167.

Yanagisawa S, Osawa T, Saito K. Assessment of Osgood-Schlatter disease and the skeletal maturation of distal attachment of the patellar tendon in preadolescent males. *Orthop J Sports Med.* 2014;2:7.

CHAPTER 41

THE ACUTELY INJURED SHOULDER

Emily M. Miller, MD, Lauren P. Oberle, MD

TOP SECRETS

- In evaluating a patient with acute shoulder pain, the mechanism of injury and age of the patient can help determine the likely diagnosis.
- In any fracture or dislocation, neurovascular status should be thoroughly assessed, and if compromised, the fracture or dislocation should be emergently reduced.

1. **What is the differential diagnosis for an acute shoulder injury?**
   - A thorough differential is dependent on an understanding of shoulder anatomy. The shoulder is a girdle consisting of four articulations: glenohumeral (GH), acromioclavicular (AC), sternoclavicular, and scapulothoracic. These articulations are supported by muscles, tendons, and ligaments.
   - Due to the small ratio of bony articulations relative to the large glenohumeral joint, the shoulder demonstrates a unique range of motion but relies heavily on dynamic stability provided by the surrounding muscles, tendons, and ligaments. This distinctive range predisposes the shoulder to injury.
   - Fractures, sprains, dislocations, and tendon and ligament tears are all common ways to injure the shoulder.
   - The focus of this chapter will be to outline the evaluation and management of acute shoulder injuries.
   - In a young patient with a direct fall onto the shoulder, the most common injuries are clavicle fractures and AC joint injuries.

2. **What imaging is useful for the acutely injured shoulder?**
   - Typical x-ray views for any acute shoulder injury include a standard AP, true AP, and axillary view.
   - In cases of diagnostic uncertainty or concern for neurovascular compromise, additional views, computed tomography (CT), or magnetic resonance imaging (MRI) may be required.

CASE

A 22-year-old lacrosse player is running midfield and collides with a player from the opposing team. He loses his balance and falls on his right shoulder. He gets up and runs to the sideline, where he complains to his athletic trainer of right anterior shoulder pain. He tries to lift his arm forward and has significant pain.

CLAVICLE FRACTURE

3. **What are the exam findings in an acute clavicle fracture, and how does this injury present?**
   Patients often appear to have a sagging shoulder. There is pain with palpation (often with crepitus) over the clavicular injury. There may be bruising, swelling, or tenting of the skin over the fracture site. There is pain with shoulder elevation.

4. **What are the best x-ray views if a clavicle fracture is suspected?**
   The acute shoulder series will typically be enough for diagnosis. For clavicle fractures, the addition of a full AP clavicle for bilateral comparison as well as 45-degree cephalic tilt view to determine displacement are useful.

5. **Will this patient require surgery?**
   Clavicle fractures are divided into three groups: medial, middle, and lateral. All nondisplaced middle fractures can be managed nonoperatively with rest and a sling for comfort. Displaced, comminuted, or fractures with >2 cm shortening should be referred to orthopedics for definitive management. Fractures of the clavicle that are lateral to the coracoclavicular (CC) ligament are at high risk for displacement and should warrant surgical referral. Recurrent clavicle fractures should also be referred for surgical intervention. Medial clavicle fractures are less common but can occur with motor vehicle accidents and are often associated with thoracic injuries; if a displaced medial clavicle fracture is identified, it can result in neurovascular injury and is considered an emergency. Complications of clavicle surgery include skin erosion, pain, and hardware breakage.

AC JOINT INJURY

6. **The case above could also result in an AC joint injury or "shoulder separation." How does an AC joint injury present?**
   Shoulder pain after a direct blow or fall onto the shoulder. On exam, there is pain to palpation over the AC joint. There is usually pain with overhead shoulder movement and pain with the cross arm test (adduction). There may be a palpable step-off deformity at the AC joint as well as referred pain to the trapezius.

7. Are there any special x-ray views that are helpful for looking at the AC joint?
   A standard shoulder series is usually adequate. An AP of the bilateral AC joints may provide a better evaluation of the widening of the coracoclavicular (CC) and acromioclavicular (AC) intervals. Weighted films are no longer recommended.

8. How are AC injuries managed? Who needs orthopedic follow-up?
   Fig. 41.1 shows the classification of AC joint injuries, and Table 41.1 outlines appropriate treatment. Nonoperative treatment consists of pain control, brief immobilization in a sling, early range-of-motion exercises, and physical therapy. Anesthetic injection can be used for acute pain control in situations when the patient needs short-term use of the arm (i.e., participation in a single game).

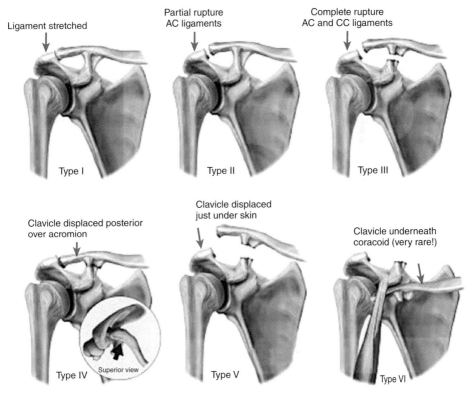

Fig. 41.1 Classification of AC injuries. (From Rockwood Jr, Charles A, et al. *Rockwood and Green's Fractures in Adults.* Vol. 3. 4th ed. Raven Publishers; 1996.)

Table 41.1 The Rockwood Classification for AC Injuries and Typical Treatments				
	AC	**CC**	**CLAVICLE DISPLACEMENT**	**TREATMENT**
Type I	Sprain	Sprain	None	Nonoperative
Type II	Tear	Sprain	<25% CC displacement	Nonoperative
Type III	Tear	Tear	25%–100% CC displacement	Usually nonoperative
Type IV	Tear	Tear	Posterior displacement of clavicle	Operative
Type V	Tear	Tear	>100% CC displacement	Operative
Type VI	Tear	Tear	Inferior displacement of clavicle	Operative

CASE

A 45-year-old left-hand-dominant painter is outside gardening. She is carrying heavy pots to her garden when she falls and lands on her outstretched left arm. She reports she heard a "pop" and felt immediate pain. She has difficulty lifting her arm and feels weak.

ROTATOR CUFF TEAR

9. **What is the common presentation of an acute rotator cuff tear?**
   Patients will complain of pain and weakness with overhead and reaching activities. Tears can occur due to progressive degenerative changes (older adults) or in the setting of trauma (younger adults).

10. **What are the exam findings?**
    Patients may have pain and/or weakness in any combination of the following directions: abduction (supraspinatus), external rotation (infraspinatus/teres minor), or internal rotation (subscapularis). Range of motion may be decreased and painful. The rotator cuff muscles are often remembered by the mnemonic SITS.

11. **What special tests are helpful?**
    Multiple exam maneuvers should be used to increase the likelihood of reaching the correct diagnosis. The Jobe test and the drop arm test (supraspinatus), resisted external rotation test and external rotation lag (infraspinatus), the Hornblower test (teres minor), bear hug, belly press, and lift-off tests (subscapularis) are commonly used (Fig. 41.2).

12. **What imaging tests are useful?**
    Standard shoulder series x-rays are recommended to rule out bony injury or dislocation. MRI, MR arthrogram, or ultrasound can provide a definitive diagnosis. It is important for the clinician to be aware that partial rotator cuff tearing is a common finding in older asymptomatic patients.

13. **Is there a way to clinically differentiate complete versus partial tears?**
    Rotator cuff tears exist on a spectrum from partial to full width and from partial to full thickness and may involve one or more tendons. As such, there is no perfect test. The described special tests can be useful in identifying tears that are large enough to cause substantial weakness. If a patient has weakness with testing, even in the absence of pain, there should be a high suspicion for a rotator cuff tear. If pain interferes with the exam, a subacromial lidocaine injection followed by a repeat exam can allow pain-free muscle activation. Be aware that injections of lidocaine may result in a false-positive tear or bursitis seen on subsequent MRI if done shortly after the injection due to the iatrogenic introduction of fluid.

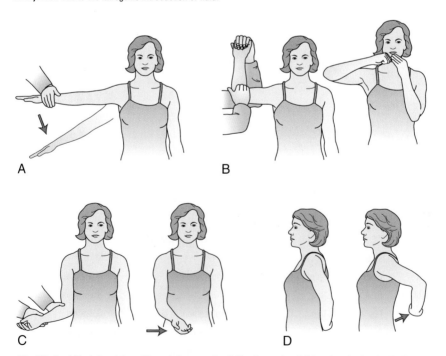

Fig. 41.2 Special tests for rotator cuff tears. A, Drop arm sign. B, Hornblower sign. C, External rotation lag. D, Lift-off test.

14. **How are tears managed?**
Most partial-thickness tears can be managed nonoperatively. Acutely, the best treatment is rest, activity modifica-tions, and NSAIDs for pain reduction, followed by supervised physical therapy. A single corticosteroid injection can be considered for pain relief; however, repetitive steroid injections should be avoided to reduce the risk of progressive tendon damage. Patients with small-medium tears can benefit from operative intervention or con-servative management with physical therapy. Patients with large, complete-thickness rotator cuff tears should be referred for prompt surgical evaluation. The decision to pursue operative versus nonoperative management should be based on factors such as the patient's age, activity level, tear size, and location.

CASE

A 72-year-old female with a history of osteoporosis is walking her dog when she slips on ice and falls onto her right arm. She has immediate pain and an inability to move the right shoulder. On examination, there is swelling and ecchymosis but no obvious deformity along the proximal upper arm.

PROXIMAL HUMERUS FRACTURE

15. **Who is likely to sustain a proximal humerus fracture?**
Proximal humerus fractures are the second most common type of shoulder fracture and are common among the elderly population. Suspect a proximal humerus fracture in a patient with osteoporosis who sustained a low-impact fall.

16. **Are there special considerations when examining patients with proximal humerus fractures?**
There are several anatomic sites on the humerus, as outlined in the Neer classification (see Fig. 41.3), where a fracture may occur. Concomitant dislocation should be ruled out. Care should be taken to perform a thorough upper and lower arm, neurovascular, and cardiothoracic examination including evaluation of axillary nerve function.

17. **What imaging views should be obtained?**
Imaging should include standing radiographs in at least three views, which must include an axillary or scapula-Y view to rule out an associated dislocation. CT may be necessary in cases of high clinical suspicion but no obvious fracture on plain radiographs.

18. **How are proximal humerus fractures managed?**
Most proximal humerus fractures can be treated conservatively with a sling and physical therapy. Simple, minimally displaced, or two-part fractures should be treated nonoperatively, but referral to orthopedic surgery can be considered for more complex fractures. However, patients with significant comorbidities or poor functional status may be better nonoperative candidates even with multipart or displaced fractures. Current data suggest

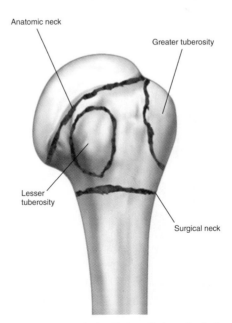

Fig. 41.3 Fracture planes in the proximal humerus. (From Sanders TG, Jersey SL. Conventional radiography of the shoulder. *Semin Roentgenol.* 2005;40(3):207–222.)

that early mobilization (within 2 weeks of injury) may improve nonoperative outcomes compared to prolonged immobilization.

19. **What are the common complications of proximal humerus fractures?**
Associated fractures and rotator cuff injuries occur in approximately 10% and 40% of proximal humerus fractures, respectively. Long-term complications include rotator cuff tears and posttraumatic osteoarthritis.

CASE

A 22-year-old right-hand-dominant male is snowboarding when he hits an edge, falls forward, and strikes his outstretched right arm on the ground. He feels his shoulder "pop out," which is followed by immediate pain over the shoulder and inability to move his shoulder. He has no history of shoulder dislocation.

GLENOHUMERAL (GH) JOINT DISLOCATION

20. **Whose shoulders are likely to dislocate?**
The shoulder is the most commonly dislocated joint, and those injured are commonly male and younger than age 40. Patients typically present as the patient above, often in the setting of trauma, sports injury, or seizure.

21. **In what directions can shoulders dislocate?**
Anterior dislocations are most common (97%), followed by posterior and inferior dislocations. Posterior dislocations classically occur in the setting of electrocution or grand mal seizure.

22. **What imaging views are helpful?**
Imaging should include standing radiographs in at least three views, which must include an axillary or scapula-Y view. Imaging should always be repeated following reduction. Additional postreduction views should include internal and external rotational AP.

23. **How are GH dislocations managed initially?**
Prompt closed reduction should be performed as soon as possible, and it should be performed immediately with any signs of neurovascular compromise. Multiple closed reduction techniques have been described (including, but not limited to, those in Figs. 41.4–41.6). Scapular manipulation and traction-counter traction have some of

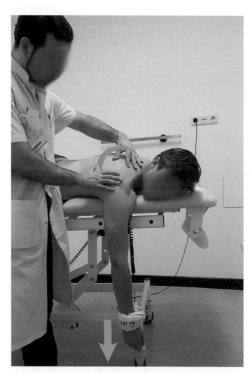

Fig. 41.4 Methods for acute shoulder reduction: scapular manipulation. (From Alkaduhimi H, van der Linde JA, Flipsen M, van Deurzen DF, van den Bekerom MP. A systematic and technical guide on how to reduce a shoulder dislocation. *Turk J Emerg Med.* 2016;16(4):155–168. Published 2016 Nov 18. doi:10.1016/j.tjem.2016.09.008. Figure 16, p.163.)

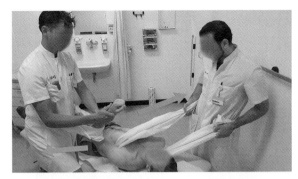

Fig. 41.5 Methods for acute shoulder reduction: traction-countertraction. (From Alkaduhimi H, van der Linde JA, Flipsen M, van Deurzen DF, van den Bekerom MP. A systematic and technical guide on how to reduce a shoulder dislocation. *Turk J Emerg Med.* 2016;16(4):155–168. Published 2016 Nov 18. doi:10.1016/j.tjem.2016.09.008. Figure 12, p.162.)

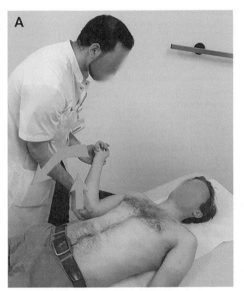
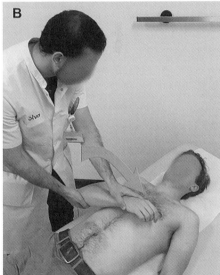

Fig. 41.6 Methods for acute shoulder reduction: Kocher method. (From Alkaduhimi H, van der Linde JA, Flipsen M, van Deurzen DF, van den Bekerom MP. A systematic and technical guide on how to reduce a shoulder dislocation. *Turk J Emerg Med.* 2016;16(4):155–168. Published 2016 Nov 18. doi:10.1016/j.tjem.2016.09.008. Figure 5, p. 159.)

the highest success rates; however, the provider should utilize whichever technique in which they are most experienced and comfortable in their setting, as most techniques have comparable success rates. Some dislocations may require sedation or, rarely, operative reduction. Intraarticular local anesthetic injection for pain control is a relatively safe alternative to other analgesics and sedation if monitoring is unavailable.

24. **What complications occur with dislocation?**
    Possible associated injuries of dislocation include injury to adjacent neurovascular and muscular structures (i.e., axillary nerve injury), Bankart lesion (breaks of the glenoid), Hill-Sachs lesions (cortical crush fractures of the humeral head; see Fig. 41.7), and chronic instability. Due to potential associated injuries, care should be taken to perform neurovascular and cardiopulmonary exams on a patient with a shoulder dislocation. There is a risk of repeat dislocation after a primary traumatic dislocation, especially in younger patients, and most occur within the first year.

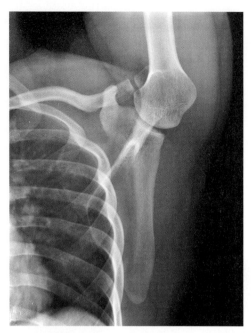

Fig. 41.7 Hill-Sachs lesion on a Stryker Notch view. (From Patel, MS. Stryker notch view radiograph. http://radiopaedia.org/cases/stryker-notch-view-radiograph. Copyright 2023 Dr Maulik S Patel and Radiopaedia.org.)

25. How should dislocations be managed long-term?
Patients with a primary GH dislocation may be considered for conservative treatment with closed reduction and short-term immobilization followed by physical therapy. Select younger, active patients should be considered for surgical management due to risk of chronic instability with conservative treatment.

KEY POINTS

1. With any shoulder trauma, dislocation, or fracture, care should be taken to complete a thorough neurovascular and cardiothoracic exam to rule out associated injury; do not forget to perform axillary nerve testing (sensation distribution over the lateral upper arm and motor function of the deltoid).
2. Nondisplaced middle clavicle fractures can be managed nonoperatively with rest and a sling for comfort.
3. With concern for shoulder fracture or trauma, ensure a Y-scapula or axillary view with initial radiographs to evaluate for concomitant dislocation.
4. Acutely, the best treatment for a low-grade AC joint injury is a sling for comfort followed by early range of motion and physical therapy.
5. Bankhart lesions (breaks of the glenoid) and Hill-Sachs lesions (cortical crush fractures of the humeral head) are common in glenohumeral joint dislocations.

Acknowledgments

The authors would like to thank Craig F. Betchart, MD and Mark Mirabelli, MD for their contributions to the first edition of this chapter.

BIBLIOGRAPHY

Alkaduhimi H, van der Linde JA, Flipsen M, van Deurzen DF, van den Bekerom MP. A systematic and technical guide on how to reduce a shoulder dislocation. *Turk J Emerg Med.* 2016;16(4):155–168. doi:10.1016/j.tjem.2016.09.008. Published 2016 Nov 18.

Alkaduhimi H, van der Linde JA, Willigenburg NW, van Deurzen DFP, van den Bekerom MPJ. A systematic comparison of the closed shoulder reduction techniques. *Arch Orthop Trauma Surg.* 2017;137(5):589–599. doi:10.1007/s00402-017-2648-4.

Belk JW, Wharton BR, Houck DA, et al. Shoulder stabilization versus immobilization for first-time anterior shoulder dislocation: a systematic review and meta-analysis of level 1 randomized controlled trials [published online ahead of print, 2022 Feb 11]. *Am J Sports Med.* 2022:3635465211065403. doi:10.1177/03635465211065403.

Davey MS, Hurley ET, Anil U, et al. Management options for proximal humerus fractures: a systematic review & network meta-analysis of randomized control trials. *Injury.* 2022;53(2):244–249. doi:10.1016/j.injury.2021.12.022.

Expert Panel on Musculoskeletal Imaging; Amini B, Beckmann NM, et al. ACR Appropriateness Criteria® Shoulder Pain-Traumatic. *J Am Coll Radiol.* 2018;15(5S):S171–S188. doi:10.1016/j.jacr.2018.03.013.

Gould FJ. An effective treatment in the austere environment? A critical appraisal into the use of intra-articular local anesthetic to facilitate reduction in acute shoulder dislocation. *Wilderness Environ Med.* 2018;29(1):102–110. doi:10.1016/j.wem.2017.09.013.

Rockwood CA, Green DP. *Rockwood and Green's Fractures in Adults.* Vol 3. 4th ed. Philadelphia, PA: Lippincott-Raven; 1996.

Schumaier A, Grawe B. Proximal humerus fractures: evaluation and management in the elderly patient. *Geriatr Orthop Surg Rehabil.* 2018;9:2151458517750516. doi:10.1177/2151458517750516. Published 2018 Jan 25.

Weber S, Chahal J. Management of rotator cuff injuries. *J Am Acad Orthop Surg.* 2020;28(5):e193–e201. doi:10.5435/JAAOS-D-19-00463.

Weiss LJ, Wang D, Hendel M, Buzzerio P, Rodeo SA. Management of rotator cuff injuries in the elite athlete. *Curr Rev Musculoskelet Med.* 2018;11(1):102–112. doi:10.1007/s12178-018-9464-5.

CHAPTER 42

FOOSH (FALL ON OUTSTRETCHED HAND) INJURIES

Marvin Dang, DO, Bret C. Jacobs, DO, MA

TOP SECRETS

1. A fall on an outstretched hand can lead to injuries of the hand, wrist, forearm, elbow, arm, and shoulder.
2. The most common fractures associated with a fall on an outstretched hand include the clavicle, elbow, and scaphoid.

1. **What are the most common upper extremity joints affected by a fall on outstretched hand (FOOSH) injury?**
   - Joints commonly affected by a FOOSH injury include the elbow, wrist, and hand.

2. **What is the most common mechanism for an upper extremity fracture in a child?**
   - A fall onto an outstretched hand while playing.
   - Children are typically more likely to have an upper extremity fracture than a lower extremity fracture.
   - The distal radius is the most commonly fractured bone.

3. **Name a risk factor that can lead to decreased bone mineral density and can increase the risk of fracture in the pediatric population after a FOOSH injury.**
   - Obesity in childhood and adolescence has been shown to decrease bone mineral density.
   - Obese and overweight children also tend to fall more frequently with activity due to balance difficulties.
   - Maintaining a healthy body weight can reduce the fracture risk from a FOOSH injury in the pediatric population.

4. **When assessing a patient with a FOOSH injury, what are the pertinent history items that need to be considered?**
   - Mechanism of injury: How did the patient land? What was the direction and magnitude of the force to the extremity?
   - History of prior injury.
   - Any other associated signs or symptoms.

5. **Name the most common pediatric fracture related to a FOOSH injury.**
   - Clavicle fractures are the most common pediatric fractures that result from a FOOSH injury.
   - The majority of these injuries occur at the middle-third of the clavicle.

6. **What x-ray views are necessary to evaluate a clavicle fracture?**
   - A dedicated clavicle series should be obtained to optimally evaluate the clavicle.
   - Additional shoulder x-rays, including anteroposterior (AP) and scapular Y views, should be obtained to evaluate for additional injuries, such as the proximal humerus and scapula.

7. **Describe treatment options for children and adults with a clavicle fracture as a result of a FOOSH injury.**
   - After diagnosing a clavicle fracture, patients can use a sling for 2–3 weeks to help with pain, if necessary. Early motion is also recommended if tolerated.
   - A figure-of-eight brace can also be used, although a sling is typically more comfortable and less cumbersome to apply.

8. **What are the indications for surgical referral for a clavicle fracture?**
   - Indications for surgical referral include open fractures, displaced fractures with skin tenting, and vascular injury.

9. **What is a joint in the shoulder that is commonly injured in a FOOSH injury?**
   - Acromioclavicular (AC) joint injuries are most often related to direct trauma to the lateral shoulder, but indirect trauma to the area can occur during a FOOSH injury.

10. **What x-ray views are necessary to evaluate an AC joint injury?**
    - Shoulder x-rays including anteroposterior (AP), lateral, and Zanca views should be obtained to evaluate for AC joint injury. The Zanca view allows the AC joint to be more clearly visualized without overlapping bone, which often occurs in the standard AP view of the shoulder.

11. Describe the treatment options for an AC injury.
    - Following the Rockwood classification system, an AC joint that is displaced by equal or less than 100%, indicated by elevation of the clavicle above the acromial border, can be treated conservatively with a sling, ice, and pain control.
    - Displacement of the clavicle above the acromion by more than 100% (or more than 75% in those requiring extensive upper extremity use, such as an athlete or laborer) will require surgical referral.

12. Which nerve needs to be assessed when evaluating a proximal humerus fracture sustained from a FOOSH injury?
    - The axillary nerve needs to be assessed with a proximal humerus fracture. Carefully assess deltoid function and sensation over the lateral aspect of the proximal humerus.
    - Any signs of neurovascular compromise necessitate urgent evaluation with an orthopedic surgeon.

13. What injury should be considered in a pediatric patient who presents with a painful elbow and decreased range of motion following a FOOSH injury?
    - Supracondylar fractures account for 60–80% of all pediatric elbow fractures, with the most common mechanism being FOOSH injury with an elbow in hyperextension.
    - Typically, these patients will have pain and swelling. Visible deformity may be present. These patients are often quite uncomfortable when a physical examination is attempted.

14. Why are supracondylar humerus fractures the most common elbow fractures in children?
    - Supracondylar humerus fractures typically occur in children aged 5–10 years because it is one of the weakest parts of the elbow joint, with thin bony architecture and ligamentous laxity.

15. Name the x-ray views necessary to evaluate for a supracondylar elbow fracture.
    - Standard elbow x-rays, including an AP and a lateral view with the elbow flexed at 90 degrees, are sufficient to visualize a supracondylar elbow fracture.
    - Comparison views to unaffected side may be helpful to diagnose subtle abnormalities.
    - Also consider imaging the shoulder and wrist for associated injuries.

16. Describe the radiographic findings that are indicative of a supracondylar fracture, even if no fracture line is clearly visible.
    - A fracture may still be present despite the absence of a clear fracture line.
    - The presence of an anterior fat pad sign, known as the "sail sign," or a posterior fat pad sign, is indicative of an intraarticular fracture with an associated effusion and hemarthrosis.

17. What is the best splint to immobilize a supracondylar fracture?
    - To immobilize a supracondylar fracture, use a long arm posterior splint with the elbow flexed to 90 degrees.

18. What are the common complications of a supracondylar humerus fracture?
    - Cubitus varus angulation can form with loss of normal carrying angle, which is mostly secondary to malreduction or loss of reduction leading to malunion.
    - Nerve injury to the radial, median nerve, and anterior interosseous nerve branches of the median nerve may occur with a supracondylar humerus fracture. This is usually a neurapraxia (impairment in nerve conduction) that will resolve within a few weeks.

19. List the three most common clinical signs to suggest a forearm shaft fracture after a FOOSH injury.
    - Visible deformity, tenderness, and decreased range of motion are the most common clinical signs to indicate a fracture.

20. What are the two common locations for fractures of the proximal radius following a FOOSH injury?
    - Fractures of the proximal radius usually occur at the radial head through the physis or just distal to the physis at the radial neck (Fig. 42.1).

21. True or False: Proximal radius fractures are among the most common elbow fractures in children.
    - False. They are among the least common elbow fractures in children. They most commonly occur in children aged 9–10 years. In adults, they make up approximately 33% of elbow fractures.

22. What four factors affect the treatment of proximal radius fractures?
    - Treatment depends on the degree of angulation, amount of displacement, age of the child, and associated fractures.

23. What degree of angulation of the radial head and neck with the radial shaft is usually acceptable for splinting and early range of motion after a proximal radius fracture?
    - Angulation up to 30 degrees can be treated conservatively.

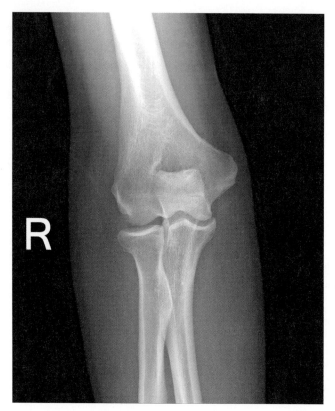

Fig. 42.1 X-ray of radial head fracture.

24. What are the indications for surgical referral for proximal radius fractures?
    • Complete displacement of the radial head, irreducible angulation over 45 degrees, or displaced Salter-Harris IV fracture.

25. What is the most common complication of proximal radius fractures treated conservatively?
    • Loss of motion—specifically, the inability to extend the elbow fully—is the most common complication with conservative therapy.

26. Describe a common injury of the distal forearm sustained by adults following a FOOSH injury
    • A Colles fracture is a fracture of the distal radius with posterior displacement of the distal fragment and is commonly seen in adults.

27. What age group has the highest incidence of distal radius fractures following a FOOSH injury?
    • Children and adolescents are at a higher risk for distal radius fractures, with higher rates in boys. Recent studies have suggested the peak age of incidence for boys is 11–14 years and 8–11 years for girls.
    • Pediatric patients are more susceptible to this injury, in part because of rapidly developing skeletal structures with smaller increases in bone mineralization.
    • Adults have a lower incidence of this fracture, but it is still the most common fracture seen in young adults.

28. What is the best imaging for diagnosis of a distal radius fracture?
    • Plain radiographs are the mainstay in diagnosing distal radius fractures.
    • Standard views should include AP, lateral, and oblique views. These views will assess ulnar variance and contour of the articular surface as well as provide visualization of the dorsal ulnar cortex.

29. Distal radius fractures from FOOSH injuries may include torus fractures or bicortical fractures. Explain the difference between a torus fracture and a bicortical fracture.
    - Torus fractures, also known as buckle fractures, are common injuries in childhood. They are incomplete cortical fractures resulting from compression along one side of the bone. They are stable fractures that can be treated conservatively with immobilization in a short arm cast or removable wrist splint for 3 weeks.
    - Bicortical fractures of the metaphysis are complete fractures through the cortex. These may include transverse, oblique, or spiral fractures and can present with significant displacement. These occur because of bending, rotational, or shear forces sustained at the wrist. Maligned displaced fractures should be reduced and splinted. Definitive treatment includes closed reduction with cast immobilization.

30. What are the indications for conservative treatment for a distal radius fracture after a FOOSH injury?
    - Indications for conservative treatment are incomplete fractures, nondisplaced complete fractures, and displaced extraarticular fractures, which can be reduced to stable fractures.

31. When should distal radius fractures be referred for surgical treatment?
    - Indications for surgical treatment are displaced extraarticular fractures with unstable reduction, displaced unstable intraarticular fractures, shortening of the distal radius by more than 2 mm, and comminuted extraarticular fractures with a small extraarticular fragment not reduced after closed reduction.

32. What are the common associated injuries related to distal radius fractures from FOOSH injuries?
    - Associated injuries can occur to the distal radius ulnar joint and triangular fibrocartilage complex. Ulnar styloid, carpal, metacarpal, or phalangeal fractures can also occur. Always be sure to assess joints above and below a fracture, as there may be associated injuries.

33. Name an important potential complication of distal radius fracture in pediatric patients.
    - Pediatric patients with distal radius fracture may experience distal radius growth arrest. Growth arrest occurs in approximately 4% of pediatric patients with a distal radius fracture.
    - If deformity persists, a corrective osteotomy can be performed after skeletal maturity is attained.

34. Following a both-bone forearm fracture of the radius and ulna, what is the accepted alignment after anatomic reduction?
    - Accepted alignment is related to the age of the patient, with not more than 10–50 degrees of angulation accepted in children less than 8 years old and 5–10 degrees of angulation accepted in children 8 years old and older.

35. What is a common complication of both-bone forearm fractures?
    - Residual loss of motion in the forearm is a common complication seen in nearly 60% of children. This complication is related to length discrepancy, residual malangulation, malrotation deformity, and narrowing of the interosseous space.

36. Name the carpal bone most commonly fractured in a FOOSH injury
    - The scaphoid is the most common carpal bone fractured in a FOOSH injury.
    - Scaphoid fractures account for 60–70% of all carpal fractures.

37. Describe common physical examination findings for a patient with a scaphoid fracture
    - Patients with a scaphoid fracture may have radial-sided wrist pain with associated swelling, along with localized tenderness over the anatomic snuffbox. The snuffbox is located on the dorsal wrist between the tendons of the extensor pollicis longus medially and the extensor pollicis brevis and abductor pollicis longus laterally.
    - Tenderness over the anatomic snuffbox is the most sensitive physical examination finding. Sensitivity ranges from 0.87 to 1.00 (Fig. 42.2).

38. How useful are plain radiographs for the diagnosis of scaphoid fracture after a FOOSH injury (Fig. 42.3)?
    - Reported sensitives for plain radiographs for scaphoid fracture range from 70–86%.
    - With clinical concern for scaphoid fracture on initial presentation, the patient should be placed in a thumb spica splint and have follow-up radiographs in 1–2 weeks.
    - If follow-up radiographs are normal and there is still high suspicion of scaphoid fracture, a computed tomography (CT) scan or magnetic resonance imaging (MRI) may be necessary to confirm the suspected scaphoid fracture.

39. Name a long-term complication of a scaphoid fracture that makes it so important to diagnose correctly.
    - Nonunion and avascular necrosis are long-term complications of a scaphoid fracture.
    - The scaphoid is susceptible to these complications because it receives its blood supply in a retrograde fashion from branches of the radial artery.

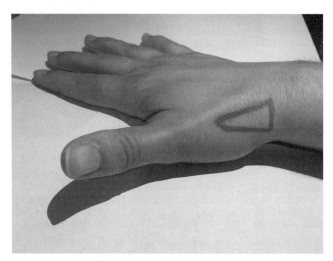

Fig. 42.2 Location of anatomic snuffbox.

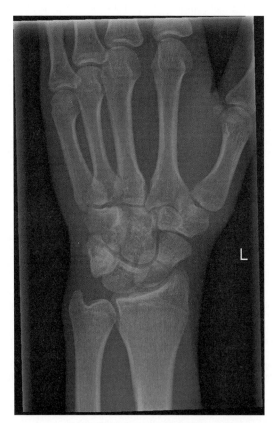

Fig. 42.3 X-ray of scaphoid fracture.

KEY POINTS

1. A fall on an outstretched hand can lead to injuries of the hand, wrist, forearm, elbow, arm, and shoulder.
2. Clavicle fractures are the most common pediatric fractures following a FOOSH injury.
3. Supracondylar humerus fractures are the most common elbow fractures in pediatric patients following a FOOSH injury.
4. The scaphoid is the most common carpal bone fractured in a FOOSH injury and may not appear on plain x-rays immediately after an injury.

Acknowledgments

The authors would like to thank Dr. Alicia Kenton for her contributions to this chapter in the previous edition.

BIBLIOGRAPHY

Arora R, et al. Pediatric upper-extremity fractures. *Pediatr Ann.* 2014;43(5):196–204.
Bae D, Waters P. Pediatric distal radius fractures and triangular fibrocartilage complex injuries. *Hand Clin.* 2006;22:43–53.
Basu S, Khan SHM. Radiology of acute wrist injuries. *Br J Hosp Med.* 2010;71(6):M90–M93.
Black W, Becker J. Common forearm fractures in adults. *Am Fam Physician.* 2009;80:1096–1102.
Kocher M, Waters P, Micheli L. Upper extremity injuries in the paediatric athlete. *Sports Med.* 2000;30:117–135.
Mallee WH, Henny EP, van Dijk CN, et al. Clinical diagnostic evaluation for scaphoid fractures: a systematic review and meta-analysis. *J Hand Surg Am.* 2014;39(9):1683–1691.
Schneppendahl J, Windolf J, Kaufmann R. Distal radius current concepts. *J Hand Surg.* 2012;37:1718–1725 (A).
Shrader MW. Pediatric supracondylar fractures and pediatric physeal elbow. *Orthop Clin North Am.* 2008;39:163–171.
Sinikumpu J, Serlo W. The shaft fractures of the radius and ulna in children: current concepts. *J Pediatr Orthop.* 2015;24:200–206.
Sirin E, Aydin N, Mert Topkar O. Acromioclavicular joint injuries: diagnosis, classification and ligamentoplasty procedures. *EFORT Open Rev.* 2018 Jul;3(7):426–433.
Taljanovic MS, Karantanas A, Griffith JF, et al. Imaging and treatment of scaphoid fractures and their complications. *Semin Musculoskelet Radiol.* 2012;16:159–174.
Tang J. Distal radius fracture: diagnosis, treatment, and controversies. *Clin Plast Surg.* 2014;41:481–499.
Tiel-van Buul MM, van Beek EJ, Borm JJ, Gubler FM, et al. The value of radiographs and bone scintigraphy in suspected scaphoid fracture: a statistical analysis. *J Hand Surg Br.* 1993;18:403–406.
Townsend D, Bassett G. Common elbow fractures in children. *Am Fam Physician.* 1996;53:2031–2041.
Zorilla S de Neira J, Prada-Canizares A, Marti-Ciruelos R, et al. Supracondylar humeral fractures in children: current concepts for management and prognosis. *Int Orthop.* 2015;39:2287–2296.

CHAPTER 43

ACUTE FINGER AND WRIST INJURIES

Heli Naik, DO, CAQSM, Thomas Trojian, MD, CAQSM, FACSM, FAMSSM, RMSK

Some of the most common acute hand and wrist injuries include scaphoid fracture, distal radius fracture, TFCC injuries, boxer's fracture (fifth metacarpal neck fracture), mallet finger, jersey finger, skiers thumb, and proximal interphalangeal (PIP) joint dislocations. This chapter reviews these injuries with emphasis on initial management and treatment.

Case: A 26-year-old tried to impress his girlfriend while ice skating and attempted to skate backward. In doing so, he slipped and fell, trying to catch himself with an outstretched hand with the wrist in extension. As a result, he presents with pain, swelling, and tenderness in the right wrist. This FOOSH (fall on an outstretched hand) injury can lead to hand or wrist injuries.

1. **How does a scaphoid fracture occur?**
   The scaphoid is the most commonly fractured carpal bone, accounting for 15% of acute wrist injuries. It often results from a force on an extended wrist, which places a tensile force at the volar scaphoid and a compression force at the dorsal scaphoid. Scaphoid fractures may also occur with a longitudinally directed axial force across the wrist.

2. **What are the physical examination findings for a patient with a scaphoid fracture?**
   Wrist range of motion is usually slightly reduced, but the pain is reproduced with circumduction. Patients will generally have pain in the anatomical snuffbox in neutral or with the wrist in ulnar deviation. Associated injuries may cause symptoms of median nerve compression.

3. **When should radiographs be used to evaluate the injury?**
   Radiographs are always indicated in the evaluation of suspected scaphoid fractures! Posteroanterior, lateral, scaphoid, and 45° pronated views help assess for a possible fracture. In addition, CT scans and magnetic resonance imaging (MRI) can be used to detect scaphoid fractures better. MRI is the most sensitive in determining fractures and ligament injuries.

4. **What if x-ray findings are negative, but the patient has snuffbox tenderness?**
   Snuffbox tenderness should be treated as a scaphoid fracture regardless of negative radiographs on the initial evaluation. Radiographs may continue to be negative at 2 weeks; further imaging is indicated if tenderness persists over the scaphoid (Fig. 43.1).

5. **When are referrals for a surgical evaluation needed?**
   Unstable fractures and proximal pole fractures are particularly at risk for nonunion, given the vascular supply, so these fractures should be referred for internal fixation. Additionally, displacement >1 mm, comminuted fractures, radiolunate angle greater than 15°, or the presence of scapholunate instability should be referred for surgical evaluation. Nondisplaced fractures may be referred for internal fixation if a quicker return to sports is required. Surgical fixation leads to 90–95% union rates. Given the risk of these fractures progressing to nonunion and subsequent pain and disability, these fractures should be managed by physicians trained to manage scaphoid fractures.

6. **What is the length and type of mobilization? (See Table 43.1.)**
   Previously they were treated with a long arm thumb spica cast/splint; however, evidence shows that a short arm cast without thumb immobilization is noninferior and just as effective in terms of nonunion rates for acute scaphoid fractures treated nonoperatively. The length of immobilization depends on the location of the fracture, with proximal fractures being the longest.

7. **What is the length of healing time? (See Table 43.1.)**
   Healing time is dependent on the location of the fracture site.

8. **What is the TFCC?**
   The triangular fibrocartilage complex is located at the ulnar side of the wrist between the ulna and the carpal bones, lunate, and triquetrum.

9. **How does a TFCC injury present, and how does an acute injury occur?**
   Ulnar-sided wrist pain is often worse with gripping +/- twisting (turning a doorknob), ulnar deviation, and pushing off with the wrist in extension. The most common mechanism of injury is a fall on an extended wrist with the forearm in pronation. Injury can also occur due to a traction injury to the ulnar side of the wrist.

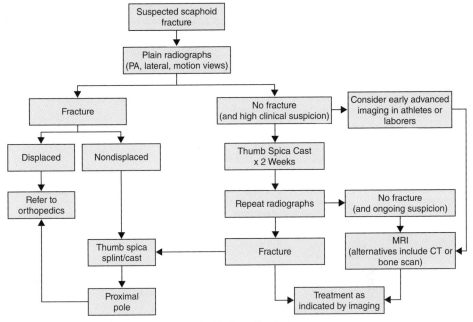

Fig. 43.1 Algorithm for snuffbox tenderness.

10. **What are the physical exam findings?**
A positive fovea sign is tenderness at the soft spot between the ulnar styloid and the flexor carpi ulnaris tendon, between the volar surface of the ulnar head and the pisiform. Pain with passive ulnar deviation is also common.

11. **Initial management of a TFCC injury.**
Immobilization with an extensor wrist brace or the more discrete TFCC brace for 2 weeks +/− a scheduled NSAID in conjunction with physical therapy for 4–6 weeks. Also, consideration for ultrasound-guided corticosteroid injections with nonoperative sports medicine.

12. **When should imaging be used to evaluate a TFCC injury?**
Suppose persistence of symptoms s/p rest and rehabilitation; imaging should be considered. Radiographs with AP, lateral, and a dynamic pronated PA grip are usually negative though the latter may show pathology. Arthroscopy is the diagnostic gold standard; however, MRI of the wrist is the most used imaging modality and has a 74–100% sensitivity.

13. **When is a surgical intervention indicated? What is the best surgical modality?**
If the patient has failed 6 weeks of nonoperative management and has persistent symptoms with limitations in using the wrist, a referral to orthopedic surgery is appropriate. Arthroscopic debridement +/− TFCC repair is considered the gold standard.

14. **What is a boxer's fracture?**
A fifth metacarpal neck fracture is a boxer's fracture due to an impaction injury with an axial load to the fifth metacarpal. Ironically, this injury is less common in boxers but more common in individuals not trained at throwing punches. Metacarpal fractures account for 40% of all hand injuries, and the fifth metacarpal is the most commonly fractured.

15. **What symptoms will a patient with a boxer's fracture have?**
Individuals often present with dorsal pain, swelling, or ecchymosis over the fifth metacarpal. Despite this, most individuals can maintain a complete functional status of the hand and fingers unless an open wound is superficial to the fracture site.

16. **What physical exam findings should someone look for with a boxer's fracture?**
Any obvious bony step-off or deformity is essential. More importantly, the clinician should assess rotational angulation of the fracture with a closed fist assessment of the distal phalanx of the fifth digit. The normal orientation of the fifth digit should have it pointing toward the scaphoid bone. The ulnar deviation may indicate further angulation of the fracture. Loss of the bony knuckle at the metacarpal phalangeal joint is frequently seen with these fractures.

Table 43.1 Treatment of Suspected/Nondisplaced Scaphoid Fractures

| | *Initial Treatment* | | | |
| | | *Fracture Location* | | |
	SUSPECTED	**DISTAL**	**MIDDLE**	**PROXIMAL**
Splint type and position	Short-arm thumb spica cast or splint	Short arm-thumb spica cast with slight wrist extension	Long arm-thumb spica cast/splint with slight wrist extension	
Follow-up	2 weeks	1–2 weeks		
Patient education	Ice and elevate for 24–48 hours Maintain finger and shoulder range of motion			
Follow-Up Care				
Splint type and position	Short-arm thumb spica cast or splint	Short arm-thumb spica cast with slight wrist extension	Long arm-thumb spica cast/splint with slight wrist extension for weeks 1–6; then short arm-thumb spica cast/splint	
Immobilization time	Until diagnosis confirmed	4–6 weeks	10–12 weeks	12–20 weeks
Healing time		6–8 weeks	12–14 weeks	18–24 weeks
Follow-up interval	Every 2 weeks until diagnosis confirmed	Every 2–3 weeks until union confirmed		
Repeat radiographic interval	Every 2 weeks until diagnosis confirmed	Every 2–3 weeks until union confirmed		
Patient education	Maintain finger and shoulder range of motion			
Indications for Orthopedics referral	Proximal pole fractures due to high risk of avascular necrosis Displaced fractures Nonunion Concern for early signs of avascular necrosis			

17. **When should imaging be used to evaluate a boxer's fracture?**
Radiographs should be ordered with any suspicion of a metacarpal fracture. Standard AP, lateral, and oblique views are the most appropriate for evaluation. Advanced imaging is generally not needed. However, a CT scan may be considered if there are multiple carpal metacarpal dislocations, a complex metacarpal head fracture, or inconclusive CMC findings.

18. **When are referrals for surgical evaluation needed for metacarpal fractures?**
Indications for surgery for a metacarpal fracture include intra-articular fractures and significant angulation greater than 40° in the fifth metacarpal (30° in the ring finger, 20° in the index, and long fingers). Other indications include rotational malalignment and multiple shaft fractures. Fractures of the base of the fifth metacarpal are inherently unstable and nearly always require internal fixation. Additionally, the clinician should promptly refer patients with evidence of ulnar nerve damage to an orthopedic surgeon. If any residual angulation is unacceptable to the patient, referral for internal fixation is indicated.

19. **How to manage a boxer's fracture?**
Nonoperative management is the initial treatment of choice for patients with stable fractures, no significant displacement, angulation, or shortening. The best method of nonoperative management for these injuries has not been universally determined; however, the initial treatment is an ulnar gutter splint. For metacarpal fractures, the clinician should place the rest in 30° of extension at the wrist, the MCP joint should be immobilized at 70–90° of flexion and remain in a cast for four weeks. Follow-up at 5–7 days should be recommended during the initial evaluation. Minimally angulated fifth metacarpal neck fractures without evidence of angulation may be adequately treated with buddy taping and a soft wrap around the hand.

20. **When can individuals return to play/regular activity after a boxer's fracture?**
Individuals typically require 4 to 6 weeks of recovery, which includes 4 weeks of immobilization. The bone will typically heal enough to return to sport by 6 weeks, although continued bone remodeling can occur for up to 1 year.

21. **How does a mallet finger occur?**
A mallet finger results from a forced flexion of the extended fingertip and occurs most commonly in sports (think the ball hitting an extended fingertip directly). The mallet finger is the most common closed tendon injury of a finger. Forced flexion of the distal interphalangeal (DIP) joint results in a disruption of the terminal extensor tendon from the dorsum of the base of the distal phalanx, +/- a bony avulsion. The long finger is the most injured.

22. **What are the symptoms of a mallet finger?**
Pain is the most common symptom that patients experience, while many will also have associated swelling. With these injuries, patients often maintain use of the hand, so there may be a delay in seeking treatment. In addition, patients often present with an "extensor lag," ranging from a 5–20° loss of extension in partial tears to over 50–60° loss of extension in complete ruptures. Physical examination shows a loss of active extension at the DIP joint while full passive extension is maintained.

23. **When should imaging be used to evaluate a mallet finger?**
The clinician should obtain the affected finger's AP, lateral, and oblique views. A pure tendon avulsion may have occurred if no apparent fracture is seen. More commonly, a small avulsion fracture may be seen. A volar sublux-ation of the distal fragment may be visualized in more complicated cases.

24. **When are referrals for surgical evaluation needed for a mallet finger?**
Indications for early surgical referral include volar subluxation of the distal phalanx, inability to fully extend the IP joint passively, avulsion fracture involving greater than 30% of the articular surface, or a swan neck deformity (hyperextension of the PIP joint and flexion of the DIP joint). Surgery may also be considered if the injury becomes chronic despite a healthy joint.

25. **How are mallet finger injuries treated?**
Most patients with a mallet finger should be treated conservatively with prolonged splinting of the DIP joint in slight hyperextension. Extension splinting of the DIP joint is used for 6–8 weeks, followed by 2–3 weeks of nighttime-only splinting. Essential to appropriate treatment is educating the patient that the DIP joint must not drop into flexion at any point in this treatment period; otherwise, the clock resets.
      The tip of the distal phalanx should be supported when the splint is being changed. Depending on the sever-ity of the lag and the time to presentation, or if a significant lag persists after the initial 6– to 8-week splinting period, some patients may require a more extended period of immobilization, up to 12 weeks. Many different splints can afford good outcomes. A stack splint, dorsal padded aluminum splints, or a volar unpadded splint can all be used for placing the DIP into a slight hyperextension.

26. **What is the typical length of injury for a mallet finger? When can individuals return to play/ regular activity?**
After the 6–12 weeks of extension splinting, individuals can start finger flexion rehabilitation, and many athletes can return to play with the injured finger in a splint. Most individuals recover fully; however, some may maintain a mild to moderate extensor lag, more common in those who presented for treatment late after the initial injury or older individuals. However, even in these cases, the patient will typically have full function of the finger.

27. **Are there any special considerations in the pediatric mallet finger?**
In the pediatric population, the growth plate is weaker than the surrounding bone but provides growth and remod-eling ability to correct an initially displaced fracture.

28. **What is a Seymour fracture?**
An often undiagnosed/overlooked injury in the pediatric population is a distal phalanx physeal fracture, which may appear as a nail bed injury. This type of fracture, a variant of a Salter Harris I and II fracture, is also known as the Seymour fracture. A mallet finger that presents with blood in the nail bed should be considered an open fracture. It is an avulsion of the proximal edge of the nail from the eponychium fold. A true lateral radiograph is required to evaluate the fracture. The difference between Seymour fracture and mallet finger is the displacement through the physis instead of the DIP joint. Late presentations of a Seymour fracture may include infection, growth arrest, or persistent deformity. Management includes debridement, irrigation, reduction, nail replacement or removal, and antibiotics. These fractures should be referred to orthopedics for ongoing management.

29. **How does a jersey finger occur?**
A jersey finger is an avulsion injury of the flexor digitorum profundus. It most commonly occurs during athletic competition, specifically tackling sports such as football or rugby. It occurs when a player is grasping an opponent who attempts to pull away, resulting in a forced extension while the DIP is held in flexion. The result is a volar avulsion of the flexor digitorum profundus tendon at the base of the distal phalanx. The ring finger is the most commonly affected finger due to it being more prominent in a grip than other fingers in 90% of patients.

30. **What symptoms will a patient with a jersey finger have?**
The patient will have pain and often swelling over the volar aspect of the distal phalanx. The finger will lie slightly extended compared to the other fingers when at rest. The patient cannot actively flex the finger at the DIP joint. The retracted tendon may be palpable along the flexor sheath. (Remember, you must isolate the DIP joint when testing FDP function by stabilizing the PIP joint and the middle phalanx and asking the patient to flex the DIP joint.)

31. **When should imaging be used to evaluate a jersey finger?**
Lateral and oblique views are always necessary to evaluate a suspected jersey finger. In addition, as with mallet fingers, radiographs are helpful to determine if there is an avulsion fracture.

32. **When are referrals for surgical evaluation needed for a jersey finger?**
Always! Prompt diagnosis with an early referral to orthopedic/hand surgery is vital to treating this injury. A jersey finger is not amenable to conservative or nonoperative treatment. Timing surgery can vary and is based on the classification of the injury, as noted in the table below.

33. **What should be done to protect a jersey finger injury from further damage?**
Unlike many other injuries, this injury typically requires an urgent surgical evaluation. Before surgery, splint the injured finger in slight flexion at the DIP and PIP joints to avoid further injury. Along with ice, medication can be helpful for pain.

34. **What is the typical length of recovery for a jersey finger injury? When can individuals return to play/regular activity?**
After surgery, it takes 2–3 months before the patient can use the hand without protection. It may take another 1–2 months before the person's hand can be used with force. Return to play (tackling sports) typically takes 4–6 months. Early rehabilitation after surgery to improve range of motion and function is vital for best outcomes.

35. **How is the jersey finger injury different in the pediatric population?**
Avulsion of the FDP does not occur in adolescents. In this population, the salter Harris IV fracture can be seen (avulsion of the metaphysis and a portion of the physis). This avulsion fragment is usually tethered at the A-4 pulley, similar to type II injuries in adults. This injury should have the DIP and PIP splinted in slight flexion and referred promptly to a hand surgeon.

36. **How does a skier's thumb (ulnar collateral ligament of the thumb) injury occur?**
A skier's (or gamekeeper's) thumb results from an injury to the UCL of the MCP joint of the thumb. The skier's thumb refers to a more acute injury, whereas a gamekeeper's thumb refers to a chronic UCL injury. The injury results from increased valgus stress (abduction), usually on a hyperextended thumb.

37. **What symptoms will a patient with UCL injury of the thumb have?**
Patients will have pain localized to the ulnar aspect of the thumb at the MCP joint (web space between thumb and index finger). They may complain of difficulty pinching or grasping objects with the thumb. Palpation of the thumb may reveal focal swelling from the torn ligament or a bony avulsion fragment. The clinician should perform stress testing of the ligament once an avulsion fracture has been ruled out with radiographs (stress testing can potentially convert a nondisplaced fracture to a displaced one). Instability may be seen with radial deviation of the thumb in neutral (indicating accessory UCL injury) or at 30° of flexion (indicating a proper UCL injury). Instability in both positions indicates a complete rupture. It is essential to test the contralateral thumb for laxity, as there is significant variation in ligamentous laxity from person to person.

38. **When should imaging be used to evaluate the UCL injury?**
Radiographs should be obtained when you suspect a UCL injury to evaluate for avulsion fractures. You should order AP, lateral, and oblique views of the thumb. Stress radiographs, and ultrasound, can also be obtained to assess stability. Ultrasound or MRI may aid in diagnosing if the exam is equivocal or if suspicion of a Stener lesion is present.

39. **What is a Stener lesion?**
Stener lesion is an avulsed UCL, with or without bony attachment, displaced above the adductor pollicus tendon and dorsal aponeurosis. This interposition of the soft tissue of the adductor aponeurosis between the torn ends of the UCL is called a Stener lesion. It prevents primary healing in cases of complete rupture of the ligament. Therefore, Stener lesions generally require surgical repair.

40. **When are referrals for surgical evaluation needed for UCL injury?**
Operative management is recommended for acute injuries with greater than 35° opening on valgus stress, fractures displaced greater than 2 mm, fractures involving greater than 20% articular surface, concern for Stener lesion, or symptomatic chronic injury. Surgical repair within 2–3 weeks provides better results than delayed reconstruction.

41. **What is done to protect the UCL injury from further damage?**
Nondisplaced avulsion and UCL injuries without joint laxity do well with nonoperative management. Therefore, they are treated initially with immobilization in a thumb Spica splint/cast, with the thumb in slight extension for 4–6 weeks.

42. **What is the typical length of injury recovery for the gamekeeper's thumb? When can individuals return to play/regular activity?**

For nonoperative cases, patients can begin rehabilitation 3–4 weeks after diagnosis. For surgical cases, immobilization is for 4–5 weeks, followed by a 1- to 2-week period with time out of the splint for a range-of-motion activity. Full return to play occurs at 6–8 weeks for surgical and nonsurgical cases; however, some authors recommend protecting the thumb from excessive abduction during work or sports with a removable splint for 2–3 months after the injury.

KEY POINTS

1. Scaphoid fractures often do not show on initial radiographs.
2. Angulation of metacarpal fractures that indicate surgical intervention varies by metacarpal.
3. Mallet fingers often are treated nonoperatively, but jersey fingers need a surgical referral.
4. UCL of thumb injuries (gamekeeper's thumb) must determine if a Stener lesion exists.

Acknowledgments

The authors would like to thank Drs. Ariel Nassim, DO, Timothy Gill, MD, and Timothy Salkauskis, MD for their contributions to this chapter in the previous edition.

BIBLIOGRAPHY

Breahna A, et al. The management of acute fracture dislocations of proximal interphalangeal joints: a systematic review. *J Plast Surg Hand Surg*. 2020;54(6):323–327.

Dias JJ, et al. Acute scaphoid fractures: making decisions for treating a troublesome bone. *J Hand Sur (Europ Vol)*. 2021;47(1):73–79.

Eiff MP, et al. *Fracture Management for Primary Care*. Elsevier Saunders; 2018.

Forli A, et al. Recent and chronic sprains of the first metacarpo-phalangeal joint. *Orthopaedics & Traumatology: Surgery & Research*. 2022;108(1):103156.

Hoyt KS, Ramirez EG. Management of hand injuries: part III. *Adv Emerg Nurs J*. 2017;39(2):86–96.

Hussain MH, et al. Management of Fifth Metacarpal Neck Fracture (Boxer's Fracture): A Literature Review. *Cureus*. 2020. https://doi.org/10.7759/cureus.9442.

Krastman P, et al. Diagnostic accuracy of history taking, physical examination and imaging for non-chronic finger, hand and wrist ligament and tendon injuries: a systematic review update. *BMJ Open*. 2020;10(11).

Leggit J, Meko C. Acute finger injuries: part II: fractures, dislocations, and thumb injuries. *Am Fam Physician*. 2006;73:827–834, 839.

Nashi N, Sandeep JS. A pragmatic and evidence-based approach to mallet finger. *J Hand Surg (Asian-Pacific Vol)*. 2021;26(3):319–332.

CHAPTER 44

THE ACUTELY SWOLLEN KNEE

Teresa Coyle, DO, Mark E. Lavallee, MD, CSCS, FACSM, FAMSSM

TOP SECRETS

1. If possible, always obtain *weight-bearing* radiographs of the knee.
2. If septic arthritis is suspected, arthrocentesis for fluid analysis followed by parenteral antibiotics and urgent referral for surgical debridement is warranted.

1. **Why is it important to be competent in evaluating an acutely swollen knee?**
   The knee is the most frequently injured joint in the body, and an acutely swollen knee is a common presentation of knee pathology in the emergency department and primary care setting. Common causes of an effusion include inflammation, infection, and structural abnormalities in the knee. Most often, the underlying etiology can be treated conservatively until seen by orthopedics or another specialist. There are, however, a few diagnoses that need immediate treatment and close observation. Therefore, it is imperative that you formulate a comprehensive differential based on the obtained history and physical. Diagnostic studies and laboratory tests can then be used to narrow and confirm the diagnosis (Fig. 44.1). This chapter will focus on common causes and management of an acutely swollen knee.

2. **What is the most useful question to ask in your history to determine the etiology of an acutely swollen knee?**
   Is the effusion traumatic or nontraumatic? Mechanism of injury is important when evaluating a traumatic knee injury. Other key components of the history include timing of swelling after an injury, localization of pain, locking, giving way, and exacerbating factors. For a nontraumatic effusion, it is imperative to ask about fevers, night sweats, night pain, weight loss, other joints involved, and social history. You will start to formulate a solid differential based on a detailed history of present illness. Refer to Table 44.1 for a broad differential diagnosis of an acutely swollen knee.

3. **In the presence of trauma, what is the most important part of the physical examination of an acutely swollen knee?**
   Neurovascular exam! Get into the habit of always starting your exam by checking distal pulses, sensation, and strength at the ankle. The popliteal artery is especially at risk in the setting of knee dislocations. If knee dislocations are not quickly identified and there is vascular compromise, a high percentage of these patients will eventually require amputation.

4. **A 17-year-old female basketball player presents to your clinic complaining of an acutely swollen knee after hearing a loud "pop" when cutting to change direction through the paint. What is the most likely diagnosis?**
   ACL rupture. ACL ruptures will typically occur after a noncontact pivoting or with hyperextension of the knee. Oftentimes a loud "pop" is heard or felt, and the patient is usually unable to continue in sports participation due to associated instability. Physical examination will reveal a positive Lachman test, anterior drawer, and, potentially, pivot shift test. X-rays are generally unremarkable; MR imaging will confirm the diagnosis. Patients should be placed in a hinged knee brace until seen by orthopedics.

5. **What is a pathognomonic sign for ACL rupture on radiographs of the knee?**
   Segond fracture: an avulsion fracture of the lateral tibial condyle (bony attachment of soft tissue structures) as a result of abnormal varus stress to the knee, combined with internal rotation of the tibia. The fracture is best seen on the AP view above the level of the fibular head (Fig. 44.2).

6. **A 45-year-old female presents to your clinic with a complaint of a swollen knee that started 2 days ago after accidentally stepping into a pothole when running a 5K. She notes pain along the posteromedial joint line, especially with getting into and out of the car. She admits to locking of the knee upon standing from a seated position. X-rays are normal. What is the diagnosis?**
   Acute medial meniscal tear. Locking of the joint, intermittent swelling, and pain with weight-bearing twisting motions are typical of a meniscal injury. On exam, the patient is generally tender along the joint line with occasional inability to fully extend the knee. The Thessaly test has a higher sensitivity and specificity in detecting a meniscal tear on exam compared to the McMurray test. X-rays typically show no acute abnormality, and MRI will confirm the diagnosis. Inability to fully extend the knee is concerning for displaced "bucket handle" meniscal tear,

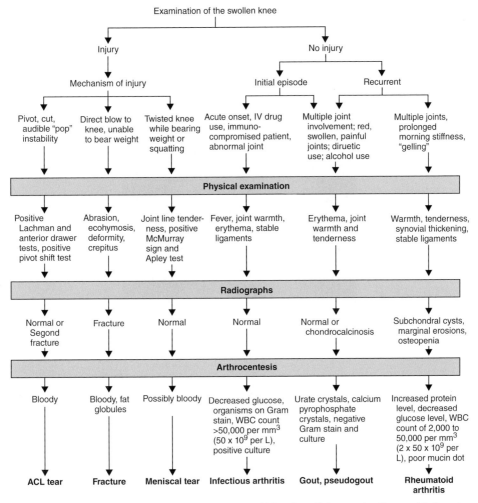

Fig. 44.1 Algorithm for the assessment of a swollen knee. (From Johnson M. Acute knee effusions: a systematic approach to diagnosis. *Am Fam Physician.* 2000;61(8):2391–2400.)

Table 44.1 Differential Diagnosis of the Acutely Swollen Knee	
TRAUMATIC	**NONTRAUMATIC**
Ligamentous injury	Osteoarthritis
Meniscal injury	Infection (lyme, bacterial, fungal, TB)
Knee dislocation	Crystal deposition
Patellar dislocation	Rheumatic disease
Intraarticular fracture	Tumor
Tendon rupture (quad/patellar)	Idiopathic synovitis/capsulitis
Prepatellar bursitis	Baker cyst
Baker cyst	

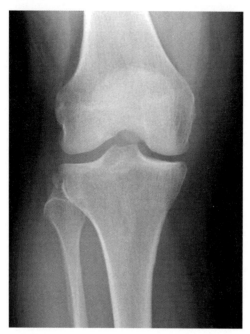

Fig. 44.2 Segond fracture with an associated ACL rupture. (Copyright 2023 Dr Gerry Gardner and Radiopaedia.org.)

and the patient should remain non–weight bearing until seen by orthopedics. Treatment of other meniscal injuries will depend on the patient's symptoms, age, comorbidities, and imaging studies.

7. **What is the most common mechanism for isolated PCL rupture?**
   A direct blow to the anterior proximal tibia with a flexed knee or a fall onto a flexed knee with the foot plantar-flexed. Most of these injuries will occur as a result of a dashboard injury in a motor vehicle accident or a high-energy collision in sport. Examination will be positive for posterior drawer test and possibly tibial sag test.

8. **How are isolated PCL injuries treated?**
   Many will be treated conservatively with protected weight bearing and therapy for range of motion and strengthening of the affected knee.

9. **What is a pathognomonic sign on radiographs for intraarticular fracture?**
   Lipohemarthrosis (fat-fluid level) is seen on the lateral view (Fig. 44.3).

10. **Who is susceptible to patellar dislocations and subluxations?**
    Patients with Down syndrome, Ehlers-Danlos syndrome, Marfan syndrome, cerebral palsy, generalized ligamentous laxity, and anatomical malalignment. Patients will generally be able to tell you that they felt their kneecap shift or slide out. On exam, patients will have a positive patellar apprehension sign and difficulty with a straight leg raise. Initial treatment should consist of immobilization of the knee.

11. **An 85-year-old male presents to your clinic complaining of progressive swelling of the left knee without injury or trauma. He describes stiffness in the morning and medial joint line pain made worse with any weight-bearing activity. What will you likely see on his weight-bearing radiographs?**
    The etiology of this patient's knee pain and swelling is osteoarthritis. His x-rays will show medial joint space narrowing with subchondral cysts and osteophyte formation. Typically, effusions secondary to osteoarthritis will reoccur after aspiration; therefore, treating the underlying cause in a progressive conservative approach is preferred. Stepwise progressive approach includes Tylenol, NSAIDs, therapy, bracing, corticosteroid injection, viscosupplementation injections for mild to moderate arthritis, and, finally, referral to a surgeon for joint replacement. Don't forget about weight loss in overweight and obese patients! One pound of weight loss results in a fourfold load reduction across a weight-bearing joint. It is reasonable to aspirate the knee if the effusion is severe enough to cause debilitation, such as limited range of motion and pain.

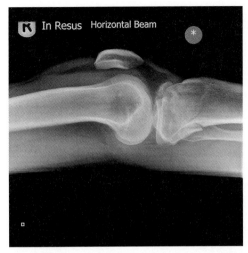

Fig. 44.3 Lipohemarthrosis with tibial plateau fracture. (Copyright 2023 Dr Jeremy Jones and Radiopaedia.org.)

12. **What are some causes of a nontraumatic, hot, painful, swollen knee?**
    Septic arthritis, gout, pseudogout, idiopathic synovitis/capsulitis, Lyme arthropathy, and rheumatoid arthritis. All of these disease entities can present with an acutely swollen knee that is erythematous, painful, and warm to the touch.

13. **What is the preferred diagnostic tool for a red, hot, painful, and acutely swollen knee?**
    Arthrocentesis to analyze the synovial fluid. Serum lab markers, including CBC, ESR, CRP, and blood cultures can be helpful in the workup of an acutely swollen knee; however, joint fluid analysis is the most sensitive investigation. Synovial fluid should be sent for the following analyses: cell count, gram stain, culture, crystals, Lyme PCR, glucose, and protein. Based on these results, a more accurate diagnosis and treatment plan can be made (Table 44.2). When possible, treatment should be withheld until joint fluid aspiration is performed.

14. **What are risk factors for a septic joint?**
    Age >60 years, diabetes, cancer, recent bacteremia, recent injury or surgical procedure, a prosthetic joint, recent history of corticosteroid injection, history of rheumatoid arthritis, renal disease, cirrhosis, and drug or alcohol abuse.

15. **What is the gold standard for diagnosing a septic joint?**
    The overall impression of an experienced clinician is the gold standard in diagnosing a septic joint. The presence of normal laboratory and radiologic studies does exclude the diagnosis of septic arthritis. If septic arthritis is suspected, advice from a musculoskeletal specialist should be sought as soon as possible, and treatment with antibiotics should not be delayed. Delayed or inadequate treatment can lead to irreversible joint damage and disability with a significant mortality rate of 11%.

16. **What is the most common bacterial pathogen in septic arthritis?**
    Staphylococci and *Streptococci* account for the majority of cases of bacterial arthritis. *Neisseria gonorrhea* is the most common pathogen in younger, sexually active individuals.

17. **What is the recommended treatment of septic arthritis?**
    IV antibiotics and debridement of the joint. Gram stain results of the joint aspirate should guide initial antibiotic choice. If the gram stain is negative but there is a strong clinical suspicion for bacterial arthritis, broad-spectrum antibiotics, such as Vancomycin and Ceftazidime, should be started until synovial fluid culture has returned.

18. **Can *Borrelia burgdorferi* be cultured in synovial fluid?**
    No; however, synovial fluid PCR testing can be used as a confirmatory test in patients with Lyme arthritis. The diagnosis of Lyme arthritis is made with a two-step serologic testing process involving an enzyme-linked immunosorbent assay, followed by confirmation with a Western blot or immunoblot test. Treatment includes 28 days of oral Doxycycline.

19. **What are the characteristic signs of crystalline arthropathy on radiographic imaging?**
    Chondrocalcinosis (Fig. 44.4).

Table 44.2 Synovial Fluid Analysis

DIAGNOSIS	COLOR	TRANSPARENCY	VISCOSITY	WBC PER mm³	PMN %	GRAM STAIN	CULTURE	PCR TEST	CRYSTALS
Normal	Clear	Transparent	High/thick	<200	<25	Negative	Negative	Negative	Negative
Noninflammatory	Straw	Translucent	High/thick	200–2000	<25	Negative	Negative	Negative	Negative
Inflammatory: crystal-line disease	Yellow	Cloudy	Low/thin	2000–100,000	>50	Negative	Negative	Negative	Positive
Inflammatory: noncrys-talline disease	Yellow	Cloudy	Low/thin	2000–100,000	>50	Negative	Negative	Negative	Negative
Infectious: Lyme Disease	Yellow	Cloudy	Low	3000–100,000	>50	Negative	Negative	Positive	Negative
Infectious: gonococcal	Yellow	Cloudy-opaque	Low	34,000–68,000	>75	Variable	Positive	Positive	Negative
Infectious: nongonococcal	Yellow-green	Cloudy	Very low	>50,000	>75	Positive	Positive	-	Negative

Credit: Horowitz D, Horowitz S. Approach to septic arthritis. *Am Fam Physician.* 2011;84(6):653–660. Table 3.

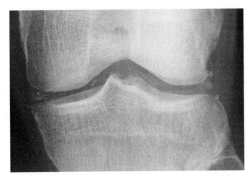

Fig. 44.4 Chondrocalcinosis seen in crystalline arthropathies. (Copyright 2023 Dr Henry Knipe and Radiopaedia.org.)

20. **How do crystals of gout and pseudogout differ?**
The urate crystals of gout appear as strongly negatively birefringent rods or needles when examined with a polarizing microscope, while calcium pyrophosphate crystals of pseudogout are weakly positively birefringent rectangles or rhomboids.

21. **What is the treatment for an acute gouty or pseudogout attack?**
NSAIDs, colchicine, or oral corticosteroids. With a diagnosis of gout, it is important to counsel the patient on dietary modifications, including alcohol restriction and decreased intake of foods high in purine.

22. **What are some common x-ray findings suggestive of rheumatoid arthritis?**
Joint space narrowing, bony erosions, and periarticular osteopenia. Severe deformity of the joint can be seen in more advanced diseases.

23. **What type of bony tumors are associated with knee effusions?**
Both benign and malignant tumors can present as knee effusions. Plain radiographs will usually rule out a bone lesion. Based on the patient's history and lesion characteristics on radiographs, further evaluation with gadolinium-enhanced MRI may be warranted.

24. **What should be on your differential for types of bony tumors?**
The most common malignant tumors are osteosarcoma, Ewing sarcoma, multiple myeloma, lymphoma, metastasis, and chondrosarcoma. The most common benign tumors are enchondromas, osteochondromas, nonossifying fibromas, osteoid osteoma, osteoblastomas, giant cell tumors, periosteal chondromas, chondromyxoid fibromas, and PVNS. Certain tumors are more likely to be found in the epiphysis, metaphysis, or diaphysis of long bones.

25. **What is PVNS?**
Pigmented villonodular synovitis is a subtype of a tenosynovial giant cell tumor that diffusely affects the soft tissue lining of joints and tendons and is slow-growing. Patients will often present with unexplained painless swelling in the affected joint. Initial x-rays will often show soft tissue swelling and bony erosion of the affected joint. MRI is the most sensitive imaging. The gold standard of treatment is surgical excision with total synovectomy of the affected joint.

26. **Do Baker cysts need to be aspirated?**
No. A Baker cyst is a benign swelling in the popliteal fossa that arises from the synovium of the knee. It is generally associated with osteoarthritis or occasionally a meniscal tear. Treatment should be directed toward the underlying cause. Unless the cyst is large enough to cause pain due to a mass effect on surrounding structures, it does not require aspiration.

KEY POINTS

1. In the absence of trauma, do not proceed initially to MR imaging of the knee.
2. Always start your knee exam by checking neurovascular status.
3. The best diagnostic tool for an acute nontraumatic knee effusion is arthrocentesis for synovial fluid analysis.
4. Detailed history and comprehensive exam are imperative when working up an acutely swollen knee.
5. Crystalline disease can coexist with septic arthritis; positive fluid analysis for crystals does not exclude infection.

BIBLIOGRAPHY

Andrade NF. Teixeira MJ, Araújo LH, Ponte CE. Knee bone tumors: findings on conventional radiology. *Radiol Bras*. 2016;49(3):182–189. doi:10.1590/0100-3984.2013.0007.

Elsissy JG, Liu JN, Wilton PJ, Nwachuku I, Gowd AK, Amin NH. Bacterial septic arthritis of the adult native knee joint: a review. *JBJS Rev*. 2020;8(1):e0059. doi:10.2106/JBJS.RVW.19.00059.

Fecek C, Carter KR. Pigmented Villonodular Synovitis. In: *StatPearls*. StatPearls Publishing; June 11, 2022.

Gupte C, St. Mart JP. The acute swollen knee: diagnosis and management. *J R Soc Med*. 2013;106:259–268.

Guyver PM, Arthur CHC, et al. The acutely swollen knee. Part two: management of traumatic pathology. *J Roy Nav Med Serv* 2014;100(2):186–192.

Guyver PM, Arthur CHC, et al. The acutely swollen knee. Part 1: management of atraumatic pathology. *J Roy Nav Med Serv*. 2014;100(1):24–33.

Horowitz D, Horowitz S. Approach to septic arthritis. *Am Fam Physician*. 2011;84(6):653–660.

Johnson M. Acute knee effusions: a systematic approach to diagnosis. *Am Fam Physician*. 2000;61(8):2391–2400.

Messier S, Gutekunst D, et al. Weight loss reduces knee-joint loads in overweight and obese older adults with knee osteoarthritis. *Arthritis Rheum*. 2005;52(7):2026–2032.

Sillanpää PJ, Kannus P, et al. Incidence of knee dislocation and concomitant vascular injury requiring surgery: a nationwide study. *J Trauma Acute Care Surg*. 2014;76(3):715.

CHAPTER 45

THE ACUTELY LIMPING CHILD

Jillian E. Sylvester, MD, CAQSM, FAAFP, Mina M. Cunningham, MD

TOP SECRETS

1. Transient synovitis is the most common cause of a limping child.
2. A child with septic arthritis will usually appear more ill than those with transient synovitis. Hip aspiration is the gold standard for diagnosis.

1. **Why is an acutely limping child a serious concern?**
   Limping is a common chief complaint, accounting for up to 4% of pediatric emergency room visits. The differential diagnosis of an acute limp in children varies by age. Most cases are benign; some are due to serious, life-threatening conditions, where delays in recognition and treatment can result in significant morbidity and mortality. A careful history and comprehensive physical examination combined with laboratory studies and imaging are often needed to arrive at a final working diagnosis (Fig. 45.1).

2. **What exactly is a limp?**
   A limp is an abnormal gait pattern that causes uneven, jerky, or painful movements. Antalgic limps are most common, caused by pain at the hip, knee, ankle, heel, or back. In this limp, the stance portion of the gait is shortened to limit the limb's contact time with the ground in an effort to reduce pain. A Trendelenburg gait occurs when weak hip abductors cause the contralateral hip to drop during the swing phase. This gait can be seen in developmental dysplasia of the hip (DDH), coxa vera, Legg-Calvé-Perthes (LCP), or slipped capital femoral epiphysis (SCFE) and can occur with or without pain.

   Spastic, short-limb, or proximal-weakness gaits are typically painless and develop over time. They may be indicative of neuromuscular disorders, hypertonicity, or leg length discrepancy.

3. **What is a normal gait pattern for a child?**
   Independent walking typically begins at 12–14 months. The initial "toddler" gait typically has a wider base, increased time in double leg stance, faster gait cadence, and often a toe-to-heel foot pattern. A child's gait matures between ages 3 and 5, and they have an adult gait pattern by age 7.

4. **What are the most common causes of pediatric hip pain?**
   The differential diagnosis for limping in children is very broad (Table 45.1). Idiopathic transient synovitis is the most common cause of pediatric hip pain in children under 10 years old, especially in boys ages 4–8. The etiology is unclear, but theories suggest a correlation with recent viral infection. This condition typically resolves in 1–2 weeks without long-term morbidity. Treatment includes rest, nonsteroidal antiinflammatory drugs (NSAIDs), and reassurance.

5. **What is the most life-threatening cause of acute limp in the pediatric patient?**
   Septic arthritis of the hip is very serious. A fast diagnosis is critical, as treatment delays increase the risk of sepsis, growth arrest, permanent loss of joint function, and osteonecrosis. Septic arthritis presents similarly to transient synovitis, although patients often appear more toxic and may be febrile. Septic arthritis can occur in all pediatric age groups. The patient may hold their thigh in a flexed and abducted position and have pain with passive movement of the hip.

6. **What is the key factor in forming the differential diagnosis for an acutely limping child?**
   Age can be very helpful in forming a differential. Table 45.2 lists some common causes of limping by age. Subtle limps can be missed until they become more pronounced, so examiners should maintain a wide differential when examining a new limp.

7. **What are the most important components of the history?**
   A careful history is crucial to help hone what is otherwise a wide differential (see Table 45.1). Mnemonics can be useful in obtaining a thorough history of events. Table 45.3 provides one such prompt. It is valuable to interview caregivers, particularly when children are too young to reliably describe events. Keep in mind to ask about family history, recent illnesses, travel history, and any previous treatments for the limp. When there is suspicion of nonaccidental trauma or sexually transmitted infection exposure, the child or adolescent should be interviewed separately.

8. **How best should the examiner initiate a physical examination, particularly in young children?**
   As young children are often apprehensive in medical settings, begin with the least painful and intimidating component. Evaluate the child's general appearance, vital signs, and resting position of their affected limb. In hip effusion, children naturally hold a flexed, abducted, and externally rotated hip position for comfort. Take care to look for bruising, erythema, or rashes. Pay close attention to the child's gait, especially how the foot strikes

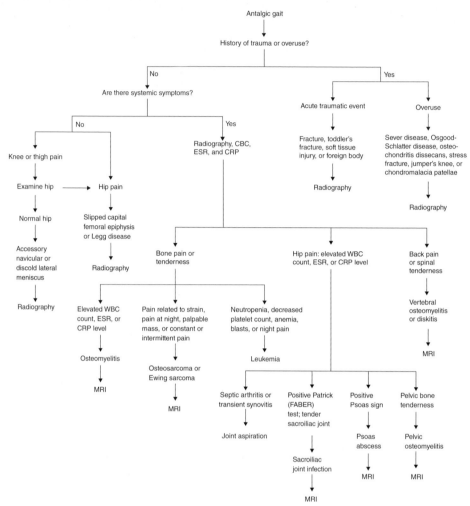

Fig. 45.1 Algorithm for approaching the acutely limping pediatric patient. (From Sawyer JR, Kapoor M. The limping child: a systematic approach to diagnosis. *Am Fam Physician.* 2009;79(3):215–224. PMID: 19202969.)

Table 45.1 Possible Causes of Limp in a Child	
Traumatic/Mechanical	Fracture, DDH, SCFE, tarsal coalition, child abuse, overuse injury, leg length discrepancy, osteochondritis dissecans, traction apophysitis, Blount disease, congenital Achilles contracture, coxa vara, osteochondrosis
Infectious	Septic arthritis, osteomyelitis, Lyme disease, psoas abscess, diskitis, appendicitis, gonococcal arthritis, myositis
Inflammatory	Transient synovitis, inflammatory arthritis, systemic lupus erythematosus, juvenile rheumatoid arthritis, Henoch-Schoenlein purpura
Vascular	Legg-Calvé-Perthes disease, osteonecrosis, sickle cell disease
Neoplastic	Leukemia, lymphoma, Ewing sarcoma, osteogenic sarcoma
Metabolic	Rickets, hyperparathyroidism
Neuromuscular	Muscular dystrophy, cerebral palsy, peripheral neuropathy

Table 45.2 Differential Diagnosis of Limping in Children by Age	
AGE GROUP	**MOST COMMON CAUSE OF LIMP**
Early Walker (up to age 3)	*Painful Limp* Septic arthritis and osteomyelitis Transient synovitis Occult trauma ("toddler's fracture") Intervertebral diskitis Malignancy Nonaccidental injury (child abuse) Foreign body in foot *Painless Limp* DDH Neuromuscular disorder Cerebral palsy Leg length discrepancy
Child (ages 4–10)	*Painful Limp* Septic arthritis, osteomyelitis, myositis Transient synovitis Trauma Rheumatologic disorders Intervertebral diskitis Malignancy Osteochondrosis (Kohler disease) Tibia Vara (Blount Disease) *Painless Limp* DDH LCP* Leg length discrepancy Neuromuscular disorder Cerebral palsy Muscular dystrophy (Duchenne)
Adolescent (age 11 to maturity)	*Painful Limp* Septic arthritis, osteomyelitis, myositis Trauma Rheumatologic disorder SCFE: acute, unstable Malignancy Overuse injury *Painless Limp* SCFE: chronic, stable* DDH/acetabular dysplasia* Leg length discrepancy Neuromuscular disorder

*Can be painful or painless.
(From Walter KD, Tassone, JC. Orthopedic Assessment. In: Nelson Essentials of Pediatrics. Marcdante KJ, Kliegman RM, eds. 7th ed. Elsevier; 2015:667–669.)

the floor, the amount of time spent in the stance phase, and the degree of motion at the ankle, knee, and hip as compared to the unaffected side. Fever, lethargy, inconsolability, inability, or refusal to bear weight, and holding their limb in a fixed position should increase suspicion for a more serious underlying condition.

9. **Describe an approach to the examination of the lower limb.**
A systematic examination of the spine, abdomen, and lower extremities decreases the chances of missed exam findings. In children with localizing symptoms, examination should not be limited to the painful joint, as pain can often be referred. Pain localized to the knee warrants careful examination of the ipsilateral hip; thigh pain can be referred from the spine.

From a supine position, expose and examine the extremity for edema, effusion, or gross deformity. Palpate the spine and affected extremity to evaluate for any focal pain. Evaluate range of motion in all joints as well as the spine. Obligate external rotation in hip flexion can be seen in SCFE. Limited hip internal rotation is concerning for

Table 45.3 SOCRATES Mnemonic for Painful Limp History

SITE	WHERE IS THE PAIN LOCALIZED? (IF APPLICABLE)
Onset	When did the limp begin and what was the child doing at that time? Was there any prior, even minor, trauma? Any change in physical activity to suggest overuse?
Character	Is the limp constant or intermittent? What kind of pain (achy, sharp, burning)?
Radiation	Does the pain radiate to other joints or other areas?
Associations	Any associated symptoms, such as fever, chills, weight loss, change in appetite, or night sweats?
Timing	What time of day does it begin? When is pain the worst? Have symptoms improved or worsened over time? Have they sought treatment for this before?
Exacerbating or Relieving factors	What activities make the limp worse (i.e., standing, jumping, bending, walking a distance)? What, if anything, makes it better? Any successful home treatments?
Severity	How would they rate the pain? How does it affect their daily life?

intra-articular pathology, including septic arthritis, LCP, and SCFE. Internal hip rotation is most easily visualized from the prone position with knees flexed to 90 degrees.

10. **Which imaging modality is the best initial test?**
Plain radiographs are the preferred first-line imaging modality. Imaging should begin with the painful joint; however, in the case of knee pain, frog-leg lateral radiographs of the hip are useful for diagnosing DDH, LCP, and SCFE.
In children under 5 with an acute limp without localizing symptoms or suspicion of infection, the American College of Radiology recommends starting with radiographs of the tibia and fibula to evaluate for occult fracture. In older children with a nonlocalized limp, imaging should begin with frog-leg lateral radiographs.

11. **Is there a role for ultrasound or MRI?**
Ultrasound is highly sensitive for detecting hip effusion but is not very sensitive for discerning among hemorrhagic, sterile, and purulent fluid accumulations. Ultrasound is also preferred when suspecting septic arthritis, as it may also facilitate hip aspiration. Magnetic resonance imaging (MRI) is highly sensitive and specific for visualizing the joint, soft tissue, and cartilage, thus making it the preferred method for diagnosing osteomyelitis and stress fractures.

12. **What clinical features help distinguish and predict septic arthritis?**
Kocher criteria are a risk stratification tool used to predict the risk of septic arthritis. When two or more of the following features are present, the risk of septic arthritis is 40%: (1) refusal to bear weight, (2) temperature >38.5°C, (3) erythrocyte sedimentation rate (ESR) >40 mm/hr or C-Reactive Protein (CRP) >20, and (4) white blood cell count (WBC) >12,000.

13. **What is the gold standard for diagnosing septic arthritis?**
Hip aspiration is the gold standard for diagnosing septic arthritis and should be performed whenever a septic joint is suspected. Aspirated fluid should be analyzed for culture/sensitivity, Gram stain, glucose, and WBC count. Treatment includes surgical drainage and/or antibiotics for a minimum of 3 weeks to cover *Staphylococcus*, *Streptococcus*, and *Neisseria* pathogens. Approximately 25% of patients will have long-term sequelae even after appropriate treatment with antibiotics.

14. **What is a toddler's fracture?**
A toddler's fracture is a spiral, oblique, nondisplaced fracture of the distal tibial shaft in children 9 months to 3 years of age. This fracture is caused by a rotational or twisting force through the tibia while on a planted foot. If the history is unclear, keep a high index of suspicion for child abuse. Plain x-ray is only 53% sensitive for detecting fracture, so bone scintigraphy can be useful degree of suspicion remains high after negative x-rays. Treatment is immobilization in a walking boot for 4 weeks.

15. **What is developmental dysplasia of the hip?**
DDH is a congenital abnormal hip development that, depending on severity, can go undetected for many years. Patients will have a painless limp, Trendelenburg gait, or waddling gait. They may also have leg shortening, abnormal skin creases in the leg, positive Galeazzi sign, and limited hip abduction. All cases of DDH should be referred promptly for orthopedic consultation.

16. **What is LCP and how is it treated?**
LCP is caused by an interruption of blood supply to the capital femoral epiphysis, causing osteonecrosis and chondronecrosis. The etiology remains unclear. It is most commonly seen in males ages 4–9 years old and can present

with a painless limp, knee pain, or lower back pain. Common physical findings include leg length discrepancy, limited abduction and internal rotation, and the presence of a Trendelenburg gait. Anteroposterior (AP) and frog-leg lateral hip radiographs are essential in LCP; MRI can confirm osteonecrosis but is often unnecessary. These children should be referred for orthopedic consultation. Initial treatment of LCP includes rest, typically with crutches, with concomitant physical therapy to help maintain range of motion.

17. **What is the most common cause of hip pain in boys older than 11 years?**
    SCFE is the most common hip disorder in early adolescence, predominantly affecting males and those of African American and Pacific Islander descent. In SCFE, the proximal femoral epiphysis slips posteriorly and inferiorly on the femoral neck through the growth plate. The peak age of diagnosis is 13 for boys and 11 for girls. Obesity is a risk factor, and it can occur bilaterally 25–40% of the time.

18. **How does SCFE typically present?**
    Children with SCFE usually present with a limp and pain in the groin, hip, thigh, or knee. On exam, the affected hip is slightly flexed and externally rotated. The hallmark of SCFE on examination is limited internal rotation of the hip. Greater limitation of internal rotation when the hip is flexed to 90 degrees is pathognomonic. No other pediatric condition has this physical finding, which makes this maneuver very useful in children with lower extremity pain.
    Radiographs should include frog-leg lateral views and AP views of both hips.

19. **How is SCFE treated?**
    Urgent orthopedic consultation is advised if SCFE is suspected. Definitive treatment is operative internal fixation, typically occurring within days of diagnosis. The child should remain non-weight-bearing until surgery. Chronic complications can develop from severe displacement, such as avascular necrosis and leg length discrepancy.

20. **What condition involves a growth disturbance of the medial tibial physis?**
    Blount disease, or tibia vara, is common in obese children between the ages of 10 and 14 but can also occur in children as young as 2 years old. More prevalent in African Americans, this condition is typically described as a chronic progressive limp and should be considered whenever evaluating a limping child. Often these children have a leg length discrepancy and tenderness at the medial tibial physis. Plain radiographs are best for diagnosis. Referral to a pediatric orthopedic surgeon is indicated for surgical intervention.

KEY POINTS

1. In a young child, knee pain is hip pain until proven otherwise.
2. Consider abuse if a child presents with a fracture after an unwitnessed trauma and the story does not match the injury pattern.
3. The differential diagnosis of an acute limp varies by age. Transient synovitis is the most common cause of a limping child.
4. SCFE is more common in boys >11 years old, and LCP is more common in boys <10 years old.
5. A child with septic arthritis will usually appear more ill than those with transient synovitis. Hip aspiration is the gold standard for diagnosis.

Acknowledgments
The authors would like to thank Dr. Eric Requa and Dr. Mark Lavallee for their contributions to this chapter in the previous edition.

BIBLIOGRAPHY
Herman MJ, Martinek M. The limping child. *Pediatr Rev.* 2015;36(5):184–197.
Hill D, Whiteside J. Limp in children: differentiating benign from dire causes. *J Fam Pract.* 2011;60(4):193–197.
Naranje S, Kelly DM, Sawyer JR. A systematic approach to the evaluation of a limping child. *Am Fam Physician.* 2015;92(10):908–916.
Payares-Lizano M. The limping child. *Pediatr Clin N Am.* 2020;67:119–138.
Thomas A, Ramachandran M. The limping child. In: Aresti NA, et al., eds. *Paediatric Orthopaedics in Clinical Practice in Clinical Practice.* Springer-Verlag; 2016:11–22.

CHAPTER 46

ANKLE SPRAINS

Charles W. Webb, DO, FAMSSM, FAAFP, CAQSM, Peter S. Seidenberg, MD, MA, FAAFP, FACSM, RMSK

TOP SECRETS

1. Imaging should only be done when the Ottawa criteria are met.
2. Cryotherapy, bracing or taping, and early mobilization are the mainstays of therapy.

1. **What is an ankle sprain?**
An ankle sprain occurs when one or more ligaments stretch beyond their limits. Ligaments serve to provide mechanical stability, directed motion, and proprioceptive information for the joint. Ankle sprains can occur laterally to the ATFL (anterior talofibular), the CFL (calcaneofibular), and PTFL (posterior talofibular) ligaments, medially to the deltoid ligament, and to the syndesmosis (high ankle sprain). Each of these can range from mild to severe, depending on how much damage there is to the ligament (e.g., stretching, partial rupture, or complete rupture). This chapter focuses on lateral and high ankle sprains.

2. **What is the classification scheme for lateral ankle sprains and the associated signs and symptoms?**
Each ligament is graded according to its individual severity of injury.
Grade I: Mild sprain resulting from ligamentous stretch without macroscopic tearing. Mild swelling or tenderness. No mechanical instability. No loss of function or motion.
Grade II: Moderate sprain resulting from partial macroscopic tearing of the ligaments. Moderate swelling, ecchymosis, and tenderness. Mild to moderate instability. Slight loss of motion. Moderate pain with weight bearing and ambulation.
Grade III: Severe sprain resulting from complete ligamentous rupture. Severe swelling, ecchymosis, tenderness, and pain. Significant mechanical instability. Loss of function and motion. Inability to bear weight.

3. **What is the incidence of lateral ankle sprains?**
Lateral ankle ligament injuries are among the most common orthopedic injuries encountered in the primary care office and emergency department.
The incidence of ankle sprains in the United States is 2.15 per 1000 person-years, with teenagers and young adults (15–19 years of age) having the highest rates, with a peak incidence of 7.2 per 1000 person-years.
No difference in the incidence of ankle sprains between men and women.
Slight preponderance in Caucasians and African Americans compared with other ethnicities.
Approximately half of acute ankle sprains occur during athletic activity, most commonly basketball.
Increased incidence in those who are near overweight and overweight (body mass index [BMI] >25).

4. **What are the risk factors for ankle sprains, both intrinsic (patient-related) and extrinsic (e.g., sports or environmental)?**
Intrinsic risk factors include limited dorsiflexion, reduced proprioception, and deficiencies in postural control/balance. In addition, the risk of sustaining an ankle sprain is increased by elevated BMI (>25); high medial plantar pressures during running (overpronation); decreased strength, coordination, and cardiovascular endurance; and anatomical abnormalities of the ankle and/or knee alignment.
The extrinsic risk factors include the type of sport (basketball, indoor volleyball, field sports, and climbing), participating on grass versus artificial turf, position played (soccer defense), wearing heels, and anatomical abnormalities of the ankle and/or knee alignment.
Girls have a higher risk for ankle sprains out of competition and boys have a higher risk when in competition.
The greatest risk factor for ankle sprain remains a previous ankle sprain that has not been appropriately rehabilitated.

5. **What are the signs and symptoms of acute ankle sprain?**
Pain, swelling, tenderness, ecchymosis, difficulty with weight bearing.

6. **What are the long-term effects of repeated ankle sprains?**
Repeated ligamentous injuries may result in chronic ankle instability (CAI), degenerative bony changes, and chronic pain. Despite initial treatment consisting of taping/bracing and physical rehabilitation, up to 40% of patients will develop CAI.

7. **What are the prognostic factors for CAI?**
Known unfavorable prognostic factors for the development of CAI are an inability to complete jumping and landing within 2 weeks after a first-time ankle sprain, deficiencies in postural control, and a lack of ankle proprioception,

with increased ligament laxity 8 weeks after ankle sprain. Other factors include sports participation at high levels, being a young male, and a BMI greater than 25.

ANATOMY

8. Describe the ligamentous anatomy of the ankle joint.
The ligamentous complexes of the ankle include the lateral, deltoid, and syndesmotic ankle ligaments, which in addition to the surrounding musculotendinous structures provide dynamic stability to the ankle joint (Fig. 46.1).

9. What comprises the lateral ligamentous complex of the ankle joint?
The lateral ankle ligamentous complex is composed of the anterior talofibular (ATFL), calcaneofibular (CFL), and posterior talofibular (PTFL) ligaments.

10. Describe the anatomy and function of the anterior talofibular ligament (ATFL)
The ATFL is a flat band that extends anteromedially from the anterior border of the lateral malleolus and inserts onto the lateral neck of the talus. It is taut in plantarflexion and loose in dorsiflexion and prevents internal rotation and adduction of the talus. It is relatively weak and has the lowest load to failure among the other lateral ankle ligaments and is thus the most commonly injured ankle ligament.

11. Describe the anatomy and function of the calcaneofibular ligament (CFL).
The CFL is a round, cord-like, extracapsular ligament that is confluent with the peroneal tendon sheath. It passes posteroinferiorly from the distal tip of the lateral malleolus and inserts onto the lateral calcaneus. The CFL is slack in plantarflexion and tense in dorsiflexion, preventing adduction of the talus within the talocrural joint.

12. Describe the anatomy and function of the posterior talofibular ligament (PTFL).
The PTFL is a capsular ligament that extends from the posteromedial aspect of the lateral malleolus and inserts onto the posterolateral aspect of the body of the talus. It has maximal tension in ankle dorsiflexion and prevents external rotation of the ankle while dorsiflexed.

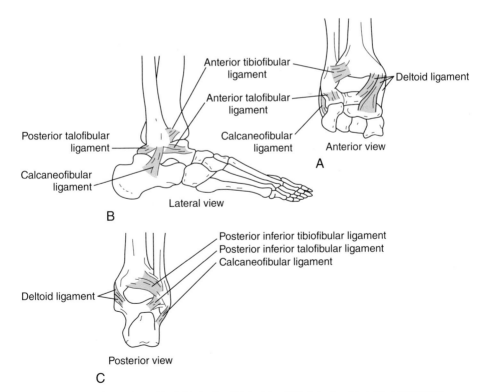

Fig. 46.1 Ligamentous anatomy of the ankle. (A) Anterior view. (B) Lateral view. (C) Posterior view. (Adapted from Pommering TL, Kluchursky L, Hall SL. *Prim Care Clin Office Pract.* 2005;32:133.)

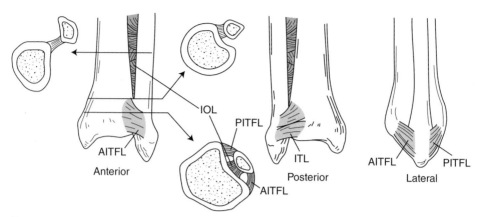

Fig. 46.2 Anterior, posterior, and lateral views (from left to right) of syndesmosis anatomy demonstrating the location and relationship of the anterior inferior talofibular ligament (AITFL), interosseous ligament (IOL), inferior transverse tibiofibular ligament (ITL), and posterior inferior tibiofibular ligament (PITFL). (Adapted from Hsu AR, Garras DN, Lee S. *Oper Tech Sports Med.* 2014;22:270.)

13. What is the syndesmosis?

The distal tibiofibular joint is a fibrous syndesmotic articulation consisting of the concave surface of the distal tibia and the convex shape of the distal fibula. The syndesmotic ligamentous complex connects the tibia and fibula through four ligamentous structures.

The interosseous ligament (IOL) extends from the fibular notch of the tibia to the medial surface of the distal fibula. It travels superiorly with the interosseous membrane running the length of the tibia and fibula and forms the principal connection between them. It is strengthened by the anterior-inferior tibiofibular ligament (AITFL) and posterior-inferior tibiofibular ligament (PITFL), which extend from the fibular notch of the tibia to the anterior and posterior surfaces of the lateral malleolus, respectively. The deep, inferior portion of the PITFL is called the inferior transverse ligament (ITL) and functions to reinforce the posterior capsule of the ankle joint (Fig. 46.2).

HIGH ANKLE SPRAIN

14. What is a high ankle sprain?

A high ankle sprain (syndesmotic injury) is a sprain of the distal syndesmotic ligaments that connect the tibia and fibula in the lower leg. They occur less frequently in the general population, comprising approximately 0.5% of ankle sprains without fracture and 13% of all ankle fractures. They occur more commonly in collision sports, including football, ice hockey, and soccer.

15. What is the classification scheme for high ankle sprains?

Several classification schemes have been developed without consensus based on the duration of symptoms, the number of ligaments involved, the level of diastasis, clinical findings, and radiographic and magnetic resonance imaging (MRI) criteria.

16. Describe stable versus unstable acute high ankle sprains.

A stable injury is characterized by a lesion to the AITFL without involvement of the deltoid ligament. An unstable ankle sprain is classified as either a latent or frank diastasis. Latent diastasis involves rupture of the AITFL with or without IOL and the deltoid ligament rupture. It can be detected on stress radiographs, MRI, and/or arthroscopic assessment. Frank diastasis involves the rupture of all syndesmotic and deltoid ligaments. It can be detected on the mortise view of standard ankle radiographs.

17. What is the mechanism for high ankle sprain?

Several mechanisms of injury have been proposed for the cause of high ankle sprains, including pronation-abduction, pronation-eversion, supination-eversion, external rotation, supination-abduction, and dorsiflexion. The typical mechanism of injury is hyper-dorsiflexion and external rotation of the foot in relation to the tibia. They are often associated with further soft tissue injury and fractures, which may lead to significant ankle instability.

18. How do you diagnose high ankle sprains?

   Clinical diagnosis is made by mechanically separating the distal tibia and fibula, stressing the syndesmosis, and causing pain. Various stress tests are used to clinically evaluate the integrity of the syndesmosis: (A) squeezing the lower leg at mid-calf (Squeeze Test); (B) having the patient cross their legs with the injured leg resting at mid-calf on the knee (Crossed-Leg Test); and (C) externally rotating the ankle with the foot dorsiflexed (Rotation Test) (Table 46.1).

19. What are the radiographic signs of syndesmotic injury?

   X-ray radiographs with anteroposterior (AP), lateral, and mortise views can be used to assess syndesmotic injury.

   Decreased tibiofibular overlap (normal >6 mm on AP view and >1 mm on mortise view).

   Increased medial gutter clear space at the distal talus and medial malleolus (normal ≤4 mm).

   Increased tibiofibular clear space at 1 cm above the tibial articulation (normal <6 mm on both AP and mortise views) or a difference >2 mm when compared to the contralateral ankle.

20. What are the long-term sequela of high ankle sprain?

   Syndesmosis injuries generally require significantly more time to heal compared with patients who have lateral ankle sprains. Early diagnosis and appropriate management are necessary to avoid long-term sequela, including reinjury, discomfort due to impingement from scar tissue, articular degeneration, increased risk of osteoarthritis, chronic instability, formation of heterotopic ossification, and deformity of the ankle joint.

DIAGNOSIS

21. What are the physical examination tests for diagnosing ankle sprains (Table 46.1).

22. What are the guidelines for obtaining ankle radiographs?

   The Ottawa Ankle Rules are guidelines indicating that x-ray studies should be obtained if there is pain in the malleolar zone and (A) bony tenderness at the distal 6 cm of the fibula, (B) bony tenderness at the distal 6 cm of the tibia, or (C) inability to take four steps immediately after injury. The Ottawa Foot Rules indicate that x-rays should be obtained if there is pain in the midfoot zone and: (A) bony tenderness at the base of the fifth metatarsal, (B) bony tenderness at the navicular bone, or (C) inability to take four steps immediately after injury (Fig. 46.3).

Table 46.1 Physical Examination Tests for Diagnosing Ankle Sprains

TESTS	DESCRIPTION	INJURY
Anterior Drawer Test	Anterior translation force applied to the ankle by grasping the plantar heel and holding the foot in neutral position (plantar flexed 10–15 degrees and slightly inverted) while stabilizing the distal leg. Anterior translation indicates a positive test.	ATFL
Talar Tilt Test	Inversion stress applied to the ankle with the foot held in neutral position and the distal leg stabilized. The degree of inversion is compared to the uninjured side.	CFL
External Rotation Test	External rotation and dorsiflexion of the foot with the knee flexed at 90 degrees and the ankle in neutral position. Pain indicates a positive test.	Syndesmotic Complex
Squeeze Test	Medial and lateral compression of the leg at the mid-calf level. Pain at the ankle indicates a positive test.	Syndesmotic Complex
Fibular Translation Test	Anterior and posterior translation force applied to the distal fibula with the tibia stabilized. Pain and increased translation of the fibula indicate a positive test.	Syndesmotic Complex
Cotton Test	Lateral translation force applied to the talus within the ankle mortise by grasping the plantar heel and stabilizing the proximal ankle. Pain indicates a positive test.	Syndesmotic Complex
Crossed-Leg Test	Having the patient cross their legs with the injured leg resting at mid-calf on the knee	Syndesmotic Complex

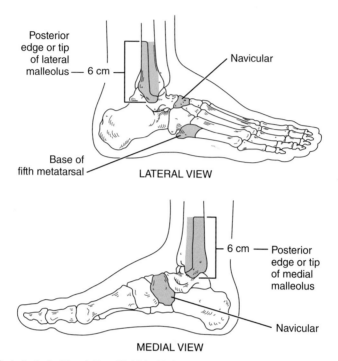

Fig. 46.3 Sites of palpation for the Ottawa Ankle and Foot Rules. Tenderness over the shaded areas warrants further radiographic evaluation. (Adapted from Seidenberg, et al., eds. *Sports Medicine Resource Manual.* W.B. Saunders; 2008:358.

TREATMENT

23. Describe the initial treatment for acute ankle sprains.
The treatment of ankle sprains in the acute phase of injury focuses on minimizing swelling, pain control, protection from further injury, and promotion of healing. The essential components of treatment include PRICEMMMS (an extension of RICE). This extension includes the use of exercise therapy for mobility and medications for pain. Otherwise, there is no solid evidence for the use of RICE alone in the treatment of acute ankle sprains.

24. What is PRICEMMMS?
Protection from further injury by restricting inversion and eversion stress (e.g., ankle bracing or taping) and employing crutches, depending on the ability of the individual to bear weight.
   Rest to avoid further exacerbation of pain.
   Ice applied to the ankle to achieve a numbing effect. Most of the evidence points to the use of ice applied to the injury for 20 minutes every 2 hours; however, when compared to a protocol of 10 minutes on, 10 minutes off, and 10 minutes on every 2 hours for 3 days while awake, this intermittent protocol demonstrated greater pain relief. Both protocols had similar pain and functional outcomes at 1 week.
   Compression aids in edema reabsorption. ACE wraps and compression stockings may be effective alone. However, studies demonstrate increased efficacy with bracing and taping combined with functional mobility.
   Elevation above the level of the heart improves venous return and decreases swelling; however, there is no conclusive evidence.
   Medications (e.g., NSAIDs, analgesics) aid in reducing pain; however, the antiinflammatory aspect of some of these medications may actually prolong healing time.
   Modalities (e.g., electrical stimulation, ultrasound) may be used for pain control, maintenance of strength, and range of motion.
   Mobilization should begin early and include active, pain-free plantarflexion and dorsiflexion.
   Strength training should begin early, focusing on the peroneal (fibularis) and gastrocnemius muscles.

25. Describe the process of functional rehabilitation in the treatment of ankle sprain.
The primary goals of rehabilitation are regaining normal function and strength while preventing future reinjury. Functional rehabilitation is an extension of traditional elements of physical therapy with the purpose of slowly

progressing the patient in a step-wise fashion from simple activities (e.g., walking or jogging) back to highly complex movement patterns that require refined levels of proprioceptive acuity (e.g., sporting activities).

26. **What are the stages of functional rehabilitation?**
Functional rehabilitation progresses through three general stages: acute, early rehabilitation, and late functional rehabilitation.

27. **Describe the acute stage of functional rehabilitation.**
The acute stage focuses on minimizing pain, promoting healing, and protection from further injury. It typically lasts 1–3 days and includes PRICEMMS.

28. **Describe the early rehabilitation stage of functional rehabilitation.**
The early rehabilitation stage focuses on early mobilization to reestablish full range of motion (e.g., ankle pumps), regain strength (e.g., resistance exercise bands), normalize neuromuscular control, restore proprioception and balance (e.g., balance board), improve endurance, and maintain cardiovascular fitness (e.g., strength training, water jogging, swimming, and cycling). It aims for a safe return to physical activity and typically lasts from several days to weeks.

29. **Describe the late rehabilitation stage of functional rehabilitation.**
The late functional rehabilitation stage includes advanced-phase rehabilitation activities that focus on regaining normal function as well as exercises specific to those performed during athletics or sports (e.g., sport-specific drills) accelerated in a gradual fashion. Lack of proper, gradual, step-wise rehabilitation places the patient at risk for recurrent and more severe ankle injury, with the potential to develop into chronic functional instability.

30. **What are some of the other commonly used therapeutic modalities and their evidence for use?**
Other treatment modalities do not always show the effect on pain, swelling, function, or quicker return to activity. Among these are therapeutic ultrasound, electrotherapy, shortwave therapy, and laser therapy. Evidence for acupuncture is inconclusive at this time, mainly because of the heterogeneity of the studies. Local vibration therapy is showing promise in a collection of small cohort studies, as well as Bioptron light therapy.

31. **What are the mechanical, functional, and degenerative causes of chronic ankle instability?**
Acute ankle sprains may lead to mechanical, functional, or degenerative deficits resulting in chronic ankle instability, persistent pain, and mechanical signs. Mechanical causes include pathologic laxity, arthrokinetic restriction, synovial changes, and degenerative changes. Functional causes include proprioception abnormalities, loss of neuromuscular control, impairment in postural control, and strength deficits. Degenerative causes include osteochondral lesions of the talus, impingement, loose bodies, painful ossicles, adhesions, chondromalacia, and osteophyte formation.

32. **How do you prevent or decrease the incidence of ankle sprains?**
Evidence suggests that well-structured preseason conditioning that focuses on agility, balance, coordination, proprioception, and flexibility decreases injury risk. Warming up should precede all intensive physical activity, and patients with sprained ankles should complete rehabilitation before resuming sport. The use of orthotics, ankle bracing/taping, or high-top shoes may prevent the recurrence of ankle sprain, while the use of proprioceptive/kinesthetic training (e.g., balance board training or equivalent) may also substantially reduce the risk and occurrence of ankle sprains.

33. **When do you refer ankle injuries?**
Indications for immediate referral include a structurally significant fracture (as opposed to small avulsion fractures), an obvious deformity, evidence of neurovascular compromise, a penetrating wound into the joint space, a sudden locking of the ankle, suspicion of grade III strain (tendon rupture), and a syndesmotic injury.

KEY POINTS

1. There are three major classifications of ligamentous ankle injuries: lateral, medial (deltoid), and syndesmotic (high) ankle sprains.
2. The ATFL is the most commonly injured ligament in lateral ankle sprains.
3. A high ankle sprain is a sprain of the distal syndesmotic ligaments that connect the distal tibia and fibula.
4. PRICEMMMS (Protection, Rest, Ice, Elevation, Medications, Modalities, Mobilization, and Strengthening) is employed during the acute phase of treating ankle sprains.
5. The evidence supports the use of cryotherapy, bracing/taping, early mobilization, pain control (with either NSAIDs or acetaminophen), and proprioceptive as well as postural training in the treatment, rehabilitation, and prevention of ankle sprains.

Acknowledgments

The authors would like to thank Dr. Duron Lee for their contributions to this chapter in the previous edition.

BIBLIOGRAPHY

Clanton TO, Matheny LM, Jarvis HC, Jeronimus AB. Return to play in athletes following ankle injuries. *Sports Health*. 2012;4(6):471–474.

Czajka CM, Tran E, Cai AN, DiPreta JA. Ankle sprains and instability. *Med Clin North Am*. 2014;98(2):313–329.

Doherty C, Bleakley C, Delahunt E, et al. Treatment and prevention of acute and recurrent ankle sprain: an overview of systemic reviews with meta-analysis. *BJSM*. 2017;51:113–125.

McCriskin BJ, Cameron KL, Orr JD, Waterman BR. Management and prevention of acute and chronic lateral ankle instability in athletic patient populations. *World J Orthop*. 2015;6(2):161–171.

Slimmon D, Brukner P. Sports ankle injuries: assessment and management. *Aus Fam Phy*. 2010;39(1):18–22.

Stasinopoulos D, Papadopoulos C, Lamnisos D, et al. The use of Biopton light (polarized, polychromiatic, non-coheret) therapy for the treatment of acute ankle sprains. *Disabil Rehabil*. 2017;39:450–457.

Tiemstra JD. Update on acute ankle sprains. *Am Fam Physician*. 2012;85(12):1170–1176.

Van Dijk CN, Longo UG, Loppini M, et al. Classification and diagnosis of acute isolated syndesmotic injuries: ESSKA-AFAS consensus and guidelines. *Knee Surg Sports Traumatol Arthrosc*. 2016;24(4):1200–1216.

Vuurberg G, Hoorntje A, Wink LM, et al. Diagnosis, treatment and prevention of ankle sprains: update of an evidence-based clinical guideline. *BJSM*. 2018;52(15):956–970.

Witt BL, Witt SL. Acute ankle sprains: a review of literature. *Osteopath Fam Physician*. 2013;5(5):178–184.

CHAPTER 47

ENVIRONMENTAL EMERGENCIES

Morgan Chambers, MD, MEd, Matthew L. Silvis, MD

COLD INJURIES

1. **What causes injuries from cold exposure?**
   Optimal thermoregulation occurs at 37°C (+/− 2°C). Heat loss occurs through radiation, conduction, convection, evaporation, and respiration. Injuries from cold exposure are due to low air temperatures, water immersion, rain, and wind, which all affect a body's ability to maintain normal temperature. They are divided into low core temperature (hypothermia), freezing (frostbite), and nonfreezing cold (chilblains, trench foot) injuries (NFCI).

2. **What are the common symptoms and signs of cold exposure injuries?**
   There are early and late signs of cold exposure injuries (see Table 47.1). There is also guidance on various degrees of frostbite (see Table 47.2).

3. **Who is at high risk?**
   Injury exposure times vary depending on the type and intensity of cold, degree of activity, protective clothing, and other individual factors.

   Type/Intensity of Cold
   Not only do the duration and severity of cold exposure (meaning the actual temperature) play an important role, but the specific climate and conditions do as well (including degree of wind, wetness, contact with other cold materials, level of altitude, and risk of hypoxia).

   Degree of Activity
   Homelessness and sports activity in inclement environments pose the greatest risk. It is important to keep in mind that athletic activities at greater risk include cold climate hiking, skiing, sledding, hang gliding, windsurfing, swimming, and ice sports.

   Other Individual Factors
   Individuals younger than 2 years or older than 60 years of age are at highest risk. Elderly persons are especially prone due to age-related decrease in the sympathetic nervous system–mediated vasoconstriction, reduced function of sweat glands, and comorbidities. Younger individuals have larger surface areas/mass ratios and exhibit greater heat loss. Specific risk factors include substance use (alcohol, smoking, drugs), medications (vasoconstrictors), psychiatric illness, malnutrition, dehydration, fatigue, sleep deprivation, and history of prior cold injury. Additionally, those with comorbid conditions affecting neural, vascular, and metabolic functioning have an increased risk in the setting of poor baseline tissue perfusion and thermal sensations as well as factors such as impaired mobility and other bodily controls.

4. **At what temperatures do cold injuries occur?**
   Hypothermia is defined as a core body temperature less than 35°C rectally (or less than 32°C tympanically, since core temperature readings may not be feasible) and occurs when heat loss exceeds heat production. Hypothermia can occur at higher temperatures, especially when clothing is wet. Frostbite is a direct freezing injury when skin freezes in water at −0.55°C and in air at <−3°C. Nonfreezing cold injuries result from exposure to cold-wet conditions that cause tissues to drop to <15°C.

5. **How should you assess and begin management for hypothermia?**
   If there is concern for hypothermia, begin by removing all wet clothing. Assess mental status, airway, and breathing. If the patient is breathing, provide oxygen, obtain vital signs, and place an intravenous (IV) line if possible. An accurate core temperature is crucial and ideally is obtained rectally with a thermometer scaled for hypothermia. The core temperature guides treatment, as indicated by the Wilderness Medical Society staging system, which ranges from mild to severe/profound. However, there is now a revised staging system, known as the Swiss Staging Model, which has been proposed for situations where obtaining an accurate core temperature is not feasible, and it ranges from stages 1–5. Both systems are outlined and discussed in Table 47.3. If there is no concern for hypothermia based on core temperature and observation, assess exposed areas and treat.

6. **What is the difference between frostnip and frostbite?**
   These injuries occur in minutes to hours and typically affect the face, ears, fingers, and toes. Frostnip is the formation of superficial ice crystals in the epidermis with no subsequent tissue damage. Mild frostbite penetrates the

Table 47.1 Common Symptoms and Signs of Cold Exposure Injuries

EARLY	LATE
Shivering	"Stumbles, grumbles, mumbles"
Numbness	Decreased or no shivering
Pain, burning	Sluggish, poor judgment, confusion
Erythema, edema, blistering	Frozen tissue (stiff to touch)
Fatigue	Shallow breathing

Table 47.2 Traditional Frostbite Grading System and Treatment Guide

INVOLVEMENT	GRADE	SIGN/SYMPTOM	APPROACH
Superficial	I	Edema, pallor, erythema Raised plaque without blistering	- NSAIDs, hydration, and wound management - Consider ^{99m}Tc scintigraphy within 48 hours
	II	Clear blisters with edema and erythema Blisters develop 6–24 hours after rewarming	- Consider Grade III/IV treatment if risk factors present
Deep	III	Hemorrhagic blisters Black eschar over a few weeks	- Rewarm within 24 hours, be cautious of reperfusion injury - Angiography or ^{99m}Tc scintigraphy, then TPA (unless contraindicated) - Follow with Grade I management - Surgery consult
	IV	Muscle and/or bone involvement; gangrene *Absence of blisters is poor for prognosis*	

dermis, and deep frostbite affects all layers of the skin with risk of permanent damage. At the correct temperature, the formation of extracellular ice crystals occurs and leads to the succession of the following steps:

Extracellular ice crystals → cellular damage → increased osmotic pressure → inflammation → thrombosis/ischemia/hypoxia → intracellular ice crystals

7. **What are the major considerations in frostbite injury?**
Remove wet, constrictive clothing and assess for hypothermia. Hypothermia treatment should take precedence. Once that is addressed or ruled out, further cold exposure should be avoided, and the injured region should be protected with a bulky splint for transport. If there is a concern for tissue refreezing, do not attempt initial thawing, as tissue necrosis may occur. If thawing is appropriate, use body heat initially followed by a 37–39°C water bath. Avoid friction and dry heat sources. Allow the extremity to air dry after the water bath. Injuries and thawing can be painful, thus adequate anesthesia should be provided. Ibuprofen can be used to prevent reperfusion injury until the affected area is fully healed. Correct hypovolemia with warm oral or IV fluids. Avoid massaging open blisters and antibiotic administration, but tetanus prophylaxis should be considered. Consider transfer for emergency care, especially when the affected area is large (see Fig. 47.1).

8. **What causes chilblain and trench foot injuries?**
Chilblains (or pernio) and trench foot (or immersion foot) are both nonfreezing injuries (Table 47.4) when tissue temperatures fall below 15°C. Prolonged water exposure or sweating from wet-cold conditions (rain, snow, immersion) causes an exaggerated inflammatory response. This causes increased vascular permeability and fluid leakage. The affected area is pale, cold, and numb and becomes cyanotic upon rewarming. Feet (wet socks, footwear) and hands are commonly affected, as well as nose and ears. Wet and constrictive clothing should be removed. Avoid weight-bearing, friction, lotions, or exposing the area to extreme heat.

9. **What is the role of radiologic studies?**
MRI angiography and ^{99m}Tc can help predict surgical margins and perfusion. This will help determine if a patient is a candidate for tissue plasminogen activator (TPA). It can also help in surgical planning, but early amputation should be avoided. Otherwise, there is no role for any imaging unless a fracture is suspected.

Table 47.3 Core Temperature Treatment Guide

CATEGORY	ESTIMATED CORE TEMPERATURE	SYMPTOMS	MANAGEMENT
Stage 1 (Swiss) **Mild (WMS)**	32–35°C (89.6–95°F)	Shivering, muscle spasms, lethargy, slurred speech, pallor, low pulse, usually normal blood pressure	- Remove wet clothing, move indoors - Passive external rewarming with blanket or wrap - Warm liquids with sugar by mouth (if able) - Active movement
Stage 2 (Swiss) **Moderate (WMS)**	28–32°C (82.4–89.6°F)	+/– shivering, cyanosis, disorientation, decreased motor skills, muscle stiffness, decreased respiration, low or irregular pulse, low blood pressure	- Rapid transport to medical facility for active core rewarming (+/– active external rewarming) - Avoid active external rewarming (fires, hot water bottles, heating pads) until active core rewarming has begun to avoid life-threatening risk of core temperature after drop - Warmed humidified oxygen if available - Warm normal saline (not LR) to 38–42°C - Monitor for arrhythmias
Stage 3 (Swiss) **Severe/Profound (WMS)**	<28°C (82.4°F)	Loss of consciousness, rigidity, pulse not palpable, depressed respirations, dilated pupils, pulmonary edema, arrhythmias	- Stage 2 management with warmed IV fluids, warmed humidified oxygen, and/or peritoneal/thoracic/gastric lavage - Monitor for ventricular fibrillation or cardiac arrest while awaiting transport - Can consider bypass
Stage 4	11.8–24°C	Apparent death	- Stage 3 management - ACLS with up to three doses of epinephrine - Consider termination of ACLS if not able to perform CPR, signs of airway obstruction, or if K+ >12.0 mEq
Stage 5	<11.8°C	Death due to irreversible hypothermia; should be rewarmed to normal core temperature before pronouncing death	

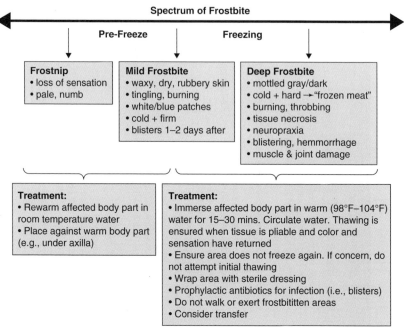

Fig. 47.1 Spectrum of frostbite.

Table 47.4 Nonfreezing Cold Injuries

	CHILBLAIN (PERNIO)	TRENCH FOOT (IMMERSION FOOT)
Etiology	Exposure at 33–60°F for 1–5 hours Pathophysiology not well understood	Exposure at 32–50°F for >12 hours Frequent and prolonged immersion of body part in cold water (typically feet)
Presentation	Local skin lesions (vesicles, bullae, plaques) typically on hands/feet Edema, erythema, cyanotic, tender, pruritic, numbness, burning, tingling, sloughing No symptom resolution with rewarming	Numbness and pale skin followed by blue and mottled skin appearance with pain Lesions turn to purple, erythematous, and edematous papules Can have long-lasting sensorimotor deficits
Management	- Wash and dry affected area - Elevate, cover with loose, warm, dry clothing; use dry bandages if needed - Avoid rapid rewarming - <u>Pain management:</u> amitriptyline more effective than NSAIDs or opioids *Usually no permanent sequelae and resolves within 2–3 weeks*	**Treatment as per chilblains with following additions:** - Apply warm packs or soak in warm water (102–110°F) for 5 minutes - Consider transfer to facility - Can consider nifedipine, vasodilators, topical corticosteroids to reduce pain and promote healing Often requires prolonged wound care as healing can take 3–6 months; tissue loss uncommon but scarring can occur

10. What is the role of TPA?

TPA can significantly reduce amputation rates, especially in Grade II-IV injuries. Contraindications include hypersensitivity, trauma, coagulopathy, anticoagulant use, stroke in the past 3 months, or BP >180/110. If no contraindications are present, TPA can be given within 24 hours of rewarming. Additional agents that have also been reported are heparin, low-molecular-weight heparin, or lloprost (vasodilator).

11. **What is the role of epinephrine pens in cold-induced urticaria?**
    Mediated by histamine, cold-induced urticaria is an allergic response to cold exposure. The response can present as hives, angioedema, or, rarely, anaphylaxis. When localized to the skin, symptoms may be controlled with oral antihistamines and low-concentration, short-term corticosteroids. Topical antihistamines can provide pruritus relief. If the reaction is anaphylaxis, epinephrine should be administered and the individual transferred to a medical facility. Treat any relevant underlying disorder if present. The only prevention known is to avoid cold exposure.

12. **What is the management of cold-induced bronchoconstriction?**
    Cold-induced bronchoconstriction causes airway surface liquid (ASL) to evaporate faster than it can be replaced, causing cooling and drying. This may trigger a reflex response of coughing and bronchial narrowing. Inhaled β2-adrenergic agonists (albuterol) can be used 15–30 minutes before exercise. In the setting of regular exercise in the cold, mast cell stabilizers (cromolyn), leukotriene receptor antagonists, and inhaled corticosteroids are capable of attenuating cold air–provoked bronchoconstriction.

13. **How do you prevent cold injuries?**
    Primarily, it is important to assess risk using clinical judgment and risk factors mentioned above and work to mitigate those factors however possible. Using other clinical tools, such as the wind chill temperature (WCT) index to estimate face frostbite risk during activity, is also important. The overall goal for prevention is to maintain core body temperature, reduce risk of contact freezing, and reduce heat loss with clothing. The following principles can be followed to achieve this:

    C – Keep the area **clean** and **covered** (cover head and neck as they are areas of high heat loss).

    O – Avoid **overheating** (remove layers as necessary).

    L – Wear **loose** clothing and in **layers** (inner [polyester], middle [wool or fleece], and outer layers [wicking fabric such as wool with wind-blocking garment]); loose clothing/footwear is important to preserve blood flow.

    D – Keep skin **dry** to prevent heat loss from moisture (waterproof outer layer; change layers such as socks and gloves frequently in cold-wet conditions).

HEAT INJURIES

14. **What causes heat injuries?**
    Exercise leads to an increased cardiac output to support blood flow to skin and muscles. The body has compensatory mechanisms in place to support tissue metabolism; however, when there is increased physiological strain and thermoregulatory mechanisms (evaporation, radiation, conduction, convection) fail, pathological events ensue leading to impaired blood flow, poor tissue metabolism, and eventually an acute phase response that triggers systemic inflammatory response syndrome resulting in cell death and central nervous system dysfunction. The spectrum of heat illness is depicted in Table 47.5. Heat edema, rash, and cramps are mild heat illnesses. Heat syncope and exhaustion are medical urgencies; heat stroke is an emergency.

15. **What are the risk factors for heat-related injuries and who is at risk?**

    Individual
    - Children, elderly, athletes
    - Obesity
    - Deconditioning
    - History of heat/febrile illness
    - Sleep deprivation/fatigue
    - Dehydration
    - Current illness
    - Comorbidities: skin disorders, sickle cell trait, cystic fibrosis, cardiovascular disease, diabetes mellitus

    Environmental
    - High temperatures, heat waves
    - Heavy clothes, equipment

    Medications/Drugs
    - Alcohol
    - Certain medication/supplement use*

    Extrinsic Pressures
    - Self-motivation to compete
    - Teammate/coach pressure to compete
    - Competition/practice structure

---

*Tricyclic antidepressants, anticholinergics, antihistamines, benzodiazepines, diarrheal agents, typical antipsychotics, antihypertensives, neuroleptics, thyroid agonists, stimulants, caffeine, diuretics.

Table 47.5 Spectrum of Heat Illnesses

CONDITION	ETIOLOGY/SIGNS/SYMPTOMS	MANAGEMENT AND COMMENTS
Heat Edema	Cause: increased interstitial fluid due to cutaneous dilation Will see swelling in dependent areas, facial flushing *Rule out organic cause of heat edema (heart/kidney failure)	Compression stockings, hydrate, and stretch. Generally, condition resolves on its own within 1–2 weeks *Diuretics will worsen the condition and deplete intravascular volume*
Heat Rash (miliaria rubra)	Cause: sweating causes clogged skin eccrine sweat glands which may predispose to infection Papulovesicular skin eruptions, typically on covered areas of skin (trunk, groin) May cause pruritus	Condition is self-limited Pruritus can be managed by topical or oral antihistamine agents Infection is managed with antibiotics based on severity
Heat Cramps (CT normal)	Cause: involuntary painful skeletal muscle contractions due to overuse and electrolyte depletion Common in patients with high sodium in sweat Muscle spasms or cramps; sweating	Fluids, electrolyte solutions with sodium IV normal saline in severe or rebound cases can be used Stretching and massaging muscles, cooling with ice
Heat Syncope (CT normal)	Cause: occurs due to orthostatic hypotension from peripheral vasodilation Weakness, faint feeling, improvement in symptoms when supine	Place patient in supine position, provide fluids
Heat Exhaustion (CT 37°C–40°C)	Cause: early multiorgan dysfunction due to hypovolemia and splanchnic vasoconstriction Headache, lethargy, hypotension, tachycardia, nausea, vomiting, +/– sweating, cold/clammy skin, oliguria, normal mental status	Remove excess clothing, elevate legs above heart, rapid cooling with ice cloths to neck, torso, axilla, and groin Hydration with cool fluids. Use IV if needed (Dextrose-0.5NS) Consider transfer to a medical facility
Heat Stroke (CT usually above 40°C)	Cause: severe thermoregulatory dysfunction leading to endotoxin leakage and multiorgan dysfunction Hypotension, tachycardia, loss of sweating, constricted pupils, warm and dry skin, oliguria, tachypnea, mental status changes, convulsions, coma *Lactic acidosis, DIC, acute renal failure, hypokalemia, and rhabdomyolysis are typically seen in exertional heat stroke	"Cool first, transport second" Remove excess clothing, elevate legs, rapid cooling with ice packs or cold towels over neck, axilla, groin (think major vessels) Apply cool water to bare skin and start fan for evaporative cooling; ice-water immersion if able Initiate IV fluids (NS) Transfer to a medical facility for possible peritoneal lavage, internal cooling, ECMO (extracorporeal membrane oxygenation), and vasopressors (dobutamine) if needed

CT, Core temperature.

16. **What is the difference between classic and exertional heat stroke?**
Classic heat stroke is environmental in origin (i.e., heat waves) and most commonly affects the elderly with predisposed medical conditions. Exertional heat stroke occurs due to dysfunction of heat dissipation, can occur in all weather conditions, and commonly affects the healthy and young.

17. **What are the signs and symptoms of heat injuries?**

Signs
- Sweating
- Decreased performance

- Lethargy
- Tachycardia
- Hypotension
- Changes in mental status

Symptoms
- Muscle cramps
- Thirst
- Vision changes
- Nausea/vomiting
- Headache
- Feeling faint/fatigue
- Unsteady gait
- Chills

18. **What are the steps to approaching an athlete with a heat illness?**
Early initiation of treatment is essential in reducing morbidity and mortality. Assess airway, breathing, and circulation (ABCs). Transport to a cooler location and initiate cooling with ice bags and/or fan mist. Assess for appropriate mentation. If mentation is appropriate, provide fluids and electrolyte replacement by mouth. If mental status is not intact, remove excess clothing, initiate rapid cooling, and alert emergency medical services (EMS). After doing so, obtain a rectal temperature by inserting a thermometer with the metal tip 1–2 inches into the rectum. Obtain vital signs, blood glucose, and sodium levels. Obtain IV access if able. Transfer the patient to a medical facility.

19. **What is the role of laboratory studies?**
The differential for heat illness is broad and includes hypoglycemia, seizures, hyponatremia, thyroid storm, neuroleptic malignant syndrome, drug ingestion, and closed head trauma. Laboratory assessment may include:
- Basic Metabolic Profile (BMP) for electrolytes, glucose, creatinine
- Complete blood count (CBC) with platelets
- Arterial blood gases (ABG) for respiratory alkalosis
- Creatine phosphokinase (CPK) for rhabdomyolysis
- Chest x-ray for pulmonary edema
- Others: lactate ($\uparrow$), calcium ($\downarrow$), phosphorous ($\downarrow$)
- Electrocardiogram and troponins for cardiac abnormalities
- Fibrinogen, fibrin-split products for disseminated intravascular coagulation (DIC)
- Liver function tests (LFTs) for hepatic injury
- Urine analysis and output (for myoglobin)

20. **What are the types of heat injuries and what is the management?**
See Table 47.5. Remember: cool if able, then transport. The goal is to lower the core body temperature to 37.5–38°C as soon as possible.

21. **What are the complications of heat stroke?**
- Seizures
- Rhabdomyolysis
- Pulmonary edema, acute respiratory distress syndrome (ARDS)
- Arrhythmias
- Hypotension
- Organ damage (liver, heart, kidney)
- DIC
Shivering and seizures can be treated with benzodiazepines. Arrhythmias often resolve with improvement in temperatures.

22. **How are heat injuries prevented?**
- Fluid and electrolyte replacement before and during exercise
- Acclimatize prior to extreme exercise
- Balanced nutrition, may need a high-sodium and high-potassium diet
- Wear temperature-appropriate clothing (loose, lightweight, light colored, moisture wicking)
- Educate civilians and athletes
- Frequent rest periods
- Reducing intensity when applicable

23. **What medications should be avoided in patients with heat-related illness?**
Avoid alpha agonists and anticholinergic agents, as they can cause peripheral vasoconstriction and prevent sweating.

24. When can an athlete return to play after suffering a heat illness?

Generally, an athlete can return after 24 hours with adequate hydration if the illness is mild. However, if suffering from heat exhaustion or heat stroke, all vital signs should be normalized, and the patient should be asymptomatic. Athletes are often instructed to wait at least 1 week after discharge from medical care before returning to play. Follow-up physical examination and laboratory testing 1 week following return to play should be considered. When returning to play, athletes should slowly increase heat exposure and the length and intensity of exercise over a 2-week period. If heat tolerance is demonstrated, they can be cleared within 2–4 weeks.

KEY POINTS

1. Severe hypothermia is a medical emergency requiring immediate transfer to a hospital.
2. In cold exposure injuries, do not allow thawed skin to refreeze, and do not use excessive heat, cold, or massage, or provide direct heat.
3. If a patient has a temperature >104°F, persistent vomiting, or altered mental status, alert emergency medical services for immediate transfer.

Acknowledgments

The authors would like to thank Dr. Ayesha Abid for her contributions to this chapter in the previous edition.

BIBLIOGRAPHY

Barrow MW, Clark KA. Heat-related illnesses. *Am Fam Phys*. 1998;58:749–756.
Brown CH, Brown MT, Tyler WB, Cruz S. Environmental factors affecting human performance. In: *Medical Manual*. International Association of Athletics Federation; 1990:1–11. [chapter 11].
Cappaert TA, Stone JA, Castellani JW, et al. National Athletic Trainer's Association position statement: environmental cold injuries. *J Athl Train*. 2008;43(6):640–658.
Casa D, Armstrong L, Kenny G, et al. Exertional heat stroke: new concepts regarding cause and care. *Curr Sports Med Rep*. 2012;11(3):115–123.
Casa D, DeMartini J, Bergeron M, et al. National Athletic Trainer's Association position statement: exertional heat illness. *J Athl TrainJournal of Athletic Training*. 2015;50(9):986–1000.
Castellani JW, Eglin CM, et al. American College of Sports Medicine expert consensus statement: injury prevention and exercise performance during cold-weather exercise. *Curr Sports Med Rep*. 2021;20(11):594–607.
Claudy A. Cold urticaria. *J Investig Dermatol Symp Proc*. 2001;6:141–142.
Corris EE, Ramirez AM, Durme DJ. Heat illness in athletes: the dangerous combination of heat, humidity and exercise. *Sports Med*. 2004;34:9–16.
Dammann GG, Boden BP. On-the-field management of heat stroke: sports medicine update. *AOSSM Newsletter (May-June)*. 2004:4–7.
Epstein Y, Yanovich RHeatstroke. *N Engl J Med*. 2019;380(25):2449–2457.
Gauer R, Meyers BK. Heat-related illnesses. *Am Fam Phys*. 2019;99(8):482–487.
Glazer JL. Management of heatstroke and heat exhaustion. *Am Fam Phys*. 2005;71:2133–2140.
Howe AS, Boden BP. Heat-related illness in athletes. *Am J Sports Med*. 2007;35(8):1384–1395.
Inter-Association Task Force on Exertional Heat Illnesses Consensus Statement. National Athletic Trainers' Association; June 2003.
Kazman JB, Heled Y, Lisman PJ, et al. Exertional heat illness: the role of heat tolerance testing. *Curr Sports Med Rep*. 2013;12(2):101–105.
Koester MC. Cold-related illness. *Sports Medicine Handbook*. National Federation of State High School Associations; 2011:40–43.
Koskela HO. Cold air-provoked respiratory symptoms: the mechanisms and management. *Int J Circumpolar Health*. 2007;66(2):91–100.
Krafczyk MA, Asplung CA. Exercise-induced bronchoconstriction: diagnosis and management. *Am Fam Physician*. 2011;84(4):427–434.
McMahon J, Howe A. Cold weather issues in sideline and event management. *Curr Sports Med Rep*. 2012;11(3):135–141.
NCAA 2014–2015. Sports Medicine Handbook. Indianapolis, IN: National Collegiate Athletic Association, www.ncaa.org. Accessed May 12, 2016.
Raducan A, Tiplica GS. Chillblains and frostbite. *J Eur Acad Dermatol Venereol*. 2013;6(1):60–64.
Rathjen NA, Shahbodaghi SD, Brown JA. Hypothermia and cold weather injuries. *Am Fam Phys*. 2019;100(11):681–686.
Roberts WO, Armstrong LE, et al. ACSM expert consensus statement on exertional heat illness: recognition, management, and return to activity. *Curr Sports Med Rep*. 2021;20(9):470–481.
US Army Research Institute of Environmental Medicine. Prevention and management of cold weather injuries. Technical Bulletin Material 508. Washington, DC: Department of the Army.

CHAPTER 48

ACUTE INFECTIOUS DISEASES AND THE ATHLETE

Ellen Maria Benitah-Bulbarelli, MD, George G.A. Pujalte, MD, FACSM, FAMSSM, FAAFP

THE COMMON COLD

1. **How does the common cold present?**
   Also known as a viral syndrome or upper respiratory tract infection (URTI), the common cold is the leading cause of missed school or workdays in the United States, often leading to missed athletic participation. Presenting symptoms typically include nasal congestion, rhinorrhea, sneezing, cough, and occasionally fever.

2. **What are the risk factors for getting the common cold?**
   Risk factors that may be concerning for more severe diseases include young age, low birth weight, prematurity, chronic disease, immunodeficiency, malnutrition, and crowding. Risk factors for athletes include traveling, close contact with teammates and opponents, indoor competition and crowding, winter months, increased psychosocial stress, and sleep disturbance. A recent study showed an increased risk for URTI in periods of rest for elite athletes, related to household illness contact.

3. **How do you diagnose and manage a common cold?**
   URTI does not typically require confirmatory testing or further workup. However, the gold standard of confirmation is viral culture, rarely indicated, except when symptoms are prolonged or worsening and other etiologies are being considered. A complete blood count (CBC) may show leukocytosis with a left shift.
   The mainstay of treatment is symptomatic management, as the symptoms typically resolve within 7–10 days. Treatment includes medications such as analgesics and antipyretics. Many agents have been studied in the treatment of the common cold; antihistamines and decongestants have proven to have the highest efficacy. However first-generation antihistamines are well known for their anticholinergic effects resulting in fatigue, dehydration, and/or heat problems. Oral decongestants can cause dehydration and hyperthermia, and there are restrictions on their use by certain sport-governing bodies (consult the World Anti-Doping Agency [WADA] website for the most up-to-date list of prohibited substances).
   A recent study from 2020 has shown that the natural enzyme cod trypsin (ColdZyme) mouth spray can reduce self-reported upper respiratory tract infection (URTI) episode duration by 3.5 days. Other studies have shown that specific probiotic strains can reduce the number of episodes, symptom severity score, and duration of URTI in athletes.
   Patients with URTI should be provided precautions, even though the course is commonly benign and self-limited, due to its significant impact on athletes' performance, preparation, and training. Additionally, more serious complications such as acute bacterial sinusitis (which occurs in 2.5% of patients after a viral URI), pneumonia, or asthma exacerbations may result. Exercise and return to play are permitted as tolerated.

SINUSITIS

4. **How does sinusitis present?**
   Patients present with significant nasal congestion, purulent nasal discharge, maxillary tooth discomfort, headaches, fever, reduction/loss of smell, and facial pain/pressure in an acute (<4 weeks), subacute (4–8 weeks), or chronic (>8 weeks) manner.

5. **How do you differentiate viral versus bacterial sinusitis?**
   Bacterial infections are less common, last longer than the usual 7- to 10-day course for a viral infection, and are associated with a history of persistent purulent rhinorrhea, severe facial pain, sinus tenderness, fever above 38°C, unilateral disease, double-sickening, and raised erythrocyte sedimentation rate (ESR)/C-reactive protein (CRP). History and physical examination are key, as further diagnostic workup is typically not indicated. Additionally, poor response to decongestants has been shown to increase the likelihood of acute bacterial sinusitis.

6. **What diagnostic tests may be helpful in diagnosing sinusitis?**
   The gold standard for diagnosis, not routine, is sinus aspirate culture (or nasopharyngeal swab cultures and polymerase chain reaction [PCR]). Computed tomography (CT) scanning is preferred over other imaging modalities if a diagnosed sinusitis does not respond to initial therapies.

7. **How is sinusitis treated?**

Antibiotics are typically indicated for acute bacterial sinusitis when symptoms have not improved over 10 days or for severe illness. Amoxicillin should be the initial choice in children and adults with uncomplicated disease for 7–10 days of treatment. Symptomatic management may also include antihistamines, decongestants, and nasal steroids, but studies have not proven efficacy to date and their use is not routinely recommended. Exercise and return to play are permitted as tolerated. Athletes with more than three episodes of rhinosinusitis per year should be referred to an otorhinolaryngologist.

PHARYNGITIS

8. **How is pharyngitis assessed?**

Acute pharyngitis is caused by an equal proportion of viral and bacterial pathogens. The most commonly treated etiology is group A streptococcus (GAS), but this only accounts for ~10% of adult cases. Centor criteria are used in an attempt to differentiate viral causes from bacterial, especially GAS. These include tender anterior cervical adenopathy, tonsillar exudates, fever by history, and absence of cough. In a large study of 206,870 patients, 7% of patients with one Centor criterion, 21% of patients with two Centor criteria, 38% of patients with three Centor criteria, and 57% of patients with four Centor criteria tested positive for GAS.

9. **What diagnostic tests may be helpful?**

Throat cultures are the gold standard of diagnosis but can take 24–48 hours to become positive and therefore are not as readily useful for same-day management. The rapid streptococcal antigen test (RSAT) is the initial test of choice and results are available in minutes.

10. **How is pharyngitis treated?**

If positive, treatment for GAS is warranted, with penicillin V being the first-line antibiotic to prevent the risk of rheumatic fever, acute glomerulonephritis, and supportive complications. Otherwise, symptomatic management is typically sufficient. Sexually active athletes may warrant suspicion and workup for gonococcal infection as a cause of pharyngitis, which is easily treatable with antibiotics. Important to remember that athletes with acute bacterial pharyngitis must be held from play and are considered contagious until treated with an antibiotic for 24 hours. After this time has passed, activity, as tolerated, is recommended.

INFECTIOUS MONONUCLEOSIS

11. **How does infectious mononucleosis present?**

More commonly known as "mono" or "the kissing disease," this illness occurs commonly at the high school and collegiate level and is spread primarily by the passage of saliva. It is caused by the Epstein-Barr virus (EBV), which can persist in the oropharynx for up to 18 months after clinical recovery. The classical presentation includes the triad of fever, tonsillar pharyngitis, and posterior cervical lymphadenopathy. Typical pharyngitis is described as white or gray exudate often accompanied by severe fatigue, head and body aches, rash, splenomegaly, and/or hepatomegaly.

12. **What diagnostic tests are useful?**

Diagnostic evaluation usually begins with the Monospot test, which detects heterophile antibodies that appear within 1 week of the onset of clinical symptoms and may persist at low levels for up to 1 year. EBV-specific antibodies are commonly used in athletes to determine the acuity of illness. Antiviral capsid antigen (VCA) immunoglobulin M (IgM) is detected early and disappears within four to six weeks. Anti-VCA IgG appears early, peaks in 2 to 4 weeks, then declines and persists throughout a patient's life. A peripheral smear, although not always warranted, will show a mild leukocytosis on occasion with a predominance of lymphocytes, with more than 10% of these being atypical.

13. **How is "mono" treated?**

Treatment is focused on supportive care (adequate nutrition, hydration, and rest).

14. **When can athletes return to play after a bout of "mono"?**

Return-to-play guidelines for athletes with primary or recurrent infectious mononucleosis have been heavily disputed and are largely based on the prevention of splenic rupture, which occurs most commonly in 1–2 per 1000 patients 4–21 days after onset of symptoms. For this reason, a gradual return to play may be started after 3 weeks by resumption of light activity. However, contact and vigorous exercise are typically prohibited for the first 4 weeks after the onset of symptoms. It is also important to ensure the athlete is afebrile and without pharyngitis, the spleen is not enlarged or painful, and liver enzymes are at baseline.

PULMONARY INFECTIONS

PNEUMONIA

15. **How does pneumonia present?**

Patients present with cough, sputum production, shortness of breath, and/or chest pain. Other associated symptoms may include malaise, anorexia, headache, myalgias, fever, and chills. Physical examination is very important in diagnosis, and vital signs will often be abnormal including fever, tachycardia, tachypnea, hypoxemia, or hypotension. The exam may reveal dullness to percussion of the chest, tactile fremitus, or egophony. Auscultation can be positive for crackles, rales, or bronchial breath sounds.

16. **What diagnostic tests may be helpful?**
The gold standard for diagnosis includes a chest radiograph showing an infiltrative lesion. Other workups may include a complete blood count (CBC) showing leukocytosis, sputum cultures with Gram stain, and urine antigens for streptococcus or legionella. Common pathogens include streptococcal pneumonia, legionella, chlamydia, and influenza.

17. **How is pneumonia treated?**
The pneumonia severity index is often used to help determine whether outpatient management is appropriate, but clinician judgment is the final word. Typically, a patient with unstable vital signs, including hypoxemia, inability to maintain hydration, or oral intake requires inpatient hospitalization. Treatment usually consists of Amoxicillin and a macrolide, such as azithromycin or doxycycline. If athletes are short of breath for extended periods of time despite adequate antibiotic therapy and resolution of other symptoms, they may have developed a transient reactive airway disease and would benefit from a short course of inhaled bronchodilator therapy. Continued fevers should warrant suspicion for other complications such as empyema, abscess, sepsis, or a secondary lung infection.

18. **When can an athlete return to play?**
Although there are few studied recommendations for return to play in these patients, the athlete should be afebrile and return to participation in a gradual and progressive fashion.

ACUTE BRONCHITIS

19. **How does acute bronchitis present?**
Bronchitis is characterized by a cough lasting for more than 10 days and up to 3 weeks and concurrent upper airway infection. Most commonly caused by a viral infection (influenza A and B virus, parainfluenza virus, respiratory syncytial virus, coronavirus, adenovirus, rhinovirus, and metapneumovirus), less than 10% of patients with bronchitis have a bacterial etiology (*Bordetella pertussis*, *Chlamydophila pneumoniae*, and *Mycoplasma pneumoniae)*. The examination is nonspecific, and patients may have pharyngeal erythema, lymphadenopathy, rhinorrhea, and, less commonly, fever. It is a clinical diagnosis and should be suspected in patients with prolonged cough after resolution of other URI symptoms. Postnasal drip, sinusitis, asthma, and GERD are often in the differential diagnosis.

20. **How is acute bronchitis treated?**
Acetaminophen, ibuprofen, and nasal decongestants are commonly used. As with pneumonia above, these patients may also develop a reactive airway disease or worsening of asthmatic symptoms and may benefit from short-term inhaled bronchodilator therapy. Exercise and return to play are permitted as tolerated.

PERTUSSIS

21. **How does pertussis (also known as "whooping cough") present?**
"Whooping cough" is caused by the gram-negative coccobacillus Bordetella pertussis and is a highly contagious infection transmitted by droplets. For this reason, it is important not to miss this diagnosis in the training room or when working with athletes in constant close contact. Athletes present with a persistent cough with URI symptoms, which may have a paroxysmal quality lasting more than 3 weeks, posttussive emesis, and/or inspiratory whooping.

22. **How is pertussis diagnosed and managed?**
Diagnosis is confirmed by nasopharyngeal culture and/or polymerase chain reaction (PCR). When clinical suspicion is high, the Centers for Disease Control and Prevention (CDC) recommends reporting and treating pertussis even prior to laboratory confirmation. Treatment, such as prophylaxis for athletes in close contact with a suspected case of pertussis, includes erythromycin. The newer macrolide antibiotics are better tolerated than erythromycin, including azithromycin (possible side effect: prolongation of the QT interval) and clarithromycin (side effects: prolongation of the QT interval and inhibition of CYP3A4). For those intolerant to macrolide antibiotics, trimethoprim/sulfamethoxazole can be prescribed.

23. **How is the spread of pertussis prevented?**
Athletes with pertussis need to be isolated from participation for 5 days from the start of treatment. Routine preventive measures in the general population are recommended by means of the Tdap vaccine for 11- to 18-year-olds who require a booster dose as well as a single dose for adults 19–64 years of age regardless of their vaccination status. After 5 days of isolation, athletes must be monitored for further complications of pertussis such as reactive airway disease, pneumonia, dehydration, weight loss, and sleep disturbances prior to returning to play.

INFLUENZA

24. **How does influenza present?**
Usually present in the winter months, athletes may complain of abrupt onset of fever, headache, myalgia, malaise, nausea, vomiting, dry cough, and/or sore throat. Physical exam findings may include minimal cervical lymphadenopathy, oropharyngeal hyperemia, eye lacrimation or redness, or dehydration.

25. **How is influenza diagnosed and managed?**
Rapid viral diagnostic tests completed with the use of nasal or throat swabs can be helpful in the outpatient setting. Influenza A and B can be treated with the neuraminidase inhibitors zanamivir and oseltamivir whereas influenza A alone can be treated with amantadine and rimantadine. Studies have shown a 2- to 3-day shortening of symptoms when these antiviral medications are given within the first 24–30 hours of symptoms. Symptomatic treatment is the mainstay of therapy for patients presenting outside of that initial 1–2 days of symptom onset and includes acetaminophen or ibuprofen, cough suppressants, and adequate sleep and hydration. To avoid the spread of influenza infection, social distancing is important, as well as not sharing household items and disinfecting common areas frequently. To avoid an outbreak in a team, early chemoprophylaxis with oseltamivir may be given to asymptomatic athletes and staff of the team after close contact with an influenza-infected person.

26. **How is influenza prevented, and when can athletes return to play?**
Vaccination is a safe method for athletes, and an annually updated influenza vaccine is important for the prevention of illness (primary prophylaxis by immunization) regardless of athletes' training sessions. Vaccines should be administered according to the season and location (northern or southern hemispheres) of competition, even to athletes previously vaccinated. Studies have shown that if athletes travel to a different hemisphere during the influenza season, the use of a second influenza vaccine would be beneficial.

Chemoprophylaxis with a neuraminidase inhibitor can be considered for close contacts and in-season sports teams when a team member tests positive for influenza.

Similar to the recommendations for pertussis, athletes with influenza should be isolated for 5 days after which they should be monitored for fever, dehydration, or dyspnea before returning to play.

If symptoms are "above the neck," such as headaches, nasal congestion, and rhinorrhea, athletes can return to light activity for 15 minutes and increase this as tolerated. If symptoms are "below the neck," such as fever, malaise, or gastrointestinal, athletes can return to play after symptoms have resolved.

Physicians should be aware of tachycardia as viral-induced myocarditis. It is possible after an upper respiratory tract infection.

Infectious disease protocols should be enforced to manage an outbreak in a sports setting. To reduce influenza outbreaks there are some recommendations proposed:
1. Vaccinate all athletes in the preseason
2. Remove shared water bottles at practice/games
3. Teach proper hygiene (no towel sharing, clean equipment regularly)
4. Provide proper locker room ventilation
5. Require hand washing prior to entry into athletic training clinics
6. If the spread occurred quickly, shut down practices/games/activities
7. If suspecting illness, provide an immediate referral to a health care provider
8. Encourage improved sleep quality and decrease sleep deprivation
9. Reduce overtraining
10. Recommend a diet focused on sufficient vitamin C and zinc consumption and vitamin D and probiotics supplementation

CARDIAC INFECTIONS

MYOCARDITIS

27. **How does myocarditis present?**
Myocarditis is an inflammatory disease of the myocardium. The most common cause of myocarditis in sports medicine is a respiratory or gastrointestinal viral illness, but this can also be caused by drug hypersensitivity, radiation, chemical agents, drugs, and allergic reactions. It is a difficult diagnosis to make, as its presentation can mimic a URTI or flulike syndrome, or athletes may simply be asymptomatic. Typical presentation includes chest pain and/or symptoms of heart failure, fatigue, palpitations, dizziness, and syncope, which may be associated with fever, malaise, arthralgias, and sudden cardiac death. Physical examination may show tachycardia, palpitations, a muffled first heart sound, and/or third heart sound, which can be associated with a mitral regurgitation murmur, edema, and pulmonary crackles. URTI symptoms may also remain.

28. **What diagnostic tests may be helpful?**
Patients present with nonspecific symptoms of fatigue, tachycardia at rest and during physical activity, muscle soreness, and reduced overall exercise capacity. When clinical suspicion is high, echocardiography is useful and may show decreased global ventricular function. Cardiac MRI can demonstrate myocardial edema and myocyte damage, as well as elevation of blood troponin (Ic or Tc) above the 99th percentile, but definitive diagnosis requires endomyocardial biopsy (EMB) with histologic evidence of mononuclear cellular infiltrates, nonischemic myocyte necrosis, and disorganized myocardial cytoskeleton. Direct detection and quantification of viral genomes in the myocardium can also be done using real-time polymerase chain reaction (PCR) techniques.

29. **How is myocarditis treated, and when can athletes return to play?**

If presuming viral myocarditis, treatment is supportive care, and most patients will recover completely. Patients can be treated with aspirin or nonsteroidal antiinflammatory drugs.

Acute human herpesvirus 6-related myocarditis has been treated with immunosuppression and antiviral agents such as ganciclovir, acyclovir, or valacyclovir. In myocarditis caused by parvovirus B19 with low viral load and no virus replication, the treatment is intravenous immunoglobulins, telbivudine, or prednisone plus azathioprine.

Heart failure has been treated with beta-blockers and angiotensin-converting enzyme inhibitors/angiotensin receptor blockers for hemodynamically stable patients. However, beta-blockers are prohibited by the World Anti-Doping Agency for some sports, including golf, shooting, and archery, due to their relieving effect on tremors.

Athletes with myocarditis are at an increased risk for heart failure, cardiomyopathies, arrhythmias, associated pericarditis, and sudden cardiac death. For this reason, it is important to withdraw these athletes from participation in sports for 6 months and only return to play once no clinical symptoms when left ventricular (LV) function and wall motion return to normal evaluated by electrocardiography (ECG), echocardiography, or cardiovascular magnetic resonance imaging (CMR). Arrhythmias should be absent on exercise tolerance testing (ETT) and ambulatory Holter monitoring. Serum markers of inflammation, troponin, and heart failure should have normalized before clearing. A postmyocarditis scar without ventricular dysfunction or arrhythmias is not a contraindication to return to sports activity, but a case-by-case evaluation should be performed. For all athletes, a follow-up examination should be performed annually.

PERICARDITIS

30. **How does pericarditis present?**

Similar to myocarditis, pericarditis is most commonly infectious or idiopathic with a similar presentation. Athletes will present with retrosternal, pleuritic chest pain, typically exacerbated by coughing, which may radiate to the back. Classically this chest pain is exacerbated when lying down and relieved by sitting forward. Fever, cough, fatigue, exertional dyspnea, myalgias, or arthralgias are not uncommon. The cardinal physical exam finding is the pericardial friction rub, and signs of cardiac tamponade may be evident in more severe cases.

31. **What diagnostic tests may be helpful?**

Multiple laboratory values may be abnormal, including elevations in erythrocyte sedimentation rate (ESR), C-reactive protein (CRP), leukocyte count, and cardiac enzymes. EKG must be obtained for initial evaluation and may show diffuse ST-segment elevation and PR depression, followed by ST-segment normalization and, subsequently, T-wave inversion. An echocardiogram is ordered to rule out pericardial effusion.

32. **How is pericarditis treated, and when can athletes return to play?**

Nonsteroidal antiinflammatory drugs (NSAIDs) or colchicine are first-line therapy for the management of pericarditis, and athletes may be treated in the outpatient setting in the absence of the following: subacute onset, leukocytosis, cardiac tamponade, fever, acute trauma, immunosuppression, large pericardial effusion, anticoagulation, or failure to respond to NSAIDs within 7 days. These athletes must be excluded from participation in all competitive sports during the acute phase, until 3 months after no evidence of effusion on echocardiogram, normalized serum inflammatory markers, normal left ventricular function, and no resting or exercise-induced frequent/complex ventricular arrhythmias detectable on 24-h ECG monitoring or exercise ECG.

ENDOCARDITIS

33. **How does endocarditis present?**

This diagnosis requires a high clinical suspicion in athletes with structural heart disease such as congenital and acquired heart valve disease (bicuspid aortic valves, mitral valve prolapse, or rheumatic heart disease), prosthetic heart valve replacement, intravenous drug use, or cardiac implanted devices. The leading cause of infective endocarditis is *Staphylococcus aureus*, including methicillin-resistant *Staphylococcus aureus* (MRSA). Fever is the most common presenting symptom and may be associated with chills, night sweats, anorexia, dyspnea, cough, chest pain, and myalgias. Physical exam may reveal mitral or aortic regurgitation murmurs and classically will reveal peripheral manifestations such as petechiae, splinter hemorrhages, Osler nodes, Janeway lesions, or Roth spots.

34. **How is endocarditis diagnosed and managed?**

Laboratory evaluation is nonspecific and may be positive for elevations in ESR and CRP and leukocytosis. The Duke criteria are commonly used for evaluating these patients with concern for infective endocarditis.

For adults with infective endocarditis with a native valve and MRSA-positive, the treatment is intravenous vancomycin or daptomycin. Adding gentamicin or rifampin to vancomycin is not recommended in patients with bacteremia or native valve infective endocarditis. Transesophageal echocardiography is preferred over transthoracic echocardiography. Valve replacement surgery is recommended if any of the following are present: large vegetation (greater than 10 mm in diameter), the occurrence of one or more embolic events during the first two weeks of therapy, severe valvular insufficiency, valvular perforation or dehiscence, decompensated heart failure, perivalvular or myocardial abscess, new heart block, or persistent fevers or bacteremia.

For adults with infective endocarditis with a prosthetic valve who are MRSA-positive, the treatment is intravenous vancomycin and rifampin, plus gentamicin. Early evaluation for valve replacement surgery is recommended.

If the athlete remains afebrile after completion of the antibiotic course, repeat blood cultures remain negative, and repeat echocardiography is performed to establish a new baseline, then they may be gradually reintroduced to competition depending on any residual aortic (AR) or mitral regurgitation (MR) as follows:

- Mild to moderate AR/MR may participate in all competitive sports
- Severe AR/MR and LV enlargement (end-diastolic diameter >65 mm) should not participate
- Symptomatic athletes with mild to moderate disease should also be excluded from the competition

BACTERIAL DERMATOSES

35. What are the common bacterial skin infections?

Impetigo, folliculitis, furuncles, carbuncles, abscesses, cellulitis, erysipelas, keratolysis, and erythrasma are among the many common skin infections affecting athletes today.

36. How are common bacterial skin infections presented, diagnosed, and treated?

Impetigo is known for its classic "honey-colored crust" lesions that typically begin as isolated vesicular or pustular lesions and progress to the mature bullous or nonbullous form. *Staphylococcus aureus* and *Streptococcus pyogenes* are the most frequent causative bacteria. These lesions are commonly mistaken for contact dermatitis such as poison ivy or acne.

IMPETIGO TREATMENT

Nonbullous impetigo first line: topical mupirocin
Bullous impetigo (for larger areas of skin infection) first line: cephalexin or amoxicillin-clavulanate
For those with penicillin allergies: azithromycin
If MRSA: trimethoprim/sulfamethoxazole or clindamycin

Folliculitis is the inflammation and infection of the superficial portion of hair follicles that typically occurs as a small pruritic pustule on an erythematous base. Most of the time the diagnosis is clinical. A confirmatory diagnosis can be made by shaving an entire lesion superficially and placing it on culture media if the condition does not resolve with treatment. Lesions are typically seen in areas of shaved skin, underneath thigh pads, or occluded areas under a bathing suit and can be pruritic, urticarial, erythematous, and mildly painful. Folliculitis is typically treated with oral antibiotics, and cephalexin or erythromycin are commonly used as first-line therapy. Topical antibacterial soaps may also help prevent a recurrence.

Furuncles, carbuncles, and abscesses are larger, more painful, erythematous, fluctuant, and circumscribed masses. An abscess is a collection of pus under the skin. When an abscess is located within the hair follicle, it is called a furuncle. An agglomerate of furuncles forms a carbuncle, which is deeper, has more communications with the skin, drains pus, and can lead to scarring. The most common sites include the groin, axilla, and posterior thighs due to friction. *Staphylococcus* and *Streptococcus* are the most common pathogens. However, *Pseudomonas aeruginosa*, *Escherichia coli*, and others have been reported as causative pathogens. First-line treatment for furuncles, carbuncles, and abscesses is incision and drainage for easily accessible lesions although warm compresses and antibiotics are intermittently used for enclosed abscesses.

Indications for oral antibiotics effective against MRSA would be lesions bigger than 5 mm, or smaller than 5 mm but did not resolve with drainage, multiple lesions, expanding cellulitis, immunocompromised patients, patients at risk of endocarditis, and/or fever.

Erysipelas and cellulitis are inflammation/infection of superficial and deep layers of the skin and are distinguished by the depth of infection. Erysipelas are restricted to the dermis with a well-demarcated plaque. Cellulitis involves the subcutaneous tissue with an ill-defined patch. They present with pain, warmth, erythema, and edema, associated with fever and chills. Lymphadenopathy may accompany these lesions. The etiology is most often group A streptococci and, less commonly, staphylococci. Diagnosis is made clinically, and treatment includes:

Non-CA MRSA first line: cephalexin
Non-CA MRSA: If penicillin allergy: azithromycin.
CA-MRSA: TMP-SMX or clindamycin.
CA-MRSA: If no improvement with oral therapy: vancomycin.

Pitted keratolysis, or "sweaty sock syndrome," presents as hyperhidrosis, malodor, and a general sliminess of the skin, with general pitting of the soles of the feet as a classic distinguishing feature. Diagnosis is clinical, and treatment always commences with frequent drying, the use of moisture-wicking synthetic socks, and antibiotic therapy with topical erythromycin or clindamycin.

Erythrasma is caused by *Corynebacterium minutissimum* and is known as the most common bacterial infection of the feet. Presents as pruritic, scaling, patchy, erythematous, and irregular plaques usually seen in the interdigital spaces of the feet. Lesions can be diagnosed under a Wood light examination with coral-red fluorescence. Multiple treatments have been used including topical fusidic acid, erythromycin, clindamycin, or miconazole, and red-light photodynamic treatment. Lifestyle changes should be emphasized, such as exercise and weight loss, personal hygiene education, and use of talcum powder for humid body areas.

37. When can athletes typically return to play?
Return-to-play guidelines are the same for most bacterial dermatoses. Return to play after 72 hours of systemic antibiotics, with no moist, oozing, or exudative lesions. All lesions must have scabs and there should have been no new onset of lesions in the past 48 hours.

METHICILLIN-RESISTANT *STAPHYLOCOCCUS AUREUS* (MRSA) INFECTIONS

38. How do MRSA infections present?
Community-acquired MRSA infections in athletes most commonly involve the skin and soft tissues, often occurring at turf-abrasion sites or other open lesions. Risk factors include skin trauma, close-contact sports, sharing of sports equipment, and poor hygiene. MRSA requires prompt treatment and monitoring as it will often progress to an abscess. For this reason, any abscess in an athlete or skin or soft tissue infection that does not respond to initial antibiotic therapy should raise concern for MRSA. Athletes can experience pyomyositis, septic arthritis mostly affecting lower extremities joints, pubic osteomyelitis presenting with pubic or hip pain and fever, and endocarditis.

39. How are MRSA infections diagnosed and managed?
Wound culture is imperative, especially when MRSA is suspected by the appearance of the lesion or by history, such as knowledge of an infected team member. Incision and drainage of any accessible abscess are usually recommended in addition to presumptive, systemic antibiotics (TMP/SMX or doxycycline/minocycline). Clindamycin is commonly used as a second-line due to potential resistance. IV vancomycin is typically used in the inpatient setting for severe infections.

40. When can athletes typically return to play?
Return-to-play guidelines are the same as for most bacterial dermatoses and range from 48 to 72 hours of systemic antibiotics with no moist, oozing, or exudative lesions and no new onset of lesions in the last 48 hours.

VIRAL CUTANEOUS INFECTIONS: HERPES SIMPLEX

41. How does herpes simplex present?
Also known as herpes gladiatorum in wrestlers or "scrumpox" in rugby players, this infection is transmitted by skin-to-skin contact, easily transmissible when associated with a superficial trauma, and causes lesions that appear as a group of vesicles that may ulcerate and leave a painful, shallow ulcer on an erythematous base. Common locations include the lips, face, hands, body (torso in wrestlers), and genitalia. When herpes gladiatorum occurs in the ophthalmic branch of the trigeminal nerve, the athlete should be treated urgently to avoid blindness from herpetic keratitis.

42. How is herpes simplex diagnosed and managed?
Diagnosis is clinical and may be confirmed by detecting herpetic deoxyribonucleic acid (DNA) via polymerase chain reaction in the fluid from the blisters or a swab of erosion or viral culture. First-line therapy includes acyclovir and valaciclovir, with the latter often being preferred for its twice-a-day dosing compared to five times daily with acyclovir.
Initial infection (HSV-1 or HSV-2): valacyclovir, famciclovir, or acyclovir for 7–10 days.
If recurrent infection, the same treatment as above for 5–7 days.
Recurrence prevention may be done using valacyclovir 500 mg/tablet by mouth daily if the most recent infection was more than 2 years ago, or three times a day throughout a wrestling season. Valacyclovir 1 gram/tablet by mouth daily should be used if the most recent infection was less than 2 years ago.

43. When can athletes typically return to play?
Athletes must complete oral antiviral treatment for at least 120 hours, must have dry lesions with a firm crust, without new lesions for at least 72 hours, and remain free of systemic symptoms for 72 hours before returning to play.

GASTROINTESTINAL INFECTIONS

VIRAL

Noroviruses are the leading cause of acute, epidemic gastroenteritis in adults and older children. Transmitted by the fecal-oral route, most outbreaks are from fecal contamination of food or water by a handler. Athletes are contagious until 48 hours after diarrhea resolves. Symptoms typically include nausea, vomiting, abdominal cramping, and diarrhea. Diagnosis is clinical, and workup is not commonly required. Treatment is supportive and can be limited to simple rehydration.

BACTERIAL

Campylobacter spp., *Escherichia coli*, *Salmonella* spp., and *Shigella* spp. are among the most common causes of bacterial, infectious diarrhea in the United States, and presenting symptoms typically include moderate to severe diarrhea, which may progress to bloody diarrhea, abdominal pain, nausea/vomiting, and fever. Transmitted by the fecal-oral route, athletes are typically contagious for 48 hours following the final episode of diarrhea. Diagnosis requires stool evaluation including culture, microscopy, Gram stain, and/or specific toxin testing. Once diagnosed, treatment varies depending on the organism, but supportive care with electrolyte-rich hydration is always the first-line treatment. Antibiotics should not be used in *E. coli* as this has not been shown to be effective and may increase the risk of hemolytic uremic syndrome. *Campylobacter* spp. infection is usually self-limited, but salmonellosis and shigellosis can be treated with trimethoprim-sulfamethoxazole or ciprofloxacin to shorten the course of illness.

Athletes should avoid fluoroquinolones because of the musculoskeletal side effect of tendon rupture. Azithromycin is preferred. Antimotility agents such as diphenoxylate and loperamide can be used in association with antibiotics.

Antibiotic prophylaxis is needed if the athlete has comorbidities such as advanced human immunodeficiency virus (HIV) infection, severe inflammatory bowel disease, or a complicated organ transplant. The use of rifaximin should be considered in such instances.

Training staff may need to observe and/or teach proper handwashing techniques if teams travel to endemic areas with poor hygiene.

FOODBORNE

Bacterial toxins, typically the culprits of "food poisoning," cause illness by the GI tract's reaction to the toxin when ingested. The most common examples include *Bacillus* spp., *Campylobacter* spp., *Clostridium* spp., *Salmonella* spp., *Shigella* spp., *Listeria* spp., *E. coli*, and *Staphylococcus* spp.; these organisms are typically responsible for the outbreaks on cruise ships. Safe practices in endemic areas include avoidance of tap water, iced drinks, or raw fruits and vegetables and only eating food served at appropriately hot temperatures. These illnesses are self-limited, but chemoprophylaxis has been used in athletes not able to miss participation; typically, ciprofloxacin is used.

Athletes diagnosed with traveler's diarrhea will return to play when they can tolerate solid foods with no residual gastrointestinal symptoms, hydration status, and no fever.

HOW TO BOOST THE IMMUNE SYSTEM IN ATHLETES

Training overload should be avoided, as overtraining is known to impair the immune system. It is important to establish a progression training load with appropriate numbers of training sessions and proper recovery, adequate sleep time and quality, a healthy diet, and lifestyle changes to reduce stress, such as meditation and breathing control.

KEY POINTS

1. When distinguishing between viral and bacterial upper respiratory tract infections, it is important to note that bacterial infections are less common, last longer than the usual 7- to 10-day course for a viral infection, and are associated with a history of persistent purulent rhinorrhea and facial pain.
2. Most acute bronchitis cases are secondary to a viral etiology; less than 10% of patients have a bacterial cause.
3. It is important to perform a culture of furuncle and carbuncle secretions and drain lesions for complete resolution.
4. Once a gastrointestinal tract infection is diagnosed, treatment varies depending on the organism, but supportive care with electrolyte-rich hydration is always the first-line treatment.
5. An infection control program to avoid the spread of infections among athletes should be established in athletic training rooms by the utilization of disinfectant products with rapid, broad-spectrum antimicrobial efficacy for skin and surfaces, and educating athletic trainers and athletes on principles of infection control. Studies show that an alcohol-based hand sanitizer along with an antimicrobial spray for hard surfaces was effective in reducing bacterial and viral load, including multidrug-resistant organisms such as methicillin-resistant *Staphylococcus aureus* (MRSA) and vancomycin-resistant enterococcus (VRE).

Acknowledgment

The authors would like to thank Dr. Ryan Cudahy of Dignity Health in San Francisco, California, for his contributions to this chapter in the previous edition.

BIBLIOGRAPHY

Amoozgar B, Kaushal V, Garsondiya B.Primary pyomyositis: contact sports as the rare risk factors. *Case Rep Infect Dis.* 2019 Jul 28;2019:5739714. doi:10.1155/2019/5739714.
Bakal DR, Kasitinon D, Kussman AL, Hwang CE. Splenomegaly from recurrent infectious mononucleosis in an NCAA Division I athlete. *Curr Sports Med Rep.* 2021;20(10):511–513. doi:10.1249/JSR.0000000000000887. PMID: 34622813.
Aldulaimi S, Mendez AM. Splenomegaly: diagnosis and management in adults. *Am Fam Physician.* 2021;104(3):271–276.

Blume K, Körber N, Hoffmann D, Wolfarth B. Training load, immune status, and clinical outcomes in young athletes: a controlled, prospective, longitudinal study. *Front Physiol.* 2018;9:120. doi:10.3389/fphys.2018.00120.

Braun T, Kahanov L. Community-associated methicillin-resistant staphylococcus aureus infection rates and management among student-athletes. *Med Sci Sports Exerc.* 2018;50(9):1802–1809. doi:10.1249/MSS.0000000000001649.

Brunetti G, Corrado D, Zorzi A. Course of acute myocarditis in athletes: does the sport pattern really matter? *Int J Cardiol Heart Vasc.* 2021;37:100911. doi:10.1016/j.ijcha.2021.100911.

Cicchella A, Stefanelli C, Massaro M. Upper respiratory tract infections in sport and the immune system response: a review. *Biology (Basel).* 2021;10(5):362. doi:10.3390/biology10050362.

Colbey C, Cox AJ, Pyne DB, Zhang P, Cripps AW, West NP. Upper respiratory symptoms, gut health and mucosal immunity in athletes. *Sports Med.* 2018;48(Suppl 1):65–77. doi:10.1007/s40279-017-0846-4.

Compagnucci P, Volpato G, Falanga U, et al. Myocardial inflammation, sports practice, and sudden cardiac death: 2021 update. *Medicina (Kaunas).* 2021;57(3):277. doi:10.3390/medicina57030277.

Davison G, Perkins E, Jones AW, Swart GM, Jenkins AR, Robinson H, Dargan K. Coldzyme Mouth Spray reduces duration of upper respiratory tract infection symptoms in endurance athletes under free living conditions. *Eur J Sport Sci.* 2021;21(5):771–780. doi:10.1080/17461391.2020.1771429. Epub 2020 Jun 30.

Delise P, Mos L, Sciarra L, et al. Italian Cardiological Guidelines (COCIS) for Competitive Sport Eligibility in athletes with heart disease: update 2020. *J Cardiovasc Med (Hagerstown).* 2021;22(11):874–891. doi:10.2459/JCM.0000000000001186. https://www.cdc.gov/epstein-barr/about-mono.html.

Fisher K, Frank E, Andrie J, Onks C. Case report of an influenza outbreak in the sports medicine setting. *Curr Sports Med Rep.* 2021;20(4):185–187. doi:10.1249/JSR.0000000000000827.

Halle M, Binzenhöfer L, Mahrholdt H, Schindler MJ, Esefeld K, Tschöpe C. Myocarditis in athletes: a clinical perspective. *Eur J Prev Cardiol.* 2020 Mar 3:2047487320909670. doi:10.1177/2047487320909670. Epub ahead of print.

Hicks J, Boswell B, Noble V. Traumatic splenic laceration: a rare complication of infectious mononucleosis in an athlete. *Curr Sports Med Rep.* 2021;20(5):250–251. doi:10.1249/JSR.0000000000000840.

Jaworski CA, Rygiel V. Acute illness in the athlete. *Clin Sports Med.* 2019;38(4):577–595. doi:10.1016/j.csm.2019.05.001. Epub 2019 Jul 27.

Keaney LC, Kilding AE, Merien F, Shaw DM, Borotkanics R, Dulson DK. Household illness is the strongest predictor of upper respiratory tract symptom risk in elite rugby union players. *J Sci Med Sport.* 2021;24(5):430–434. doi:10.1016/j.jsams.2020.10.011. Epub 2020 Oct 24.

Kleynhans J, Treurnicht FK, Cohen C, et al. Outbreak of influenza A in a boarding school in South Africa, 2016. *Pan Afr Med J.* 2019;33:42. doi:10.11604/pamj.2019.33.42.16666. Published 2019 May 21.

Krzywański J, Kuchar E, Pokrywka A, et al. Safety and impact on training of the influenza vaccines in elite athletes participating in the Rio 2016 Olympics. *Clin J Sport Med.* 2021;31(5):423–429. doi:10.1097/JSM.0000000000000808.

LaBelle MW, Knapik DM, Arbogast JW, Zhou S, Bowersock L, Parker A, Voos JE. Infection risk reduction program on pathogens in high school and collegiate athletic training rooms. *Sports Health.* 2020;12(1):51–57. doi:10.1177/1941738119877865. Epub 2019 Oct 29.

Mascaro V, Capano MS, Iona T, Nobile CGA, Ammendolia A, Pavia M. Prevalence of *Staphylococcus aureus* carriage and pattern of antibiotic resistance, including methicillin resistance, among contact sport athletes in Italy. *Infect Drug Resist.* 2019;12:1161–1170. doi:10.2147/IDR.S195749. Published 2019 May 7.

McIntosh C, Clemm HH, Sewry N, Hrubos-Strøm H, Schwellnus MP. Diagnosis and management of nasal obstruction in the athlete: a narrative review by subgroup B of the IOC Consensus Group on "Acute Respiratory Illness in the Athlete". *J Sports Med Phys Fitness.* 2021;61(8):1144–1158. doi:10.23736/S0022-4707.21.12821-X. Epub 2021 Jun 22.

Morse D, Vangipuram R, Tyring SK. Painful lesions on the arms of a teenage wrestler. *Eur J Intern Med.* 2019;60:e1–e2. doi:10.1016/j.ejim.2018.05.011. Epub 2018 May 10.

Patel AR, Oheb D, Zaslow TL. Gastrointestinal prophylaxis in sports medicine. *Sports Health.* 2018;10(2):152–155. doi:10.1177/1941738117732733. Epub 2017 Sep 27. PMID: 28952896; PMCID: PMC5857727. https://www.aafp.org/afp/2013/1015/p507.html.

Pelliccia A, Solberg EE, Papadakis M, et al. Recommendations for participation in competitive and leisure time sport in athletes with cardiomyopathies, myocarditis, and pericarditis: position statement of the Sport Cardiology Section of the European Association of Preventive Cardiology (EAPC). *Eur Heart J.* 2019;40(1):19–33. doi:10.1093/eurheartj/ehy730.

Peterson AR, Nash E, Anderson BJ. Infectious disease in contact sports. *Sports Health.* 2019;11(1):47–58. doi:10.1177/1941738118789954. Epub 2018 Aug 14.

Pujalte GGA, Costa LMC, Clapp AD, Presutti RJ, Sluzevich JC. More than skin deep: dermatologic conditions in athletes. *Sports Health.* 2023;15(1):74–85. doi:10.1177/19417381211065026. Epub ahead of print. https://www.merckmanuals.com/professional/dermatologic-disorders/bacterial-skin-infections/furuncles-and-carbuncles.

Sylvester JE, Buchanan BK, Paradise SL, Yauger JJ, Beutler AI. Association of splenic rupture and infectious mononucleosis: a retrospective analysis and review of return-to-play recommendations. *Sports Health.* 2019;11(6):543–549. doi:10.1177/1941738119873665. Epub 2019 Sep 24.

Thompson PD, Dec GW. We need better data on how to manage myocarditis in athletes. *Eur J Prev Cardiol.* 2020 Mar 31:2047487320915545. doi:10.1177/2047487320915545. Epub ahead of print.

CHAPTER 49

WHEN TO IMAGE FOR SPORTS-RELATED COMPLAINTS

Heath C. Thornton, MD, Jeremy Swisher, MD

TOP URGENT CARE SECRETS

1. Utilization of validated imaging guidelines (i.e., Ottawa ankle/knee rules, Pittsburgh rules for knee trauma, Canadian C-spine Rule) can reduce unnecessary imaging.
2. Identification of specific fractures around the knee on x-ray can help in diagnosing other ligamentous and meniscal pathology only seen with advanced imaging.

1. **In an acutely injured athlete, what should I look for to decide if x-ray imaging might be needed?**
   Focal swelling, point tenderness over bony prominences or growth plates, positive tap or percussion test, gross deformity, inability to move a joint, and traumatic mechanism of injury are all signs of potential fracture. Any concern for fracture would justify proceeding with radiographic imaging. A good rule of thumb when acquiring plain radiographs is two views for long bones and three views for joints. Weight bearing radiographs can also be useful for evaluation of the joint space.

2. **Are there any special views I should consider for pediatric injuries given growth plates and ossification centers?**
   In addition to the area of concern, contralateral imaging for pediatric injuries will allow comparison of the injury to the patient's "normal." This can help in determining if the epiphyseal plates or ossification centers are asymmetric. Any asymmetry that correlates with injury and/or tenderness on exam may justify treatment and follow-up.

3. **A middle-aged adult sustains an injury to their ankle. They are unable to bear weight immediately after the event. Upon evaluation in the office, they are still unable to walk four steps but have no tenderness on palpation of the foot or ankle. Are there guidelines that can help determine if imaging is indicated after a foot or ankle injury?**
   The Ottawa ankle rules (Table 49.1) were created to encourage judicious use of radiography in acute midfoot and ankle injuries. These rules can be useful in ruling out fractures due to their high sensitivity: 97.2% sensitivity, 7.8% specificity, 13.9% positive predictive value, and 95% negative predictive value. Weight bearing inability appears to be the highest reliable marker with a 93% negative predictive value.

4. **In what scenarios do the Ottawa ankle rules not apply?**
   These rules should not be applied to patients less than 5 years old or ankle injuries greater than 10 days old. The rules should also not be applied to patients with intoxication, skin injuries, head injuries, or decreased sensation in the lower extremities.

5. **Ottawa rules are negative, but the patient has a positive Tib-Fib Squeeze test on examination. Is imaging indicated?**
   Compression of the tibia and fibula together at the mid-calf resulting in pain in the ankle is highly indicative of syndesmotic injury. Dorsiflexion of the foot with external rotation that elicits similar pain is another provocative test for this condition. Plain radiographs are required due to the association of this injury with joint instability. In addition to standard AP, lateral, and mortise views, one should obtain a weight-bearing AP view and a stress view. If diastasis is seen, an orthopedic surgery referral is needed. Greater than 5.3 mm of diastasis of the tibiofibular clear space (AP view) has a sensitivity of 82% and specificity of 75% for syndesmotic injury. Tibiofibular overlap can also be used and is normal when greater than 6 mm on AP view and 1 mm on mortise view.

6. **A patient presents with an acute knee injury. Is there a decision rule that can be used to guide whether imaging is needed to rule out acute fracture?**
   Both Ottawa knee rules and Pittsburgh knee rules can be used to decide whether to obtain imaging in acute knee injury (Table 49.2). Pittsburgh knee rules have been found to have a sensitivity of 99–100% with slightly better specificity than the Ottawa rules. In a systematic review and meta-analysis in 2009, the Ottawa knee rules were found to have high sensitivity (99%) and adequate specificity (46%) for children over 5 years of age. The Pittsburgh criteria were originally described in patients of all ages.

7. **What exclusion criteria exist for the Ottawa and Pittsburgh knee rules?**
   Decision rules for imaging in knee injuries should not be applied to patients with skin injuries surrounding the knee, multiple injuries, injuries greater than 1 week old, altered consciousness or intoxication, head injury, decreased sensation in the lower extremities, or history of previous surgery or fracture on the affected knee.

Table 49.1 Ottawa Ankle Rules	
ANKLE SERIES IF ANY CRITERIA BELOW ARE MET	**FOOT SERIES IF ANY CRITERIA BELOW ARE MET**
• Bony tenderness of the distal 6 cm of the posterior edge of the lateral malleolus • Bony tenderness of the distal 6 cm of the posterior edge of the medial malleolus	• Bony tenderness of the base of the fifth metatarsal • Bony tenderness of the navicular bone
Inability to bear weight for four steps both immediately following the injury and upon presentation to the physician's office or emergency room	

Table 49.2 Comparison of Ottawa and Pittsburgh Criteria	
OTTAWA KNEE RULES	**PITTSBURGH KNEE RULES**
One or more of the following: • Age >55 years • Tenderness of patella • Tenderness over fibular head • Limited knee flexion to 90 degrees • Inability to bear weight	Blunt trauma or fall plus either of the following: • Age <12 or >50 years • Inability to bear weight

8. **What fractures seen on plain films of the knee are concerning for an associated ligament and/or meniscal injury requiring further evaluation with MRI?**
Segond fracture, reverse Segond sign, Stieda fracture, tibial spine fracture, fibular head avulsion fracture (Arcuate sign), and posterior tibial plateau fracture.

9. **A 28-year-old runner comes into your office complaining of focal pain in their left shin that has been worsening over the past few weeks. They recently signed up to run a 10k a few months from now and have been ramping up both running intensity and frequency. What injury are you most concerned for and what is the next step in diagnosis?**
This patient potentially has a stress fracture of the tibia if focal bony tenderness is found on exam. Plain radiographs are the initial imaging of choice, but they typically will be normal in the first 2–3 weeks and have a sensitivity of 56% and a specificity of 96%. The lateral x-ray for tibial stress fractures may show the "dreaded black line," which is highly suspicious for stress fracture. When clinical suspicion remains high with normal radiographs, MRI is the next imaging modality of choice. MRI is the most sensitive (99%) and specific (97%) test. The most common sites for stress fractures include the tibia, fibula, femoral neck, and metatarsal bones. Upper extremity stress fractures are less common but could be seen in the humerus (baseball or tennis) and ribs (rowing).

10. **A patient presents after a traumatic event with the inability to move the left arm and severe pain. On exam, his arm is held in adduction and internal rotation. You suspect anterior shoulder dislocation. What imaging test do you obtain to confirm the diagnosis?**
Plain radiograph is used to verify the diagnosis and rule out associated humeral and glenoid fractures. Anteroposterior (AP), axillary, and lateral scapular views should be obtained. A single axillary view after attempted reduction can be used to confirm the anatomic alignment of the joint.

11. **Is there a role for radiographic imaging in the suspected elbow dislocation?**
Obvious deformity and swelling at the joint and malposition of the extremity are clinical signs that suggest dislocation after traumatic injury. To assess direction of dislocation and potential concomitant fractures prior to closed reduction, AP and lateral x-rays of the elbow can be a useful modality. After reduction, repeat x-rays should be obtained to verify reduction and assess for postreduction coronoid process fractures.

12. **Can imaging be a useful tool in the diagnosis of concussion?**
Concussion is a clinical diagnosis. Structural neuroimaging will be normal in patients with concussions and is not necessary for diagnosis. Imaging may be indicated to evaluate for more serious traumatic brain injury in patients with certain symptoms such as repeated vomiting, prolonged loss of consciousness, or a severe mechanism of injury. One could use the Canadian Head CT rules (Table 49.3) to evaluate the need for imaging in patients over 16 years of age. If between the ages of 2 and 16, the PECARN rules may be applied. If you are concerned for a cervical spine injury in the setting of evaluating a concussion, you can utilize the Canadian C-Spine Rules (Box 49.1) to assess the need for imaging.

Table 49.3 Canadian Head Computed Tomography Rules: Risk Factors

HIGH-RISK FACTORS	MEDIUM-RISK FACTORS
Glasgow Coma Scale Score <15 at 2 hours after injury	Amnesia before impact >30 minutes
Any sign of basilar skull fracture: • Hemotympanum • Raccoon eyes • Cerebrospinal fluid otorrhea or rhinorrhea • Battle sign	Dangerous mechanism: • Pedestrian struck by motor vehicle • Occupant ejected from motor vehicle • Fall from 3 or more feet or down five stairs
Suspected open or depressed skull fracture	
Two or more episodes of vomiting	
Age 65 or older	

BOX 49.1 Canadian C-Spine Rules

- Is there any high-risk factor that mandates radiography?
  - Age 65 years or older
  - Dangerous mechanism
  - Fall from 1 m (or five stairs)
  - Axial load to the head (e.g., diving accidents)
  - Motor vehicle collisions at high speed (>100 km/h)
  - Motorized recreational vehicle accident
  - Ejection from a vehicle
  - Bicycle collision with an immovable object
  - Paresthesias in extremities
- Is there any low-risk factor that allows safe assessment of range of motion? Patients who do not have any of the following low-risk factors should be radiographed and are not suitable for range of motion testing:
  - Simple rear-end motor vehicle collision
  - Sitting position in emergency department
  - Ambulatory at any time since injury
  - Delayed onset of neck pain
  - Absence of midline C-spine tenderness
  - Range of motion testing
  - Is the patient able to actively rotate the neck 45 degrees to the left and right (regardless of pain)? If so, imaging is not indicated.

Data from Stiell IG, Wells GA, Vandemheen KL, et al. The Canadian C-spine rule for radiography in alert and stable trauma patients. *JAMA.* 2001;286(15):1841.

13. If you are concerned about a facial fracture, what type of imaging is most useful?
    Computed tomography is superior to conventional radiography and magnetic resonance imaging (MRI) in detecting facial fractures.

14. Are there any other resources to help in deciding when imaging is appropriate?
    The American College of Radiology has published guidelines for practitioners to help determine the appropriateness of imaging for various conditions. These can be found online at: https://www.acr.org/Clinical-Resources/ACR-Appropriateness-Criteria.

15. What are the most common high-yield MSK injuries that would be appropriate for point-of-care ultrasound (POCUS) in an urgent care setting?
    POCUS can be useful for assessing a number of soft tissue injuries and other musculoskeletal pathology. Given the time constraints of a busy clinic, utilizing the "Yes/No" clinical questions approach for POCUS promotes the efficient use of this tool. This imaging modality can also be useful for guiding injections or aspirations of many of the joints that present to urgent care. Some of the most useful applications in this setting are listed in Table 49.4.

Table 49.4 High-Yield POCUS

UPPER EXTREMITY HIGH-YIELD POCUS	LOWER EXTREMITY HIGH-YIELD POCUS
• **Shoulder:** Tendonitis, tendinosis, or tear of the rotator cuff muscles. Most commonly, could assess the supraspinatus. • **Elbow:** UCL tear or laxity, common flexor tendons, ulnar nerve entrapment. • **Hand/Wrist:** Ganglion cyst vs. abscess, mallet finger, jersey finger	• **Hip:** Evaluate for hip effusion in the anterior synovial recess, which is anterior to the femoral neck. • **Knee:** Can be used to identify tendonitis or tendon rupture of the patellar or quadriceps tendon, confirming intraarticular effusion, degree of injury to MCL or LCL, identify parameniscal cysts (suggesting meniscal tear), as well as a Baker cyst. • **Ankle:** ATFL, Achilles tendon rupture, and stress fractures in the foot.

KEY POINTS

1. There are several imaging guidelines that can assist in the decision to obtain radiographic imaging for ankle, knee, and neck injuries.
2. Ottawa ankle rules do not apply to patients less than 5 years old or ankle injuries greater than 10 days old.
3. In general, imaging is not indicated in the setting of concussion unless the criteria for Canadian Head CT Rules are met.
4. After reduction of a dislocation, radiographic imaging is generally recommended to evaluate for associated fractures.
5. Point-of-care ultrasound is an excellent tool for high-yield, "Yes-No" clinical questions in MSK injuries. These can include identifying tendon ruptures, effusions, bursitis/ganglion cysts, and acute ligamentous injuries.

Acknowledgments

The authors would like to thank coauthors Lindsay Smith and Crystal Higginson for their contributions to this chapter in the previous edition.

BIBLIOGRAPHY

Alidina S, Alidina J, Souza F, Kalandiak S, Subhawong TK. Radiographic evaluation of elbow fractures. *Semin Musculoskelet Radiol.* 2021;25:529–537.

Alzuhairy AK. Accuracy of Canadian CT Head Rule and New Orleans Criteria for Minor Head Trauma: a systematic review and meta-analysis. *Arch Acad Emerg Med [eCollection].* 2020;8(1):e79. https://www.ncbi.nlm.nih.gov/pmc/articles/PMC7682632/. Accessed September 30, 2022.

American College of Radiology. ACR Appropriateness Criteria. Available at: https://www.acr.org/Clinical-Resources/ACR-Appropriateness-Criteria. Accessed June 6, 2022.

American Medical Society of Sports Medicine. AMSSM Sports Ultrasound Online Didactics. Available at: https://www.amssm.org/SportsUltrasound.php. Published 2015. Accessed September 30, 2022.

Cheung TC, et al. Diagnostic accuracy and reproducibility of the Ottawa Knee Rule vs. the Pittsburgh Decision Rule. *Amer J of Emerg Med.* 2013;31(4):641–645.

French CN, et al. Ultrasound in sports injuries. *Clinics in Sports Med.* 2021;40(3):801–819.

Gaillard F, Rasuli B. Segond fracture. Radiopaedia.org. Available at: https://radiopaedia.org/articles/segond-fracture?lang=us. Published 2010 (last revision July 2021). Accessed September 30, 2022.

Herman L. A 20-year perspective on the Ottawa Ankle Rules: are we still on solid footing? *JAAPA.* 2021;34(7):15–20.

Kellett JJ, et al. Diagnostic imaging of ankle syndesmosis injuries: a general review. *J Med Imaging Rad Onc.* 2018;62(2):159–168.

Knipe H, Bell D. Distal tibiofibular syndesmostic injury. Radiopaedia.org. Available at: https://radiopaedia.org/articles/distal-tibiofibular-syndesmosis-injury?lang=us. Published 2019 (last revision November 2021). Accessed September 30, 2022.

Lee CH, Tan CF, Kim O, Suh KJ, Yao M, Chan WP, Wu JS. Osseous injury associated with ligamentous tear of the knee. *Can Assoc Radiol J.* 2016;67(4):379–386.

Vijayasankar D, Boyle A, Atkinson P. Can the Ottawa knee rule be applied to children? A systematic review and meta-analysis of observational studies. *Emerg Med J.* 2009;26(4):250–253.

CHAPTER 50

WOUND ASSESSMENT, BURNS, AND ANIMAL BITES

John A. Park, MD, Lilia Reyes, MD, FAAP

WOUND ASSESSMENT

1. **Why does wound assessment matter?**
   Traumatic wounds are a common presenting complaint in acute care centers. Nearly 12 million wounds are treated in US emergency departments annually, with about one-third of those in patients under the age of 18. Wound care accounts for approximately 10% of all procedures performed in emergency departments, with literally millions more wounds assessed yearly that do not require procedural intervention.

   Each wound is different, necessitating individualized treatment based on clinical assessment. Without appropriate treatment, patients with acute wounds may suffer complications such as poor healing and infections.

2. **How do we begin wound assessment?**
   In assessment of any patient in the acute care setting, patient resuscitation and stabilization always take precedence and should proceed according to pediatric advanced life support (PALS) and advanced trauma life support (ATLS) protocols. Assuming the patient is stable and requires only management of minor wounds, assessment may progress. Careful history taking and examination are essential to the appropriate assessment and treatment of wounds. Documentation should include the mechanism described by the family as well as a clear description of the wound and an assessment of whether or not the wound is consistent with the mechanism described by the caregiver.

3. **What types of wounds may be appropriately treated in the urgent care setting?**
   - Appropriate: minor cuts, lacerations, and abrasions.
   - Not appropriate: any penetrating, complex, or severe traumatic injury should be referred to an emergency department (ED) for definitive management after ensuring patient stability for transfer. Any wounds concerning for nonaccidental trauma should also be referred to the ED.

4. **What are the goals of wound management?**
   - Establishing hemostasis
   - Minimizing the risk of infection
   - Optimizing cosmetic results
   - Returning function to normal
   - Minimizing pain

5. **Are there different types of wounds?**
   - Abrasions: caused by force applied in opposite directions that scrapes away layers of skin or underlying tissue.
   - Lacerations: wounds where there is a separation between tissues. Different types of force can generate different subtypes.
   - Cuts: caused by shearing forces in injuries such as knife wounds, which are often "cleaner" in appearance with sharp edges or margins.
   - True lacerations: caused by compressive or tensile forces and often have somewhat rough, jagged, or torn edges and may be associated with contusion.
   - Puncture wounds: penetrating injuries with a small surface opening and depth that cannot be directly visualized. Susceptible to infection because of the enclosed environment, caused by a combination of forces.
   - Avulsions: tissue is separated either completely or nearly so from its base. Caused by shearing and tensile forces.
   - Burns: result in wounds (will be discussed separately).
   Wounds may be a combination of these types.

6. **What details of the patient history are key to wound assessment?**
   - How did this happen and what has happened since?
   - When did this happen?
   - Where did this happen? (Any exposure to soil, natural bodies of water, or animals or insects that bite can cause wounds that are at increased risk of infection.)
   - Immunization and immune status
   - Does the story make sense and fit with the presenting injury? (If it does not or if there is any doubt, appropriate steps to investigate nonaccidental injury should be taken.)

7. **What aspects of exam should be focused on?**
   - Examination using clean or sterile gloves and other protective measures such as mask and eye shield.
   - Exam should be conducted in a well-lit area, and additional lamps may be necessary for best visualization of the injury.
   - Measures to control bleeding should be taken and then exam repeated once bleeding is controlled to ensure blood does not obscure any findings.
   - Note the extent of injury, any visible contamination, and damage to nearby structures.
   - Neurovascular status in the form of distal perfusion as well as motor and sensory function are important to note and document before the use of any anesthetics.

8. **A 17-year-old male patient presents with a laceration of the left hand that occurred 2 days ago. He states that he wants it "sewn up" so that it will heal faster. Is this laceration too old to be sutured?**
   - There is no absolute time period for when a wound is too old for surgical repair.
   - Studies have demonstrated that many wounds may be closed safely up to 24 hours after injury, and this is used as a "golden period" for repair.

9. **A 5-year-old male patient presents with a laceration to the scalp that is bleeding profusely. How can bleeding be controlled?**
   - Apply direct pressure gently but firmly over the wound.
   - Elevate the wound if it is on an extremity.
   - Suturing or stapling of highly vascular areas may be useful for persistent bleeding.
   - Epinephrine, either locally injected into the surrounding soft tissue at a bleeding site or applied topically in a preparation such as LET (Lidocaine, Epinephrine, and Tetracaine) gel, may help with hemostasis through vasoconstriction.

10. **A 13-year-old female patient presents for treatment of a laceration on her foot. You decide it requires closure with sutures, but she refuses to allow this, stating she is afraid it will hurt. How can her pain be controlled?**
    - Pain control for minor injuries is often well achieved using local methods such as topical gels or injectable solutions.
    - Generally, these methods should be coincidentally given with epinephrine to decrease systemic effects and prolong localized exposure to the medication.
    - Medications such as benzodiazepine given orally, intravenously (IV), intramuscularly (IM), or intranasally (IN) may be useful for anxiolysis as well, particularly prior to attempting wound repair.

11. **Do all lacerations need to be repaired?**
    No. Remembering our goals of wound management, sometimes these are best served by leaving a wound to heal by secondary intent. Many wounds should not be repaired because they will heal well on their own, repair may significantly increase the risk of infection, or for other reasons. The first rule in medicine is to do no harm, so repair should only be performed if necessary.

12. **When are antibiotics indicated?**
    There is no absolute guide for when antibiotic prophylaxis is indicated; however, antibiotics should generally be given for complicated wounds such as:
    - Bites
    - Open fractures
    - Tendon or joint involvement
    - Obvious infection or high risk for infection such as exposure to soil, bodies of fresh water, or other contaminants. Absent contaminants, many providers will also consider wounds distally on extremities as likely to become infected with those on the face and scalp as unlikely to become infected.

13. **A 7-year-old male patient presents after stepping on a nail in the backyard. Does he require tetanus immunization or immunoglobulin?**
    See Table 50.1.

BURN MANAGEMENT

14. **What burns can be managed in an urgent care setting?**
    Children younger than 5 years account for 18% of burns presenting to care in the United States. Of these, the majority are minor, covering <10% of the total body surface area, and the predominant type of injury is a scald. Minor superficial burns are appropriate for treatment in the acute or urgent care setting; however, those affecting larger areas, greater depths, or with other associated injuries should be referred to advanced care centers.

Table 50.1 Tetanus Vaccines and TIG for Wound Management

AGE (YEARS)	VACCINATION HISTORY	CLEAN, MINOR WOUNDS	ALL OTHER WOUNDS
0–6	Unknown or not up-to-date on DTaP series based on age	DTaP	DTaP TIG
	Up-to-date on DTaP series based on age	No indication	No indication
7–10	Unknown or incomplete DTaP series	Tdap and recommend catch-up vaccination	Tdap and recommend catch-up vaccination TIG
	Completed DTaP series AND <5 years since last dose	No indication	No indication
	Completed DTaP series AND ≥5 years since last dose	No indication	Td, but Tdap preferred if child is 10 years of age
11 years and older (*if pregnant, see footnote)	Unknown or <3 doses of tetanus toxoid-containing vaccine	Tdap and recommend catch-up vaccination	Tdap and recommend catch-up vaccination TIG
	3 or more doses of tetanus toxoid-containing vaccine AND <5 years since last dose	No indication	No indication
	3 or more doses of tetanus toxoid-containing vaccine AND 5–10 years since last dose	No indication	Tdap preferred (if not yet received) or Td
	3 or more doses of tetanus toxoid-containing vaccine AND >10 years since last dose	Tdap preferred (if not yet received) or Td	Tdap preferred (if not yet received) or Td

From http://emergency.cdc.gov/disasters/disease/tetanus.asp.

15. How are burns classified?

Burns are generally classified or grouped according to three characteristics: depth of affected tissue, percent of total body surface area affected, and cause of injury (thermal, chemical, electrical, etc.). These classifications are in turn used to determine the severity of a burn and aid in triage toward appropriate treatment (Table 50.2).

Burns are often assigned a "degree" according to the depth of affected tissue. Burns affecting only the epidermis are considered first degree or superficial, and those affecting dermis as well as epidermis are considered second degree or partial thickness. Burns that damage or destroy all layers of skin are called third degree or full thickness. Some clinicians also consider burns damaging tissue deep to the skin as fourth degree. Burn wounds can change dramatically over the first several days after initial injury and appear more severe than on initial presentation. This occurs in spite of the burn process being arrested and is thought to be part of the pathophysiology of burns.

Table 50.2 Burn Classification

	SUPERFICIAL OR FIRST DEGREE	PARTIAL THICKNESS OR SECOND DEGREE	FULL THICKNESS OR THIRD DEGREE
Tissue depth affected	Epidermis only	Epidermis and dermis	Epidermis, dermis, and below
Sensation	Painful	Painful	Diminished
Appearance	Erythematous, hyperemic, intact skin	Blistered, disrupted skin	Skin layers destroyed; deep tissue exposed

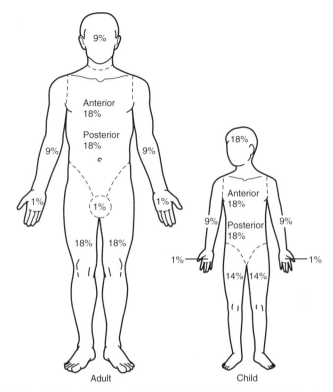

Fig. 50.1 The rule of nines. (From Ciottone, GR. Ciottone Disaster Medicine. 1st ed. Elsevier/Saunders; 2005.)

16. **A 2-year-old girl presents to your urgent care with burns to her forearms and the upper portion of her anterior chest wall after pulling her mother's coffee mug from the counter. How would you estimate the percent of total body surface area affected?**
    Determining the percentage of body surface area affected can be difficult, and although there are many methods utilized by clinicians to estimate this, there is no perfect method. The "rule of nines" (Fig. 50.1) is a widespread method and perhaps the oldest in use but is applicable to older pediatric patients and adults. This boils down to each body area roughly equaling a multiple of 9% of the total body surface area (TBSA). This is slightly more complex in children than in adults, as various body parts comprise differing percentages of body surface area in children as compared to adults; for example, the head is proportionally much larger in children. Another method used to estimate BSA is the Lund Browder charts (Fig. 50.2). Similar to the charts illustrating the rule of nines, the charts show percentages of BSA occupied by various body areas. A third way to quickly estimate BSA is by using the palm and fingers of the patient's hand to represent approximately 1% of BSA (Fig. 50.3) and multiplying the burn area out from this. No method of BSA estimation is perfect, and clinical judgment should be used in this process.

17. **A 5-year-old male patient presents to care after spilling a cup of hot tea in his lap. After exposing the affected area, you note burns encompassing the anterior thighs as well as the genitalia and suprapubic area. The burns cover approximately 2–3% of the boy's TBSA. Is it appropriate to treat this boy as an outpatient?**
    The American Burn Association sets forth criteria for burns necessitating admission as follows:
    1. Partial-thickness burns covering greater than 10% of total body surface area
    2. Burns involving the face, hands, feet, genitalia, perineum, or major joints
    3. Third-degree burns
    4. Electrical burns
    5. Chemical burns
    6. Inhalation injury
    7. Burns in patients with complicating medical disorders
    8. Burns with concomitant trauma where the burn poses the greater threat to life
    9. Burns in children at hospitals without qualified pediatric providers and facilities
    10. Burns in patients who will require special supportive services or interventions

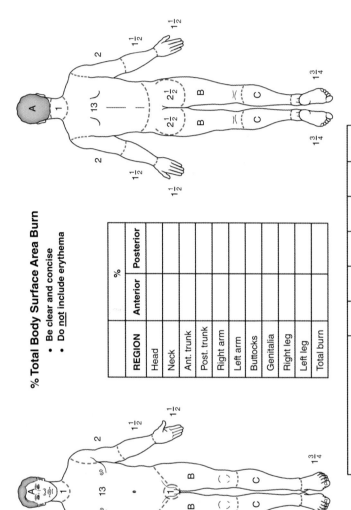

% Total Body Surface Area Burn

- Be clear and concise
- Do **not** include erythema

REGION	% Anterior	Posterior
Head		
Neck		
Ant. trunk		
Post. trunk		
Right arm		
Left arm		
Buttocks		
Genitalia		
Right leg		
Left leg		
Total burn		

AREA	Age 0	1	5	10	15	Adult
A = $\frac{1}{2}$ OF HEAD	$9\frac{1}{2}$	$8\frac{1}{2}$	$6\frac{1}{2}$	$5\frac{1}{2}$	$4\frac{1}{2}$	$3\frac{1}{2}$
B = $\frac{1}{2}$ OF ONE THIGH	$2\frac{3}{4}$	$3\frac{1}{4}$	4	$4\frac{1}{2}$	$4\frac{1}{2}$	$4\frac{3}{4}$
C = $\frac{1}{2}$ OF ONE LOWER LEG	$2\frac{1}{2}$	$2\frac{1}{2}$	$2\frac{3}{4}$	3	$3\frac{1}{4}$	$3\frac{1}{2}$

Fig. 50.2 Lund Browder (LB) Chart. The shape of the burn is drawn onto the chart, excluding simple erythematous areas. Each area is assigned a value of the body surface area percentage, which is entered into the table and the total body surface area affected is then calculated. (Redrawn from Hettiaratchy S, Papini R. Initial management of a major burn: II—assessment and resuscitation. *BMJ*. 2004;329:101.)

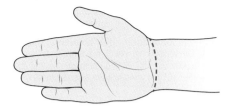

Fig. 50.3 Palm and fingers represent 1% of total body surface area. (From Magee DJ. Orthopedic physical assessment. 7th ed. St. Louis: Saunders; 2021.)

18. **What comprises the initial outpatient burn care?**
    - Cooling works to help mitigate further injury as well as decrease pain. Irrigation of the wound with room-temperature saline or sterile water is effective. Caution should be used with ice, as it may cause further thermal injury.
    - Clothing, jewelry, and debris should be removed from the burn area.
    - The wound should be cleaned with a mild antiseptic, such as chlorhexidine, and irrigated.
    - Blisters are somewhat controversial, with some evidence both for and against rupturing any blisters and removing devitalized tissue. The blister can function as a biodressing, but it has also been reported that devitalized tissue can serve as a nidus for infection.
    - Antibiotic ointment (such as bacitracin or Silvadene) should be applied to the wound.
    - Nonadhesive dressing should be applied to the wound; if this is unavailable, mesh gauze may be used instead. The wound should then be padded and wrapped with further gauze.
    - If wounds involve the digits of the hand or foot, each digit should be padded and wrapped separately.
    - Some burn wounds may be in areas such as the face that make them difficult to dress. In this case, it is acceptable to apply antibiotic ointment in place of dressing and instruct patients to wash the area a few times a day to keep the wound clean, reapplying the ointment after each cleansing.
    - If possible, the wound should be kept elevated to minimize edema.

19. **A 2-year-old male patient with no past medical conditions presents to care with burns on his chest and abdomen. He was reaching up to grab a bowl of hot soup off a table and spilled it on himself after dropping the bowl. He is crying and minimally consolable by his parents, and you note a blistered burn about the size of the patient's hand on his torso. After exposing and then cooling the burned area with sterile saline, what is the next step in appropriately treating this patient?**
    Analgesia is a critical component in the treatment of burn wounds. The pain associated with minor burns is often quite severe, and manipulating the wound in the process of examining and dressing it can make this pain worse. It is often appropriate to use opiate medication for pain control during this process. Intravenous, intramuscular, and intranasal medications should be utilized for their rapid onset and potency of pain control. Oral therapy often takes too long to take effect, limiting the practicality of its use. Local nerve blocks may also be utilized where practical to provide adequate pain control. It is also important to consider pain control after the patient is discharged home.

HUMAN AND ANIMAL BITES

20. **What makes a cat bite more prone to causing a wound infection?**
    It causes a deep puncture wound, making it difficult to irrigate, thus subjecting it to having a high infection rate. In a series done in Austria, they were able to observe a six times higher infection rate in cat bites (48.5%) versus dog bites (7.7%) in this study.

21. **What are the indications for antibiotics in the setting of an animal bite?**
    Human and cat bites through the dermis
        Bites closed prematurely
        Bites more than 8 hours old with significant crush injury or edema
        Potential damage to bones, joints, or tendons
        Bites to hands and feet
        Patients with increased risk of infection
        Signs of infection within 24 hours

22. The common pathogens in animal bites, in order of prevalence, are:
    Pasteurella species, staphylococci, streptococci, and anaerobic bacteria.

23. What are the antibiotic options for children after an animal bite?
    Amoxicillin-clavulanate 20 mg/kg (amoxicillin component) two times daily (max 875 mg amoxicillin/125 mg cla-
    vulanic acid per dose). If allergic to penicillin, TMP-SMX (trimethoprim-sulfamethazole) 4–5 mg/kg (trimethoprim
    component) per dose twice daily (max 160 mg trimethoprim per dose) PLUS Clindamycin 10 mg/kg three times a
    day (max 450 mg per dose).

24. How many cases of rabies have occurred in the United States after the suspected animal
    has been observed during the 10-day period?
    No case of human rabies in the United States has been attributed to a dog, cat, or ferret that has remained healthy
    throughout the standard 10-day period of confinement after exposure.

25. A 10-year-old patient was playing basketball with his friends in his driveway when a
    neighborhood pitbull bit him. The patient has a deformity in the right distal wrist region with
    an overlying 3-cm laceration and another 5-cm laceration on his left biceps region. The dog
    is unknown to patient and parents. What do you recommend to the family regarding rabies
    vaccine and immunoglobulin?
    In the United States, postexposure prophylaxis consists of a regimen of one dose of immune globulin and four
    doses of rabies vaccine over a 14-day period. Rabies immune globulin and the first dose of rabies vaccine should
    be given by the health care provider as soon as possible after exposure. Additional doses of the rabies vaccine
    should be given on days 3, 7, and 14 after the first vaccination. Human rabies immune globulin (HRIG) is dosed at
    20 IU/kg.

26. A 3-year-old patient is brought to the emergency department for evaluation of a bite mark
    on her arm. The caregiver reports that the bite mark is from a classmate in daycare that
    occurred earlier in the day. On exam, the child has an ovoid mark with teeth markings on
    the right radial region without a break in the skin. How can you tell the difference between
    an adult bite and a child bite on exam?
    The measurement of the intercanine distance of the bite will distinguish human adult bites (3.0–4.5 cm being
    adult human; 2.5–3.0 cm being child or small adult; and less than 2.5 cm, being child's deciduous teeth). How-
    ever, this is based on orthodontic data and has not been validated in clinical practice.

27. Human bite wounds tend to become infected with which bacterial species?
    Staphylococcus aureus, *Streptococcus* spp., and *Eikenella corrodens*.

28. Why is it recommended to obtain an x-ray on patients after a dog bite, especially on bites
    on the extremities?
    Dogs have large, dull teeth and powerful jaws that are capable of inducing a significant amount of damage due to
    a crush injury. Larger dogs are able to deliver a bite force of greater than 450 pounds per square inch, capable of
    perforating light sheet metal.

SPIDER, SCORPION, BEE, AND SNAKE BITES

29. What characterizes this spider (Fig. 50.4) as being potentially poisonous?
    They can be identified by the hourglass pattern (red or orange in color) on the ventral aspect of their shiny, black
    abdomen. It is located primarily in the Southwest United States. Only female black widow spiders are dangerous.

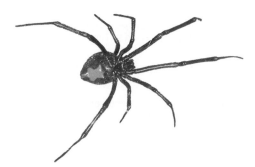

Fig. 50.4 Female black widow spider with a red hourglass marking on the underside of her abdomen. (From Habif TP. Clinical Dermatology: A Color Guide to Diagnosis and Therapy. 5th ed. McGraw-Hill Companies; 2010:581–634.)

30. **How can a black widow spider bite be identified?**
The classic *Latrodectus* envenomation starts with a localized reaction that is generally minimal. The bite site quickly develops into a pale central area with surrounding erythema, producing a "target" or "halo" lesion.

31. **What are the expected symptoms after a black widow spider envenomation?**
Cholinergic symptoms such as salivation, diaphoresis, tachycardia, hypertension, and bronchorrhea can peak a few hours after the bite. Severe abdominal pain can be seen often. The abdominal pain and associated rigidity of widow spider envenomation can often be mistaken for a surgical abdominal process such as appendicitis.

32. **An 8-year-old patient was brought to the ED by his mother approximately 3 hours after sustaining a black widow spider bite to his right second toe. It is suspected that the spider was in a shoe that the patient put on. The mother had brought the spider to the ED, where it was identified as a female black widow. The patient complained of severe pain that began in the foot and then progressed to the leg, lower back, abdomen, and chest.**
Initial vital signs are blood pressure, 134/92 mmHg; respiratory rate, 26 breaths/min; heart rate, 130 beats/min; temperature, 97.8°F; pulse oxygen saturation, 96% on room air. The patient appeared to be in distress secondary to pain and was diaphoretic. The abdomen was rigid, and the patient exhibited diffuse guarding. The lungs were clear, and findings on cardiac examination were normal. There was mild erythema of the right second toe, but there were no identifiable puncture marks. While in the ED, the patient began to complain of difficulty breathing.
    What would be your treatment for this patient?
    This patient is displaying grade 3 *Latrodectus* spider envenomation (Table 50.3) and would benefit from antivenin treatment. A single vial (2.5 mL) of Antivenin Latrodectus mactans should be infused intravenously during a 20-minute period.

33. **A 12-year-old patient reports obtaining a spider bite on the dorsum of the left hand 3 days ago while doing chores in the barn. The wound has a blue/black central area with concentric rings of pallor and erythema. Aside from pain at the site, there are no further symptoms. The parents happened to take this picture (Fig. 50.5) of the spider with their smartphone. The mother and patient ask what type of spider this is and if there is any further treatment.**
This is a brown recluse (*Loxosceles*) spider, which is best identified by its violin-shaped mask marking. Treatment is usually supportive care and local wound management.

Table 50.3 Grading Scale for *Latrodectus* Spider Envenomations	
GRADE	**SIGNS AND SYMPTOMS**
1	Normal vital signs, no systemic symptoms, local pain at the bite site
2	Muscular pain in bitten extremity, extension of pain to the chest or abdomen, local diaphoresis at bite site/extremity, normal vital signs
3	Generalized muscle pain to back, chest, and abdomen; diaphoresis distant from bite site/extremity; hypertension/tachycardia; nausea/vomiting; headache

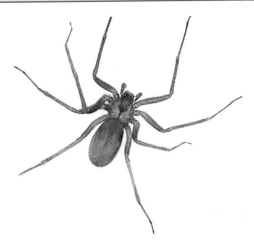

Fig. 50.5 The brown recluse spider. A dark, violin-shaped marking is located on the spider's back. (From Habif TP. Clinical Dermatology: A Color Guide to Diagnosis and Therapy. 5th ed. McGraw-Hill; 2010:581–634.)

34. **A 5-year-old patient is rock hunting with their siblings while on vacation in the Southwest. The patient is brought to the nearest urgent care center because of an acute change in their behavior after rock hunting. The patient is complaining of difficulty breathing, and the father reports that the child has "dancing eyes." You immediately suspect that your patient has been bitten by what arthropod?**
Common symptoms of a scorpion bite include local pain, restlessness, hyperactivity, roving eye movements, and respiratory distress. Treatment is mostly supportive care. Sedative-anticonvulsants can be used to treat hyperactivity, convulsions, and agitation. An equine-derived antivenom made with Fab2 antibodies (Anascorp) can be used for treatment of envenomation by *Centuroides sculpturatus.*

35. **An 8-year-old patient is brought to an urgent care center after being stung by a bee. They complain of an itchy throat. On exam, there is some expiratory wheezing, and the bite site has some erythema and swelling. What should be the first intervention?**
This patient is experiencing an anaphylactic reaction to the bee sting and should be given epinephrine 1:1000 solution 0.01 mL/kg (max 0.3 mL) intramuscularly x 1. Afterwards, the patient may be given antihistamines IV/PO and steroids IV/PO. These patients should be sent to the nearest hospital for a recommended 24-hour observation.

36. **Why does a pediatric patient seem to exhibit severe snakebite envenomation as compared to an adult?**
Because children receive a larger dose of venom per kilogram as compared to adults.

37. **Which pit viper snakes are considered part of the *Crotalid* family and can account for up to 90% of venomous snakebites in the United States?**
Rattlesnakes, cottonmouths, and copperheads.

38. **A 17-year-old patient presents to the emergency department 2 hours after being bitten by a rattlesnake while hiking with friends. The patient presents with a left lower extremity wound with erythema and edema from the ankle to the knee with palpable pedal pulses. They report that the wound was originally located at the ankle but the reaction has progressed quickly to the knee. The park ranger splinted the extremity, and the patient was brought via advanced life support (ALS) ambulance having received 50 mcg of Fentanyl with some relief of pain upon arrival to the emergency department. Upon arrival, the patient reports that they are beginning to feel pain in the left thigh. What are your next steps in the management of this patient?**
Assess the patient's vital signs; if there is evidence of shock, begin with resuscitation with normal saline 20cc/kg according to PALS (Pediatric Advanced Life Support) recommendation. Treat pain with narcotic analgesia. Keep extremity splinted and elevated. Obtain labs such as CBC with platelets, prothrombin time, fibrinogen, urine analysis, type and screen, as well as electrolytes. Our patient is exhibiting grade 3 envenomation (Table 50.4) and would benefit from treatment with Crotalidae Polyvalent Immune Fab (CroFab). The initial dose is 4–6 vials of antivenom diluted in 250 mL of crystalloid. The initial dose may be repeated in 1 hour if no arrest of progression of reaction and return to normal coagulation profile are observed.

39. **What are the indications for CroFab?**
Pit viper envenomations, grades moderate to severe, within 4 hours
    Significant local reaction
    Coagulation abnormalities
    Cardiovascular instability
    Of note, there is a 20% risk of hypersensitivity (anaphylaxis) and a 23% risk of serum sickness in giving patients CroFab.

40. **A 16-year-old male presents after being bitten by a red, black, and yellow striped snake. What type of snake is this?**
The animal described could be a coral snake, various species of which can be found in many southern and western areas of the United States, and their bites can be dangerous. There are also many look-alikes for these snakes that are fairly harmless, such as the king snake. A helpful way to pick out coral snakes found in the United States is to look at the banding of color, and "if red touches yellow, it can kill a fellow," meaning the animal is probably a coral snake. Note that the yellow bands can be pale and appear white.

Table 50.4 Crotalidae Envenomation Grading	
GRADE	**SYMPTOMS**
Minimal	Local swelling and pain without progression
Moderate	Swelling and pain beyond the site of injury with some systemic or laboratory findings
Severe	Severe local, systemic, and laboratory findings

41. **What symptoms could a patient bitten by a coral snake display?**
The local wound may progress to extremity paresthesia and weakness. Over a period of hours, the patient may develop malaise, nausea, fasciculations, diplopia, difficulty speaking or swallowing, and generalized weakness.

42. **How are coral snake bites treated?**
Coral snake venom is a potent neurotoxin that can provoke paralysis leading to respiratory failure. Fortunately, there are very few of these bites in the United States per year, and they account for less than 1% of all US snake-bites. Additionally, the coral snake has very short fangs that often fail to adequately penetrate through clothing and achieve envenomation. Coralmyn is an antivenom similar to CroFab that can be used to treat coral snake bites; however, due to the rarity of these bites, it is also rare and difficult to obtain. Any suspected coral snake bite should be emergently referred to advanced care.

MARINE ENVENOMATIONS

43. **A 17-year-old patient was swimming in shallow waters. The patient suddenly feels a sharp pain in the leg. They note the animal swim away and it appears to be a stingray. The patient comes to shore and is brought to your UrgiCare with a 10-cm laceration on the right leg. How would you manage this wound?**
At the scene, the wound should be irrigated with cold salt water, as this can remove much of the venom. Remnants of the integumentary sheath from the stingray's spine should be removed if they can be seen in the wound. The extremity should be placed in hot water (40–45°C [104–113°F]) for 30–90 minutes. After soaking, the wound should be reexplored, debrided again if necessary, and closed. Pain relief is best achieved with narcotics. Tetanus prophylaxis should be considered, and prophylactic antibiotics are not needed.

44. **An 8-year-old patient was playing in the ocean with siblings on a Florida shore. They saw a shiny "squishy" fish with long legs. The patient picked up the fish and within a few minutes began to cry because they were having a burning and painful sensation on the right hand. The nearest UrgiCare is within an hour, and the patient begins to have nausea with vomiting. The right hand has erythema extending to the forearm that is pruritic. You suspect a jellyfish sting. What would you do next for this patient?**
The sting is often caused by nematocysts located on jellyfish. These nematocysts release a toxin that caused the symptoms in our patient. The unexploded nematocysts can be inactivated with topical application for 30 minutes of 3–10% of aqueous acetic acid, a slurry of baking soda (50% wt/vol), or meat tenderizer (papain). Papain should not be left on for more than 15 min. Though it is the best disarming agent in jellyfish stings, vinegar is ineffective in Portuguese man-of-war stings. These stings should be washed out with sea water or normal saline. The affected limb should be immobilized. General supportive measures for more systemic reactions can include oral antihistamines, oral corticosteroids, and opiates for pain.

FISH AND SHELLFISH POISONING

45. **What are the two main clinical syndromes seen with seafood poisoning?**
There are two main clinical syndromes seen with seafood poisoning:
gastrointestinal symptoms with neurotoxic symptoms and histamine-like fish poisoning.

46. **A 16-year-old patient on vacation in the Caribbean with the family presents to an urgent care center about 1 hour after having a fish dinner at a restaurant. The patient reports having a dish with fresh snapper and within the hour began having a metallic taste in the mouth along with profuse vomiting and diarrhea. What kind of seafood poisoning is this patient presenting with?**
The patient is presenting with signs of ciguatera fish poisoning, which is the commonest cause of seafood poisoning. Tropical reef fish such as snappers, groupers, mackerel, and moray eels are common examples. Early symptoms are a burning mouth sensation or a metallic taste 45 minutes after ingestion. Acute gastroenteritis symptoms may follow after about 1–6 hours of ingestion and can last for up to a week. After about 24 hours distinct neurologic symptoms may occur such as perioral paresthesia, cold allodynia or dysesthesia of the extremities, weakness, ataxia, arthralgia, and myalgia.

47. **A college-aged student went out with friends for a sushi dinner. The patient had tuna sashimi and immediately began having a tingling feeling on their lips, tongue, and mouth. They began to have severe abdominal pain, flushing, urticaria, and sweating, along with profuse diarrhea and vomiting within 30 minutes of ingestion. The patient's friends called 911, and the patient was brought to your ED via EMS. How would you manage this patient's symptoms?**
This patient is displaying symptoms of scombroid poisoning, which would respond to epinephrine, anti-H1 histamine blockers, adrenergic β2 agonist bronchodilators, and fluid replacement as needed.

KEY POINTS

1. Appropriate wounds to manage in urgent care are minor cuts, lacerations, and abrasions.
2. The what, when, where, and why (accidental vs. nonaccidental) of wound occurrence are key pieces of a history.
3. Pain control and anxiolysis are important considerations for treating injured pediatric patients.
4. It is important to assess the percent of total body surface area that burns occupy, which can be done by various methods including the "rule of nines," the "hand method," and Lund Browder charts.
5. After the initial ABCs, treatment for bites and stings should start with identifying the probable offending species and targeting therapy based on the types of envenomation or injury they cause.

BIBLIOGRAPHY

American Academy of Pediatrics. Red Book Online. http://aapredbook.aapublications.org.

American Burn Association. http://www.ameriburn.org/.

Bryan P. Black Widow Spider Envenomation. *Utox Update*. 2002;4(3).

Centers for Disease Control and Prevention. http://www.cdc.gov/.

FDA.gov. FDA Approves First Scorpion Sting Antidote.

Goldstein EJ. Management of human and animal bite wounds. *J Am Acad Dermatol*. 1989;21:1275.

Goto C, Feng S. Crotalidae polyvalent immune fab for the treatment of pediatric Crotaline envenomation. *Ped Emergency Care*. 2009;25(4):273–282.

Hodge III D. Environmental Emergencies, Radiological Emergencies, Bites and Stings. In: Fleisher GR, Ludwig S, eds. *Textbook of Pediatric Emergency Medicine*. 7th ed. Philadelphia: Wolters Kluwer/Lippincott Williams & Wilkins; 2016:718–760.

Jaindl M. Management of bite wounds in children and adults: an analysis of over 5000 cases at a level I trauma centre. *Wien Klin Wochenschr*. 2015(Dec 11).

Kemp A. Can we identify abuse bites on children? *Arch Dis Child*. 2006 Nov;91(11):951.

Kliegman R, Nelson WE. *Nelson Textbook of Pediatrics*. Philadelphia: Elsevier/Saunders; 2011.

Offerman S. The treatment of black widow spider envenomation with Antivenin Lactrodecuts Mactans: a case series. *Perm J*. 2011;15(3):76–81.

Roberts JR, Custalow CB, Thomsen TW, Hedges JR. *Roberts and Hedges' Clinical Procedures in Emergency Medicine*. 6th ed. Philadelphia: Elsevier/Saunders; 2014. http://www.cdc.gov/rabies/location/index.html.

Warrell D. Venomous bites, stings, and poisoning: an update. *Infect Dis Clin N Am*. 2019;33:17–38.

LACERATION REPAIR

Ruby F. Rivera, MD, Michele J. Fagan, MD

CHAPTER 51

TOP SECRETS

1. In young children in whom suture removal may be a challenge, it is reasonable to use absorbable suture material for facial and scalp lacerations.
2. Align the vermillion border first for lip lacerations involving the vermillion border.

1. **A 3-year-old female presents with a forehead laceration. What are important details that one must pay attention to when assessing the laceration?**
There are several factors that can affect incidence of infection, delayed wound healing, and scar formation:
   Laceration factors – mechanism of injury, wound age, possibility of foreign body, contamination, cosmetic significance of the wound, extent of the wound, neurovascular or tendon injury.
   Individual factors – determination of allergies (e.g., to local anesthetics, antibiotics, or latex), underlying medical history/disease state (diabetes mellitus, obesity, peripheral arterial disease, malnutrition [protein, vitamin C deficiency], chronic renal failure, use of steroids or other immunosuppressive agents, tendency to form keloids, connective tissue disorders), status of tetanus immunization.

2. **How and why are bites managed differently?**
Bite wounds are at higher risk of infection because of the polymicrobial nature of the oral cavity of humans/animals.
   For simple lacerations due to dog bites on the face, trunk, arms, or legs as well as lacerations caused by cat bites on the face, given the cosmetic importance of this region, primary closure is utilized. Lacerations closed primarily should be clinically uninfected and ideally <24 hours old (facial lacerations) or <12 hours old (sites other than the face). Debridement and irrigation should be performed prior to closure. Subcutaneous sutures should be avoided or used sparingly, as these can function as a nidus for infection. Tissue adhesive should not be used.
   Wounds left open to heal by secondary intention should be debrided, irrigated copiously, dressed, and evaluated daily for signs of infection. Such wounds are crush injuries, puncture wounds, cat bite wounds (nonfacial), wounds involving the hands and feet, wounds ≥12 hours old (≥24 hours old on the face), wounds in immunocompromised hosts, and wounds in patients with venous stasis.

3. **What is the concept of the "golden period," a traditional belief that there is a time interval within which lacerations should be closed primarily?**
The optimal length of time between injury and laceration repair has not been clearly defined. In patients without risk factors for poor wound outcome, most simple lacerations that are small (e.g., <5 cm in length), do not have gross contamination, and are not located on the lower extremities can be closed up to 12–18 hours from the time of injury with low risk of infection. Closure beyond 12 hours after injury should be avoided for large wounds (longer than 5 cm in length), contaminated wounds, or lacerations in individuals with risk factors. Wounds that are closed more than 18 hours from the time of injury, especially those involving the distal extremities, should be treated with antibiotic prophylaxis.

4. **When is primary closure of open lacerations suggested?**
Wounds that are clean and uncontaminated with little tissue loss may undergo primary closure up to 12–18 hours from the time of injury. Wounds of the head and neck may be closed up to 24 hours after injury because of the rich vascular supply of the face and scalp.

5. **When is delayed closure (or tertiary closure) indicated?**
Delayed primary closure is used for contaminated or infected wounds, wounds that present after the safe period for primary closure, and select bite wounds (crushing, avulsion).
   Delayed primary closure consists of initial cleaning and debridement of the wound followed by up to a 5-day waiting period prior to wound closure. Oral prophylactic antibiotics are sometimes prescribed to further diminish the risk of infection in wounds that will not be immediately closed.
   At the time of closure, additional debridement may be needed. Referral to a wound expert is advised.

6. **Does one need to use sterile gloves when performing suture repair?**
The use of nonsterile gloves does not increase the risk of wound infection.

7. **When should one consider radiographic images?**
   If one suspects a fracture, a joint disruption, or a foreign body (FB), then radiographic imaging should be considered. A detailed history, exploration with visualization of the base of the wound, and radiography reduce the risk of missing a foreign body but do not eliminate the possibility that one is present. Fragments of glass and metal if larger than 2 mm usually can be identified on plain radiography. Studies show that ultrasound is better at detecting plastic, wood, and glass, depending on the operator's ability and other confounding factors. Patients should always be told of the possibility of a retained foreign body and what symptoms they should look for.

8. **When should a foreign body be removed?**
   Identifying and removing foreign bodies is important because retained foreign bodies increase the risk of delayed wound healing and infection; however, one must consider location: intraarticular, intravascular, or proximity to vital structures.

9. **What should be done about surrounding hair?**
   Hair need not be removed unless it interferes with wound closure. Lubrication to comb the hair away from wound margins or clipping the hair rather than shaving is preferred, as shaving causes small dermal wounds that allow bacteria to penetrate deeper structures and can potentially cause infection. Eyebrows should not be clipped or shaved because they serve as a landmark during repair. In addition, eyebrow growth is unpredictable.

10. **What type of fluid solution should be used for irrigating a wound?**
    Isotonic (normal) saline is frequently used for irrigation of uncomplicated wounds. Tap water has been shown to be an acceptable alternative solution without an increased risk of wound infection. Hydrogen peroxide, povidone iodine scrub solution, and chlorhexidine should not be used because it might be toxic to wound tissue. For contaminated traumatic wounds, a 1:10 dilute solution of 10% povidone-iodine solution may be used.
    The area should be anesthetized prior to irrigation. Warming the fluid may also decrease discomfort during wound irrigation.

11. **How much fluid and pressure should be used to irrigate a wound?**
    The volume depends on the location and mechanism of injury. Highly vascular areas require less volume (i.e., 100 cc/cm) for a clean, uncomplicated laceration. Larger volumes may be needed for contaminated wounds. Irrigation should be continued until all visible particulate matter has been removed. Adequate pressure (5–8 psi) may be obtained by using a 60-mL syringe with a 19-gauge catheter. Commercially available splash guards that attach to a syringe or on top of saline bottles are reported to generate 4–15 psi. Pierced intravenous bags and plastic bottles should not be used for irrigation, as they do not achieve adequate pressure.

12. **What can be done to reduce pain associated with lidocaine injection?**
    - Use a small-gauge needle (27G).
    - Buffer with sodium bicarbonate (1 ml 8.4% sodium bicarbonate: 9 ml lidocaine).
    - Slow the rate of injection.
    - Warm the local anesthetic.
    - Preanesthetize with topical anesthetic.
    - Infiltrate the anesthetic through the edge of the wound.

13. **What topical anesthetics are available?**
    Topical anesthetics have the advantage of being administered without using a needle and help reduce pain associated with the injection of local anesthetic. There are two topical anesthetics available for laceration repair: lidocaine, epinephrine, tetracaine (LET) and tetracaine, adrenaline, cocaine (TAC). TAC has fallen out of favor because it is expensive and contains cocaine. Both LET and TAC are contraindicated for use on mucous membranes, as this may result in systemic absorption. LET should not be used on end organs such as the tip of the nose, ear, digits, or penis. Other topical anesthetics include a eutectic mixture of local anesthetic (EMLA), which contains lidocaine and prilocaine in a cream base, and liposomal lidocaine (LMX). Both are currently approved for use on intact skin and are helpful prior to venipuncture, intravenous (IV) placement, portacath access, and incision and drainage.
    Dripping approximately 3–5 mL of injectable lidocaine onto mucosal wounds for oral mucosa laceration repair is a new and needle-less approach. Local anesthesia is achieved after approximately 5 minutes.

14. **What are the components of LET and how is it used?**
    LET contains 4% lidocaine, 0.1% epinephrine, and 0.5% tetracaine. It can be mixed with methylcellulose gel or as a solution. About 1–3 mL can be mixed with methylcellulose to make a gel, which then can be applied over the wound and secured with gauze or occlusive dressing (i.e., Tegaderm or OpSite for about 20–30 minutes). It can also be applied by placing the solution on a cotton ball, which is then applied over the wound for about 20 minutes. Duration of action is 45–60 minutes. If no blanching is observed, application can be repeated until blanching occurs. Many patients still require a subsequent local lidocaine injection or field block.

15. A 9-year-old boy comes in with a scalp laceration after hitting his head on a wall while running. There was no loss of consciousness, and on exam he has a 4–5-cm superficial laceration on the right parietotemporal area. What are the options for closure of this laceration?

Primary closure is preferred for scalp laceration through the dermis. The wound is anesthetized and irrigated, and options for wound closure include:
- Staples are particularly useful in children.
- Hair apposition technique (Fig. 51.1) involves hair on each side of the scalp being twisted together and then secured with tissue adhesive. This technique is ideal for lacerations that are linear, nonstellate, and <10 cm and in patients with hair >2 cm. Hemostasis is not achieved by this technique, so it should not be used in wounds with significant bleeding.
- Simple interrupted sutures can be used if staples are not available or if hemostasis is required. Absorbable sutures may be used, especially in young children.

16. If the scalp laceration extends into the galea aponeurotica, why is it important to repair the galea?

The scalp consists of five layers: skin, superficial fascia, galea aponeurotica, loose areolar tissue, and pericranium. The galea aponeurotica anchors the frontalis muscle; thus, failure to repair galeal lacerations in the frontal scalp may result in abnormalities in facial expression.

17. What are tissue adhesives, and what are the indications for their use?

Tissue adhesives provide an alternative method for wound closure that is painless, fast, and does not require a follow-up visit for removal. The most common components of tissue adhesives are 2-octyl-cyanoacrylate (Derma-bond, Surgiseal) and n-2-butyl-cyanoacrylate (Histoacryl Blue, Periacryl). The 2-octyl-cyanoacrylate is preferred because of its plasticity and flexibility. Tissue adhesives are liquid monomers that undergo an exothermic reaction

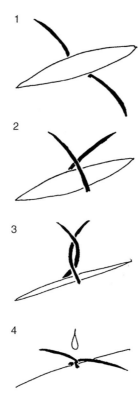

Fig. 51.1 Hair apposition technique. Strands of hair on each side are twisted and a drop of glue is applied. (From Hock MO, Ooi SB, Saw SM, et al. A randomized controlled trial comparing the hair apposition technique with tissue glue to standard suturing in scalp laceration (HAT study). *Ann Emerg Med.* 2002;40:19–26.)

upon exposure to a moist surface (skin), changing to a polymer that forms a strong tissue bond. The wound edges are approximated, and two to three layers of tissue adhesive are applied. Indications for the use of tissue adhesives include:

- Superficial lacerations
- Length <5 cm
- Low wound tension
- Good wound approximation
- After placement of deep sutures to close the skin
- Nailbed lacerations

18. **What are the contraindications for using tissue adhesives?**
    - Over joints
    - Bite wounds
    - Eyebrows, hairy areas
    - Mucous membranes
    - Complex wounds (e.g., stellate wounds, crush injuries)
    - Wounds with increased risk of infection (e.g., puncture wounds, contaminated wounds)

19. **What are the complications with tissue adhesive use?**
    - Infection, especially if the tissue adhesive goes into the wound or if the wound was not adequately cleaned.
    - Adhesion of the eye if tissue adhesive gets into the eye. The eye should be protected when using glue near the eye by covering it with gauze impregnated with petroleum. If the tissue adhesive causes adhesion of the eyelids, ophthalmic antibiotic ointment can be applied over the area and manual traction gently applied to open the eye. Ophthalmology should be consulted if this fails to open the eye.
    - Glove sticking near site of laceration

20. **How do I decide which suture material to use?**
    There are two types of suture material: absorbable and nonabsorbable. Absorbable sutures are used for deep and subcutaneous repair; nonabsorbable sutures are used to repair superficial skin. However, absorbable sutures (fast-absorbing gut) may be used for closure of facial lacerations, especially in children where suture removal can be a challenge. Table 51.1 shows suture material selection by site and depth of laceration.

21. **When can adhesive tapes (Steri strips) be used?**
    - Old contaminated wounds such as dog bites on extremities
    - Superficial, straight lacerations that barely extend through the dermis in areas with low tension
    - Superficial lacerations including flaps in individuals with thin skin (e.g., elderly or those on corticosteroids)
    Adhesive tapes should not be used in hairy areas, naturally moist areas (i.e., axilla, palms of hands, soles of feet), and over joints.

22. **When should an intraoral laceration be repaired?**
    - When the wound is gaping and is likely to trap food particles
    - Tongue lacerations:
      - When the laceration is greater than 1 cm in length and extends into the muscular layers of the tongue
      - When the laceration creates a large flap or continues bleeding
      - Deep lacerations on the lateral border of the tongue
      - Lacerations that may cause dysfunction if healed improperly (anterior split tongue)
    - Lacerations that involve the Stenson duct should be referred to an oral surgeon. Deep laceration of the cheek anterior to the ear may cause injury to the Stenson duct. On physical examination, bloody discharge may be seen on the buccal mucosa at the level of the second maxillary molar.

23. **A 15-year-old boy comes in with a lip laceration involving the vermillion border. What is the most important consideration in the repair of this laceration?**
    Lacerations involving the vermillion border require repair to be done correctly to preserve cosmetic appearance and lip function. As shown in Fig. 51.2, it is important to align the vermillion border first before the rest of the laceration is repaired.

24. **When should a subungual hematoma be drained?**
    One should trephinate subungual hematomas that are acute, less than 24–48 hours old, not spontaneously draining, associated with intact nail folds, and painful. Nail removal and primary repair of the laceration are recommended in the event of disruption of the nail matrix (nail fold) or if the nail is partially avulsed. Trephination is easily done by using an electric cautery device or by boring a hole through the nail using a needle. A heated paper clip should not be used, as most paper clips are made of aluminum and are difficult to heat sufficiently to penetrate the nail. Anesthesia is usually not needed prior to trephination.

Table 51.1 Wound Closure Type per Anatomic Site

ANATOMIC SITE	LAYER	CLOSURE TYPE	ALTERNATIVES
Scalp	Deep[a]	4-0 Polyglactin 910[b]	4-0 Polyglycolic acid[c]
	Skin	Staples	5-0 Vicryl Rapide
			4-0 Nylon, polypropylene
Face	Deep	5-0 Polyglactin 910	5-0 Polyglycolic acid
	Skin	6-0 Nylon[d]	6-0 Polypropylene[e]
		Wound adhesive (pediatrics)[f]	5-0 Fast-absorbing gut, Vicryl Rapide
Ears	**Skin**	**6-0 Nylon**	**6-0 Polypropylene**
Lip	Muscle/subcutaneous	5-0 Polyglactin 910	5-0 Polyglycolic acid
	Skin	6-0 Nylon	6-0 Polypropylene, Vicryl Rapide
Intraoral	**Mucosa**	**5-0 Chromic gut**	**4-0 Polyglactin 910**
Tongue	Mucosa	4-0 Chromic gut	4-0 Polyglycolic acid
Eyelid	Skin	**6-0 Nylon**	**6-0 Polypropylene**
Neck	Deep	5-0 Polyglactin 910	5-0 Polyglycolic acid
	Skin	5-0 Nylon	5-0 Polypropylene
Trunk	Deep	**4-0 Polyglactin 910**	**4-0 Polyglycolic acid**
	Skin	**4-0 Nylon**	**4-0 Polypropylene, staples[g]**
Arm/forearm	Deep	4-0 Polyglactin 910	4-0 Polyglycolic acid
	Skin	4-0 Nylon	4-0 Polypropylene
Hand	Skin	**5-0 Nylon**	**5-0 Polypropylene, Vicryl Rapide (pediatrics)**
Leg	Deep	3-0 Polyglactin 910	3-0 Polyglycolic acid
	Skin	4-0 Nylon	4-0 Polypropylene staples[g]
Foot	Skin	5-0 Nylon	5-0 Polypropylene
Penis	Skin	5-0 Nylon	5-0 Polypropylene
Scrotum	Skin	**5-0 Chromic gut**	**5-0 Polyglactin 910**
Introitus	Labia majora	5-0 Nylon	5-0 Polypropylene
	Labia minora	5-0 Chromic gut	5-0 Polyglactin 910
	Vagina	5-0 Chromic gut	5-0 Polyglactin 910

[a]Subcutaneous layer.
[b]Polyglactin 910 (Vicryl).
[c]Polyglycolic acid (Down).
[d]Nylon (Ethilon, Dermalon).
[e]Polypropylene (Prolene).
[f]Children.
[g]Avoid weight-bearing surfaces.
(From Trott A, ed. *Wounds and Lacerations: Emergency Care and Closure*. 4th ed. Philadelphia: Elsevier Saunders; 2012:90 [Table 8.3]).

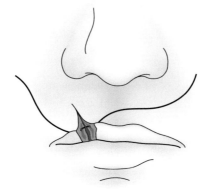

Fig. 51.2 Lip laceration Involving the vermillion border. The vermillion border should be aligned first. (From Trott A, ed. *Wounds and Lacerations: Emergency Care and Closure.* 4th ed. Elsevier Saunders; 2012:154 (Fig. 12.15).)

25. **If a fingertip is completely cut off, how should the amputated part be taken care of?**
    - Gently clean the amputated part with water (preferably saline).
    - Cover it in moistened sterile gauze.
    - Put it in a watertight bag.
    - Place the bag on ice.
    - Do not put the amputated part directly in ice, to avoid further damage.

26. **When should a hand surgeon be consulted?**
    - Finger fractures (other than tuft fractures)
    - Extensive nail bed injury
    - Infected wounds
    - Fingertip injuries with associated tendon injuries
    - Amputation with significant bone exposure

27. **When should nasolacrimal duct injury with eyelid laceration be suspected?**
    - Excessive tearing
    - Lacerations medial to the puncta are highly suspicious of canalicular injury.

28. **When should eyelid lacerations be referred to an ophthalmologist?**
    - Ptosis in the presence of horizontal upper lid laceration suggests involvement of levator palpebral muscle.
    - Lid trauma with tissue avulsion
    - Periorbital fat exposure
    - Full-thickness laceration
    - Wounds through tarsal plate
    - Eyelid margin laceration

29. **When are sutures removed?**
    The timing of suture removal depends on the anatomic location of the wound (Table 51.2).

30. **A 33-year-old painter comes in with a puncture wound to the thumb sustained from a high-pressure paint gun. He complains of mild pain, and on physical exam there is a puncture wound on the volar aspect of the proximal phalanx. How should this be managed?**
    High-pressure injuries occur due to forceful injection of paint, grease, and liquids through a small high-pressure nozzle. Initially, the patient may be asymptomatic or have mild pain and minimal external injury. However, these materials can cause inflammatory responses and spread throughout the tissues. Delays in diagnosis and management can lead to significant morbidity. Management includes radiographs, broad-spectrum antibiotics, and prompt consultation with a hand surgeon.

31. **A child comes in having stepped on a sharp object a few days ago. When should one be concerned?**
    - Symptoms that are progressive over several days
    - Pain with passive movement
    - Joint swelling
    - Crepitus

Table 51.2 Recommended Intervals for Removal of Percutaneous (Skin) Sutures

LOCATION	DAYS TO REMOVAL
Scalp	6–8
Face	3–5
Ear	4–5
Chest/abdomen	8–10
Back	12–14
Arm/leg*	8–12
Hand*	8–10
Fingertip	10–12
Foot	12–14

*Add 2–3 days for joint extensor surfaces.
From Trott A, ed. *Wounds and Lacerations: Emergency Care and Closure.* 4th ed. Philadelphia: Elsevier Saunders; 2012:289 [table 22.1].

- Purulent discharge
- Systemic illness
- Pain out of proportion to the exam
  Complications following puncture wounds include cellulitis, abscess, septic arthritis, tenosynovitis, necrotizing soft tissue infection, and osteomyelitis. The probability of wound infection is increased with deeper puncture wounds, delayed presentation (>24 hours), penetration through a rubber-sole shoe (known to inoculate pseudomonas), retained foreign bodies, and contaminated wounds. Diabetes mellitus is a risk factor for serious infection following a puncture wound.

32. **A 20-year-old patient comes in having stepped on a nail. Is the tetanus vaccine indicated?**
    Tetanus prophylaxis depends on the patient's immunization history and the type of wound (Table 51.3). Tetanus-prone wounds include those contaminated with dirt, soil, feces, or saliva; puncture wounds; crush injuries; missile injuries; avulsions; burns; and frostbite. Patients with tetanus-prone wounds and unknown or <3 doses of tetanus immunization should be given tetanus vaccine and tetanus immune globulin. If the patient has had three or more doses of tetanus immunization and the last dose is more than 5 years prior, a tetanus vaccine should be given. Patients with human immunodeficiency virus (HIV) or other severe immunodeficiency with tetanus-prone wounds should be given tetanus immune globulin regardless of tetanus immunization.

33. **A 9-year-old boy comes in with a deep laceration on the lateral aspect of the knee after a bicycle accident. What are the concerns prior to wound repair?**
    Periarticular lacerations raise concern for joint involvement. A delay in diagnosis may lead to septic arthritis. Plain x-rays may be obtained to check for fractures, dislocations, or free air in the joint. The presence of air in the joint clinches the diagnosis. A saline load test or CT scan may be needed if the x-ray is negative and there is concern for joint involvement. Urgent orthopedic consultation is required with penetrating intraarticular wounds.

Table 51.3 Tetanus Prophylaxis

	INDICATIONS FOR TETANUS PROPHYLAXIS				
PRIOR TETANUS TOXOID DOSES	**Clean, Minor Wounds**		**All Other Wounds**		
	TETANUS VACCINE[a]	**TIG**	**TETANUS VACCINE**[a]	**TIG**	
Unknown or <3	Yes	No	Yes	Yes	
≥3, last <5 years ago	No	No	No	No	
≥3, last 5–10 years ago	No	No	Yes	No	
≥3, last ≥10 years ago	Yes	No	Yes	No	

[a]DTaP preferred under age 7 years; Tdap preferred over Td for children ≥ 7 years if patient is underimmunized or hasn't received Tdap previously; otherwise, either one is acceptable.
From Sheets L. Immunoprophylaxis. In: Anderson CC, Kapoor S, Mark TE, eds. The Harriet Lane Handbook. 23rd ed. Philadelphia, PA: Elsevier Inc; 2024:447.

34. **When should one give prophylactic antibiotics?**

Several studies failed to show any benefit for prophylactic antibiotics after laceration repair; however, most excluded certain patient populations, i.e., immunocompromised patients and those with wounds that are considered at high risk for infection such as crush injuries, bites, those involving tendons, cartilage, bones, or joints. Antibiotics may be considered for older wounds, human bites, dog bites, cat bites, crush injuries, contaminated wounds, wounds involving tendons, cartilage, bones or joints, and intraoral lacerations.

35. **What antibiotics are prescribed for prophylaxis?**

First-generation cephalosporins cover for *Staphylococcus aureus* and *Streptococcus pyogenes*. For patients with penicillin allergy, clindamycin or azithromycin may be used.

Clindamycin or trimethoprim-sulfamethoxazole if methicillin-resistant *S. aureus* is a concern.

Amoxicillin-clavulanic acid is the antibiotic of choice for dog and cat bites (contains *Pasteurella multocida, Staphylococcus,* and *Streptococcus*) as well as human bites (to cover for *Eikenella corrodens, Staphylococcus,* and *Streptococcus*). Clindamycin plus trimethoprim-sulfamethoxazole can be given as an alternative if a patient is allergic to penicillin.

36. **How should wounds be bandaged after repair?**
- Cover the wound for 24–48 hours with a semiocclusive nonadherent dressing and either antibiotic cream or simple petroleum jelly to maintain a moist clean environment.
- Wounds that are closed with tissue adhesives should remain uncovered. Antibiotic ointment should not be used, as this may loosen the tissue adhesives.
- Elevate to decrease swelling.
- If a joint is involved, immobilize the joint with a bulky dressing or splint.
- Apply compression dressing to wounds with potential for hematoma.
- Gentle washing with mild soap and water after 48 hours

37. **A 20-year-old female patient has a laceration on her right lower leg requiring repair with sutures. She wants to know if she can use topical vitamin E or aloe vera to help minimize scar formation.**

Vitamin E has been implicated in minimizing scar formation through its antioxidant effects. Topical onion extract gel is thought to improve scar formation through its antiinflammatory and antibacterial properties. However, there is little clinical evidence for the use of topical vitamin E, topical onion-based extract gel (Mederma), or aloe vera to minimize scar formation.

38. **What are the signs of a wound infection?**
- Worsening pain and tenderness
- Erythema
- Warmth
- Swelling
- Discharge
- Fever
- Streaking

39. **An anxious 7-year-old boy has a facial laceration. What are the ways in which to decrease distress associated with the repair procedure?**
- Apply topical anesthetic prior to the procedure.
- Explain the procedure using developmentally appropriate terms.
- During the procedure, find a position of comfort and restraint (i.e., having the patient sit on parent's lap with the parent able to secure arms).
- Use distraction techniques such as videos.

40. **When should we allow wounds to heal by granulation (secondary intention) after appropriate cleaning?**
- Contaminated with debris that cannot be removed
- Infected tissue
- Noncosmetic wounds that come to medical attention late
- Animal bites in noncosmetic locations
- Deep puncture wounds that cannot be irrigated well
- Patients with risk factors (immunocompromised, peripheral artery disease, diabetes mellitus)
- Superficial wounds involving only the epidermis that will heal well

41. **When should a surgical subspecialist be consulted?**
- Wounds with significant tissue loss
- Severely contaminated wounds
- Tendon, nerve, or vessel damage
- Open fracture, amputation, joint penetration

- Laceration over site of fracture
- Compression between two rollers that causes delayed damage
- Ear lacerations with significant cartilage involvement or tissue loss
- High-pressure paint/grease gun injury
- Strong concern about cosmetic outcome

KEY POINTS

1. Repair lacerations of the galea aponeurotica to avoid abnormalities in facial expressions.
2. Align the vermillion border first for lip lacerations involving the vermillion border.
3. Eyebrows should not be shaved, as hair growth is irregular and the eyebrows serve as important facial landmarks.
4. In young children in whom suture removal may be a challenge, it is reasonable to use absorbable suture material for facial and scalp lacerations.
5. Open wounds involving the metacarpophalangeal joints sustained from punching the mouth should be treated as human bites.

BIBLIOGRAPHY

Bond MC, Willis GC. Risk management and avoiding legal pitfalls in the emergency treatment of high risk orthopedic injuries. *Emerg Med Clin North Am.* 2020;38:193–206.

Bord S, Khuri CE. High risk chief complaints: abdomen and extremities. *Emerg Med Clin North Am.* 2020;38:499–522.

Drendel AL, Ali S. Ten practical ways to make your ED painless and more child-friendly. *Clin Pediatr Emerg Med.* 2017;18(4):242–255.

Edwards S, Parkinson L. Is fixing pediatric nailbed injuries with medical adhesive as effective as suturing? *Pediatr Emerg Care.* 2019;35:75–77.

James V, Jia Heng TY, Yap QV, Ganapathy S. Epidemiology and outcome of nailbed injuries managed in children's emergency department, a 10-year single center experience. *Pediatr Emerg Care.* 2022;38(2):e776–e783.

Lammers RL, Aldy KN. Principles of wound management. In: Roberts JR, Custalow CB, Thomsen TW, eds. *Roberts and Hedges' Clinical Procedures in Emergency Medicine and Acute Care.* Philadelphia, PA: Elesevier; 2019:621e–654e.

Mankowitz SL. Laceration management. *J Emerg Med.* 2017;53(3):369–382.

Navanandan N, Renna-Rodriguez M, DiStefano MC. Pearls in wound management. *Clin Pediatr Emerg Med.* 2017;18(1):53–61.

Nickerson J, Tay ET. Dripped lidocaine: a novel approach to needleless anesthesia for mucosal lacerations. *J of Emerg Med.* 2018;55(3):405–407.

Otterness K, Singer A. Updates in emergency department laceration management. *Clin Exp Emerg Med.* 2019;6(2):97–105.

CHAPTER 52

FRACTURE AND DISLOCATION REDUCTIONS

Shenel A. Heisler, DO, Daniel M. Fein, MD

TOP SECRETS

- Ensure use of appropriate analgesia during reductions of any dislocation or fracture.
- A mallet finger should be splinted in complete extension for 8 weeks, and the patient should follow up with a hand surgeon.
- Hyperpronation and supination-flexion are both acceptable mechanisms for reduction of a nursemaid's elbow.

1. **When is an emergent reduction of a fracture or dislocation indicated?**
   Most fractures and dislocations can be reduced in a nonemergent fashion in the urgent care center, splinted and sta-bilized for future reduction, or, in the case of certain fractures, not require reduction. However, if there are any signs of neurovascular compromise, emergent reduction is indicated. Symptoms of neurovascular compromise include absent or diminished pulses, cyanosis, pallor, and/or loss of sensation or motor function distal to the fracture.

2. **A 17-year-old has not been able to close their mouth since yawning 1 hour ago. What are mechanisms for this injury?**
   Mandibular dislocation can occur after prolonged or extreme mouth opening or following a direct blow to the jaw with an open mouth. Both mechanisms stretch the ligaments, allowing the mandibular condyles to move anterior to the articular eminence. The dislocation can be either unilateral or bilateral.

3. **Why is sedation useful prior to reduction of a mandibular dislocation?**
   In addition to providing anxiolysis and analgesia, sedation helps overcome muscle spasms that prohibit the patient from closing their mouth. Benzodiazepines may be particularly helpful in this respect.

4. **How does one reduce a mandibular dislocation?**
   After wrapping their thumbs in gauze for protection, the provider should apply downward pressure to the molars. Backward pressure to the chin or molars may also be required. This allows the condyles to slip below the articular eminence and back into the mandibular fossa.

5. **What postreduction care is indicated for this patient?**
   The patient should be counseled to eat a soft diet and should follow up with otolaryngology or a maxillofacial surgeon.

6. **A 20-year-old presents after sustaining an injury to their left shoulder while playing basketball during an attempt to block a shot. Radiographs confirm an anterior shoulder dislocation. How does an anterior shoulder dislocation most commonly occur?**
   Anterior shoulder dislocations are most often caused by sudden external rotation of the shoulder while in abduc-tion (e.g., getting hit on the volar aspect of the arm while reaching for a loose ball).

7. **What complications can occur during a shoulder dislocation?**
   A Bankhart lesion occurs when the inferior labrum is avulsed from the glenoid rim. A Hill-Sachs lesion occurs when the posterior aspect of the humeral head sustains trauma as it strikes the anterior glenoid rim. Rotator cuff tears are also common.

8. **Which nerve is at risk of injury from a shoulder dislocation? How does one test its function?**
   The axillary nerve is at risk, and its function is tested by assessing deltoid muscle strength and sensation over the lateral aspect of the shoulder.

9. **How do I best provide analgesia for reduction of a dislocated shoulder?**
   In addition to providing the patient with either oral or parenteral analgesia as soon as possible, additional medica-tion may be necessary for the reduction itself, as it can be a painful procedure that requires significant force. Choices for procedural analgesia include conscious sedation, intravenous analgesia, intraarticular lidocaine, or an interscalene nerve block.

10. **How does one administer an interscalene block prior to shoulder reduction?**
    An ultrasound probe is used to identify the carotid artery as an anatomical marker. Moving laterally across the neck, the anterior and middle scalene muscles are located, after which the brachial plexus is visualized in between the two muscles. Continuing to use ultrasound guidance, lidocaine (up to 5 mg/kg) is injected around the site of the brachial plexus.

11. **What are some common mechanisms to reduce an anterior shoulder dislocation?**
    There are many different mechanisms available for reduction of a shoulder dislocation. They include (but are not limited to) external rotation, scapular manipulation, and traction–countertraction.

12. **How does one reduce a shoulder using the external rotation method?**
    The patient lies supine or sits supported with the affected arm completely adducted and elbow flexed to 90°. The elbow is then supported while the arm is slowly rotated externally. The arm is then slowly flexed at the shoulder. The technique is completed by rotating the shoulder internally. Relocation may occur during either external or internal rotation.

13. **Describe the scapular manipulation method of anterior shoulder dislocation reduction.**
    The patient lies prone with the affected arm dangling off the side of the bed. A weight is taped or strapped to the affected wrist to provide axial traction, or a second clinician can manually provide traction. The inferior aspect of the ipsilateral scapula is pushed medially, toward the spine, while the superior aspect is rotated laterally, away from the spine (Fig. 52.1).

14. **What is the traction–countertraction method of shoulder reduction?**
    The patient is placed supine with the affected arm abducted and elbow flexed to 90 degrees. A sheet is wrapped around the clinician's waist and the affected forearm while the clinician stabilizes the forearm. A second clinician places a sheet around the waist and the patient's trunk immediately below the axilla. The clinicians both lean backward, providing slow, steady traction (and countertraction), until reduction is achieved (Fig. 52.2).

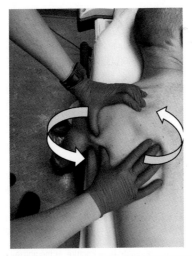

Fig. 52.1 Scapular manipulation to reduce an anterior shoulder dislocation. The inferior aspect of the scapula is rotated toward the spine while the patient is lying in the prone position.

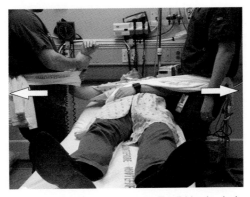

Fig. 52.2 Traction–countertraction to reduce an anterior shoulder dislocation. The clinicians lean backward, providing steady traction until reduction is achieved.

15. **How do I know that my reduction was successful?**
Reduction of a dislocated shoulder is not subtle. There is usually an audible "clunk" as the humeral head returns to the glenoid fossa. Additionally, the shoulder regains its normal contour, and the patient has decreased pain and increased range of motion.

16. **What should I do after successful reduction of a dislocated shoulder?**
Patients are at risk of redislocation, as the integrity of the rotator cuff is compromised after a dislocation. The arm should be placed in a sling and the patient should have a follow-up with an orthopedic surgeon.

17. **When is reduction of an anterior dislocation contraindicated?**
Reduction of an anterior shoulder dislocation is contraindicated if there is an associated fracture.

18. **A 3-year-old is brought to your urgent care center for a right arm injury. The child's mother was holding their hand when the child tripped and fell and has not moved the arm since. On exam, the arm is immobile in slight flexion and pronation. What injury did this child likely sustain?**
Radial head subluxation ("Nursemaid's elbow") is the most common joint injury in children less than 5 years of age, frequently resulting from traction on an outstretched and slightly pronated hand. This causes displacement and entrapment of the annular ligament at the radial head. The child typically presents with the affected arm slightly flexed and pronated with a refusal to use the affected arm.

19. **What are options for reduction of a nursemaid's elbow?**
The two options for reduction are:
   a. Supination-flexion: the arm is held in flexion at the elbow with the provider's thumb over the radial head and the other hand holding the patient's hand. Applying mild longitudinal traction, the provider then supinates the forearm while flexing at the elbow.
   b. Hyperpronation: the affected arm is stabilized at the elbow with the provider's thumb over the radial head and the other hand holding the patient's hand. Applying mild longitudinal traction, the hand is hyperpronated (Fig. 52.3).

20. **How do you know if you are successful in reducing a nursemaid's elbow?**
In either technique, the provider may feel a click when the reduction is successful. As this is not always the case, the provider should observe the child to ensure function returns.

21. **Is one reduction method preferable to the other?**
There is evidence that hyperpronation results in fewer first-attempt failures than supination-flexion (Krul); however, both are commonly accepted methods of reduction.

22. **How long after reduction should return of function be expected?**
Function typically returns rapidly, within the first 10–15 minutes after reduction. This may take longer for a more remote injury.

23. **What should the provider do if function does not return within a reasonable time frame?**
If the history and physical exam are convincing for a nursemaid's elbow, the initial maneuver may be reattempted or the alternate maneuver may be employed. If repeated attempts are unsuccessful or the diagnosis is not certain, the provider should consider imaging to evaluate for a fracture. In the absence of another injury, the arm should be placed in a sling and the child referred for outpatient orthopedic follow-up.

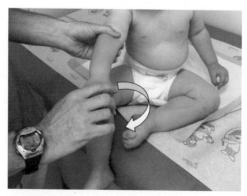

Fig. 52.3 Hyperpronation for reduction of a nursemaid's elbow. The forearm is slowly rotated into hyperpronation, with the stabilizing hand situated to feel the reduction at the radial head.

24. A 26-year-old playing goalie during soccer went to block an incoming ball; however, the ball bounced off the tip of his finger, resulting in significant pain and an obvious deformity. An x-ray shows a dorsal dislocation of the proximal interphalangeal (PIP) joint. What is the nomenclature used for finger dislocations?
The distal aspect of the finger is described relative to the proximal aspect. For example, in a dorsal dislocation of the PIP joint, the distal and middle phalanges are located dorsal to the proximal phalanx.

25. What is the proper analgesia for reduction of finger fractures or dislocations?
Proper analgesia can typically be obtained by performing a digital nerve block.

26. How is a digital nerve block performed?
A classic digital nerve block involves the injection of local anesthetic without epinephrine into the web spaces on both sides of the digit immediately distal to the metacarpophalangeal (MCP) joint. This should provide anesthesia for the entire digit, as the dorsal and palmar digital nerves run alongside the phalanx traversing the web spaces.

27. How do I reduce a dislocated interphalangeal (IP) joint?
Reduction of a dislocated IP joint begins with application of longitudinal traction of the dislocated phalanges. Dorsal dislocations are reduced with subsequent hyperextension of the dislocated phalanx with gentle pressure at the dorsal aspect of the base of the dislocated phalanx, pushing it back into place. Volar dislocations are reduced with hyperflexion of the dislocated phalanx with gentle pressure at the volar aspect of the base of the dislocated phalanx, pushing it back into place. Lateral dislocations are reduced with radial or ulnar pressure in the direction that will move the distal phalanx back to the midline.

28. What are the common complications of an IP joint reduction?
Complications are rare when reducing IP joints; however, it is possible that there is an inability to reduce the dislocation. This is more common with volar dislocations, as the dislocated phalanx can get entrapped in the extensor tendons. Inadequate stabilization can lead to recurrent dislocation.

29. How do you reduce a dorsally dislocated MCP joint?
Reduction of a dorsal MCP joint dislocation can typically be reduced by flexing the wrist to relax the flexor tendon, hyperextending the digit, and applying volar pressure on the dorsal aspect of the proximal phalanx.

30. How is a finger splinted after reduction of a dislocation or fracture?
The key to splinting a finger is the location of the dislocation or fracture. For fractures that were reduced, stabilization of the joints proximal and distal to the fracture is necessary. For dislocations, it suffices to stabilize the joint that was reduced. Fractures of the distal or middle phalanges and dislocations of the distal IP joint are stabilized with a finger splint. Proximal phalanx fracture reductions and proximal IP joint or MCP reductions require stabilization of the proximal IP and MCP joints, which can be obtained with an ulnar or radial gutter splint, volar splint, or thumb spica, depending on the digit involved.

31. What should be done after splinting the reduction?
Obtain postreduction films to ensure proper alignment and have the patient follow up with a hand surgeon.

32. What is a mallet finger? Why is it important to recognize it?
A mallet finger is caused by avulsion of the extensor tendon that inserts on the base of the distal phalanx. It results in an inability to extend the distal phalanx and occurs in association with a Salter-Harris I or II fracture in a child or a Salter-Harris III fracture in adolescents. While the fracture does not typically need reduction, it is crucial to splint the distal phalanx in full extension to slight hyperextension for 8 weeks.

33. A 34-year-old comes to the urgent care center after punching a wall with a closed fist. The distal ulnar aspect of the hand is swollen and tender. An x-ray shows an angulated fracture of the neck of the fifth metacarpal with volar angulation of the metacarpal head. How does one reduce a boxer's fracture?
The first step is providing adequate analgesia, typically with a hematoma block or an ulnar nerve block. Once adequate analgesia is obtained, the fifth digit is flexed to 90° at the MCP joint. Reduction is performed by applying pressure to the dorsal aspect of the metacarpal proximal to the fracture and upward pressure to the volar aspect of the metacarpal distal to the fracture. Alternatively, if the MCP and PIP joints are both flexed to 90 degrees, dorsally angled pressure can be applied at the PIP joint while volarly directed pressure is applied to the fifth metacarpal proximal to the fracture (Fig. 52.4).

34. How do you splint a reduced boxer's fracture?
A reduced boxer's fracture is immobilized with an ulnar gutter splint.

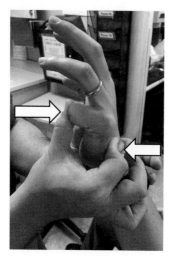

Fig. 52.4 Reduction of a boxer's fracture. Pressure is applied to the PIP joint, which is flexed to 90 degrees with simultaneous pressure to the dorsal aspect of the proximal fifth metacarpal.

35. **A 15-year-old at bat during a baseball game swings at the ball and develops an abrupt onset of right knee pain and inability to bear weight. On your exam, the knee is edematous, and the patella appears to be laterally displaced. What physical exam findings are suggestive of this injury?**
    Patients with patellar dislocation typically present with the knee held in slight flexion, edema of the knee, and tenderness along the medial patellar retinaculum at the medial superior aspect of the patella. If not spontaneously reduced, the laterally displaced patella is clinically evident.

36. **Is sedation indicated for reduction of patellar dislocation?**
    Depending on the patient, sedation may be needed for reduction. At times, the injury will reduce spontaneously after administration of a benzodiazepine alone.

37. **How does one reduce a lateral patellar dislocation?**
    Hold the ipsilateral hip in flexion with the upper leg stabilized by an assistant. Slowly extend the knee, applying gentle medial pressure to the patella.

38. **What is the "apprehension test"?**
    In the apprehension test, the provider holds the knee slightly flexed while applying lateral pressure to the patella. The test is positive if the patient expresses pain or anxiety that the patella will dislocate, either verbally or by sudden contraction of the quadriceps. This indicates that the patient had a patellar dislocation that has spontaneously reduced.

40. **Why is postreduction imaging indicated for these patients?**
    Postreduction x-rays are required to rule out a concomitant fracture of the lateral femoral condyle or medial patellar facet.

41. **What postreduction care is indicated for this patient?**
    The patient should be placed in a knee immobilizer and referred for orthopedic follow-up in approximately 1 week.

KEY POINTS

1. A benzodiazepine can be used to overcome muscle spasms in mandibular dislocations, greatly facilitating reduction.
2. Reduction of an anterior shoulder dislocation can be accomplished by many different maneuvers; however, they can be painful and require appropriate analgesia.
3. Reduction of a dislocated phalanx requires longitudinal traction and pressure at the base of the dislocated phalanx, gently pushing it back into place.
4. Mallet finger is often associated with a Salter-Harris type II/III fracture. Though it does not typically require reduction, it is crucial to splint the distal phalanx in full extension to slight hyperextension for 8 weeks.
5. Patellar dislocations may reduce spontaneously prior to presentation; this can be assumed if the patient becomes anxious when lateral pressure is applied to the patella.

Acknowledgments

The authors would like to acknowledge the work of Dr. Maya Haasz on the previous version of this chapter.

BIBLIOGRAPHY

Aronson PL, Mistry RD. Intra-articular lidocaine for reduction of shoulder dislocation. *Pediatr Emerg Care.* 2014;30:358.

Childress MA, Olivas J, Crutchfield A. Common finger fractures and dislocations. *American Family Physician.* 2022;105(6):631–639.

Cutts S, Prempeh M, Drew S. Anterior shoulder dislocation. *Ann R Coll Surg Engl.* 2009;91(2).

Gunaydin YK, Katirci Y, Duymaz H, et al. Comparison of success and pain levels of supination-flexion and hyperpronation maneuvers in childhood nursemaid's elbow cases. *Am J Emerg Med.* 2013;31:1078.

Johnson FC, Okada PJ. Reduction of common joint dislocations and subluxations. In: King C, Henretig FM, eds. *Textbook of Pediatric Emergency Procedures.* 2nd ed. Wolters Kluwer; 2008:962–990.

Krul M, van der Wouden JC, Kruithof EJ, van Suijlekom-Smit LWA, Koes BW. Manipulative interventions for reducing pulled elbow in young children. *Cochrane Database of Systematic Reviews.* 2017(Issue 7) Art. No.: CD007759.

Liwei Y, Wenwei D, Zeting W, et al. Ultrasound-guided interscalene block versus intravenous analgesia and sedation for reduction of first anterior shoulder dislocation. *Am J Emerg Med.* 2022;56:232–235.

Mailhot T, Lyn ET. Hand. In: Mar JA, ed. *Rosen's Emergency Medicine.* 8th ed. Elsevier-Saunders; 2014:534–569.

CHAPTER 53

SPLINTING AND CASTING

Rachel Rothstein, MD, MPH, Ellen Szydlowski, MD

TOP SECRETS

1. Indications for transfer to the ED include open or displaced fractures, neurovascular emergencies, compartment syndrome, or any fracture with skin tenting or compromise.
2. Children may not exhibit the classic "4 Ps" (pallor, paresthesias, pulseless, pain with passive stretch) of compartment syndrome. The earliest signs are the "3 As" (increased agitation, anxiety, analgesic requirement).

1. **What are the purposes of immobilization?**
   - Decrease pain
   - Mechanical stabilization
   - Prevent contractures
   - Decrease further injury

2. **How do splints and casts differ?**
   See Table 53.1.

3. **What are the layers (inner to outer) of a splint?**
   - Stockinette
   - Undersplint material (e.g., Webril) (Fig. 53.1B)
   - Plaster or fiberglass (Fig. 53.1C, D)
   - ACE bandage

4. **Does immobilization require sedation?**
   Nondisplaced fractures do not require sedation for casting. Patients may benefit from pain control during manipulation. Displaced fractures requiring closed reduction and casting may require procedural sedation unless local anesthesia with a hematoma block is possible.

Table 53.1 Splints vs. Casts

	DEFINITION	INDICATIONS	DISADVANTAGES	COMPLICATIONS
Splint	Noncircumferential Applied in a position of function Preformed or manufactured	Sprains Salter-Harris Type I Closed, nondisplaced fractures Temporary immobilization pending cast placement Lacerations crossing joints or involving tendons	Noncompliance	Motion at injury site, leading to displacement or reduction loss Suboptimal pain control Contact dermatitis Skin breakdown Pressure sores Infection Thermal injury Neurovascular injury Compartment syndrome
Cast	Circumferential Applied in a position of function Plaster or fiberglass	Closed, nondisplaced, or reduced fractures	Additional costs Higher school and work absenteeism Discomfort from poor fit Water avoidance Hygiene challenges Delayed return to activities	Thermal injury Neurovascular injury Compartment syndrome Contact dermatitis Skin breakdown Pressure sores Infection Joint stiffness Muscle atrophy Removal injuries Incarcerated objects

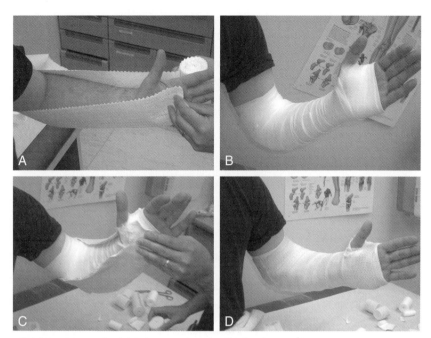

Fig. 53.1 Webril (B) and plaster splint (A, C, D) for a sugar tong wrist splint. (From Mazzola T. Splinting and casting. In: Seidenberg P, Beutler A (eds): The Sports Medicine Resource Manual. Philadelphia: Saunders; 2008, Fig. 16-3.)

5. When is ED transfer indicated?
   - Open or displaced fractures
   - Neurovascular emergencies
   - Compartment syndrome
   - Hip, knee, sternoclavicular, elbow dislocations
   - Amputations
   - Fractures with skin tenting or compromise
     Splint the injury and provide pain control before transfer.

6. What are the different methods of immobilization?
   Tables 53.2–53.3.

7. Can open fractures be managed with splinting?
   Open fractures generally require OR washout and reduction. Prior to transfer, irrigate and splint the wound and provide antibiotics and tetanus prophylaxis if indicated. Nail bed lacerations with an underlying fracture are not usually considered open fractures and can be managed in the ED.

8. What is a dreaded complication of forearm fractures?
   Compartment syndrome usually presents within 48 hours of an injury and is most commonly associated with tibia, forearm, and supracondylar fractures. Children may not exhibit the classic "4Ps" (pallor, paresthesias, pulseless, pain with passive stretch). Rather, the earliest signs are the "3As" (increased agitation, anxiety, analgesic requirement). If suspected, remove constrictive dressings, elevate the limb to the level of the heart, and obtain an orthopedic consultation.

9. Which splints are utilized for wrist injuries?
   - Volar (Fig. 53.2) or dorsal splint
   - Length: proximal fingers to proximal forearm
   - Width: as wide or slightly wider than the forearm surface

Table 53.2 Upper Extremity Immobilization (see "Indications" Column in Table 53.1)

Splinting

Dorsal Aluminum Foam Splint	Distal phalangeal fractures
Buddy Taping	Proximal or middle phalangeal fractures
Radial Gutter Splint	Second or third metacarpal fracture Corresponding proximal or middle phalangeal fractures
Ulnar Gutter Splint	Fourth or fifth (i.e., Boxer) metacarpal fracture Corresponding proximal or middle phalangeal fractures
Thumb Spica Splint	Scaphoid and lunate fractures Thumb phalangeal and first metacarpal fractures Jammed or dislocated thumb
Velcro Splint	Buckle fractures
Volar Splint	Soft tissue injuries of hand or wrist Carpal bone fractures (excluding those noted elsewhere) Lunate or perilunate dislocations Second through fifth metacarpal head fractures Distal radius or ulna fractures
Forearm Sugar-Tong Splint	Distal radius or ulna fractures
Double Sugar-Tong Splint, Long Arm Posterior Splint	Distal humerus, supracondylar, or condylar fractures Olecranon fractures Elbow dislocations
Simple Sling	Proximal humeral, humeral shaft, or clavicular fractures
Coaptation Splint	Proximal humeral or humeral shaft fractures (displaced)
Figure-of-Eight Splint	Clavicular fractures

Casting

Short Arm Cast	Greenstick fractures Distal radius fractures
Short Arm Cast Thumb Spicca	Scaphoid fracture Snuffbox tenderness
Long Arm Cast	Displaced radius or ulna fractures following reduction Radial head or neck fractures Concurrent radius and ulnar fractures Monteggia fractures Elbow fractures or dislocations Patients who cannot comply with a short arm cast

10. **How does treatment of pediatric femur fractures vary by age?**
    Nonoperative management with hip spica casting is preferred in young children. Older children often require intramedullary rod fixation.

11. **What is the proper splint for ankle sprains?**
    - CAM boot or preformed splint
    - Posterior short leg splint (Fig. 53.3B), then stirrup splint (Fig. 53.3A)
        - Length: fibular head around the heel to below the medial knee
        - Width: half the circumference of the lower leg

Table 53.3 Lower Extremity Immobilization (see "Indications" Column in Table 53.1)

Splinting

Buddy Taping	Toe fractures
Postoperative Shoe	Fifth metatarsal fracture at tuberosity or styloid avulsion fracture
Cam Boot	Fifth metatarsal fracture at tuberosity or styloid avulsion fracture Tibia spiral fracture (i.e., Toddler's) Ankle sprains
U-Splint (aka Stirrup/ Sugar-Tong Splint)	Distal fibula and tibia fractures Ankle dislocations following reduction Severe ankle sprains
Posterior Ankle Splint	Distal fibula and tibia fractures Fifth metatarsal fracture at proximal diaphysis (i.e., Jones)
Posterior Knee Splint	Angulated fractures around the knee Temporary immobilization of injuries prior to operative repair Injuries in extremities too large for a knee immobilizer
Knee Immobilizer	Ligamentous and soft tissue injuries of the knee Tibial plateau fractures Reduced patellar/knee dislocations
Posterior Long Leg Splint	Proximal tibia and tibial shaft fractures Distal femur fractures Soft tissue injuries around the knee

Casting

Short Leg Cast	Ankle fractures Achilles tendon injuries Hindfoot and midfoot injuries Fifth metatarsal fracture at proximal diaphysis (i.e., Jones)
Long Leg Cast	Tibia or fibula fractures
Hip Spica Cast	Femur fractures

Adapted From: Chudnofsky CR; Alexandre V; Children's Hospital of Philadelphia.

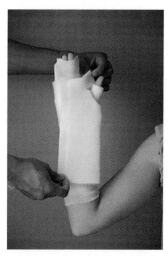

Fig. 53.2 Volar wrist splint. (From Cromer DA. Splinting and casting. In: Rynders SD, Hart JA (eds): Orthopedics for Physician Assistants. Philadelphia: Saunders; 2013:373.)

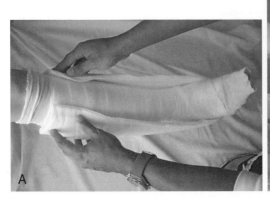

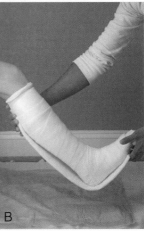

Fig. 53.3 A, Sugar tong ankle splint (stirrup). B, Posterior ankle splint. (From Cromer DA. Splinting and casting. In: Rynders SD, Hart JA (eds): Orthopedics for Physician Assistants. Philadelphia: Saunders; 2013:379–381.)

KEY POINTS

1. Splinting is a potential treatment for nondisplaced closed fractures or sprains.
2. Splints can improve stabilization and decrease pain pending transfer for definitive care.
3. Open or displaced fractures, neurovascular emergencies, compartment syndrome, and fractures with skin tenting or compromise require ED transfer.

Acknowledgements

Thank you to Dr. Todd A. Mastrovitch and Dr. Yashas Nathani for their contributions to this chapter in the previous edition.

BIBLIOGRAPHY

Alexandre V, Hodax JD. Splinting and Casting Techniques. In: Hodax J, Eltorai A, eds. *The Orthopedic Consult Survival Guide.* Springer; 2017:25–39.

Children's Hospital of Philadelphia. Emergency Department Clinical Pathway for Children with a Suspected Extremity Fracture. Available at: https://www.chop.edu/clinical-pathway/fracture-extremity-suspected-clinical-pathway. Published 2022. Accessed July 6, 2022.

Children's Hospital of Philadelphia. Emergency Department Clinical Pathway for the Evaluation/Treatment of Children with Suspected Long Bone Open Fracture. Available at: https://www.chop.edu/clinical-pathway/suspected-long-bone-open-fracture-clinical-pathway. Published 2020. Accessed July 6, 2022.

Chudnofsky CR, Chudnofsky AR. Splinting Techniques. In: Roberts JR, ed. *Roberts and Hedges' Clinical Procedures in Emergency Medicine and Acute Care.* Elsevier; 2019:1027–1055.

Cromer DA. Splinting and Casting. In: Rynders SD, Hart JA, eds. *Orthopedics for Physician Assistants.* Saunders; 2013:373.

Mazzola T. Splinting and Casting. In: Seidenberg P, Beutler A, eds. *The Sports Medicine Resource Manual.* Saunders; 2008; Figure 16-3.

Nemeth BA, Halanski MA, Noonan KJ. Cast and Splint Immobilization. In: Waters PM, Skaggs DL, Flynn JM, eds. *Rockwood and Wilkins' Fractures in Children.* Wolters Kluwer; 2020:40–65.

Runyon RS, Doyle SM. When is it ok to use a splint versus cast and what remolding can one expect for common pediatric forearm fractures? *Curr Opin Pediatr.* 2017;29(1):46–54.

Selbst S. *Pediatric Emergency Medicine Secrets.* 3rd ed. Elsevier; 2015.

Shirley ED, Maguire KJ, Mantica AL, et al. Alternatives to traditional cast immobilization in pediatric patients. *J Am Acad Orthop Surg.* 2020;28(1):e20–e27.

CHAPTER 54

ABSCESS INCISION AND DRAINAGE

Ee Tein Tay, MD, Nicolas Delacruz, MD

1. **What is a skin abscess?**
   An abscess is a contained cavity filled with purulent fluid and usually surrounded by inflamed deep subcutaneous tissue.

2. **What causes a skin abscess?**
   Abscesses are usually caused by gram-positive cocci, commonly *Staphylococcus aureus* and group A *Streptococcus*. There is now an increase in community-acquired methicillin-resistant *Staphylococcus aureus* (CA-MRSA). Gram-negative bacteria may cause skin abscesses in the buttock and axilla. Infections may occur when the skin barrier is disrupted and bacteria enter the open wound.

3. **What does a skin abscess look like?**
   The skin may appear fluctuant (fluid-filled), tender, indurated, and erythematous. There may be an area of skin disruption, such as a punctum or laceration. A "point" may be visible in some abscesses.

4. **What is the difference between an abscess and cellulitis?**
   Cellulitis is a skin infection that usually involves the epidermis, dermis, and superficial subcutaneous tissues and does not have an organized cavity; abscesses have an organized fluid-filled cavity and involve deeper subcutaneous tissues.

5. **How can I tell the difference between an abscess and cellulitis on physical exam?**
   Both the skin surrounding abscesses and the skin surrounding cellulitis may be indurated, but abscesses will usually feel fluctuant on physical exam. Often, it may be difficult to differentiate by visualization and palpation.

6. **Is there a role for ultrasound when evaluating an abscess?**
   Point-of-care ultrasound has been found to be 90–97% sensitive and 67–83% specific in detecting skin abscesses and has been shown to improve accuracy in abscess diagnosis. Ultrasounds can also be used to measure the size of an abscess, detect loculations, and evaluate surrounding structures, such as lymph nodes or blood vessels (Fig. 54.1).

7. **Will discharge be present when examining for an abscess?**
   If an abscess erupts, discharge may be present. Discharge may not necessarily be present during examination.

8. **What is the treatment for an abscess?**
   The treatment of choice is incision and drainage of an abscess. Antibiotics alone, needle aspiration of the abscess, and mechanical unroofing of the "point" of an abscess all have high rates of treatment failure.

9. **What type of pain relief is used for incision and drainage?**
   Topical anesthetics can be used to promote drainage through maceration, but local anesthesia is best achieved with lidocaine infiltrate. A "field block" is often injected around the wound of an abscess. Injecting into the wound may not provide adequate local anesthesia. Often, lidocaine is injected over the area of the abscess where the incision is expected to be made.

10. **How is incision and drainage of an abscess performed?**
    After proper local anesthesia is achieved, the wound is cleansed with an antiseptic solution. Incision of the abscess along the area of maximum fluctuance is performed by using an #11-blade scalpel through the dermis. The length of the incision depends on the size of the abscess. Once the incision is performed, pressure is applied to the surrounding tissue to express the abscess fluid from the incision site.

11. **Is wound irrigation necessary in the incision site?**
    Although some providers recommend irrigating the wound after incision to "clean out" the wound, irrigation of an abscess has not been shown to improve wound healing.

12. **How do I know if there are septations or loculations within the abscess?**
    Ultrasounds can potentially detect septations or loculations, but they may not be clinically detectable on physical exam. A hemostat is inserted into the incised wound to explore and break apart any septations and loculations.

13. **Are wound cultures performed from the abscess fluid?**
    Routine swabbing is not recommended for immunocompetent patients without risk factors. Some providers perform wound cultures to survey local resistance patterns or to determine type of antibiotic use.

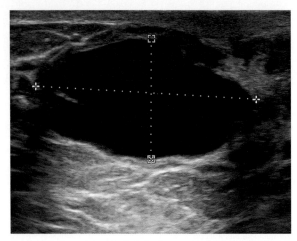

Fig. 54.1 The hypoechoic region indicates the presence of abscess on ultrasound.

14. **Are blood cultures necessary in a patient with an abscess?**
Blood cultures are generally not obtained in immunocompetent patients with skin infections unless patients have serious or complicated soft tissue infections from surgical or traumatic wounds or require further surgical intervention. The emergence of CA-MRSA increases patients' risks of developing other types of infections such as pneumonia, but the incidences of bacteremia are generally low for both immunocompetent patients and patients with CA-MRSA.

15. **Does the incision site need to be closed up after the procedure?**
Wound healing by secondary intention is generally favored, as previous studies have not found a difference in wound healing between primary versus secondary closure following an abscess incision and drainage.

16. **Is wound packing necessary after the incision and drainage?**
Wound packing following incision and drainage has not been found to impact drainage failure rates or recurrence rates of an abscess; thus, it is not favored by most providers. Wound packing has been used to assist in wound debridement and to avoid fluid reaccumulation. Packing is removed within 24–48 hours, and the wound is reassessed then.

17. **What is a wound "stent"?**
It is the insertion of a strip of iodoform or Penrose drain into the wound to keep the wound open to promote drainage after the incision and drainage. Its use and impact on wound healing are debatable.

18. **What is a loop drain?**
A loop drain is the insertion of a rubber vessel loop into the wound and tunneled to a distal healthy tissue and tied to form a loop following incision, drainage, and irrigation of the abscess. The loop remains in place to promote further drainage and is removed between 3 and 10 days. While this is a novel technique, early studies have shown higher healing rates than traditional incision and drainage methods with wound packing.

19. **When is procedural sedation necessary during an incision and drainage?**
Procedural sedation may assist in performing incision and drainage in patients who may not be cooperative with the procedure. Sedation is often performed in pediatric patients or patients with large abscesses requiring aggressive manipulation.

20. **What medications are often used for procedural sedation during an abscess incision and drainage?**
This is generally up to the preference of the provider. Options include ketamine, propofol, or benzodiazepines in oral, intranasal, or intravenous forms.

21. **When should consultants be called for abscess drainage?**
Incision and drainage for simple skin abscesses are generally performed by clinicians in an urgent care setting. Subspecialists such as otolaryngologists may be consulted for abscesses involving the face and neck. A gynecology consult may be warranted for patients with abscesses involving the genitalia, such as a Bartholin gland cyst. In patients with deep and complex lesions, lesions involving the breast, or perianal abscesses, consultation with general surgery may be necessary.

22. **Should patients receive antibiotics after incision and drainage?**
    The decision to provide antibiotics after incision and drainage is controversial. The 2014 guidelines provided by the Infectious Diseases Society of America state that mild abscesses should be treated with incision and drainage alone without antibiotic use. Antibiotics were originally recommended only for patients with systemic infections, those who are immunocompromised, those with multiple abscesses, extremes of ages, or lack of response to incision and drainage.

    These recommendations are being challenged by new evidence. A recently published meta-analysis demonstrated that providing systemic antibiotics after incision and drainage more than doubled clinical cure rates. Providers should consider the use of antibiotics while balancing the risks of side effects and adverse events.

23. **Which types of antibiotics should be given if the decision were to give antibiotics after incision and drainage?**
    If antibiotics are chosen, medications effective against MRSA should be selected. Previous studies have not found any difference in clinical improvement in patients who received antibiotics for coverage against MRSA versus antibiotics for traditional skin flora or placebo, except in patients less than 1 year of age presenting with fever and abscess.

24. **Should topical antibiotics be given for abscess treatment?**
    Topical antibiotics are not helpful in abscesses that require draining.

25. **When should patients with abscesses be hospitalized?**
    Admission may be warranted in patients who appear toxic with systemic symptoms such as fever, diabetic patients, and those who are immunocompromised. Patients with lymphangitis and concomitant rapidly spreading cellulitis should also be hospitalized for intravenous antibiotics.

KEY POINTS

1. Incision and drainage are the treatment of choice for abscesses.
2. Providers should consider administering systemic antibiotics that provide coverage against MRSA to patients after incision and drainage of skin abscesses.
3. Wound packing after incision and drainage has no impact on wound improvement.

BIBLIOGRAPHY

Barbic D, Chenkin J, Cho DD, Jelic T, Scheuemeyer FX. In patients presenting to the emergency department with skin and soft tissue infections, what is the diagnostic accuracy of point-of-care ultrasonography for the diagnosis of abscess compared to the current standard of care? A systemic review and meta-analysis. *BMC Open.* 2017;7(1):e013688.

Chinnock B, Hendey GW. Irrigation of cutaneous abscesses does not improve treatment success. *Ann Emerg Med.* 2016;67(3):379–383.

Gespari RJ, Sanseverino A, Gleeson T. Abscess incision and drainage with or without ultrasonography: a randomized controlled trial. *Ann Emerg Med.* 2019;73(1):1–7.

Gottlieb M, DeMott JM, Hallock M, Peksa GD. Systemic antibiotics for the treatment of skin and soft tissue abscesses: a systematic review and meta-analysis. *Ann Emerg Med.* 2019;73(1):8–16.

Gottlieb M, Schmitz G, Peksa GD. Comparison of the loop technique with incision and drainage for skin and soft tissue abscesses: a systematic review and meta-analysis. *Acad Emerg Med.* 2021;28(3):346–354.

Lake JG, Miller LG, Fritz SA. Antibiotic duration, but not abscess size, impacts clinical cure of limited skin and soft tissue infection after incision and drainage. *Clin Infect Dis.* 2020;71(3):661–663.

Mellick L. *Pilonidal abscess emergency incision & drainage* [Video]. YouTube. https://youtu.be/u1lysff7StM. April 8, 2020.

Menegas S, Moayedi S, Torres M. Abscess management: an evidence-based review for emergency medicine clinicians. *J Emerg Med.* 2021;60(3):310–320.

Schmitz GR, Gottlieb M. Managing a cutaneous abscess in the emergency department. *Ann Emerg Med.* 2021;78(1):44–48.

CHAPTER 55

FOREIGN BODY REMOVAL

Roselyn A. Appenteng, MD, Thuy L. Ngo, DO MEd

TOP SECRETS

1. Successful foreign body removal requires thoughtful preprocedural planning, including the choice of immobilization and the use of local anesthetic or sedation in appropriate scenarios.
2. Factors that affect the method and urgency of removal of a foreign body include the type of material (e.g., button battery versus food item), location, risk of further injury to surrounding tissue, long-term sequelae, and potential for infection.
3. Firm immobilization, behavior management (e.g., pain control or anxiolysis), and good lighting will aid in nasal, ear, or skin foreign body removal in children.
4. A thorough exam is warranted to avoid missing foreign bodies in contralateral orifices or in the absence of a witnessed ingestion or aspiration.
5. Button batteries in any cavity or two high-powered magnets ingested or present across the nasal septum are medical emergencies and require immediate removal.
6. Suspect foreign body aspiration in a toddler to preschool-aged child who was last seen with a small, hard object and has a sudden onset of cough, choke, wheeze, drooling, or inability to tolerate oral secretions.

EAR AND NASAL FOREIGN BODIES

1. **What makes foreign body removal unique in the pediatric patient?**
   The provider must accommodate for the maturity level and behavior of the child in obtaining a history and seek input from the parent on the child's ability to tolerate a minor procedure. The provider must explain the procedure to both the parent and the child in language that they can both understand. A referral to an otolaryngologist may be warranted if the likelihood of success is low based on the initial evaluation of the patient.

2. **What behavioral or immobilization techniques can assist in procedures on an uncooperative child?**
   The child may remain in the parent's lap while giving the parent straightforward instructions on how to assist while holding the child. An alternative method is laying the child down, swaddling the arms and legs with a bedsheet in a papoose, with an assistant or parent gently immobilizing the trunk and head. Additionally, cervical collar placement can be considered to assist with immobilizing the head.

3. **Should medications be used for ear or nasal foreign body removal?**
   Acetone, ethanol, or isopropyl alcohol can be used as insecticides to help kill a live insect and decrease discomfort in the ear. Alternatively, 1–2% nonviscous lidocaine can also be instilled into the ear to assist with anesthesia or to drown insects if present. This practice should be avoided if a tympanic membrane perforation is suspected or if the foreign body may expand. For example, vegetables or batteries, whole or fragment, may expand in the presence of a liquid. Vasoconstrictors (e.g., oxymetazoline nasal spray) may reduce nasal mucosal swelling and improve success. Limit medication use with button batteries to avoid an increased risk of alkaline caustic exposures.

4. **Is sedation appropriate for pediatric foreign body removal?**
   Anxiolysis with intranasal midazolam (0.2–0.5 mg/kg; maximum dose 10 mg/dose), is the preferred strategy for minor pediatric procedures. It has a faster time of onset (5–10 minutes) in comparison to oral midazolam, which is typically dosed at 0.5 mg/kg (maximum dose 20 mg/dose) with a time onset of 20–30 minutes. A single dose of intranasal midazolam does not induce moderate sedation and therefore does not require cardiorespiratory monitoring; however, pulse oximetry may be used if institutional protocol dictates.

5. **Is there a noninvasive method to remove a foreign body from the nose?**
   The "mother's kiss" or "parent's kiss" is a positive pressure technique that is a noninvasive option. The parent occludes the unobstructed nostril with a finger and applies positive pressure by creating a mouth-to-mouth seal and blowing air into the patient's mouth to dislodge the foreign body. Alternatively, a bag-valve mask can be used to apply positive pressure via the mouth instead of the parent. These methods can also advance the foreign body proximally, improving visibility and enabling removal via forceps or curette.

6. **When is irrigation indicated for foreign body removal?**
   Irrigation is contraindicated for nasal foreign body removal due to the risk of aspiration. Irrigation with warm tap water or saline through the soft catheter of a butterfly cannula or an angiocath with the needle removed can flush a foreign body from the auditory canal. Irrigation should be avoided with organic matter that can swell or injure the tympanic membrane, including button batteries.

7. **When can tissue adhesive (glue) be used to aid foreign body removal?**
   Tissue adhesive, such as Dermabond or cyanoacrylate "superglue," is useful for round, rigid, or smooth objects (e.g., beads) that are difficult to grasp in the ear. The foreign body must be dry and easily visualized. A drop of tissue glue is placed on a cotton swab stick and applied to make contact with the foreign body. Wait several seconds for the glue to dry, then the object can be extracted. To avoid further trauma to the ear, take caution not to drip tissue adhesive into the ear canal or push the object deeper.

8. **How can a Foley catheter be used to remove foreign bodies from the nose?**
   Apply lubricating jelly or viscous lidocaine jelly to a small Foley catheter bulb (e.g., 6–8 French), slide the catheter along the floor of the nare past the foreign body, then inflate the balloon and sweep the object out of the nose. Ensure the balloon inflates properly prior to placement in the nare (Figs. 55.1A-1D). If possible, place the child in a lateral position to decrease the risk of aspiration. The Katz extractor, which has a thinner Foley attached to a syringe, was also designed for nasal foreign bodies and can be used if available.

9. **When are forceps appropriate for foreign body removal?**
   Forceps are appropriate for materials that can be both easily visualized and grasped. Avoid the use of forceps with materials that can easily fragment. Additionally, they can push round objects more distally. Potential complications associated with the use of forceps include canal and mucosal abrasions and epistaxis. Other complications, such as septal perforation, are associated with the specific type of foreign body (e.g., button battery).

10. **When is a nasal foreign body a medical emergency?**
    Button batteries in any cavity (e.g., ear, nose, or esophagus) require immediate removal, due to the risk of liquefaction necrosis, secondary to the battery current discharged when adjacent to mucosal tissue. In addition, corrosion of the battery can result in release of alkaline material. Two magnets across the nasal septum require emergent removal due to the risk of pressure necrosis.

11. **What are the indications for referral to otolaryngology for removal?**
    Indications for referral include the need for sedation, development of granulation tissue, signs of trauma including penetration through the septum, ungraspable or inadequately visualized foreign body, sharp objects, objects abutting the tympanic membrane or wedged in the medial external auditory canal, or unsuccessful extraction attempt.

12. **When are antibiotics needed?**
    Antibiotic coverage is not routinely required after extraction of the acute foreign body unless there are signs of concomitant infection such as otitis externa, cellulitis, or sinusitis. A thorough exam of bilateral ears and nares must be performed to avoid missing a secondary foreign body as well as an occult infection.

FOREIGN BODY INGESTION OR ASPIRATION

13. **What is the typical profile of a foreign body ingestion or aspiration in a child or adolescent?**
    The typical profile of a foreign body ingestion or aspiration is a toddler to preschool-aged child who was eating or playing with hot dogs, grapes, peanuts, seeds, raw carrots, popcorn, coins, toy parts, button batteries, magnets, or balloons and has sudden onset of choking or respiratory distress. Children less than 6 years of age account for the significant majority of foreign body ingestions, and coins are the most common culprits. Adolescent ingestions are often intentional with the intent to harm or mimic trends online.

14. **What are symptoms of foreign body aspiration or ingestion?**
    Symptoms of a foreign body in the oropharynx or esophagus can include vomiting, throat pain, drooling, dysphagia, odynophagia, globus or pricking sensation, and decreased oral intake. Children with foreign bodies in the airway may have cough, stridor, choking or gagging, cyanosis, wheeze, or respiratory distress. However, some ingestions or aspirations may not be immediately symptomatic. Therefore, having a high index of suspicion is key, especially in the absence of a reliable witness.

15. **What are x-ray findings of an aspirated foreign body?**
    Radiography can be useful for identifying radiopaque foreign bodies. However, it is not as reliable with radiolucent objects such as wood. Secondary signs of an aspirated foreign body may be found on inspiratory and expiratory chest x-rays or bilateral decubitus views in the uncooperative child. The foreign body causes air trapping, leading to ipsilateral hyperinflation and mediastinal shift to the contralateral side, or segmental hyperlucency or atelectasis. In addition, chest x-rays may demonstrate infiltrates. Sensitivity and specificity ranging between 35–66% and 50–93%, respectively, have been reported for chest x-rays. Additionally, anterior-posterior and lateral neck films may be warranted for upper airway obstruction. The gold standard for visualization of an aspirated foreign body is bronchoscopy.

16. **When is a foreign body aspiration or ingestion considered an emergency?**
    Emergent endoscopic removal is indicated for any foreign body aspiration, or an ingested object with a high risk for perforation, gastrointestinal bleeding, bowel ischemia, obstruction, or toxicity (Table 55.1). Endoscopic removal is indicated for esophageal foreign bodies. This includes coins, button batteries, multiple magnets, and impacted food. A single, high-powered magnet ingestion is managed expectantly with serial x-rays and

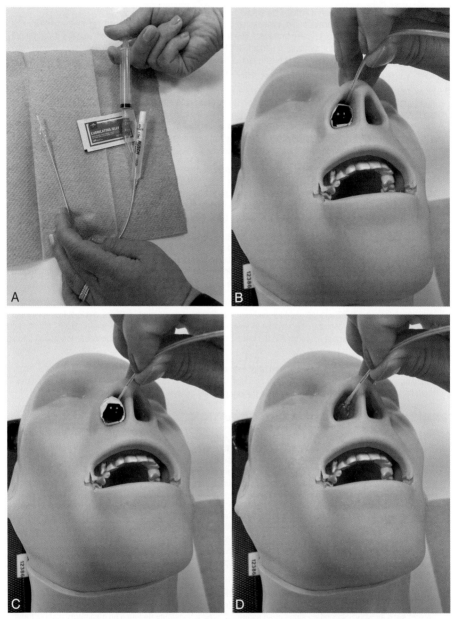

Fig. 55.1A-1D A bead in a mannequin removed with an 8-Fr Foley catheter. Foley balloon inflation verified prior to placement. If the bead has a hollow hole, the Foley may be threaded through the hole prior to balloon inflation to aid in removal.

removing all nearby magnet sources at home. However, multiple attached magnets can appear as a single magnet. Therefore, it is important to ascertain the number of magnets as accurately as possible with anterior-posterior and lateral x-rays.

The North American Society for Pediatric Gastroenterology, Hepatology, and Nutrition (NASPGHAN) Endoscopy Committee recommends removal of gastric button batteries if the child's age is <5 years and if the button battery is ≥20 mm, or in cases where repeat x-ray in 48 hours for ≥20 mm or 10–14 days if <20 mm and the button battery has failed to pass in the stool. Endoscopic removal is recommended if the patient is symptomatic or if the foreign body is retained in the stomach. The Poison Control Center conservatively recommends repeat x-rays for batteries >15 mm

Table 55.1 Indications for Urgent Endoscopic Removal of a Foreign Body Ingestion[a,b]

- Severe respiratory distress
- Signs of abdominal obstruction or inflammation (fever, abdominal pain, or vomiting)
- Objects containing heavy metals that cause toxicity (e.g., lead, iron)
- Soft tissue swelling is seen in the pharyngeal space on neck x-ray
- Object in esophagus or stomach
  - Button battery or sharp object
  - Signs of esophageal obstruction (e.g., drooling, inability to tolerate secretions dysphagia)
  - Long object >4 cm, sharp, high-powered magnet, multiple magnets
- Object in stomach or duodenal bulb
  - Long object >4 cm, sharp, high-powered magnet, multiple magnets, superabsorbent polymer
  - Button battery, if symptomatic

[a]Indications adapted from the clinical report of National Association of Pediatric Gastroenterology, Hepatology and Nutrition endoscopy committee.
[b]Indications adapted from UpToDate: Foreign bodies of the esophagus and gastrointestinal tract in children.

in the stomach after 4 days for <6 years. Management of low-risk objects (e.g., coins) in the stomach includes weekly x-rays to ensure passage. Coins retained in the stomach at 4 weeks may warrant elective endoscopic removal. Any symptomatic foreign body requires emergent removal. Long objects >4 cm are unlikely to progress past the duodenum and/or the ileocecal valve, and objects with a diameter of >25 mm are unlikely to clear the pylorus and may warrant urgent removal. Lastly, superabsorbent polymers can become obstructive when they increase in size in a moist environment.

FOREIGN BODIES IN THE SKIN

17. **What is the first step in any foreign body removal from the skin?**
   All foreign body removal from the skin warrants universal precautions for the provider, including gloves and a face shield as indicated, sterilization of the wound, local anesthesia if indicated, and routine wound care afterward.

18. **Before removal of a foreign body in the skin, what must the provider examine?**
   The provider should determine whether the object has injured deeper structures such as bone, tendon, fascia, or vasculature, via direct visualization and probing as indicated (with good anesthesia), performing a thorough neurovasculature exam, and obtaining an x-ray if indicated. Radiolucent objects may not be identifiable on x-ray; point-of-care ultrasound can have utility in this scenario.

19. **What are common fishhook removal techniques?**
   There are four common techniques for fishhook removal. The advance-and-cut technique is generally the most successful: grasp the hook with a needle driver and rotate the hook to emerge the barb out of the skin, proximally creating an exit wound. Use wire cutters to cut the barb, then remove the hook from the entry site (Figs. 55.2A-2D). Other options include the string yank (which requires technical experience), retrograde removal (for barbless or superficial hooks), or the needle cover technique (superficial hooks). Local anesthetic can be helpful, particularly for deeply embedded hooks. Ensure that the wound site is adequately cleaned. Providers must use caution to avoid self-inflicted injury with the hook, and eye protection is strongly recommended.

20. **What are the common techniques for splinter removal?**
   A visible wood or plant-based splinter that is parallel to the skin should be removed with caution because simply grasping and pulling can lead to fragmentation. Set a 30-minute time limit for the procedure to avoid excess tissue damage or trauma if the object is not found. If the splinter is small and superficial, it may be removed using an 18-gauge needle to gently disrupt the skin over the splinter, then grasp the splinter with forceps. For the deeper, parallel object, use a scalpel to make an incision over the object, or, if perpendicular, make an elliptical incision around the object; the core of tissue containing the object is then removed.

21. **What is the technique to remove a tick?**
   Both a suture lasso and tweezer or forceps methods have been described. The tick's head is grasped firmly by forceps, as close to the skin as possible, and constant, vertical traction is applied. Avoid detaching mouthparts when the tick is removed. An attempt should be made to remove retained mouthparts. However, if unsuccessful, avoid multiple attempts at removal and allow the skin to heal. With any technique, caution should be taken to avoid causing the tick to salivate and regurgitate at the attachment site.

22. **Should chemoprophylaxis be started after tick removal?**
   Chemoprophylaxis with a single dose of doxycycline to prevent Lyme disease in endemic areas may be considered. Additionally, the CDC recommends a single 200-mg dose of doxycycline for adults and 4.4 mg/kg for children (<45 kg), if doxycycline is not contraindicated, to reduce the risk of acquiring Lyme disease after a high-risk

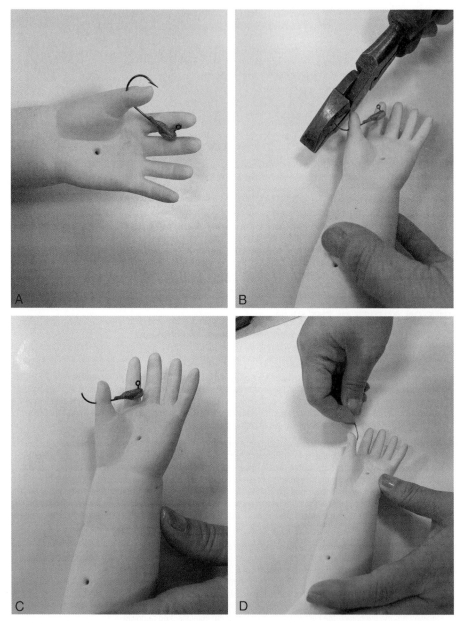

Fig. 55.2A-2D Fishhook removal in a mannequin by the advance-and-cut method.

tick bite: the child is in a highly endemic region, the bite is within 72 hours, the tick is identifiable as *I. scapularis*, estimated attachment is ≥36 hours, or if the tick is engorged.

23. **What vaccinations should be up to date for patients with skin foreign bodies?**
For all foreign bodies in the skin, ensure that the patient's tetanus vaccination is up to date. For children who have minor clean wounds, a tetanus vaccine should only be administered if their vaccination status is unknown or they have received <3 doses. However, children with ≥3 vaccine doses should receive a tetanus vaccine if ≥10 years after their last vaccine. If the wound is contaminated or significant, including puncture wounds, a vaccine should be administered if <3 doses previously obtained or ≥5 years if the patient has a prior history of ≥3 doses.

Table 55.2 Indications for Prophylactic Antibiotics After High-Risk Skin Puncture Wounds[a,b]

- Grossly contaminated puncture wounds (e.g., organic matter, dirt, water organisms, fishhook injuries)
- Immunocompromised host (e.g., immunodeficiency, immunosuppression, diabetes mellitus)
- Retained organic foreign body
- Deep wounds (including close proximity to bone, joint, tendons, or cartilage)
- Plantar punctures through an intact sole
- Evidence of cellulitis

[a]Indications adapted from UpToDate: Infectious complications of puncture wounds.
[b]Indications adapted from Enzler et al. article (2011) on Antimicrobial Prophylaxis in Adults.

Table 55.3 Prophylactic Oral Antibiotic Selection After Skin Puncture Wounds[a,b,c]

- Coverage of skin flora (*S. aureus* and beta-hemolytic streptococci):
  - Cephalexin OR clindamycin
- If dirty, contaminated wound, consider:
  - Trimethoprim/sulfamethoxazole OR clindamycin
- Exposure to water organisms[c]:
  - Levofloxacin[d] OR doxycycline (*Vibrio* species coverage) for brackish or saltwater exposure
  - Levofloxacin OR ciprofloxacin for freshwater exposure
  - Levofloxacin AND metronidazole for sewage or soil contaminants
- Plantar puncture wound (include coverage for *P. aeruginosa*):
  - Levofloxacin OR ciprofloxacin (with cephalexin)

[a]Indications adapted from UpToDate: Infectious complications of puncture wounds.
[b]Indications adapted from Enzler et al. article (2011) on Antimicrobial Prophylaxis in Adults.
[c]Adapted from Noonberg 2005 on the Management of extremity trauma and related infections occuring in the acquatic environment.
[d]Caution is advised if treating children with fluoroquinolones due to rare adverse risk of tendon inflammation or rupture. Advise limited strenuous physical activity and discontinuation at the first sign of musculoskeletal pain or tingling.

24. **Are antibiotics indicated for a skin puncture wound?**
    A 3- to 5-day course of prophylactic antibiotics should be considered for injuries that are at high risk for infection (Table 55.2). Oral antibiotic selection (Table 55.3) should cover gram-positive skin flora and expand coverage for aquatic organisms in fishhook injuries, gram-negative and anaerobes in dirty wounds, and pseudomonas in punctures through a shoe sole.

KEY POINTS

1. Adequate preparation, visualization, and immobilization of the child are crucial in extracting a foreign body.
2. Nasal foreign bodies can be removed with positive pressure, tissue adhesive, Foley catheter, or forceps.
3. Ear foreign bodies can be removed with irrigation, tissue adhesive, or forceps.
4. Extraction attempts should cease in the event of any tissue damage or inability of the patient to tolerate the procedure.
5. Medical emergencies include button batteries in any cavity or two magnets across the nasal septum. Both require immediate removal.
6. Otolaryngology referral for nonemergent foreign bodies is frequently appropriate.
7. Suspect foreign body aspiration in a child who is a toddler to preschool age, was last seen with a small, hard object, and has sudden onset of cough, choke, or wheeze.
8. Chest x-ray with foreign body aspiration can show air trapping and hyperinflation on the affected side.
9. Obstructive or caustic material in the esophagus warrants emergent removal.
10. Low-risk ingested objects can be managed expectantly.
11. Set a 30-minute time limit for the procedure to avoid excess tissue damage or trauma.
12. Tetanus should be up to date for all skin puncture wounds.
13. Antibiotic prophylaxis is indicated for high-risk skin punctures.

Acknowledgments

The authors would like to thank Drs. Therese L. Canares and Anne O'Connor for their contributions to this chapter in the previous edition.

BIBLIOGRAPHY

Ahmad KH, Kamal Y, Lone AU. Fish hook injury: removal by "push through and cut off" technique: a case report and brief literature review. *Trauma Mon.* 2014;19(2):e17728. doi:10.5812/traumamon.17728.

Antonelli PJ, Ahmadi A, Prevatt A. Insecticidal activity of common reagents for insect foreign bodies of the ear. *The Laryngoscope.* 2001;111(1):15–20. https://doi.org/10.1097/00005537-200101000-00003.

Baddour LM, Brown AM. Infectious complications of puncture wounds. UpToDate Web site. https://www.uptodate.com/contents/infectious-complications-of-puncture-wounds?csi=e0468549-26af-4f26-9f4d-78d46cabca93&source=contentShare. Updated 2022. Accessed August 14, 2022.

Centers for Disease Control and Prevention. Tick removal. https://www.cdc.gov/ticks/removing_a_tick.html. Updated 2022. Accessed September 5, 2022.

Centers for Disease Control and Prevention. Tickborne diseases of the United States. https://www.cdc.gov/ticks/tickbornediseases/tick-bite-prophylaxis.html. Updated 2019.

del Cura JL, Aza I, Zabala RM, Sarabia M, Korta I. US-guided localization and removal of soft-tissue foreign bodies. *Radiographics.* 2020;40(4):1188–1195. https://doi.org/10.1148/rg.2020200001.

Dwyer D. Foley catheter technique for nasal foreign body removal in children. *Emerg Med Australas.* 2015;27(5):495–496. https://doi.org/10.1111/1742-6723.12481.

Fasseeh NA, Elagamy OA, Gaafar AH, et al. A new scoring system and clinical algorithm for the management of suspected foreign body aspiration in children: a retrospective cohort study. *Ital J Pediatr.* 2021;47(1):194–199. doi:10.1186/s13052-021-01147-9.

Gammons M, Salam G. Tick removal. *Am Fam Physician.* 2002;66(4):643–645.

Gilger MA, Jain AK. Foreign bodies of the esophagus and gastrointestinal tract in children. UpToDate. https://www.uptodate.com/contents/foreign-bodies-of-the-esophagus-and-gastrointestinal-tract-in-children?csi=c2852863-b814-45e5-8587-1a3a71d86799&source=contentShare. Updated 2022. Accessed August 14, 2022.

Grigg S, Grigg C. Removal of ear, nose and throat foreign bodies: a review. *Aust J Gen Pract.* 2018;47(10):682–685. doi:10.31128/AJGP-02-18-4503.

Gummin DD, Mowry JB, Beuhler MC, et al. 2020 Annual Report of the American Association of Poison Control Centers' national poison data system (NPDS): 38th annual report. *Clin Toxicol.* 2021;59(12):1282–1501. https://doi.org/10.1080/15563650.2021.1989785.

Jayachandra S, Eslick GD. A systematic review of paediatric foreign body ingestion: presentation, complications, and management. *Int J Pediatr Otorhinolaryngol.* 2013;77(3):311–317. https://www.sciencedirect.com/science/article/pii/S0165587612006519. https://doi.org/10.1016/j.ijporl.2012.11.025.

Jungbauer WN, Shih M, Nguyen SA, Clemmens CS. Comparison of pediatric nasal foreign body removal by care setting: a systematic review and meta-analysis. *Int J Pediatr Otorhinolaryngol.* 2022;158:111162. https://www.sciencedirect.com/science/article/pii/S0165587622001239. https://doi.org/10.1016/j.ijporl.2022.111162.

Kadish HA, Corneli HM. Removal of nasal foreign bodies in the pediatric population. *Am J Emerg Med.* 1997;15(1):54–56. https://www.sciencedirect.com/science/article/pii/S0735675797900498. https://doi.org/10.1016/S0735-6757(97)90049-8.

Kalan A, Tariq M. Foreign bodies in the nasal cavities: a comprehensive review of the aetiology, diagnostic pointers, and therapeutic measures. *Postgrad Med J.* 2000;76(898):484–487. doi:10.1136/pmj.76.898.484.

Kiger JR, Brenkert TE, Losek JD. Nasal foreign body removal in children. *Pediatr Emerg Care.* 2008;24(11). https://journals.lww.com/pec-online/Fulltext/2008/11000/Nasal_Foreign_Body_Removal_in_Children.13.aspx.

Kramer RE, Lerner DG, Lin T, et al. Management of ingested foreign bodies in children: a clinical report of the NASPGHAN endoscopy committee. *J Pediatr Gastroenterol Nutr.* 2015;60(4):562–574. doi:10.1097/MPG.0000000000000729.

Lane RD, Schunk JE. Atomized intranasal midazolam use for minor procedures in the pediatric emergency department. *Pediatr Emerg Care.* 2008;24(5):300–303. doi:10.1097/PEC.0b013e31816ecb6f.

Loh WS, Leong JL, Tan HK. Hazardous foreign bodies: complications and management of button batteries in nose. *Ann Otol Rhinol Laryngol.* 2003;112(4):379–383. doi:10.1177/000348940311200415.

McCormick S, Brennan P, Yassa J, Shawis R. Children and mini-magnets: an almost fatal attraction. *Emerg Med J.* 2002;19(1):71–73. doi:10.1136/emj.19.1.71.

McLaughlin R, Ullah R, Heylings D. Comparative prospective study of foreign body removal from external auditory canals of cadavers with right angle hook or cyanoacrylate glue. *Emerg Med J.* 2002;19(1):43–45. doi:10.1136/emj.19.1.43.

Mehdi I, Parveen S, Choubey S, Rasheed A, Singh P, Ghayas M. Comparative study of oral midazolam syrup and intranasal midazolam spray for sedative premedication in pediatric surgeries. *Anesth Essays Res.* 2019;13(2):370–375. doi:10.4103/aer.AER_182_18.

Moran GJ, Talan DA, Abrahamian FM. Antimicrobial prophylaxis for wounds and procedures in the emergency department. *Infect Dis Clin North Am.* 2008;22(1):117–143. https://www.sciencedirect.com/science/article/pii/S0891552007001195. https://doi.org/10.1016/j.idc.2007.12.002.

Na'ara S, Vainer I, Amit M, Gordin A. Foreign body aspiration in infants and older children: a comparative study. *Ear Nose Throat J.* 2020;99(1):47–51. https://doi.org/10.1177/0145561319839900.

National Capital Poison Center. National Capital Poison Center button battery ingestion triage and treatment guideline. Poison Control: National Capital Poison Center. https://www.poison.org/battery/guideline. Updated 2018. Accessed September 5, 2022.

Noonburg GE. Management of extremity trauma and related infections occurring in the aquatic environment. *J Am Acad Orthop Surg.* 2005;13(4):243–253. doi: 13/4/243 [pii].

Oliva S, Romano C, De Angelis P, et al. Foreign body and caustic ingestions in children: a clinical practice guideline. *Digestive and Liver Disease.* 2020;52(11):1266–1281. https://www.sciencedirect.com/science/article/pii/S1590865820303741. https://doi.org/10.1016/j.dld.2020.07.016.

Orobello NC, Dirain CO, Kaufman PE, Antonelli PJ. Efficacy of common reagents for killing ticks in the ear canal. *Laryngoscope Investig Otolaryngol.* 2018;3(6):492–495. doi:10.1002/lio2.217.

Oyama LC. Foreign bodies of the ear, nose and throat. *Emerg Med Clin North Am.* 2019;37(1):121–130. https://www.sciencedirect.com/science/article/pii/S0733862718300968. https://doi.org/10.1016/j.emc.2018.09.009.

Pansini V, Curatola A, Gatto A, Lazzareschi I, Ruggiero A, Chiaretti A. Intranasal drugs for analgesia and sedation in children admitted to pediatric emergency department: a narrative review. *Ann Transl Med.* 2021;9(2):189–5177. doi:10.21037/atm-20-5177.

Prats M, O'Connell M, Wellock A, Kman NE. Fish hook removal: case reports and a review of the literature. *J Emerg Med.* 2013;44(6):e375–e380. https://www.sciencedirect.com/science/article/pii/S073646791201582X. https://doi.org/10.1016/j.jemermed.2012.11.058.

Purohit N, Ray S, Wilson T, Chawla OP. The 'parent's kiss': an effective way to remove paediatric nasal foreign bodies. *Ann R Coll Surg Engl.* 2008;90(5):420–422. doi:10.1308/003588408X300966.

Red Book 2021: Report of the committee on infectious diseases. Elk Grove Village: American Academy of Pediatrics; 2021. http://ebook-central.proquest.com/lib/jhu/detail.action?docID=6639842.

Şahin AR, Hakkoymaz H, Taşdoğan AM, Kireçci E. Evaluation and comparison of tick detachment techniques and technical mistakes made during tick removal. *Ulus Travma Acil Cerrahi Derg.* 2020;26(3):405–410. doi:10.14744/tjtes.2020.59680.

Scholes MA, Jensen EL. Presentation and management of nasal foreign bodies at a tertiary children's hospital in an American metro area. *Int J Pediatr Otorhinolaryngol.* 2016;88:190–193. https://www.sciencedirect.com/science/article/pii/S0165587616302221. https://doi.org/10.1016/j.ijporl.2016.07.016.

Schulze SL, Kerschner J, Beste D. Pediatric external auditory canal foreign bodies: a review of 698 cases. *Otolaryngol Head Neck Surg.* 2002;127(1):73–78. https://doi.org/10.1067/mhn.2002.126724.

Sink JR, Kitsko DJ, Mehta DK, Georg MW, Simons JP. Diagnosis of pediatric foreign body ingestion: clinical presentation, physical examination, and radiologic findings. *Ann Otol Rhinol Laryngol.* 2016;125(4):342–350. https://doi.org/10.1177/0003489415611128.

Stephenson AL, Wu W, Cortes D, Rochon PA. Tendon injury and fluoroquinolone use: a systematic review. *Drug Saf.* 2013;36(9):709–721. https://doi.org/10.1007/s40264-013-0089-8.

Taşkınlar H, Bahadır GB, Erdoğan C, Yiğit D, Avlan D, Naycı A. A diagnostic dilemma for the pediatrician: radiolucent tracheobronchial foreign body. *Pediatr Neonatol.* 2017;58(3):264–269. doi: S1875-9572(16)30240-6 [pii].

Thabet MH, Basha WM, Askar S. Button battery foreign bodies in children: hazards, management, and recommendations. *BioMed Research International.* 2013;2013:846091. doi:10.1155/2013/846091. https://europepmc.org/articles/PMC3725977?pdf=render.

Upreti L, Gupta N. Imaging for diagnosis of foreign body aspiration in children? *Indian Pediatr.* 2015;52(8):659–660.

Wright CC, Closson FT. Updates in pediatric gastrointestinal foreign bodies. *Pediatr Clin North Am.* 2013;60(5):1221–1239. https://www.sciencedirect.com/science/article/pii/S0031395513000837. https://doi.org/10.1016/j.pcl.2013.06.007.

Zavdy O, Viner I, London N, et al. Intranasal foreign bodies: a 10-year analysis of a large cohort, in a tertiary medical center. *Am J Emerg Med.* 2021;50:356–359. https://www.sciencedirect.com/science/article/pii/S0735675721006859. https://doi.org/10.1016/j.ajem.2021.08.045.

Zerella JT, Dimler M, McGill LC, Pippus KJ. Foreign body aspiration in children: value of radiography and complications of bronchoscopy. *J Pediatr Surg.* 1998;33(11):1651–1654. https://www.sciencedirect.com/science/article/pii/S0022346898906017. https://doi.org/10.1016/S0022-3468(98)90601-7.

CHAPTER 56

DENTAL AND ORAL COMPLAINTS AND PROCEDURES

Selena Hariharan, MD, MHSA, Cindy D. Chang, MD

DENTAL INJURIES

1. **In pediatric dental trauma, why is it important to distinguish between primary and permanent teeth?**
   Management strategies and treatment differ depending on whether the injured tooth is a primary or permanent tooth. Improperly distinguishing can result in damage to the permanent tooth.

2. **A 5-year-old male presents with a dental injury. Your examination reveals a child with an isolated avulsion of his left maxillary central incisor. His mother has the tooth with an intact root in a cup of cold milk. You recall that reimplantation should be performed immediately for avulsed permanent teeth but not for primary teeth. How do you make the distinction of whether an injured tooth is a primary or permanent tooth?**
   - Primary teeth
     - Will erupt in a typical pattern depending on the age of the child
     - Central incisors will erupt as early as 6–8 months of age; all primary teeth should be present by 3 years of age.
     - Mandibular teeth tend to erupt earlier than their maxillary counterparts.
     - A full complement of primary teeth consists of 10 mandibular and 10 maxillary teeth.
   - Permanent teeth
     - Similarly, permanent teeth erupt in a typical pattern depending on the age of the child, typically starting at 5–6 years of age.
     - Central incisors and first molars are the first permanent teeth to erupt, with a full complement of permanent teeth erupted by 16 years of age.
     - A full complement of permanent teeth consists of 16 mandibular and 16 maxillary teeth.
   - Answer
     - In this case, given the patient's age, the tooth is most likely a primary tooth, and avulsed primary teeth should not be reimplanted. This family should be reassured with recommendations for good oral hygiene.
     - Use the age of the child to help you determine whether the injured tooth is primary or permanent.
       - ALL teeth in children less than 5 years of age are primary.
       - Children 5–12 years of age have mixed dentition; use caution when treating dental injury.
       - ALL teeth in children older than 13 years of age are permanent.
     - Primary teeth are smaller compared to permanent teeth.
     - The occlusive surface of primary teeth is smooth as opposed to ridged.
     - When in doubt, ask the parents to help distinguish between primary and permanent teeth.

3. **What are the various injuries to primary dentition and how are they managed?**
   - **Fractures** can be classified based on the Ellis classification system.
     - Enamel fracture (Ellis class I fracture): fracture through the enamel ONLY
       - **Treatment:** file down sharp edges if present.
     - Enamel-dentin fracture (Ellis class II fracture): fracture through the enamel and dentin
       - **Treatment:** apply sealant with glass ionomer.
     - **Crown fracture with exposed pulp (Ellis class III fracture):** fracture through the enamel and dentin WITH exposure of the pulp
       - **Treatment:** preserve pulp vitality by applying a layer of calcium hydroxide. Tooth extraction is an alternative treatment option.
     - **Crown-root fracture:** fracture involving the enamel, dentin, and root structure. The pulp may or may not be exposed. Fragments of tooth may be loose but still attached.
       - **Treatment:** emergent pediatric dental referral for possible fragment removal or tooth extraction
     - **Root fracture:** fracture involving the enamel, dentin, and root structure. If coronal fragment is displaced, pulp may be exposed.

- **Treatment:** emergent pediatric dental referral. If coronal fragment is not displaced, repositioning with splinting can be considered. Otherwise, tooth may need to be extracted.
  - **Alveolar fracture:** involving the alveolar bone, usually associated with mobility and dislocation of multiple adjacent teeth with malocclusion
    - **Treatment:** emergent referral to a dentist or oral surgeon for reduction, stabilization, and splinting
- Other dentoalveolar trauma
  - **Avulsion:** complete displacement of a tooth from its socket
    - An avulsed primary tooth should NOT be reimplanted, to reduce the risk of further injury to the permanent tooth successor.
    - The apex of the root of the primary tooth lies in close proximity to the permanent tooth germ.
    - Common sequelae can include discoloration and hypoplasia of the permanent tooth.
    - In young children, consider radiographs of the chest/abdomen to rule out aspiration of an avulsed tooth if it cannot be found.
  - **Concussion:** tooth is tender to touch but not mobile, and there is no evidence of gingival bleeding.
    - **Treatment:** supportive care, soft diet, observation, routine dental follow-up
  - **Subluxation:** tooth is tender to touch with increased mobility and evidence of gingival bleeding but still within its socket without displacement; "loose tooth."
    - **Treatment:** gentle mouth care with a soft brush, soft diet, supportive care, observation, and routine dental follow-up
  - **Extrusive luxation:** tooth is partially displaced out of its socket, appears elongated, tender to touch, increased mobility, gingival bleeding.
    - **Treatment** (depending on degree of displacement):
      - **If <3 mm,** can be carefully repositioned or left to spontaneously align
      - **If >3 mm or concern for aspiration risk,** consider tooth extraction or emergent referral to a pediatric dentist.
  - **Intrusive luxation:** apex of the tooth is displaced into the socket either through the labial bone plate (apical tip can be visualized and the tooth appears shorter) or impinging on the developing tooth bud (apical tip cannot be visualized).
    - **Treatment:**
      - **If intruded through the labial bone plate,** tooth can be left for spontaneous repositioning.
      - **If apex is displaced into the developing tooth bud,** tooth should be extracted. Consider emergent referral to a pediatric dentist.
  - **Lateral luxation:** displacement of tooth in either palatal, lingual, or labial direction
    - **Treatment:** soft diet, observation, supportive care, and allow for spontaneous repositioning as long as there is no malocclusion present
    - Gentle repositioning is warranted if there is occlusal interference.
    - No evidence for prophylactic antibiotics in the treatment of luxation injuries

4. What is good anticipatory guidance following dental trauma?
   - Brush teeth with a soft-bristled toothbrush.
   - Use alcohol-free 0.1% chlorhexidine gluconate topically as an oral rinse or apply with a cotton swab twice daily for 1 week to prevent plaque and debris.
   - Soft diet for 10 days
   - Restrict use of pacifiers or sucking of digits/fingers.
   - Avoid flossing.
   - Avoid contact sports.
   - Pain management with acetaminophen and ibuprofen
   - Watch for signs of infection: fever, redness, swelling, and pain.

5. How are fractures in permanent teeth managed and treated?
   - **Enamel fractures:** if tooth fragment is available, it can be bonded to the tooth. Otherwise, the sharp edges of the tooth can be filed down for patient comfort.
   - **Enamel-dentin fractures:** cover exposed dentin with glass ionomer, composite resin, and calcium hydroxide paste.
   - Emergent pediatric dental referral within 72 hours should be considered for **enamel-dentin-pulp fractures, crown-root fractures, root fractures, and alveolar fractures.** This will be important in preserving pulp vitality, continued root development, preventing apical periodontitis, and a positive cosmetic outcome.

6. How are dentoalveolar injuries managed and treated in permanent teeth?
   - **Concussion:** no treatment necessary
   - **Subluxation:** no treatment necessary, although a flexible splint can be placed to stabilize the tooth for patient comfort
   - **Extrusive and lateral luxation:** gently reposition tooth back into its socket; stabilize the tooth with a flexible splint on facial side with 1–2 teeth in either direction of the affected tooth with available periodontal material.
   - **Intrusive luxation:** if only slightly intruded (<3 mm), can allow for eruption with close follow-up to monitor for movement in case orthodontic repositioning is required. If severely intruded (>7 mm), may require surgical repositioning. Emergent pediatric dental referral would be necessary.

- **Avulsion:** one of the most serious dental injuries to permanent teeth, as the prognosis is dependent on actions taken promptly after the injury takes place
  - Immediate reimplantation is the treatment of choice in most situations and may ultimately save the tooth.
  - Primary teeth should NOT be reimplanted; only permanent teeth.
  - Dry time of greater than 60 minutes results in irreversible damage to the periodontal ligament cells and decreases the likelihood of tooth viability.
  - Pick up the tooth by the crown.
  - Do NOT touch the root.
  - If the tooth is dirty, wash with saline briefly before reimplantation.
  - Do NOT scrub the tooth.
  - Gently reimplant the tooth into its socket.
  - Instruct the patient to bite down on a piece of dry gauze to hold it in position.
  - If reimplantation is not possible, store the tooth in a glass of milk or other storage medium (there are several commercially available balanced solutions, including pediatric electrolyte rehydrating solutions).
  - If the patient is conscious and can follow instructions, the tooth can be stored inside the patient's lip or cheeks using saliva as the storage medium.
  - Tap water should NOT be used.
  - A flexible splint is then placed to stabilize the reimplanted tooth.
  - Consider prophylactic antibiotics and tetanus:
    - Penicillin VK or amoxicillin for children under 12 years of age
    - Doxycycline for children older than 12 years of age
  - Chlorhexidine rinses and a soft diet recommended
  - Pediatric dental follow-up for possible root canal in 7–10 days

7. A 16-year-old male presents to urgent care after sustaining a dental injury while playing basketball. On examination, he is revealed to have a fracture of his left mandibular lateral incisor. It is tender to palpation but not mobile and without any bleeding. You notice that the fracture involves the enamel and the dentin without pulp exposure. What is the appropriate treatment for this patient?
   - This patient has an Ellis II classification dental fracture of a permanent tooth. This type of injury requires application of calcium hydroxide paste for patient comfort and to maintain pulp vitality as well as dental follow-up within 48 hours.
   - Application of calcium hydroxide paste:
     - Mix equal parts of calcium hydroxide base paste with catalyst paste on a padded surface until you achieve a uniform color.
     - Dry the tooth with cotton roll immediately before application.
     - Apply with applicator directly on surface of dentin or exposed pulp of tooth.
     - Apply a thin layer of calcium hydroxide paste (1 mm in thickness).
     - Calcium hydroxide paste will harden in 2–3 minutes.

8. A 14-year-old female presents to urgent care after sustaining a dental injury during soccer practice. On examination, she is found to have an extruded right maxillary lateral incisor. The tooth still appears to be in its socket, is relatively stable, and is elongated about 3 mm. It is tender to palpation and mobile with some gingival bleeding. What is the appropriate treatment for this patient?
   - This patient has a minor extrusion injury of a permanent tooth. This type of injury requires gentle repositioning of the tooth back into its socket followed by stabilization with a flexible splint and dental follow-up within 48 hours.
   - **Splinting:**
     - Adjust the length of the flexible splint so that it extends one tooth on either side of repositioned tooth.
     - Apply etchant and bonding solution on surface of teeth.
     - Place a dab of composite on the center of teeth to be bonded.
     - Position wire on the composite.
     - Allow composite to set.
     - Add additional composite to cover terminal ends of the wire.
     - Smooth the composite so there are no rough surfaces to irritate the soft tissue.

9. A 5-year-old female presents to urgent care after falling off a trampoline and sustaining multiple dental injuries. On examination, she is found to have significant extrusion of both her maxillary central incisors with gingival bleeding and tenderness to palpation. They are extremely mobile with the root visible. They are elongated about 5 mm. What is the appropriate treatment for this patient?
   - The patient has significant extrusion of two primary teeth that appear to be very unstable and can put her at risk for aspiration. In this case, extraction of both teeth is warranted with dental follow-up within 48 hours. Since the teeth are significantly extruded, take a dry gauze, grasp the crown, and pull.

- **Tooth extraction:**
  - Prepare patient with adequate local anesthesia.
  - Elevate the gingival soft tissue attachment.
  - Luxate the tooth with small and large straight elevators.
  - Apply forceps to the crown of the tooth.
  - Continue to luxate the tooth with forceps in a buccolingual direction with slight rotation until removed from socket.

10. A 15-year-old male presents to urgent care after being assaulted on his way home from school. He reports being punched in the face. On examination, he has multiple subluxed incisors, but his dentition is otherwise intact. He denies any malocclusion. He has multiple (<1 cm) superficial lacerations to his buccal mucosa as well as a 1-cm laceration of his tongue that does not involve the lateral border. Bleeding is well controlled. What is the appropriate treatment for this patient?
    - The patient has multiple subluxed permanent teeth that appear stable within their socket without malocclusion. No intervention is required, but placement of a flexible splint for patient comfort is an option.
      Buccal mucosal and gingival lacerations:
    - Minor lacerations in these areas heal very well without intervention.
    - Suture repair should be considered for gaping wounds (>2 cm) or if flaps of tissue are present. For the repair, use absorbable sutures such as 5-0 chromic gut.
    - The patient in this scenario does not need suture repair.
      Tongue lacerations:
    - Minor lacerations to the tongue also heal very well without intervention.
    - Suture repair should be considered for the following situations: gaping wounds (check with the tongue extended), large lacerations (>1.5 cm), active bleeding, flaps of tissue present, involvement of muscle and involvement of the border of the tongue (particularly the tip of the tongue).
    - Anesthetize with local infiltration without epinephrine.
    - Control the tongue by grasping with dry gauze or throwing a suture through the tip of the tongue and pulling on the suture.
    - Close with absorbable sutures such as chromic gut.

11. A 5-year-old male presents to urgent care after falling with a pencil in his mouth. He initially cried out in pain and spit out some blood. Since then, he has been calm and playful, is in no acute distress, and the bleeding has stopped. The parents brought the pencil with them. Your examination reveals a puncture wound just lateral to the right tonsillar pillar that is 1 cm in diameter but of unclear depth. There is no active bleeding and no other injuries. What is the appropriate management of this patient?
    - The patient has a puncture wound in an area that puts him at risk for injury to his carotid artery and/or jugular vein. He appears stable and is not actively bleeding, but he should still be referred to a pediatric emergency department for otolaryngology consultation and further imaging, which may include angiography, computed tomography angiogram (CTA), or magnetic resonance imaging arteriogram/venogram (MRA/MRV).
    - Signs of vascular injury include expanding hematoma of the neck or pharynx, continued bleeding, diminished pulses in the neck, and neurologic changes.
    - It is VERY important to rule out a retained foreign body within the puncture wound. In the case here, be sure to inspect the pencil to ensure that it is intact. Otherwise, surgical exploration of the wound may be necessary.
    - Plain radiographs may NOT be helpful to rule out foreign bodies such as pencils or sticks.
    - Children with minor puncture wounds to the central portion of the palate can be sent home with routine mouth care.

DENTAL INFECTIONS

12. Where do dental infections originate?
    Most dental infections occur secondary to cavities or after trauma. They may also be a consequence of periodontal (gum) infection, pericoronitis (inflammation of the soft tissue around a partially erupted tooth, usually the wisdom teeth), or a postoperative complication.

13. Who usually suffers from dental infections?
    Dental infections are most common in healthy people, though they are more severe in chronically ill or immunocompromised individuals.

14. During anatomy, I remember there being a lot of confusing anatomic parts around this area. How can I possibly approach a differential diagnosis?
    - It is helpful to divide the face into sectors.
    - The upper face is the orbits and surrounding structures; maxillary and ethmoid sinuses, ears and surrounding structures, upper buccal areas, and maxillary teeth.

- The lower face is the mandibular teeth; lower buccal area; and sublingual, submental, and submandibular regions.
- The neck is everything below the submandibular triangle and above the clavicle.
- First, look at the sector and then at the structures within the sector (e.g., soft tissue, muscle, salivary glands, lymph nodes, mucus, bone, skin, or teeth) to determine the origin of infection.

15. **A 21-year-old patient presents to urgent care complaining of excruciating tooth pain. He has been to his dentist repeatedly, and a dental exam and radiographs failed to reveal the cause of his pain. He even had a root canal. He is now on your examining table stating he refuses to leave without an answer. He notices the pain is aching and diffuse and worse when he chews. How will you approach the differential?**
    - Not all tooth pain is odontogenic. A careful history and physical can often differentiate nonodontogenic pain referred to the teeth. In this case, pressing on a trigger point on the cheek reproduced the pain, and he was discharged with a muscle relaxant and a referral to physical therapy.
    - Other diagnoses on the differential include neuropathic pain (e.g., trigeminal neuralgia, herpes, injury), idiopathic pain, neurovascular headache, sinus disease, atypical acute myocardial event, psychogenic pain (including drug-seeking behavior), and ubiquitous "others" such as malignancy, temporal arteritis, rheumatologic disease, and bone disease

16. **A 2-year-old with speech delay is brought to urgent care by her father just prior to closing because she refuses to sleep. With her speech delay, she cannot tell him the source of her discomfort. Not wanting to miss closing time, he has not given her any pain medicine. She is afebrile but did not eat dinner. She is, however, sucking on her bottle with vigor. You are convinced she is going to have an ear infection and are disappointed to note her ears are normal. What is another potential and common source for her pain and what are the clues in the history?**
    - Overlooking the fact that this is a chapter on dental complaints, dental caries is a common source of infection and pain in children.
    - Caries is caused by a continuous process of bacteria and nutrients interacting and creating fluctuations in pH on the surface of the teeth. These fluctuations result in changes in the surface mineralization of the tooth. If the net mineralization change is a loss, then caries eventually forms.
    - Clues to a dental source of pain for this child are refusing to eat (pain with mastication); pain when lying down (referred pain to the ears); and still drinking from a baby bottle and using it at night (baby bottle caries). If you take a close look at what is in the bottle, it is likely to be milk, juice, or soda.
    - For tonight, you can offer pain control with acetaminophen or ibuprofen, give recommendations for oral hygiene, ensure there is not an evolving dental abscess, facial cellulitis, or airway involvement, and provide a referral for dental care

17. **An adolescent female presents complaining of tooth pain. She has a dentist, but it is Saturday, and she does not want to wait to be seen on Monday. When you look in her mouth, you notice diffuse gingivitis and an area of purulence above her canine. She has no facial swelling, erythema, or fever and can tolerate oral intake. How should this patient be treated? Does she need to be transferred from urgent care to an emergency department?**
    - As this patient does not have any systemic symptoms or evidence of facial cellulitis at this time, she can be treated in urgent care as long as the family will ensure follow-up with her primary physician or, preferably, her dentist.
    - The noted abscess should be incised and drained.
    - Anesthesia can be achieved using a nerve block (to be reviewed in a later section) or a topical or locally injected anesthetic if the abscess is localized and circumscribed.
    - The patient should be discharged on antibiotics and antibacterial mouthwash. She does not need to be transferred to an emergency department for further evaluation.

18. **What antibiotics should the patient from question 17 be prescribed?**
    - Dental infections are usually polymicrobial and a mix of aerobic and anaerobic bacteria.
    - The aerobic bacteria are overwhelmingly some variety of *Streptococcus*.
    - The anaerobic pathogens are multiple and varied.
    - First-choice antibiotics for uncomplicated dental infections are penicillin, cephalosporin, tetracycline, or clindamycin after taking into consideration age, allergies, and previous drug history.
    - She can also be discharged with a mouthwash such as chlorhexidine swish and spit.
    - The most common bacteria in oral cavity are:
        - When a baby is born, the bacteria in the mouth are mostly aerobic.
        - The teeth provide a surface for anaerobes to proliferate.
        - As dental hygiene diminishes and cavities increase, acidic bacteria increase.
        - There are gram-positive cocci, most importantly streptococci, peptostreptococci, and staphylococci.

- There are gram-negative cocci that are less recognized: *Veillonella, Neisseria,* and *Branhamella.*
- There are gram-positive rods collectively known as diphtheroids and branched filaments known as the *Actinomyces* species.
- There are anaerobes: *Bacteroides, Capnocytophaga, Eikenella, Fusobacterium.*
- An organism specific to juvenile periodontitis is *Aggregatibacter actinomycetemcomitans.*
- Finally, there are a variety of spirochetes, fungi, yeast, viruses, and protozoa.
- These organisms usually live in harmony, but when the oral environment gets out of balance, any one or several of them adhere to the mucous membranes, overcome host defenses, and create an infection.

19. Should the patient from question 17 have radiographs done at this visit?
   For uncomplicated dental caries or an abscess without deep tissue spread, radiographs are not needed.

20. The adolescent from question 17 returns Sunday night complaining of eye pain and a fever of 101°F. Her cheek is swollen and warm. She did not fill the prescription for the penicillin you gave her, as she had a school event last night and slept in this morning. What do you do now?
   - She should be transferred to an emergency department for further evaluation, imaging, and admission.
   - Risks of dental infections that spread along facial and fascial planes include facial cellulitis, periorbital cellulitis, orbital cellulitis, airway compromise, mediastinitis, intracranial infections, and death.

21. Should you do any imaging of the patient from question 17 at urgent care prior to transfer?
   - There is a role for imaging in dental infections, though not in this case, as the eye pain and rapid progression of fever suggest urgent transfer and initiation of therapy will benefit the patient most.
   - Computed tomography (CT) and magnetic resonance imaging (MRI) are considered the gold standard for soft tissue imaging for facial cellulitis or abscess.
   - Plain x-ray films are effective in diagnosing dental caries and local trauma that may be a source of infection but are relatively ineffective for diagnosing infection or inflammation in soft tissue.
   - Dental experts rely on a panoramic x-ray, which also is good at delineating bony abnormalities but is not effective at diagnosing soft tissue infection.
   - CT and MRI machines are prohibitive in urgent care centers; however, ultrasound is increasingly being used to effectively diagnose soft tissue infections of odontogenic origin.

22. Fortunately, when you call for follow-up of the patient from question 17, the doctor on the night shift tells you a CT in the emergency department showed periorbital cellulitis but no orbital cellulitis. You ask, "What is the protocol for treatment of such patients?"
   - These patients are admitted for intravenous antibiotics (either a penicillin derivative or clindamycin, depending on previous therapy and medical history).
   - Dental or oromaxillofacial surgery is consulted as an inpatient.
   - The infected tooth (or teeth) is extracted.

23. Are the characteristics of bacterial odontogenic infections changing significantly?
   - A study compared patients hospitalized with odontogenic infections in the 1980s and the 1990s.
   - Patient characteristics did not change.
   - Bacteria isolated in the 1990s were more likely to show emerging resistance to commonly used antibiotics.
   - When possible, responsible antibiotic stewardship and narrow spectrum use are recommended to prevent further resistance.

24. An adolescent male presents with fever, trismus, and a firm, tender neck swelling originating in the submandibular space. When you are finally able to coax him to open his mouth, you notice his tongue is elevated and resting on a firm, tender, sublingual mass. What is your concern?
   - This description should immediately raise concern for Ludwig angina, a potential airway emergency.
   - Ludwig angina is an infection of the submandibular, submental, and sublingual spaces.
   - It was first fully described by Wilhelm Friedrich von Ludwig in 1836 and recognized as frequently fatal.
   - The term "angina" was added because it gave a feeling of suffocation.
   - Dental infection is usually the cause.
   - Preventive care and antibiotics have reduced mortality significantly.

25. What should you do?
   - First, ensure the patient's airway is intact and arrange for critical care transport if available; use ALS if critical care is not available.
   - If the airway is not intact, the patient must be intubated. This should be considered a difficult airway, and consider using video laryngoscopy, airway adjuncts, and avoiding sedatives and muscle relaxants. Due to the massive neck edema and distortion of the anatomy in Ludwig angina, even airway experts are often unsuccessful. While tracheostomy was once considered standard, with the advancements in available airway technology this is no longer the case.

- If the child is stable, establish intravenous access and start broad-spectrum antibiotics, as the infection is polymicrobial.
- The adolescent male in question 25 is successfully transferred to a tertiary care hospital, where he is intubated by an otolaryngologist in the operating suite. The infection was surgically drained, he received intravenous antibiotics for several weeks, and he had extensive dental extractions done.

26. A 10-year-old girl presents to urgent care with a fever of 104°F. She recently had dental work done and has been complaining of continued tooth pain for the last 5 days. Her mother treated her fever with acetaminophen and ibuprofen, but over the last 6 hours she noted her daughter had developed vomiting, rigors, and pallor and was increasingly difficult to arouse. On your exam, her heart rate is 140 beats per minute, her blood pressure is 75 systolic over 30 diastolic, and she is ill-appearing and very sleepy. The only time she seems to wake up and respond is when you palpate the left side of her neck, when she cries, and when you percuss her left lower molars. What are you thinking?
    - You most likely wish you had drawn a different schedule for the month!
    - Since that did not happen, your mind reaches into its far recesses, and you recall reading a case study about Lemierre syndrome. However, as you recall, Lemierre syndrome is usually the consequence of pharyngitis and not dental infection.
    - After stabilizing the patient by treating her sepsis with aggressive fluid resuscitation, broad-spectrum antibiotics, respiratory support, and transfer to a pediatric center with a critical care unit, you take a moment to read about Lemierre syndrome.
    - Dental infections account for only about 2% of cases, but it is a virulent complication.
    - An oropharyngeal infection causes septic thrombophlebitis of the internal jugular vein and, ultimately, hematogenous spread of the infection via septic emboli, resulting in multisystem abscesses and organ failure.
    - Common presenting symptoms are fever, chills, rigors, and sore throat that progress to trouble swallowing and trismus due to deep neck space infection. Ultimately, symptoms of distal infection develop, such as chest pain, tachypnea, and tachycardia. Finally, if unrecognized, the patient will develop severe sepsis and die. Mortality has diminished significantly since the advent of penicillin. Death is often due to mediastinitis.
    - Patients may also develop intracranial infections from the septic emboli.
    - In urgent care, while awaiting transfer of this patient, ultrasound may detect jugular thrombosis. However, ultrasound lacks the diagnostic certainty of contrast CT or MRI and should not be used as the sole diagnostic modality. Further, the attempt to image the internal jugular in urgent care should not delay aggressive resuscitation or transfer of the patient.
    - Treatment ultimately consists of sepsis management, antibiotics, controlling the airway, and surgical debridement.

27. What are other common complications of pediatric dental infections?
    - The jaw bone structure makes children more prone to osteomyelitis and subsequent facial deformity.
    - The permanent teeth can be damaged.
    - Tetracyclines commonly used in dental infections can cause tooth discoloration and hypoplasia in the developing teeth of both small children and fetuses.
    - Abscesses are more likely to create a fistula to the skin that necessitates repeated surgery and results in permanent deformity.

28. A 13-year-old girl presented to urgent care complaining of tooth pain. She has multiple caries but no evidence of abscess, facial cellulitis, or systemic symptoms. The family does not feel that ibuprofen is providing adequate pain control, and you are uncomfortable prescribing narcotics for this family who presents frequently with various complaints of pain. You decide to offer a dental nerve block instead. What are the various approaches?
    - Infraorbital nerve block
        - Anesthetizes the anterior and middle superior alveolar nerves by the infraorbital foramen denervating the anterior maxillary teeth
        - The patient should be partially or fully reclined.
        - The infraorbital foramen is in line with the pupil when the patient is looking forward. Palpate the supraorbital and infraorbital notches. About 0.5 cm below the infraorbital notch, there is a depression. Retracting the upper lip, insert the needle with the syringe of local anesthetic anterior to the first premolar and direct the tip toward the depression without entering the foramen to avoid nerve damage.
        - Potential complications include excessive advancement into the orbit, improper angle of insertion, prevention of adequate anesthesia, and nerve damage as a result of direct damage from needle puncture.
    - Inferior alveolar nerve block
        - Anesthetizes all the mandibular teeth, the skin of the chin and the lower lip, and usually the tongue on the side of the block
        - The block is placed in the mandibular sulcus.

- To inject, picture the inside of the mandible as a rectangle. Draw a horizontal line through the rectangle marked by the occlusal plane of the teeth and a vertical line marked by the midpoint of the rectangle. Where these intersect is the point of injection.
- Grasp the ramus of the mandible with the thumb inside the mouth and the finger behind the ramus of the mandible, approach the nerve from the opposite side of the mouth over the primary molars, and inject.
- Potential complications include nerve damage and excessive pain.

KEY POINTS

1. If immediate reimplantation of an avulsed permanent tooth is not possible, it should be stored in a suitable culture media such as cold milk.
2. Most lacerations of the buccal mucosa, gingiva, and tongue heal well without intervention.
3. Penicillin, clindamycin, and tetracyclines provide appropriate antimicrobial activity against the most common oropharyngeal bacteria.
4. If a dental infection is localized and there are no systemic symptoms of disease, the patient can be treated with oral antibiotics, antimicrobial mouthwash, and pain control. If there are systemic symptoms of disease, the patient should be stabilized and transferred to a medical center with the ability to admit the patient and manage potential airway and cardiovascular compromise.
5. Dental pain can be managed with oral pain medications or with a dental block that targets nerve groups that include the affected tooth.

Acknowledgments

Dr. Cindy Chang and Dr. Selena Hariharan would like to thank the late Dr. Steven Chan for his contribution to this chapter.

BIBLIOGRAPHY

Andersson L, Andreasen JO, Day P, et al. International Association of Dental Traumatology guidelines for the management of traumatic dental injuries: 2. Avulsion of permanent teeth. *Dent Traumatol.* 2012;28(2):88–96.

Bassiony M, Yang J, Abdel-Monem TM, Elmogy S, Elnagdy M. Exploration of ultrasonography in assessment of fascial space spread of odontogenic infections. *Oral Surg Oral Med Oral Pathol Oral Radiol Endod.* 2009;107:861–869.

Diangelis AJ, Andreasen JO, Ebeleseder KA, et al. International Association of Dental Luxations Traumatology guidelines for the management of traumatic dental injuries: 1. Fractures and of permanent teeth. *Dent Traumatol.* 2012;28(1):2–12.

Heimdahl A, Nord CE. Treatment of orofacial infections of odontogenic origin. *Scand J Infect Dis Suppl.* 1985;46:101–105.

Kassutto Z, Helpin ML. Orofacial anesthesia techniques. In: Henretig FM, King C, eds. *Textbook of Pediatric Emergency Procedures.* Baltimore: Williams & Wilkins; 1997:713–723.

Pedigo RA. Dental emergencies: management strategies that improve outcomes. *Emerg Med Pract.* 2017 Jun;19(6):1–24. Epub 2017 Jun 1.

Malmgren B, Andreasen JO, Flores MT, et al. International Association of Dental Traumatology guidelines for the management of traumatic dental injuries: 3. Injuries in the primary dentition. *Dent Traumatol.* 2012;28(3):174–182.

Noy D, Rachmiel A, Levy-Faber D, Emodi O. Lemierre's syndrome from odontogenic infection: review of the literature and case description. *Ann Maxillofac Surg.* 2015;5:219–225.

Thikkurissy S, Rawlins JT, Kumar A, Evans E, Casamassimo PS. Rapid treatment reduces hospitalizations for pediatric patients with odontogenic-based cellulitis. *Am J Emerg Med.* 2010;28:668–672.

Topazian RG, Goldberg RH. *Odontogenic Infections and Deep Fascial Space Infections of Dental Origin.* 2nd ed. WB Saunders; 1987.

Yatani H, Komiyama O, Matsuka Y, Wajima K, Muraoka W, Ikawa M, Heir GM. Systematic review and recommendations for nonodontogenic toothache. *J Oral Rehabil.* 2014;41:843–852.

CHAPTER 57

ANALGESIA AND SEDATION

R. Blake Windsor, MD

CASE 1

A 10-year-old boy with a history of sickle cell disease presents to urgent care for pain in his right lower leg. He describes the pain as severe (Numeric Rating Scale [NRS] 9/10), "sharp and throbbing," and his parent reports that this is similar to his typical vaso-occlusive episodes. He has not had fevers, dyspnea, cough, limp, or joint swelling. His labs reveal anemia and reticulocytosis. He is intermittently crying, guarding his right leg, and limps during attempts to ambulate.

1. **What is pain?**
   Pain is a complex sensory and emotional experience. It is unpleasant by definition and inherently subjective. *Nociception* is the neural sensation of tissue damage and is associated with activation of the sympathetic nervous system. Clinicians often assess a patient's *pain* and assume that the intensity of pain is proportionate to the degree of tissue injury. This is not the case. Understanding that the severity of tissue injury, and thus the degree of *nociception* (sensation of injury), is not the same as the intensity of *pain* felt is key to understanding more complex and chronic pain conditions. In response to tissue injury and nociception, people exhibit physiologic protective behaviors including sympathetic activation and classically described behaviors (such as lying completely still with peritonitis or writhing with visceral pains).

   In contrast, *pain* is a more complex experience that includes the sensation (*nociception*) as well as higher-level cortical activity involving attention, associations cortices, fear, and emotional centers. To put it another way, the intensity of pain felt is a better indicator of the brain's need to *protect* the body than it is the degree of *injury* a patient experiences and is often affected by the biopsychosocial context including past experiences, fears, and the meaning of the pain.

   The typical goal of the urgent care environment is to assess *nociception* to aid diagnosis and treatment. The astute urgent care clinician will take a history of the presenting illness, characterize the nature of a painful complaint including the intensity that is reported using a validated scale as well as other qualities of the pain experience, interpret vital signs to look for signs of sympathetic activation, and, as part of their physical exam, make observations about the behaviors demonstrated to infer the degree of tissue injury (or nociception).

2. **What are various age-appropriate ways to measure pain?**
   Many validated scales exist to measure nociception or pain behaviors.
   - FLACC: a commonly used pain scale for infants, children, and people with cognitive impairment who have trouble communicating. FLACC is an abbreviation and mnemonic for **F**aces, **L**egs, **A**ctivity, **C**ry, and **C**onsolability. Each section is scored 0–2 for a possible total of 10 points. This scale observes automatic protective behaviors in patients who are unable to describe their experience and is extrapolated to a 10-point scale.
   - Wong-Baker FACES scale: an instrument validated for children as young as 3 years, as well as children and adults with cognitive delay. Six faces (scores of 0–5) of progressive discomfort are displayed, and patients pick the face that corresponds to their pain. To extrapolate the scale, the score is doubled to create a 10-point scale.
   - Numeric Rating Scale (NRS): the most commonly used self-report scale; patients pick a number on a scale from 0 ("no pain") to 10 ("the worst pain imaginable"). This is validated in children as young as 5 years who have a concept of numbers (i.e., "5 is larger than 1"), but should be understood in a developmental context for both children and adults.

3. **What is the difference between acute and chronic pain?**
   Pain can be divided into acute pain and chronic pain. Acute pain is defined by self-limited pain of <3 months' duration that is closely related to tissue injury. Chronic pain is defined as pain lasting longer than 3 months, or longer than expected for the degree of injury. The approaches to acute and chronic pain differ, and an in-depth approach to treating chronic pain is beyond the scope of this chapter. Acute pain related to an injury in a patient with chronic pain can be one of the more challenging and nuanced aspects of urgent care.

4. **How can classifying pain help guide treatment?**
   Pain descriptors and patterns can help discern the underlying injury. There are many taxonomies of pain; however, they are broadly classified as *nociceptive, neuropathic,* and *nociplastic.* Nociceptive pain is pain associated with tissue injury (e.g., surgery or fracture), inflammation (e.g., rheumatoid arthritis), or tumor. Neuropathic pain is classified to highlight altered nervous system activity due to a known or suspected injury to the peripheral or central nervous system (e.g., amputation, diabetic neuropathy, spinal cord injury). *Nociplastic* pain is the term to describe pain arising from functional changes to the nervous system that can lead to pain despite no clear tissue injury.

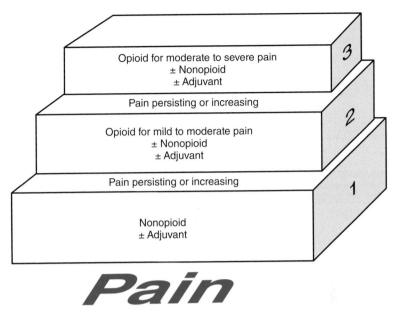

Fig. 57.1 World Health Organization (WHO) pain relief ladder for adults. A useful strategy is to continue weak analgesics when stepping up to stronger medications. Weak analgesics can be scheduled to reduce the need and total dose of opioids.

These pains are not exclusive, and patients, as a common example, can have both nociceptive and nociplastic types of pain. For instance, a patient with irritable bowel syndrome (IBS) may also have appendicitis, and the nociplastic changes of IBS may make the pain felt from appendicitis to be a more intense and unpleasant experience.

In general, antiinflammatories and tissue-based treatments are typically effective for nociceptive pain, antineuropathic agents are fairly effective for neuropathic pain, and opioids are *not* very effective for nociplastic pain at typical doses.

5. **What is the general approach to acute pain?**
   Acute pain is best treated with medications that target the underlying cause of pain. Effective treatments include nonsteroidal antiinflammatory drugs (NSAIDs), acetaminophen, local anesthetics, general anesthetics, muscle relaxants, and opioids. The World Health Organization (WHO) pain ladder (Fig. 57.1) is an effective framework for treating acute and cancer-related pain. For pain with a predictable trajectory, scheduled dosing of nonopioid medications is preferred. These strategies can help prevent opioid use or reduce total opioid doses if they are required. This concept is called *opioid-sparing strategies*.

6. **How do NSAIDs work?**
   NSAIDs inhibit the enzyme cyclooxygenase (COX), which produces prostaglandins that contribute to inflammation. This causes pain by sensitizing nerve terminals to injury. Thus, NSAIDs are useful for decreasing inflammation and are generally considered weak analgesics. COX-1 and COX-2 are differentially produced. Most tissues constitutively produce COX-1, and COX-2 is induced by inflammation.

   It is increasingly recognized that the inflammatory response is important for tissue healing after injury. Overriding an appropriate and innate healing mechanism by the use of antiinflammatories has demonstrated consequences in preclinical models. Routine use of antiinflammatories to treat symptoms of injury and inflammation is increasingly discouraged unless those symptoms are bothersome and insufficiently managed with nonpharmacologic strategies.

7. **What are the differences between NSAIDs?**
   NSAIDs are more similar than they are different. Nonselective NSAIDs have similar predictable side effect profiles based on their COX-2/COX-1 inhibition. Also, NSAIDs differ in their duration of action. COX-2 inhibitors ("Coxibs") were designed to minimize the long-term side effect profile of this medication class but unfortunately were associated with a possible increase in the risk of myocardial infarction and thrombotic strokes with prolonged use. The only COX-2 inhibitor currently approved for use in the United States is celecoxib.

8. **What are the principal adverse effects of long-term NSAID therapy?**
   The frequency of side effects is often associated with COX-2/COX-1 inhibition (Table 57.1):
   - Gastrointestinal (GI) effects: gastritis, peptic ulcer disease (Table 57.2), diarrhea, GI hemorrhage

Table 57.1 Select COX-2/COX-1 Ratios (Higher Value Indicates Higher Proportion of COX-2 Inhibition)

Celecoxib	30
Meloxicam	18
Ibuprofen	1.5
Naproxen	0.7
Indomethacin	0.02

Table 57.2 Cumulative Prevalence of GI Ulcers after 12 Weeks of NSAID Therapy Without GI Protection

Celecoxib (200 mg bid)	8.5%
Naproxen (500 mg bid)	40.7%
Ibuprofen (800 mg tid)	28.5%

bid, Twice a day; *GI,* gastrointestinal; *NSAID,* nonsteroidal antiinflammatory drug; *tid,* three times a day.

- Renal effects: decreased renal blood flow, decreased glomerular filtration rate (GFR), salt and water retention, acute papillary necrosis, chronic interstitial nephritis, hypertension
- Hematologic effects: inhibition of platelet aggregation, increased bleeding time
- Pulmonary effects: bronchospasm
- Hepatic effects: elevated aspartate aminotransferase/alanine aminotransferase (AST/ALT), drug-induced hepatitis
- Idiopathic reactions: vasomotor rhinitis, angioedema, hypotension, drug-induced rash

9. **Which is the best NSAID to use?**
   - No NSAID is clearly better than another, although subtle differences may make one more preferable for a specific reason. Table 57.3 lists typical doses and useful notes about select NSAIDs. Factors that influence choice include route of administration, desired dosing interval, COX selectivity, and special considerations.
   - Intravenous (IV) ketorolac is potent, and therapeutic doses are often described as producing analgesia equivalent to typical doses (10 mg or 0.1 mg/kg) of IV morphine. This is accompanied by a higher-than-typical adverse effect profile, and use should not exceed 5 days.

10. **How is acetaminophen different from typical NSAIDs?**
    Acetaminophen has an unclear mechanism of action and a different elimination and side effect profile from NSAIDs. However, it also contains both analgesic and antipyretic activity. It can be safely used in combination with all NSAIDs.

11. **What side effects are associated with acetaminophen?**
    Acetaminophen is not associated with the GI or renal effects of NSAIDs. The most concerning side effect is hepatotoxicity. Acetaminophen-induced hepatotoxicity can be life-threatening. It is influenced by dose, duration of use, and comorbid conditions such as hepatic disease or malnutrition.

12. **What are the safe dose ranges for acetaminophen?**
    Acetaminophen is safe and effective at doses of 650–1000 mg every 4–6 hours in adults and 10–15 mg/kg for infants and children. Rectally administered acetaminophen should be dosed as 15 mg/kg due to reductions in bioavailability. The maximum recommended daily dose is 4 g/day for adults and 75 mg/kg/day for infants and children with attempts to keep doses to no more than 3 g/day in adults and 60 mg/kg for infants and children.

13. **What are toxic doses of acetaminophen?**
    Toxicity depends on multiple factors, including dose, duration of use, and comorbid conditions. Single-dose toxicity is unlikely at doses below 7.5–10 g for adults or 150 mg/kg for infants and children. Chronic administration can produce toxicity at any dose at or above the maximum recommended daily dose.

14. **What diseases influence acetaminophen toxicity?**
    Comorbid conditions that decrease hepatic glucuronidation (i.e., liver disease, malnutrition, or alcoholism) and states of induced cytochrome P-450 (i.e., alcoholism, medications) lead to increased production of NAPQI. NAPQI is a toxic metabolite that can lead to oxidative hepatic injury. In these states, the daily acetaminophen dose should be reduced or avoided entirely.

Table 57.3 Suggested Dosing and Useful Notes for Common NSAIDs

DRUG	DOSE (MG/KG)	DURATION	ROUTES	NOTES
Ibuprofen	400–800 mg (4–10 mg/kg)	4–8 h	IV, PO	PO form is inexpensive and available OTC May have ceiling effect at 600 mg in adults For use >6 months old
Naproxen	250–500 mg (5 mg/kg)	8–12 h	PO	Inexpensive often started with a loading dose in adults
Diclofenac	50 mg (1 mg/kg)	8 h	PO, TOP	Inexpensive; often used with a loading dose in adults Topical gel available
Ketorolac	15–30 mg IV, 60 mg IM once (0.5 mg/kg IV or 0.1 mg IM once)	8 h	IV, IM, PO	Potent analgesic; use for <5 days PO generally used only for IV continuation May have ceiling effect at 15 mg IV (0.25 mg/kg IV) Consider 50% dose reduction in critical illness For use >8 months and 8 kg
Indomethacin	25–75 mg (0.5–1 mg/kg)	6–12 h	PO	Max dose of 200 mg/day for adults, 4 mg/kg for children Use in children is limited; alternative use is preferred
Meloxicam	5–10 mg (0.125 mg/kg)	24 h	PO	Capsules and tablets are not interchangeable, even if dose is equal
Celecoxib	100–200 mg 10–25 kg: 50 mg 25–50 kg: 100 mg	12–24 h	PO	Best GI profile and use with platelet disorders May increase risk of thrombosis and myocardial infarction

IM, Intramuscularly; *IN*, intranasally; *IV*, intravenously; *NSAIDs*, nonsteroidal antiinflammatory drugs; *OTC*, over the counter; *PO*, orally; *TOP*, topical.

15. When are opioids indicated?

Opioids, a useful and versatile class of medications, are broadly indicated for surgical conditions, trauma, procedural sedation, cancer-related pain, and severe pain. In general, opioids are indicated for *nociception* refractory to nonopioid management including severe injuries that may impact important physiologic functions (e.g., rib fractures) but generally are not indicated for *pain* in the absence of known or suspected injury. Unfortunately, opioid prescriptions have increased due to multiple factors and have resulted in an epidemic of substance abuse disorders and deaths.

16. What general guidelines should be followed when prescribing opioids?

Opioids are best prescribed when there is a clear endpoint to their use, and routine use should be limited to 3–5 days with a single point of contact (such as urgent care). Increasingly, state law may set limits on opioid prescriptions and knowledge of these local regulations is critical.

Opioids are not first-line therapy for chronically painful conditions except in palliative care or atypical conditions. Multimodal therapies should be used whenever possible to limit opioid doses to the minimal effective dose.

17. What are opioid-sparing strategies?

Strategies include maximizing multimodal therapy, such as scheduling use of acetaminophen, NSAIDs, topical therapies, and disease-specific therapies (i.e., muscle relaxants for muscle spasms or anticonvulsants for neuropathic pain). If needed for longer-term therapy, opioids are best prescribed by clinicians with continuity of care and advanced training in evidence-based practice and opioid monitoring.

18. What does PRN mean?

PRN is a Latin abbreviation that stands for *pro re nata* (loosely translated "as the circumstances arise"). In practice, it often means "Pain Received Nothing." Telling patients to take an over-the-counter analgesic "as needed" often results in a medication not being taken. A useful strategy is to tell patients to take a weak analgesic on a schedule for a few days and to use an opioid "as needed." This strategy can reduce opioid use.

19. **How do opioids work?**
Major opioids bind to opioid receptors, primarily mu-, kappa-, and delta-receptors. These are located both centrally (spine and brain) as well as peripherally and are responsible for the analgesic, euphoric, and adverse effects of opioid medications.

20. **What are the differences between opioids?**
Major opioids are agonists of their receptors. Newer opioids have been developed that are partial agonists, mixed agonists/antagonists, and antagonists. Combination agonist and antagonist products are also available in an attempt to limit substance abuse. Mu agonists should be used if analgesia is the primary goal (i.e., procedural sedation or surgical process). Partial agonists/antagonists typically provide less analgesia and should be used for patients with moderate pain that does not respond to conservative therapy, for patients with relative contraindications to opioid use (including substance abuse history), or in an attempt to limit typical opioid adverse effects. Most partial agonists/antagonists have limited use in children and generally should be avoided.

Of important note, the Federal Drug Administration labels products containing codeine and tramadol as *absolutely contraindicated* in patients under age 12, as well as patients under age 18 who are obese, have obstructive sleep apnea, respiratory disease, or after tonsillectomies, and nursing mothers. These are listed as *relatively contraindicated* in all other patients under 18.

21. **What are some of the expected effects of opioids?**
   - CNS: analgesia, mood changes (positive or negative), sedation
   - Eyes: miosis
   - Respiratory: respiratory depression, hypercapnia
   - Cardiac: hypotension, bradycardia (high doses)
   - GI: nausea, vomiting, delayed gastric emptying, constipation
   - Skin: pruritus
   - Urinary: urinary retention

22. **Is any major opioid better?**
No particular opioid is inherently superior or stronger than another. Medications vary in potency, but when dosed appropriately (Table 57.4), they typically provide equal analgesia. Patients with frequent opioid exposures often express preferences, most often due to adverse effect profiles. This is thought to be due to complex interactions between an individual's opioid receptor subtypes and the opioid's selectivity for those subtypes. Additionally, certain opioids have clear advantages in select situations.

23. **What is opioid tolerance?**
Chronic administration of opioids can lead to tolerance. Tolerance is defined as the need for an increased dose of medication to achieve the same effect. Tolerance develops to all effects of opioids except constipation. Patients may or may not have miosis if taking their usual dose of opioids.

24. **How is tolerance different than dependence?**
Tolerance is a prerequisite for dependence. Tolerance demonstrates neurologic changes that reduce the inhibitory effects of the opioid dose. Dependence is the state where abrupt discontinuation leads to rebound neurologic excitation and development of a withdrawal syndrome. Opioid dependence does not indicate addiction or substance abuse.

25. **How are opioids dosed when someone is opioid tolerant?**
Knowing the patient's history of opioid exposure is helpful. If that information is unavailable, one option is to start at the upper range of usual dosing and reassess every 5–10 minutes (for IV morphine and hydromorphone) until captured. When patients demonstrate tolerance to the analgesic effects of opioids, they are typically also tolerant to respiratory depression.

26. **Why do opioids cause respiratory depression?**
Opioids act directly on the brainstem to affect respiration. The respiratory rhythm is the most sensitive and leads to an initial hypopnea with increased tidal volume. With higher doses, the tidal volume also decreases and leads to apnea. Opioids also shift the sensitivity of the medullary chemoreceptors to CO_2 and lead to hypercapnia. Natural sleep and coadministration of medications, such as benzodiazepines and other sedatives, can potentiate respiratory depression. Pain and stimulation can reduce respiratory depression.

27. **How is iatrogenic opioid-induced respiratory depression treated?**
Treatment depends on context. With oversedation and hypopnea in an otherwise stable patient, stimulating the patient is the first treatment. Low-dose naloxone can be titrated to increase respiratory rate without affecting analgesia. An ampule of 0.4 mg of naloxone is diluted with 10 mL of saline, and 0.04–0.08 mg (1–2 mL) is given every 1–2 minutes to the desired effect. To achieve the same effect in children, 0.01 mg/kg of naloxone can be given every 2 minutes to the desired effect. Naloxone typically lasts 20–40 minutes, and respiratory depression may return as the naloxone is eliminated. Close monitoring is required.

28. **How is opioid-induced constipation treated?**
Opioids act on intestinal smooth muscle to decrease peristalsis. Because of this, stool softeners are not an appropriate monotherapy to prevent constipation. Promotility agents, such as senna, bisacodyl, and lactulose, are

Table 57.4 Suggested Dosing and Useful Notes for Common Opioids

SELECT MEDICATIONS	Usual Starting Doses and Intervals for Analgesia in Opioid-Naïve Patients		NOTES
	CHILDREN <50 KG	CHILDREN >50 KG AND ADULTS	
Morphine	IV: 0.05–0.1 mg/kg every 2–4 h PO: 0.3 mg/kg every 4 h	IV: 2.5–5 mg every 2–4 h PO: 10–30 mg every 4 h	Traditional initial choice for opioids. Contraindicated in renal failure due to accumulation of toxic metabolite.
Hydromorphone	IV: 0.01–0.02 mg/kg every 2–4 h PO: 0.04–0.08 mg/kg every 4 h	IV: 0.2–1 mg every 2–4 h PO: 2–4 mg every 4 h	More rapid onset of CNS effects (analgesia, sedation) compared to morphine. Evidence of better adverse effect profile is mixed. Safer for use in renal failure.
Fentanyl	IV: 0.5–2 mcg/kg every 30–60 min 2 mcg/kg as initial load	IV: 25–50 mcg every 30–60 min 100 mcg as initial load	Considered hemodynamically neutral. Rapid onset of 2–3 minutes. Can be dosed intranasally for rapid analgesic load prior to IV access. For children, dose volume should not exceed 1 mL per nostril. Transbuccal, sublingual, and trans-dermal forms also available.
Oxycodone	PO: 0.1–0.2 mg/kg every 3–4 h	PO: 5–10 mg every 3–4 h	Good choice for opioid rotation. Possibly enhanced effect on visceral pain due to increased kappa agonism.

CNS, Central nervous system; *IN,* intranasally; *IR,* immediate release; *IV,* intravenously; *PO,* orally.

the mainstay of treatment because they improve peristalsis. Softeners, such as polyethylene glycol, docusate, or magnesium hydroxide, can be added.

CASE 2

An 8-year-old girl presents to urgent care for wrist pain and deformity after a fall during soccer practice. X-ray reveals a greenstick fracture with 30-degree angulation. Orthopedics is consulted and recommends closed reduction and immobilization.

29. **What is the general approach to procedural sedation?**
    Most importantly, sedation should be performed only by a clinician experienced in airway management. A safe sedation requires a clinician capable of intervening as necessary and dedicated to monitoring the patient's safety, pain, and anxiety. Reversal medications, oxygen, and airway equipment should be immediately available.

30. **What equipment is needed for procedural sedation?**
    A helpful mnemonic for setting up a room for sedation is "SOAP-ME."

    S: Suction
    O: Oxygen source (including face mask, nonrebreather)
    A: Airway equipment (including bag-mask and endotracheal tube)
    P: Pharmacy (sedation medications, reversal agents, code medications)
    M: Monitors (cardiac monitor, oximetry, capnography)
    E: Equipment for procedure (fluoroscopy, peripherally inserted central catheter [PICC])

31. **What are the special considerations for pediatric sedation?**
    Pediatric sedation requires appropriately sized equipment. This is especially true of airway equipment, particularly mask size, and multiple endotracheal tube or laryngeal mask airway sizes. Children receive weight-based dosing of medications. Comorbid conditions, such as craniofacial abnormalities, genetic syndromes, and viral infections, are relatively common in children who require sedation and need special consideration.

32. **What are the red flags for procedural sedation?**
    - Craniofacial abnormality or high-risk airway on examination
    - History of difficult sedation or airway

Table 57.5 Suggested Dosing and Useful Notes for Common Procedural Sedation Medications

MEDICATION	DOSE	ONSET/DURATION	NOTES
Midazolam	IN: 0.5 mg/kg (max 10 mg) PO: 0.5 mg/kg (max 20 mg) IV: Max 2 mg/dose 6 mo–5 y: 0.05–0.1 mg/kg/dose 6–12 y: 0.025–0.05 mg/kg/dose >12 y: initial 2 mg/dose, titrate with 1 mg prn	IN: 1–3 min/60 min PO: 15–30 min/60–90 min IV: 1–3 min/45–60 min	Peak IN/IV effect after 20 minutes May cause paradoxical effect in children Given over 10–20 seconds
Fentanyl	IN: 2 mcg/kg (max 100 mcg/dose) IV: Max 100 mcg/dose 1–2 mcg/kg/dose q3 min prn	IN: 3–5 min/30 min IV: 2–3 min/30 min	Give over 10–20 seconds
Ketamine	IV: Initial dose of 1–2 mg/kg/dose (max 100 mg/dose), repeat with 0.5 mg/kg (max 50 mg/dose) q5–10 min prn IM: 4–5 mg/kg/dose, repeat 2–4 mg/kg after 10–20 min	IV: 0.5–1 min/5–15 min IM: 3–5 min/15–30 min Recovery: 60–150 min	Dissociative anesthetic with all or no response May cause laryngospasm, hallucinations, vocalization, recovery agitation Contraindicated in obstructive hydrocephalus, active respiratory infection, poorly controlled asthma
Propofol	IV Induction: 0–4 y: 2 mg/kg 5–10 y: 1.5 mg/kg >10 y: 1 mg/kg* Maintenance: 50–200 mcg/kg/min to effect	IV: <1 min/5–15 min	Associated with hypotension, bradycardia, apnea, and infusion pain For infusion pain: apply tourniquet proximal to IV, give lidocaine 1% IV 1 mg/kg (max 25 mg), remove after 60 seconds, and flush with propofol bolus

IN, Intranasally, *IV,* intravenously, *PO,* oral.
*May require additional 0.5 mg/kg bolus every 60–90 seconds for induction.

- Active vomiting or severe, uncontrolled gastroesophageal reflux disease (GERD)
- Active viral upper respiratory infection
- Obstructive sleep apnea
- Symptomatic asthma
- Young age or history of extreme prematurity

33. **What are the typical medication doses for procedural sedation?**
Typical doses and useful notes are listed in Table 57.5.

CASE 3

A 25-year-old man presents to urgent care after a crush injury to the nail of his right index finger. He is in significant pain, with a nail matrix laceration, and has developed a subungual hematoma. There is no neurovascular compromise and x-rays reveal no fracture.

34. **How do local anesthetics provide analgesia?**
Local anesthetics bind to sodium channels most tightly in the open and inactivated states. When deposited into tissue near a nerve, the local anesthetic diffuses across the hydrophobic cell membrane and inactivates the sodium channel.

35. **What is the maximum total dose of select common local anesthetics?**
Table 57.6 provides basic dosing information for some commonly used local anesthetics. Local anesthetic toxicity is extremely rare in the urgent care setting as most nerve blocks require only a few milliliters of anesthetic. However, when injecting infants or with multiple planned injections, attention to the total dose is crucial.

Table 57.6 Basic Dosing and Useful Notes for Commonly Used Local Anesthetics

MEDICATIONS	ONSET	DURATION	TOXIC DOSE
Lidocaine 1% (10 mg/mL)	1–2 min	1–1.5 h	4.5 mg/kg
Lidocaine 1% with 1:100,000 epinephrine	1–2 min	2–6 h	7 mg/kg
0.25% bupivacaine (2.5 mg/mL)	5 min	2–8 h	2 mg/kg
0.2% ropivacaine (2 mg/mL)	5 min	2–8 h	3 mg/kg

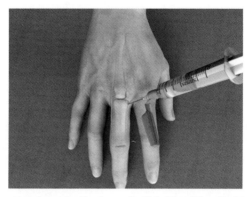

Fig. 57.2 Traditional digital nerve block. Prepare the skin using an antiseptic technique. Using a 25-, 27-, or 30-g needle, the needle is advanced to bone and withdrawn a few millimeters as shown. One or 2 mL of local anesthetic is injected into the dorsal and volar surfaces of the finger. A similar process is performed on the opposite side of the finger to numb both palmar nerves. Traditionally, epinephrine should not be used when injecting digits. (From: Thomsen TW, Setnik GS: Digital Nerve Block, Figure 7. Procedure Consult [serial online]. 2008. Available at: http://www.proceduresconsult.com/medical-procedures/digital-nerve-block-EM-053-procedure.aspx. Accessed July 26, 2016.)

36. **What does local anesthetic toxicity look like?**
    Local anesthetics are nonselective sodium channel blockers and can also affect myocytes and CNS neurons. Local anesthetic toxicity can be life-threatening. CNS effects generally occur first, including tinnitus, drowsiness, altered taste, seizures, altered mental status, and coma. Cardiac effects include increased tachycardia, T-wave changes, P-R interval and QRS duration, reentrant tachyarrhythmias, ventricular arrhythmias, and torsades de pointes.

37. **How is local anesthetic toxicity treated?**
    Local anesthetic toxicity can be very challenging to treat. Strategies include maintenance of airway, breathing, and circulation using advanced cardiovascular life support and pediatric advanced life support protocols, as well as benzodiazepines for seizures. Intralipid 20% is used as an "antidote." It is thought to function as a hydrophobic "sink" and sequester the local anesthetic. It is administered at 1.5 mL/kg over 1 minute, followed by an infusion of 0.25 mL/kg/min. Boluses can be repeated every 3–5 minutes.

38. **What equipment is needed for local anesthetic infiltration?**
    Syringe, large-bore drawing needle, injection needle (25, 27, or 30 gauge), local anesthetic of choice, antiseptic.

39. **What are the special considerations for local anesthetics?**
    Buffered lidocaine at a mixture of 1 mL of 8.4% bicarbonate to 10 mL of lidocaine can reduce injection pain. Additionally, warming lidocaine to body temperature reduces the burning sensation. Accidental intravascular administration of local anesthetic should be avoided by careful aspiration prior to injection. It is a medical maxim never to inject lidocaine with epinephrine into the ears, fingers, penis, or toes, although this has recently been called into significant question by multiple studies.

40. **What are the common nerve blocks performed in urgent care?**
    Common nerve blocks in urgent care are the digital nerve block (Fig. 57.2), infraorbital nerve block (Fig. 57.3), and mental nerve block (Fig. 57.4). These blocks are useful because they are painful locations with clear nerve territories. An effective nerve block can eliminate the need for procedural analgesia, although procedural anxiolysis may still be needed for younger or needle-phobic patients. The infraorbital and mental nerve blocks are particularly useful for repair of the vermillion border because injection of local anesthetic into the damaged lip can make repair of the vermillion border extremely challenging.

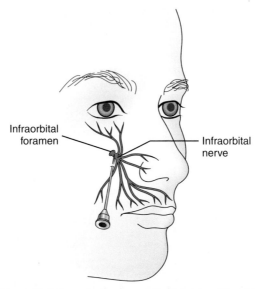

Infraorbital
foramen

Infraorbital
nerve

Fig. 57.3 Extraoral infraorbital nerve block. Prepare the skin using an antiseptic technique. Using a 25-, 27-, or 30-g needle, insert the needle as shown. After a negative aspiration, 1–2 mL of local anesthetic is injected. This block produces analgesia to the face in the region shown. It is especially useful for upper lip lacerations because local infiltration can affect the repair of the vermillion border. (From: Waldman, S. Infraorbital nerve block, Figure 17-3. In: Waldman S (ed): *Atlas of Interventional Pain Management*. 4th ed. Elsevier Saunders; 2015:61–64.)

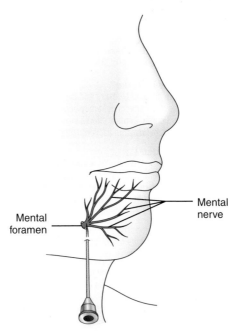

Mental
nerve

Mental
foramen

Fig. 57.4 Extraoral mental nerve block. Prepare the skin using an antiseptic technique. Using a 25-, 27-, or 30-g needle, insert the needle as shown. After a negative aspiration, 1–2 mL of local anesthetic is injected. This block produces analgesia to the face in the region shown. It is especially useful for lower lip lacerations because local infiltration can affect the repair of the vermillion border. (From: Waldman, S. Mental nerve block, Figure 19-3. In: Waldman S (ed): *Atlas of Interventional Pain Management*. 4th ed. Elsevier Saunders; 2015:68–71.)

KEY POINTS

1. Distinguishing acute from chronic pain and categorizing pain mechanisms can help drive treatment choices.
2. Multimodal treatments should always be used to treat pain without opioids or to reduce the opioid to the minimum required dose.
3. The WHO analgesic ladder is an effective treatment approach for acute and cancer-related pain.
4. Scheduling weak analgesics for a few days around an injury can improve pain control and reduce the need for opioids.
5. Procedural sedation should be performed by a clinician experienced in managing airways, and with appropriate emergency equipment and medications immediately available.

BIBLIOGRAPHY

Berde CB, Sethna NF. Analgesics for the treatment of pain in children. *N Engl J Med.* 2002;14:347.

Birmingham B, Buvanendran A. Nonsteroidal anti-inflammatory drugs, acetaminophen, and COX-2 inhibitors. In: Benzon H, Raj PP, Rathmell JP, et al., eds. *Practical Management of Pain.* 5th ed. Mosby; 2014:553–568 697–715.

Busse JW, Sadeghirad B, et al. Management of acute pain from non-low back, musculoskeletal injuries: a systematic review and network meta-analysis of randomized trials. *Ann Intern Med.* 2020;173(9):730–738.

Chand A. Pain management in the emergency department. In: Benzon H, Raj PP, Rathmell JP,et al., eds. *Practical Management of Pain.* 6th ed. Mosby; 2023:1034–1038.

Copenhaver D, Hoss R, Cortazzo MH, Vuong I, Fishman SM. Major opioids and chronic opioid therapy. In: Benzon H, Raj PP, Rathmell JP, et al., eds. *Practical Management of Pain.* 6th ed. Mosby; 2023:689–702.

Eidinejad L, Bahreini M, Ahmadi A, et al. Comparison of intravenous ketorolac at three doses for treating renal colic in the emergency department: a noninferiority randomized controlled trial. *Acad Emerg Med.* 2021;28(7):768–775.

Feldon L, Walter C, Harder S, et al. Comparative clinical effects of hydromorphone and morphine: a meta-analysis. *Br J Anaest.* 2011;3:107.

World Health Organization: *WHO's Pain Relief Ladder.* Available at: http://www.who.int/cancer/palliative/painladder/en/. Accessed July 26, 2016.

CHAPTER 58

MENTAL HEALTH URGENCIES

Jodi Brady-Olympia, MD

1. A 14-year-old male with no significant past medical history presents to your urgent care center with a 6-month history of daily headaches and poor appetite. His parents are concerned because he has become more "withdrawn" recently, spending much of his day in his room alone, playing on his computer. On exam, he is sullen, unengaging, and says he "doesn't want to talk about it." His vital signs and physical exam are unremarkable. What signs and symptoms may lead you to consider depression in a child or adolescent?
   - Isolation or withdrawing from friends and family
   - Loss of interest in things they previously enjoyed
   - Changes in sleep patterns (i.e., hypersomnia or insomnia)
   - Decline in school grades or performance
   - Somatic complaints: headaches, abdominal pain, chest pain
   - Change in appetite: loss of appetite, weight loss or weight gain
   - Irritability

2. What other conditions must be considered when suspecting a diagnosis of depression?
   - Psychiatric conditions: anxiety, eating disorders, ADHD, substance or alcohol use
   - Endocrine: hypo- or hyperthyroidism, Addison disease, Cushing disease
   - Hematologic: anemia, oncologic process
   - Insomnia

3. What is an essential element to obtaining a psychosocial history in an adolescent?
   In talking with an adolescent, it is necessary to discuss confidentiality. When a medical provider discusses confidentiality at the onset of the visit, adolescents are more likely to disclose information about sensitive topics. In addition, when confidentiality is not discussed, the adolescent is more likely to forgo care or not disclose the information.

4. What is a "conditional" discussion of confidentiality?
   Confidentiality is best discussed with the adolescent and family/guardian at the start of the encounter. The idea that confidentiality is "conditional" means that there are situations in which confidentiality will be breached. Under these circumstances, disclosure is required by law, such as abuse or homicidal ideation, or when the provider has concern for risk or harm to the adolescent such as suicidal ideation or high-risk behavior.

5. What are some of the risk factors for suicide attempt in adolescents?
   - Male gender
   - Age >16 years
   - Homosexual orientation
   - Parental mental health problems
   - Family history of suicide or suicide attempts
   - History of physical or sexual abuse
   - Previous suicide attempt
   - Mood disorder
   - Substance use
   - Pathologic internet use
   - Access to firearms or lethal means
   - Poor social support
   - Bullying
   - Recent psychosocial stressor(s)

6. You are working at your local urgent care center, with patients presenting for both medical as well as mental health complaints. You have learned that many patients who present to an emergency department for a suicide attempt have previously sought care in primary care, urgent care, or an emergency department for nonsuicidal concerns in the weeks or months leading up to their suicide attempt
   You consider what suicide screening tools are commonly used in acute care settings and if you should be using one of these tools to identify patients at increased risk for suicide.

In 2020, suicide was the third leading cause of death among children aged 10–14 years, following unintentional injury. Among 15- to 24-year-olds, it was the third leading cause of death following unintentional injury and homicide.

Two of the most commonly used tools to identify patients at increased risk for suicide in the emergency department include the Ask Suicide-Screening Questions (ASQ) and the Columbia-Suicide Severity Rating Scale (C-SSRS). These tools can be used in a variety of acute care and primary care settings.

The Ask-Suicide Screening Questions have a sensitivity of 96.9% and a specificity of 87.6% in patients presenting to a pediatric emergency department. Answering yes to one or more of the four questions is considered a positive screen.
1. In the past few weeks, have you ever felt that your family would be better off if you were dead?
2. In the past few weeks, have you wished you were dead?
3. In the past week, have you been having thoughts about killing yourself?
4. Have you ever tried to kill yourself?

7. **An 11-year-old female is brought to the urgent care clinic by her mother. The daughter has been complaining of stomachaches over the past 2 weeks since starting school. She is eating very little at lunch and cries every morning before leaving for school. She has never expressed any concerns about body image but says she is just not hungry. What signs may a child present with when exhibiting anxiety?**
- School avoidance or refusal
- Avoidance of social situations or activities
- Somatic complaints (headache, chest, or abdominal pain)
- Restlessness, nail biting, or hair pulling
- Declining school performance, inattentiveness
- Decreased appetite

8. **What should your differential diagnosis include when considering a child presenting with anxiety?**
- Psychiatric conditions: separation anxiety disorder, childhood-onset social phobia or social anxiety disorder, generalized anxiety disorder, agoraphobia and specific phobias, selective mutism, posttraumatic stress disorder, panic disorder, psychosis
- Acute painful conditions
- Central nervous system: trauma, tumor, meningitis/encephalitis
- Cardiac: dysrhythmias, shock states/dehydration
- Respiratory: acute asthma, hypoxia
- Endocrine: hyperthyroid
- Ingestions and exposures

9. **What toxidromes may present as acute psychiatric conditions?**
- Anticholinergic toxidrome: "Red as a beet, dry as a bone, blind as a bat, mad as a hatter, and hot as a hare."
  - Fever, tachycardia, cardiac arrhythmias
  - Hypertension
  - Delirium, psychosis, convulsions, coma
  - Mydriasis
  - Flushed, dry skin
- Amphetamine/cocaine toxidrome: fever, tachycardia, hypertension; hyperactive, delirious; tremors, myoclonus, psychosis; seizures; mydriasis; sweaty
- Opiate toxidrome: bradycardia, bradypnea, hypotension, hypothermia, euphoria to coma, hyporeflexia, pinpoint pupils
- Organophosphate toxidrome
  - Bradycardia to tachycardia
  - Tachypnea
  - Confusion, coma, convulsion, muscle fasciculations, weakness to paralysis
  - Miosis, blurry vision, lacrimation
  - Sweating
  - Salivation, bronchorrhea, bronchospasm, urinary frequency, diarrhea
- Neuroleptic malignant syndrome: fever, axial muscular rigidity, autonomic instability/shock, altered consciousness
- Serotonin syndrome: use of SSRI, agitation, stupor, myoclonus, hyperreflexia, diaphoresis, shivering, tremor, diarrhea, incoordination, fever

10. A 15-year-old female presents to your urgent care center with her mother because of a 3-month history of daily abdominal pain. She denies fever, vomiting, or diarrhea. She has lost approximately 15 pounds over the past 3 months, admitting that she has "no appetite." She has been seen by her pediatrician several times and has an extensive workup, including blood tests and computed tomography (CT) scans, all reported as normal. She was healthy prior to the onset of pain. Social history reveals that her parents are recently divorced. Her physician's exam is unremarkable. You have a suspicion for an eating disorder. In addition to your physical exam, what initial studies should be ordered?
    - Comprehensive metabolic panel (including electrolytes, blood urea nitrogen [BUN], creatinine, glucose, and liver function tests [LFTs])
    - Calcium, magnesium, and phosphorus levels
    - Complete blood count
    - Thyroid function testing (thyroid-stimulating hormone [TSH] and free thyroxine [free T4])
    - Electrocardiogram (EKG)
        Hypokalemic hypochloremic metabolic alkalosis may be seen with vomiting while hypophosphatemia may be seen with refeeding syndrome. A complete blood count may demonstrate anemia or leukopenia. An EKG may demonstrate significant sinus bradycardia. Normal lab and EKG results do not exclude the diagnosis of an eating disorder.

11. What other conditions should be considered in an adolescent presenting to urgent care with weight loss?
    - Endocrine: hyperthyroidism, glucocorticoid insufficiency, diabetes mellitus
    - Gastrointestinal: inflammatory bowel disease, celiac disease, peptic ulcer disease
    - Neoplastic: central nervous system tumor or other malignancies

12. What are the medical indications for direct referral to the emergency department and consideration of inpatient hospitalization for eating disorders and other psychiatric conditions?
    - Acute food refusal
    - Acute medical complications such as syncope or seizures
    - Uncontrolled binging and purging
    - Failure of outpatient treatment
    - <75% mean BMI for age and gender
    - Physiologic instability
        - Heart rate <50 bpm during the daytime, <45 bpm at night
        - Orthostatic blood pressure changes
        - Poor extremity perfusion with prolonged capillary refill
        - Weak/thread or strong/bounding pulses
        - Hypothermia (body temperature <96°F or 35.6°C)
        - Hypotension (90/45 mm Hg)
    - Acute mental status changes or focal neurologic findings
    - EKG abnormalities
    - Electrolyte disturbances: hypophosphatemia, hypokalemia, hypoglycemia
    - Moderate to severe dehydration
    - Psychiatric emergencies: homicidal or suicidal ideations, significant psychosis, severe depression
    - Concern for toxic ingestion or exposure
    - Social or family instability

13. A 17-year-old female presents to your urgent care center with her 16-year-old sister with complaints of lower abdominal pain and vaginal bleeding. She admits to having unprotected sex and is worried that she may be pregnant or have a sexually transmitted infection. Do you need to contact her guardian?
    Circumstances in which an adolescent can consent to their own health care in most states include:
    - Testing and treatment for sexually transmitted infections, including human immunodeficiency virus (HIV)
    - Contraceptive counseling and services
    - Prenatal care
    - Evaluation and treatment for substance use
    - Evaluation and treatment for mental health care
    - Life-threatening emergency care
    - Judicial bypass
    - Mature minor (i.e., married, pregnant, has a child, finically independent and not living at home, active duty in the military)
        Keep in mind that laws may vary from state to state, such as the minimal age necessary for an adolescent. Remember to check the laws governing your specific state of practice. (Guttmacher Institute. www.guttmacher.org)

14. A 16-year-old female presents to your urgent care center with a 1-month history of headache. While in the waiting room, she begins to experience shaking in her arms and legs, despite being able to follow commands and nod "yes" and "no" to questions. You are able to stop the seizure by merely holding the extremity. When you place her arm over her face, she avoids hitting herself when you drop her arm. What is likely going on?

She is most likely exhibiting a pseudoseizure. Associated with a conversion disorder, pseudoseizures are commonly seen in adolescent females and are typically nonrhythmic and prolonged. Pseudoseizures may be generalized or focal. The adolescent may be able to communicate with words or sounds, follow commands, and have purposeful movements during the event. Injury to the patient, urinary and bowel incontinence, and postictal states are rare. Anticonvulsants are unnecessary in the management of pseudoseizures.

Conversion disorder is an involuntary, stress-related condition where the patient presents with an alteration of physical functioning that does not correspond to a recognizable medical condition. Examples of conversion disorders include pseudoseizures, syncope, psychogenic cough, and paralysis/paresthesia of the extremities.

KEY POINTS

1. Underlying medical conditions must be considered in a child or adolescent presenting to urgent care with depression or anxiety.
2. In most circumstances, adolescents are able to consent for themselves when presenting for testing and treatment of sexually transmitted infections.
3. Normal labs, weight, and EKG do not exclude the diagnosis of an eating disorder.
4. Substance abuse, medication overdose, and alcohol intoxication must be considered in a child or adolescent presenting with a change in mental status.
5. There are certain circumstances in which confidentiality may be breached, including when disclosure is required by law, such as with abuse or homicidal ideation, or when the provider has concern for risk or harm to the adolescent such as suicidal ideation or high-risk behavior.

BIBLIOGRAPHY

Alrisi K, Alnasif N, Nazeer A, Shareef J, Latif F. Risk of suicide in children and adolescents in the emergency department-is universal screening the answer? *Arch Dis Child.* 2023 Mar 16:archdischild-2022-325122. doi:10.1136/archdischild-2022-325122. Epub ahead of print.

American Psychiatric Association. *Diagnostic and Statistical Manual of Mental Disorders.* 5th ed. (DSM-5). Arlington, VA: APA; 2013.

DeVylder JE, Ryan TC, Cwik M, Wilson ME, Jay S, Nestadt PS, Goldstein M, Wilcox HC. Assessment of selective and universal screening for suicide risk in a pediatric emergency department. *JAMA Netw Open.* 2019;2(10):e1914070. doi:10.1001/jamanetworkopen.2019.14070.

Ford CA, Millstein SG, Halpern-Felsher BL, Irwin CE. Influence of physician confidentiality assurances on adolescents' willingness to disclose information and seek future health care: a randomized controlled trial. *JAMA.* 1997;278:1029–1034. https://www.guttmacher.org/.

Horowitz LM, Bridge JA, Teach SJ, et al. Ask Suicide-Screening Questions (ASQ): a brief instrument for the pediatric emergency department. *Arch Pediatric Adolesc Med.* 2012;166(12):1170–1176.

Maslow GR, Dunlap K, Chung RJ. Depression and suicide in children and adolescents. *Pediatr Rev.* 2015;36(7):299–310.

Mehler PS, Anderson K, Bauschka M, Cost J, Farooq A. Emergency room presentations of people with anorexia nervosa. *J Eat Disord.* 2023;11(1):16.

Mientkiewicz L, Grover P. Adolescent confidentiality and consent in an emergency setting. *Pediatr Emerg Care.* 2022;38(12):697–699. http://www.cahl.org.

Scudder A, Rosin R, Baltich Nelson B, Boudreaux ED, Larkin C. Suicide screening tools for pediatric emergency department patients: a systematic review. *Front Psychiatry.* 2022;13:916731.

Shain B. Committee on adolescence: suicide and suicide attempts in adolescents. *Pediatrics. (June).* 2016.

WISQARS (Web-based Injury Statistics Query and Reporting System). Injury Center. CDC.

CHAPTER 59

TOXICOLOGY

Christopher Pitotti, MD, FACEP, Laurie Seidel Halmo, MD, FAAP

TOP SECRETS

1. Acetaminophen concentrations prior to 4 hours from ingestion are unreliable for predicting clinical outcomes and need for antidote.
2. Activated charcoal is the primary decontamination method in the urgent care setting and may still benefit a patient hours after ingestion.

QUESTIONS/ANSWERS

1. **Describe five common toxidromes.**
   See Table 59.1.
   A toxidrome (a portmanteau of "toxic syndrome") can be influenced by polypharmacy, individual pharmacodynamics, and variable absorption kinetics. As such, many toxicology patients present with signs and symptoms that do not fit into a classic toxidrome.

2. **How long from an ingestion can you administer activated charcoal?**
   If a patient presents with a recent overdose that can be adsorbed to activated charcoal (AC) and has no contraindications such as sedation or unprotected airway, it is safe to administer AC, even beyond 1–4 hours. In most cases, AC is the only indicated decontamination method indicated in urgent care. Delays will limit time for effective adsorption and may result in needing an antidote or hospitalization. Multidose-activated charcoal has been shown to reduce serum concentrations for some drugs even 24 hours after ingestion.

3. **What tests are helpful in the evaluation of an unknown ingestion?**
   History and clinical findings should guide test selection. Most toxicologic testing is unnecessary in the urgent care setting given the likelihood of transfer for antidote or observation. Screen for acetaminophen and salicylate

Table 59.1 Most Common Toxic Syndromes

TOXIDROME	COMMON SIGNS/ SYMPTOMS	COMMON CAUSES	COMMON TREATMENTS
Anticholinergic	Dry flushed skin, mydriasis, agitated delirium with mumbling, slight elevation in temperature, urinary retention, tachycardia, seizures	Antihistamines, antipsychotics, tricyclic antidepressants, atropine and scopolamine, plants such as jimson weed	First line: benzodiazepine In consultation with a poison center: physostigmine
Opioid	Miosis, sedation, respiratory depression, decreased gut motility	Opiates/opioids Clonidine mimics opioid toxidrome (and can cause hypotension)	First line: naloxone 0.1–2 mg IV based on symptoms or IN/IM
Sedative/ Hypnotic	CNS depression, hyporeflexia, neutral to slightly decreased HR and BP Respiratory depression in large overdose or in combination	Benzodiazepine, ethanol, barbiturates	First line: supportive care Flumazenil only to avoid intubation after benzodiazepine overdose
Serotonin Syndrome	Agitation, tremor, hyperreflexia with clonus, ocular clonus, diaphoresis, altered mental status, hyperthermia, tachycardia	SSRI, SNRI, MDMA	First line: benzodiazepine May administer other GABA-agonists or dexmedetomidine
Sympathomimetic	Agitation, diaphoresis, hypertension, hyperthermia, tachycardia, mydriasis	Amphetamines ("meth" and MDMA), pseudoephedrine, cocaine, caffeine can overlap	First line: benzodiazepines

exposure in all patients in whom self-harm or intentional ingestion is suspected. Glucometry, renal, and liver function test abnormalities can prompt an urgent intervention, but common urine drug screens rarely change management acutely except in pediatric patients with altered mental status. Electrocardiography may detect characteristic toxicity, and an x-ray may identify pill burden or foreign body, but both are not sensitive enough to exclude a clinically important ingestion.

4. **What poison gas exposure is often confused with seasonal influenza?**
Mild carbon monoxide (CO) exposure commonly presents with headache, fatigue, and nausea. It often presents simultaneously in multiple household members in the early winter, and pets may also be affected. The provider who suspects CO should administer 100% oxygen via a facemask, high-flow nasal cannula, or CPAP while continuing the workup and alerting poison control and local officials to identify a source.

5. **Which patients presenting after acetaminophen ingestion require transfer to the emergency department for antidote administration?**
Use the **Rumack-Matthew nomogram (Fig. 59.1)** to determine if n-acetylcysteine is necessary for **acute** ingestions. Beware: acetaminophen concentrations earlier than 4 hours from ingestion do not correlate with clinical outcome, so a 4-hour or later concentration must be obtained. If the time of ingestion is unknown, or if repeated super-therapeutic ingestions are suspected and either elevated AST, ALT, or acetaminophen concentrations are detected, initiate therapy.

6. **What is the clinical presentation of salicylate toxicity?**
See Table 59.2.

7. **How can you recognize a toxic alcohol ingestion? What causes the anion gap?**
Toxic alcohols, namely methanol, ethylene glycol, and diethylene glycol, may present similarly to ethanol intoxication, but often history will be the best chance of identifying this ingestion in the UCC due to the lack of osmolality or specific testing. Toxic alcohols may be found in many household products including denatured alcohol, antifreeze, and brake fluid. It is the charged metabolite that is indirectly detected with an elevated anion gap, which may take hours to be detectable. Calcium oxalate crystals, abnormally high lactate, and impaired renal function may signal a recent ethylene glycol ingestion. Methanol presents with milder clinical intoxication and possible visual deficit (late).

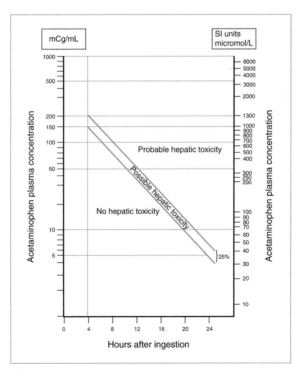

Fig. 59.1 The Rumack-Matthew nomogram. (From: Latham MD. Toxicology. In: Kleinman K, McDaniel L, Molloy M, eds. The Harriet Lane Handbook. Elsevier; 2021:52–60.)

Table 59.2 Common Presentation of Salicylate Toxicity	
Neurologic	Tinnitus or hearing deficit, confusion, delirium, coma
Gastrointestinal	Nausea, vomiting, abdominal pain
Pulmonary	Hyperventilation early, pulmonary edema
Dermatologic	Diaphoresis, hyperthermia
Cardiovascular	Tachycardia, late cardiovascular instability
Laboratory:	Early: mixed respiratory alkalosis and anion gap metabolic acidosis. Acute kidney injury and rhabdomyolysis may also be seen

Note: Chronic salicylism, usually in older adults, is often initially misdiagnosed as sepsis and can occur at lower serum concentrations of salicylic acid.

8. **What commonly prescribed UTI medications are known to cause methemoglobinemia, and how would you manage it?**
   Phenazopyridine is classic for causing methemoglobinemia; other common causes are benzocaine, dapsone, and recreational drugs like amyl nitrate. Pulse oximetry will be inaccurate even after administering the antidote, methylene blue. If the patient is asymptomatic, just observation is likely indicated. If the methemoglobin concentration is significantly elevated (>30%) or the patient is symptomatic, treatment with methylene blue is indicated.

9. **What common drugs are known to cause QRS widening on an EKG in overdose? What are important EKG findings in toxicology?**
   Drugs that affect cardiac sodium channels or gap junctions can influence QRS duration, namely tricyclic antidepressants, local anesthetics (including cocaine), some antiarrhythmics, and bupropion. Many medications prolong QTc (reference crediblemeds.org), which can precipitate Torsades de pointes. Digoxin can cause the "digoxin effect" (the "Salvador Dali" sign) in therapeutic use; in overdose, digoxin presents with a variety of arrhythmias for which slow atrial fibrillation and bidirectional ventricular tachycardia are fairly specific.

10. **Which antiemetic should be avoided in patients with a known prolonged QTc?**
    Most common antiemetics are associated with QTc prolongation, including droperidol, ondansetron, metoclopramide, and prochlorperazine, so alternate therapies (e.g., low-dose lorazepam) are encouraged.

11. **What chronically used drug can present with intractable nausea and vomiting with symptoms that get better in a hot shower?**
    Cannabis or cannabinoid-containing products, particularly when used frequently, can lead to cannabinoid hyperemesis syndrome (CHS). CHS patients typically use cannabis products at least weekly and present with intractable nausea and vomiting that classically improves with a hot bath or shower but is often refractory to traditional antiemetics. Limited evidence supports the use of topical capsaicin cream applied to the abdomen for symptom relief; dopamine antagonists such as haloperidol have also reportedly been effective. The most effective treatment for long-term symptom relief is complete abstinence from cannabis.

12. **What medications are known to cause dystonic reactions, and how should you manage these?**
    Dystonic reactions are classically associated with dopamine antagonists and represent the most acute-onset form of extrapyramidal symptoms. Although dystonic reactions are more common with first-generation antipsychotics than second-generation antipsychotics, any drug that antagonizes dopamine receptors can precipitate dystonia (see Table 59.3). Many commonly used antiemetics such as promethazine, prochlorperazine, and metoclopramide are also dopamine antagonists and thus can precipitate dystonia. Anticholinergic agents such as diphenhydramine or benztropine are the treatment of choice, as they restore the dopamine-choline imbalance that is thought to precipitate acute dystonia.

13. **How much ibuprofen is needed for serious toxicity, and how would it present?**
    Ingestions of less than 100 mg/kg ibuprofen in children under 6 years old or of less than 3 grams in teenagers and adults are highly unlikely to cause serious toxicity and are generally considered benign. Ingestions of over 400 mg/kg in children under 6 years of age or of over 6 grams in teenagers and adults pose a risk of serious toxicity, which may manifest with vomiting, significant CNS depression, seizures, apnea, metabolic acidosis, and acute kidney injury. Ingestions of between 100–400 mg/kg in young children or 3–6 grams in teens and adults may present with milder forms of toxicity, such as less significant CNS depression, less severe degrees of metabolic acidosis, and less significant kidney injury.

14. **What class of noninsulin antihyperglycemic is known to cause delayed hypoglycemia?**
    Sulfonylureas such as glipizide and glyburide function as insulin secretagogues, meaning they cause insulin release irrespective of the patient's blood glucose concentration. As such, ingestion of sulfonylurea in a person without baseline hyperglycemia can lead to significant hypoglycemia. Though the onset of hypoglycemia after sulfonylurea ingestion often occurs within 8 hours of ingestion, there are reports of hypoglycemia first occurring

Table 59.3 Commonly Used Dopamine Antagonists

FIRST-GENERATION ANTIPSYCHOTICS	SECOND-GENERATION ANTIPSYCHOTICS	OTHER DOPAMINE ANTAGONISTS USED FOR NAUSEA/VOMITING
Chlorpromazine	Aripiprazole	Metoclopramide
Droperidol	Clozapine	Promethazine
Fluphenazine	Lurasidone	
Haloperidol	Olanzapine	
Loxapine	Paliperidone	
Perphenazine	Quetiapine	
Prochlorperazine	Risperidone	
Thioridazine	Ziprasidone	

much later after ingestion, including several cases of onset 12–24 hours after ingestion. As such, all patients with nontherapeutic sulfonylurea ingestions require prolonged observation to monitor for possible delayed-onset hypoglycemia.

15. **What common cold medications are abused? Which one could cause serotonin syndrome when combined with an SSRI or other serotonergic drugs?**
Over-the-counter cough and cold medications are easily accessible, inexpensive, and legal, all of which make them appealing to recreational substance users. Many of these products contain **diphenhydramine**, which—when ingested in supratherapeutic doses—leads to anticholinergic toxicity including hallucinations and risk of seizures and QRS prolongation leading to life-threatening dysrhythmias. Other products contain **dextromethorphan**, an NMDA receptor antagonist and serotonin reuptake inhibitor that—in high doses—can produce euphoria and hallucinations but also can cause serotonin syndrome, particularly when combined with other serotonergic medications.

16. **Overdose of what opioid is unlikely to cause respiratory depression in adults but may in children?**
Buprenorphine is increasingly being used to treat opioid use disorder. As a partial agonist, it is extremely unlikely to cause respiratory depression in adults; however, respiratory depression in young children after accidental, exploratory buprenorphine ingestion has been reported. The ingestion of a single tablet or sublingual film is sufficient to cause respiratory depression in a young child severe enough to require naloxone administration (see Table 59.4 for a list of common medications that can cause severe toxicity in a young child even after a single tablet ingestion). Young children with buprenorphine ingestions require a prolonged observation period.

17. **Which spider is found throughout the United States and can cause a medically significant envenomation?**
Black widow spiders (*Latrodectus* species) are found in dozens of countries across the world; in the United States, they are found in every state except Alaska. A small wheal and flare reaction at the bite site sometimes

Table 59.4 One Pill Can Kill: Common Pharmaceuticals With Significant Toxicity After Single-Dose Ingestion in Young Children

Benzonatate
Beta blockers
Calcium channel blockers
Clonidine
Cyclic antidepressants
Diphenoxylate/atropine (Lomotil)
Opioids, including partial agonists like buprenorphine
Sulfonylureas

occurs, though often the bite site goes unnoticed as the skin changes are minimal. The clinical manifestations of envenomation range from local pain at the bite site to severe pain and muscle cramping that may be distal from the bite site. Antivenom is highly effective at rapidly and completely reversing these symptoms; if antivenom is not available, supportive care with analgesics and benzodiazepines for muscle spasms is recommended.

18. **What are the clinical manifestations of brown recluse spider envenomation?**
Brown recluse spiders are found in the south and central United States. There are three primary clinical syndromes that can occur after envenomation: (1) a localized urticarial response to the bite site; (2) a more extensive cytotoxic reaction that presents as an ulcer that necroses and forms an eschar; and (3) systemic loxoscelism, which occurs primarily in children 24–72 hours after envenomation and presents with fevers, chills, nausea, vomiting, and arthralgias, and is associated with hemolysis, disseminated intravascular coagulation, and rhabdomyolysis. Management of all three clinical syndromes is supportive and should include wound care, tetanus prophylaxis, and analgesics as needed. Prophylactic antibiotic use is not recommended.

19. **What mushroom is potentially lethal and presents with delayed (>6 hours) nausea and vomiting?**
Most fatalities following mushroom ingestions are associated with cyclopeptide-containing mushrooms such as some *Amanita* species (particularly *Amanita phalloides*), *Galerina* species, and *Lepiota* species. Differentiating these highly toxic mushrooms from less toxic or nontoxic species is challenging and typically requires consultation with a mycologist. As such, clinicians treating patients who are ill after mushroom ingestion typically must proceed without knowing the species involved. A good general rule of thumb is that while many mushrooms contain GI irritants that will cause nausea, vomiting, and diarrhea after ingestion, these symptoms are classically delayed for many hours or days after ingestion of a highly toxic cyclopeptide-containing mushroom, whereas they typically occur earlier (within 6 hours) after ingestion of less dangerous, non-cyclopeptide-containing mushroom species.

20. **Ingestion of what foreign body must be removed immediately when lodged in the esophagus, even if there are currently no symptoms?**
Button batteries are often accidentally swallowed and sometimes get lodged in the esophagus of young children. When this occurs, esophageal tissue maintains contact with both sides of the button battery, completing the electrical circuit. This leads to hydrolysis at the battery's negative pole, causing tissue damage within minutes. If allowed to proceed, the damage can progress to the point of causing esophageal perforation or an aortoesophageal fistula, which can lead to life-threatening hemorrhage. As such, children presenting to urgent care with a button battery in the esophagus must be emergently transferred to a facility where a gastroenterologist or surgeon can endoscopically remove the battery as soon as possible. Honey (for children >12 months old) or sucralfate may be given to mitigate tissue damage while awaiting battery removal.

KEY POINTS

1. Always report suspected toxic exposures to the poison control center by calling 1-800-222-1222 and initiate transfer for ill-appearing overdoses to the emergency department immediately.
2. Screen for acetaminophen and salicylate exposure in all patients in whom self-harm or intentional ingestion is suspected.
3. The dose makes the poison; large or massive exposures to seemingly innocuous substances may require transfer to the emergency department.
4. Many common toxicologic therapies such as activated charcoal, naloxone, and n-acetylcysteine can and should be started in the urgent care setting prior to transfer to a higher level of care.

BIBLIOGRAPHY

Akinkugbe O, James AL, Ostrow O, Everett T, Wolter NE, McKinnon NK. Vascular complications in children following button battery ingestions: a systematic review. *Pediatrics*. 2022;150(3):e2022057477. doi:10.1542/peds.2022-057477.

Anfang RR, Jatana KR, Linn RL, Rhoades K, Fry J, Jacobs IN. pH-neutralizing esophageal irrigations as a novel mitigation strategy for button battery injury. *Laryngoscope*. 2019;129(1):49–57.

Buckley NA, Whyte IM, O'Connell DL, Dawson AH. Activated charcoal reduces the need for N-acetylcysteine treatment after acetaminophen (paracetamol) overdose. *J Toxicol Clin Toxicol*. 1999;37(6):753–757.

Gavioli EM, Guardado N, Haniff F, Deiab N, Vider E. The risk of QTc prolongation with antiemetics in the palliative care setting: a narrative review. *J Pain Palliat Care Pharmacother*. 2021;35(2):125–135.

Glatstein M, Carbell G, Scolnik D, Rimon A, Hoyte C. Treatment of pediatric black widow spider envenomation: a national poison center's experience. *Am J Emerg Med*. 2018;36(6):998–1002.

Hall AH, Smolinske SC, Conrad FL, et al. Ibuprofen overdose: 126 cases. *Ann Emerg Med*. 1986;15(11):1308–1313.

Hall AH, Smolinske SC, Stover B, Conrad FL, Rumack BH. Ibuprofen overdose in adults. *J Toxicol Clin Toxicol*. 1992;30(1):23–37.

Holstege CP, Eldridge DL, Rowden AK. ECG manifestations: the poisoned patient. *Emerg Med Clin North Am*. 2006;24(1):159–177, vii.

Klein-Schwartz W, Stassinos GL, Isbister GK. Treatment of sulfonylurea and insulin overdose. *Br J Clin Pharmacol*. 2016;81(3):496–504.

Lewis K, O'Day CS. *Dystonic Reactions*. In: *StatPearls* Treasure Island (FL) 2022.

Loden JK, Seger DL, Spiller HA, Wang L, Byrne DW. Cutaneous-hemolytic loxoscelism following brown recluse spider envenomation: new understandings. *Clin Toxicol (Phila)*. 2020;58(12):1297–1305.

Rumack BH, Matthew H. Acetaminophen poisoning and toxicity. *Pediatrics*. 1975;55(6):871–876.

Sorensen CJ, DeSanto K, Borgelt L, Phillips KT, Monte AA. Cannabinoid hyperemesis syndrome: diagnosis, pathophysiology, and treatment—a systematic review. *J Med Toxicol*. 2017;13(1):71–87.

Tan JL, Stam J, van den Berg AP, van Rheenen PF, Dekkers BGJ, Touw DJ. Amanitin intoxication: effects of therapies on clinical outcomes – a review of 40 years of reported cases. *Clin Toxicol (Phila)*. 2022:1–15.

Toce MS, Burns MM, O'Donnell KA. Clinical effects of unintentional pediatric buprenorphine exposures: experience at a single tertiary care center. *Clin Toxicol (Phila)*. 2017;55(1):12–17.

CHAPTER 60

TRAVEL MEDICINE

Sandra K. Schumacher, MD, MPH, CTropMed, Jeffrey I. Campbell, MD, MPH

1. **What are VFRs, and why is this population at particular risk of acquiring travel-related illness?**

   VFRs (visiting friends and relatives) are individuals who travel to visit relatives or friends, which often involves a return to the individual's country of origin. VFRs tend to have a higher incidence of travel-related infectious diseases (e.g., VFRs are eight times more likely to be diagnosed with malaria than are tourist travelers). Many VFRs assume immunity against infectious diseases in their home countries; however, immunity has often waned by the time of travel. Also, ≤30% of VFRs have a pretravel health care encounter, so these travelers may lack awareness of risk. Furthermore, many may travel to higher-risk destinations while staying in homes that lack health amenities frequently available to foreign tourists, such as bed nets and safe food and water.

2. **In a returning traveler who is sick, what illnesses might you suspect based on duration of time since travel?**

   Time since potential exposure can help identify illness in returning travelers. COVID-19, chikungunya, dengue, Japanese encephalitis, enteric fever, influenza, and spotted fever Rickettsial illnesses often have an incubation period of <2 weeks. Hepatitis A and E often have an incubation of 2–6 weeks; enteric fever may also be seen during this time period. Hepatitis B, amebic liver abscesses, schistosomiasis, leishmaniasis, and tuberculosis often have an incubation of >6 weeks. Although malaria typically presents within 2 weeks of travel, symptoms may not develop until months after return (98% of *Plasmodium falciparum* infections present within 3 months of travel; however, almost 50% of *P. vivax* infections present after 30 days of travel and may not be seen until 12 months after return). Human immunodeficiency virus (HIV) may present at any time.

3. **What special concerns do health care workers face when practicing abroad?**

   Health care workers who spend time abroad in health care settings may face health risks less prevalent in the United States, as well as decreased access to effective treatment while abroad. Risk is largely dependent upon the specific environment in which the health care worker operates. Specific considerations include increased exposure to bloodborne pathogens such as hepatitis B and HIV, highly contagious diseases such as measles and tuberculosis, and epidemics such as cholera. Health care workers should consider bringing postexposure prophylaxis antiretrovirals with them for potential HIV exposure. Health care workers also may experience unique psychological stress related to their work.

4. **What causes cholera and how is it treated?**

   The bacterium causing cholera, *Vibrio cholerae,* is typically acquired from untreated, contaminated water, but it can also be transmitted through food (especially seafood). The characteristic symptom is a diffuse, "rice-water" secretory diarrhea that may lead rapidly to hypovolemia. Treatment focuses on rehydration with oral rehydration solution and/or intravenous fluids; antibiotics, including macrolides, fluoroquinolones, or tetracyclines, may reduce symptom duration and fluid requirements but do not obviate the need for aggressive rehydration. In mid-2016, the FDA approved Vaxchora, a live, attenuated vaccine for the prevention of cholera caused by serogroup 01 in people 2–64 years old.

5. **What is the meningitis belt?**

   The meningitis belt is an area of sub-Saharan Africa where meningococcal meningitis is hyperendemic (Fig. 60.1), most notably during the dry season (December–June). Although meningococcal outbreaks are most common in the meningitis belt, outbreaks can occur worldwide (notably, the Hajj pilgrimage to Saudi Arabia has been associated with outbreaks). Transmission occurs person-to-person by close contact with saliva or respiratory secretions. The six major *Neisseria meningitidis* serogroups are A, B, C, W, X, and Y; serogroup A predominates in the meningitis belt. At-risk travelers are recommended to receive a quadrivalent meningitis vaccine, which protects against serogroups A, C, W, and Y. Those aged 10–25 years may also be vaccinated with a serogroup B meningococcal vaccine series.

6. **What causes travelers' diarrhea, and how can it be prevented and treated?**

   Travelers' diarrhea is the most common travel-related illness and occurs worldwide, especially in most of Asia, Mexico, Central and South America, Africa, and the Middle East. Bacterial pathogens are the typical cause, led by enterotoxigenic *Escherichia coli.* Prevention centers on good hand hygiene, avoiding ice and tap water in endemic areas, and eating well-prepared foods. Oral hydration is key in the treatment of travelers' diarrhea. Indications for antibiotic use include more than four unformed stools daily, fever, or blood or mucus in the stool. In adults, fluoroquinolone is often prescribed empirically; azithromycin is recommended for children, pregnant women, and travelers to Asia (where quinolone-resistant *Campylobacter* is prevalent).

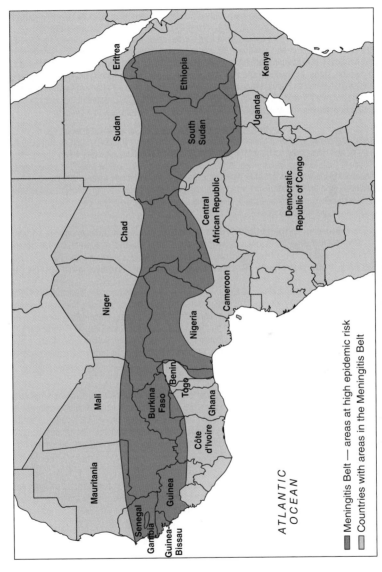

Fig. 60.1 The Meningitis Belt. (https://wwwnc.cdc.gov/travel/yellowbook/2020/travel-related-infectious-diseases/meningococcal-disease#4670.)

■ Meningitis Belt — areas at high epidemic risk

☐ Countries with areas in the Meningitis Belt

7. **What causes ciguatera, and what are the symptoms of ciguatera?**
Reef fish (such as barracuda) predate on ciguatoxin-producing dinoflagellates. These fish may then accumulate the toxin and pass it to humans when eaten. Ciguatera typically presents with gastrointestinal symptoms starting 3–24 hours after eating a toxin-laden fish but may include more severe symptoms such as hypotension and bradycardia as well as neurologic and psychiatric symptoms such as paresthesias, hot/cold reversal, and hallucinations. Symptoms usually last a few days but may persist up to 4 weeks; treatment is primarily supportive. Ciguatera toxin-containing fish do not smell or appear unusual, and neither cooking nor freezing destroys the toxin. There is no clinical testing for ciguatera.

8. **A patient presents to urgent care with facial flushing, diarrhea, and respiratory distress shortly after eating at a sushi restaurant. What likely caused this acute illness?**
Scombroid, also known as histamine toxicity from fish, causes up to 40% of seafood-related foodborne illnesses in the United States and is common worldwide. Illness occurs when bacteria, proliferating in poorly refrigerated fish, convert the amino acid histidine into histamine. Symptoms result from consuming histamine and present like an allergic reaction, starting between 5 and 60 minutes after eating contaminated fish. Classically, patients may describe contaminated fish as tasting bitter, peppery, or metallic, but concentrations of histamine needed to produce symptoms are much lower than concentrations needed to affect taste. Treatment is usually not necessary, although antihistamines may be helpful, and possibly epinephrine if anaphylaxis is a concern.

9. **What vector-borne diseases should travelers be wary of, and what transmits them?**
Vector-borne diseases are infections transmitted by the bite of infected arthropods, such as mosquitoes, ticks, triatomine bugs, and fleas. They account for more than 17% of all infectious diseases. Vector-borne illnesses worldwide include malaria (*Anopheles* mosquitoes); dengue, chikungunya, yellow fever, Rift Valley fever, and Zika (*Aedes* mosquitoes); Japanese encephalitis, lymphatic filariasis, and West Nile fever (*Culex* mosquitoes); Rickettsial diseases and Lyme (ticks); American trypanosomiasis (triatomine bugs); African trypanosomiasis (tsetse flies); leishmaniasis (sandflies); and onchocerciasis (blackflies). Many of these diseases are preventable by limiting exposures to their respective vectors.

10. **An adult who returned to the United States from Kenya 1 week ago presents to your office with an intermittent fever, headaches, and body aches. He did not seek travel counsel before traveling and said he had multiple mosquito bites during his trip. You find he is anemic as well. What potentially life-threatening infectious illness should you be certain to exclude?**
Malaria is found in over 100 countries, is caused by the *Plasmodium* parasite, and is transmitted by *Anopheles* mosquitoes, which bite humans (thereby transmitting the parasite) at dusk and during the night. An experienced laboratorian can distinguish between the four most common disease-causing *Plasmodium* species—*P. falciparum, P. vivax, P. malariae,* and *P. ovale*—based on their appearance on a blood smear. *P. falciparum* is typically associated with severe malaria, and *P. vivax* and *P. ovale* can develop dormant liver stages. Most cases of malaria are curable. However, malaria causes more than 400,000 annual deaths globally, primarily among children <5 years old.

11. **How can malaria be prevented?**
Travelers to malaria-endemic areas can reduce the chances of infection by taking prophylactic medications before, during, and after their trip. Prophylactic medications include doxycycline, mefloquine, chloroquine, and atovaquone-proguanil; the choice of which medication to take should account for local resistance patterns in the traveler's destination. Other methods of prevention include sleeping under bed nets, staying in well-screened areas at night, properly using mosquito spray, avoiding standing water, and wearing long-sleeved shirts and long pants at night to cover skin and avoid mosquito bites.

12. **What is yellow fever?**
Yellow fever is a syndrome caused by the yellow fever virus, which is found in certain parts of South America and Africa (Figs. 60.2 and 60.3) and spread via bites of infected *Aedes* mosquitoes. Yellow fever can cause fever and flu-like symptoms, jaundice, hemorrhage, multiple organ failure, and death (in 20–50% of serious cases).

13. **What are the indications and contraindications for yellow fever vaccination?**
The yellow fever vaccine is a live, attenuated virus vaccine that is given in a single injection to people 9 months to 59 years old traveling to an area of risk (as outlined in the CDC's *Yellow Book*) or traveling to a country with an entry requirement for the vaccination. Anyone <6 months old or with a life-threatening allergy to any component of the vaccine, including eggs, should not get the vaccine. Additional relative contraindications to yellow fever vaccination include ages 6–9 months old, ≥60 years old, having a weakened immune system, having had a thymectomy or thymic disorder, being pregnant, or breastfeeding. Protection against yellow fever lasts for a lifetime after vaccination.

14. **What is Japanese encephalitis, and who should be vaccinated against it?**
Japanese encephalitis virus (JEV) is a *Culex* mosquito-transmitted arbovirus and is the primary cause of encephalitis in East Asia. The majority of individuals infected with JEV are asymptomatic, and fewer than 1% of JEV

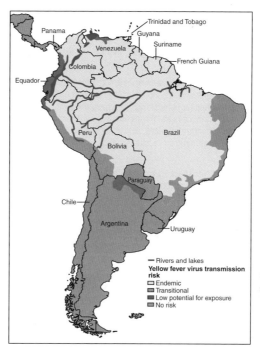

Fig. 60.2 Areas with risk of yellow fever virus transmission in South America. (https://www.cdc.gov/yellowfever/maps/south_america.html.)

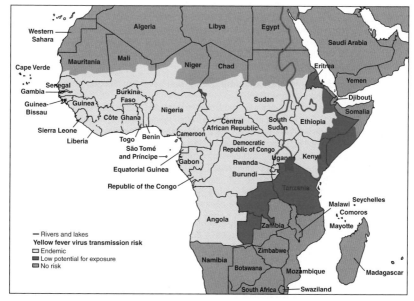

Fig. 60.3 Areas with risk of yellow fever virus transmission in Africa. (http://www.cdc.gov/yellowfever/maps/africa.html.)

infections result in symptomatic neuroinvasive disease. However, when neurologic disease does occur, it is usually quite severe, with a high case fatality rate and neurologic sequelae occurring in 30–50% of survivors. The CDC recommends JEV vaccination for long-term (≥1 month) travel to endemic areas or short-term travel if the traveler is visiting an endemic area and participating in activities that will increase exposure to JEV-bearing mosquitoes (e.g., camping, hiking, or farming).

15. **What postexposure prophylaxis steps should be taken after a potential rabies exposure?**
    After a potential rabies exposure, bite wounds should be cleaned thoroughly with soap and water; suturing should be avoided if possible unless required for hemostasis. For exposed individuals who did not receive preexposure vaccination, postexposure prophylaxis consists of rabies immune globulin injected at the wound site (prior to suturing, if closure is required) and intramuscularly, as well as four doses of the rabies vaccine. Individuals who completed the three-dose preexposure rabies vaccination series should receive two additional booster doses of the vaccine if exposed.

16. **How can travelers protect themselves from tetanus?**
    Tetanus typically occurs when wounds are contaminated with dirt or soil containing the bacterium *Clostridium tetani*. The CDC recommends tetanus booster vaccinations prior to travel to areas where access to health services may be limited. When a potential exposure occurs (e.g., a laceration or a dog bite), the patient should receive a booster vaccine if the last booster was ≥5 years prior and at least three previous tetanus doses were obtained, if the patient received an unknown amount of doses, or if the patient received less than three doses regardless of time since the last dose. Human tetanus immune globulin should also be given if less than three previous tetanus doses were obtained, and the wound is considered dirty or major.

17. **When should infant travelers be vaccinated against measles, mumps, and rubella (MMR), and how does MMR vaccination affect the timing of other vaccinations?**
    The first dose of the MMR vaccine is typically administered to children between 12 and 15 months old. However, infants between the ages of 6 and 11 months who travel to areas where these diseases remain prevalent should receive the first MMR dose prior to departure. Children ≥12 months old should receive two doses of the vaccine, separated by 28 days. If the MMR vaccine is given prior to 12 months of age, this dose typically does not count toward the MMR series, and the child must get two doses of MMR after turning 1 year old. The MMR vaccine is a live vaccine, and administration of another live vaccine should occur either on the same day as MMR or ≥28 days later (≥30 days later if yellow fever vaccine) to ensure immunogenicity.

18. **Where is polio found, and when is vaccination indicated?**
    Although most people infected with polio are asymptomatic, this enterovirus can famously cause paralysis. Despite massive global polio vaccination campaigns, polio has not been eradicated. Only two countries (Afghanistan and Pakistan) continue to have endemic polio. However, wild poliovirus still circulates in a number of countries. The CDC recommends that travelers to any country where wild-type polio was found to be circulating in the previous 12 months protect themselves by being fully vaccinated against polio, including a single lifetime polio vaccine booster for adults. The World Health Organization posts up-to-date booster recommendations for countries with wild poliovirus.

19. **In addition to handwashing and consuming only well-prepared foods, how can travelers protect themselves from hepatitis A?**
    Hepatitis A virus is transmitted fecal–orally via contaminated water and food or from close contact with someone who is infected. Young children infected with the virus are often spared severe symptoms but can shed the virus, and the two-dose series hepatitis A vaccination is a part of the routine vaccinations for young children. Because of lack of exposure in the United States, many older children and adults born in the United States lack natural immunity to the virus, and so can acquire this infection if exposed. The CDC recommends the two-dose series hepatitis A vaccination for travelers to endemic areas. Contraindications to the vaccine include age <12 months and an allergy to a component of the vaccine. Individuals who cannot or opt not to receive the vaccine, including travelers <12 months old, can instead receive immune globulin, which confers protection against the virus for up to 5 months. The duration depends upon the dose of immune globulin given.

20. **What vaccines protect against typhoid, and how effective are they?**
    Enteric fever (also known as typhoid fever) is caused by *Salmonella* serovar Typhi bacteria and is transmitted fecal–orally by consumption of contaminated food or water. Two typhoid vaccines, an oral version (Ty21a, a live, attenuated vaccine) and an injected version (ViCPS, an inactivated vaccine), are available commercially in the United States. The oral vaccine is administered in four doses (1 pill every other day for a week), is approved for children ≥6 years old, and requires redosing after 5 years. The injected vaccine is approved for children ≥2 years old and requires redosing after 2 years. Studies of these vaccines have shown efficacy rates of 50–80%; vaccination therefore does not eliminate the need to avoid potentially contaminated food or water.

21. **How can altitude sickness be prevented?**

    Altitude sickness is divided into three syndromes: acute mountain sickness, high-altitude cerebral edema, and high-altitude pulmonary edema. Individuals with a history of altitude sickness and those who rapidly ascend to 2500 meters or higher are at particular risk for altitude sickness. To help prevent altitude sickness, individuals should be advised to ascend gradually, avoiding going directly from low altitude to more than 2750 meters sleeping altitude in a single day. Once above 2750 meters, individuals should increase their sleeping altitude no more than 500 meters per day and plan an extra day for acclimatization every 1000 meters. Acetazolamide may assist acclimatization, potentially by acidifying the blood, which results in compensatory increased respirations and oxygenation.

22. **What are useful websites that provide accurate, current information about travel-related health risks?**

    Regularly updated online resources that are of particular relevance are:

    - The CDC's *Health Information for International Travel* (the *Yellow Book*) provides detailed assistance for health care providers and comprehensively summarizes pre-, during, and posttravel health concerns and their management.
      See https://wwwnc.cdc.gov/travel/page/yellowbook-home for more information.
    - The US State Department publishes travel notifications and travel-related policies that are up-to-date and country-specific.
      See https://travel.state.gov/content/travel/en.html for more information.

KEY POINTS

1. VFRs (visiting friends and relatives) tend to have a higher incidence of travel-related infectious diseases than other tourists.
2. Health care workers face special concerns when working abroad.
3. Many illnesses, mostly infectious in origin, are associated with travel but can often be prevented.
4. It is crucial to inquire about the countries traveled to, time of travel, travel activities, and basic health status to determine what illnesses need to be considered in a returning traveler who is sick.
5. There are many websites that provide accurate, current information about travel-related health risks.

BIBLIOGRAPHY

Centers for Disease Control and Prevention. Vaccines. Medicines. Advice. http://wwwnc.cdc.gov/travel/; accessed December 4, 2022.
Centers for Disease Control and Prevention. *Yellow Book.* https://wwwnc.cdc.gov/travel/page/yellowbook-home; accessed November 10, 2023.
Kimberlin DW, Barnett ED, Lynfield R, Sawyer MH, eds. *Red Book.* 32nd ed. Elk Grove Village, IL: American Academy of Pediatrics; 2021.
World Health Organization. http://www.who.int/en/; accessed December 4, 2022.

CHAPTER 61

DIAGNOSTIC IMAGING: GENERAL CONCEPTS

Jonathan L. Mezrich, MD, JD, MBA, LLM, Sean Lisse, MD

TOP SECRETS

1. Position of acquisition and lung volumes can impact the size and appearance of cardiomediastinal structures on a chest x-ray.
2. When looking for fractures, be aware that ringed structures (e.g. forearm, lower leg, pelvis and mandible) typically disrupt in two places, so always look for a second fracture/dislocation.
3. Shoulders most commonly dislocate anteriorly.
4. Imaging of the contralateral extremity can be helpful for comparison in assessing for subtle fractures or separations.
5. An elbow joint effusion may suggest an occult injury, particularly in pediatric patients.

WHAT TYPES OF IMAGING MIGHT YOU USE IN URGENT CARE?

There are several different ways you can generate images of the body, which fall into a few broad categories: ultrasound, MRI, nuclear medicine, and x-ray-based. X-ray-based can be further broken down into radiographs (x-rays), computed tomography (CT or CAT scan), and fluoroscopy. Ultrasound and MRI do not use ionizing radiation and thus do not have any risk of DNA damage. Nuclear medicine studies and all x-ray-based modalities carry a risk of DNA damage, although whether the risk is negligible or substantial varies from study to study. Because radiography is the most common modality used in the urgent care setting, this will be the focus of this chapter.

1. **What is diagnostic radiography?**
   Radiography (commonly just called "x-ray") is an imaging technique whereby x-rays are produced by a source and shine through the patient toward a detector. A certain portion of the x-rays are absorbed by the body; exactly how much depends on the density of the subject. "Radiodense" things such as bones, foreign bodies, and orthopedic hardware absorb more x-rays, and lower-density things such as soft tissues, fat, fluid, and air absorb fewer x-rays. The result is a two-dimensional image of the patient generated by the remaining x-rays that reach the detector. Radiography is generally the staple of urgent care imaging and is the first imaging step for many clinical concerns. Radiographs are cheap, fast, and relatively low in radiation. A discussion of all uses of radiography would be extensive and impossible to distill into a single chapter; the following is a sample of common pathology seen on x-ray that one might find in the urgent care setting, as well as some pearls to consider that may aid in interpretation.

2. **Chest radiographs.**
   Perhaps the most common imaging performed during an urgent care visit is the chest radiograph.

2a. **How do you approach a chest radiograph?**
   Position, gravity, lung volumes. When looking at a chest radiograph, the first step of analysis is to be aware of the projection and positioning. Most common are the "frontal" (facing toward or away from the detector) and "lateral" (facing at a right angle to the detector) positions. In each of these positions, it is important to know which part of the patient is closest to the detector. For example, a frontal radiograph can be obtained in the anterior-to-posterior (AP) projection or posterior-to-anterior (PA) projection. The PA projection positions the heart closer to the detector, lessening the magnifying effect of distance (imagine putting your thumb on the end of a flashlight and looking at the huge thumb shadow on the wall, vs. the shadow of your thumb nearly against the wall). The patient's position relative to gravity is also important. Air moves away from gravity and fluid down toward gravity. You can use this fact when looking for small amounts of fluid or air in the chest or abdomen. Lung volumes are also important; low volumes can make the heart appear larger and lung markings appear more prominent. By convention, a chest radiograph is presented as if the patient is standing in front of you, facing you, but the technologist will also mark the patient's right or left side.

2b. **What anatomy can be seen on a normal chest x-ray?**
   A chest x-ray provides a flat, two-dimensional picture of the thoracic structures, including the lung fields, heart, portions of the airway, pulmonary vasculature, aorta, and ribs (see Fig. 61.1). It usually also involves some of the upper abdomen and lower neck.

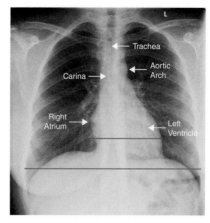

Fig. 61.1 Annotated Normal PA chest radiograph.

2c. What approach does one use when reviewing a chest radiograph?

Because of the many structures present on a chest radiograph, a systematic approach is useful. A common, if simple, mnemonic taught in medical schools is the "ABCD" approach.

A: Airway

B: Breathing

C: Cardiovascular/cardiomediastinal

D: "Disability"

E: Everything else)

The "A" stands for airway (the trachea, carina, right and left main bronchus – see arrows in Fig. 61.1). In the urgent care setting, the airway may move/bend from external pressure or may be internally blocked. The "B" stands for breathing, looking at the lung fields. You assess for denser areas such as a pneumonia (Fig. 61.2), atelectasis, or pleural effusions, or for less dense areas like pleural air ("pneumothorax," Fig. 61.3). Pulmonary edema is also a common lung finding, manifesting early as thickening of the lung markings and progressing to hazy pulmonary opacification or even full "white-out."

The "C" stands for cardiovascular; the cardiomediastinal silhouette is composed of the heart, aorta, and other large chest vessels. A widened mediastinum may suggest a mass, bleeding, or enlarged vessels – but be careful! As we've already learned, the heart and mediastinum will often be magnified by position or distorted by low lung volumes. Air in the mediastinum (pneumomediastinum) or lower neck can suggest tracheal or esophageal injury. A quick gauge of heart size can be made by dividing it by the distance between the inner portions of the ribs at the widest part of the lungs (horizontal lines in Fig. 61.1), the cardiothoracic ratio. If the heart is more than half the width of the ribs, it may be enlarged. The heart size is often larger in normal infants, though! A large heart on a radiograph is a nonspecific finding but may suggest dilated chambers, pericardial effusion, or other

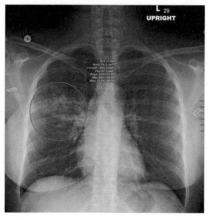

Fig. 61.2 Right upper lobe pneumonia.

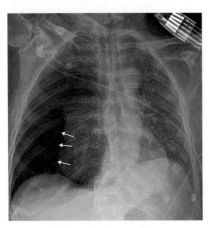

Fig. 61.3 Right pneumothorax.

cardiac abnormality. Unless explained, cardiomegaly on x-ray needs more investigation such as an echocardiogram (specialized heart ultrasound typically performed by cardiologists). The "D" stands for "disability," (i.e., the bones). The ribs, thoracic spine, and clavicles should be evaluated for fractures; bony changes related to metabolic and neoplastic diseases may also be visible. Finally, "E" stands for "everything else"; in particular, lines and tubes should be assessed, as well as any changes to overlying soft tissues (e.g., air, swelling, foreign bodies). Don't forget to look at the visualized upper abdomen, lower neck, and chest wall!

3. Musculoskeletal injuries.

3a. **How can radiographs help in musculoskeletal injuries? When are they less useful?**
Bones are dense, and thus radiographs are usually the best first choice for diagnosing fractures and dislocations. On the other hand, muscles, cartilage, ligaments/tendons, blood, and swelling can all be of similar density; sprains, strains, and bruises are harder to see via radiography. It is therefore not uncommon to follow up an x-ray with imaging in another modality (MRI or ultrasound) to assess for non-bony injury.

3b. **What are some common musculoskeletal injuries seen in the urgent care setting?**
Fracture patterns are nearly infinite in their variety, but some patterns are so common that they are always worth looking for, and some even have their own eponyms.
   a. Case #1: A patient comes in complaining of right-hand pain after punching a door in frustration. What kind of injury might he have sustained?
   Answer: "Boxer's" fracture. This is a transverse, usually angulated fracture in the distal shaft/neck of the fifth (or fourth) metacarpal bone of the hand (Fig. 61.4). A Boxer's fracture typically occurs when an individual punches a solid, immovable object, such as a wall, with a clenched fist. (It is actually rarely seen in individuals with significant boxing experience; experienced martial artists use their first two knuckles for striking!)

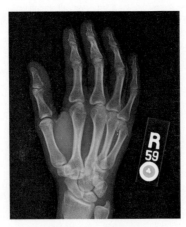

Fig. 61.4 Boxer's fracture.

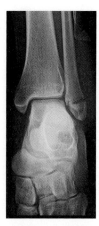

Fig. 61.5 Ankle fracture.

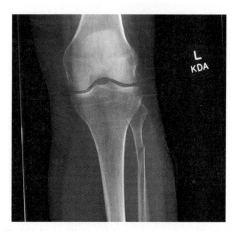

Fig. 61.6 Proximal fibular neck fracture (same patient as Fig. 61.5).

b. Case #2: A patient comes in having twisted her left ankle tripping off a curb. She has ankle/leg pain and swelling, and cannot put weight on that extremity. A left ankle radiograph was obtained. What is demonstrated?

Answer: The radiograph (Fig. 61.5) shows a fracture of the lateral malleolus (distal fibula) with intraarticular extension of the fracture to the lateral aspect of the ankle mortise joint. Additionally, there is mild widening of the medial clear space between the medial malleolus and talus, suggestive of an associated injury to the deltoid ligament of the ankle.

Fracture found! Should we look anywhere else?

Answer: Yes, you should obtain imaging of the proximal tibia/fibula.

See Fig. 61.6.

A "Maisonneuve" fracture is a combination of a fracture of the proximal fibula and an unstable ankle injury (defined as a widening at the ankle mortise secondary to ligamentous or syndesmotic injury). It is caused by a pronation and external rotation mechanism, driving the foot upward into the fibula. The tibia/fibula and associated syndesmosis form a ring; like other rings in the body, this tends to disrupt in more than one location, with forces from the ankle injury most commonly being translated up the fibular shaft. In the above case, a subsequent radiograph of the proximal fibula revealed a subtle nondisplaced fracture.

When interpreting musculoskeletal imaging, it is important to be cognizant of the concept that rings tend to break or dislocate in two places, as there are multiple rings found throughout the human skeleton. For instance, the radius and ulna form a ring between the wrist and elbow and will therefore often fracture with an associated dislocation at either the wrist or elbow (see e.g., Fig. 61.7, Monteggia fracture – an ulnar shaft fracture with radial head dislocation). Other rings within the body include the bony pelvis (you may see pelvic fractures accompanied by joint disruption at the sacroiliac joints or pubic symphysis) and the mandible.

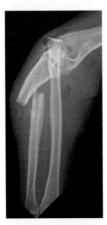

Fig. 61.7 Monteggia fracture/dislocation.

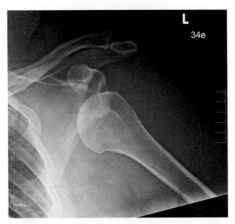

Fig. 61.8 Anterior shoulder dislocation.

c. Case #3: A patient presents having fallen onto his left shoulder and now is unable to raise his left arm. A shoulder radiograph is obtained. What does the imaging show?

Answer: Anterior shoulder dislocation (Fig. 61.8). This is the most common shoulder dislocation and frequently occurs in high-energy forced abduction, external rotation, and extension of the shoulder. Crush deformity of the posterolateral humeral head, as subtly suggested in Fig. 61.8, is known as a Hill-Sachs defect and represents a commonly associated injury. Associated chip/crush injuries to the glenoid rim (not seen here) are termed *Bankart lesions* and are also common.

What are the various shoulder dislocations that can occur, and which is the most common?

The anterior shoulder dislocation is by far the most common shoulder dislocation, representing approximately 95% of shoulder dislocations. Posterior dislocation is less common, seen in less than 4% of all shoulder dislocations, and occurs when the humeral head is forced posteriorly in internal rotation while the arm is abducted. This tends to occur in the setting of strong muscular contractions such as those in seizures or electrocution. Inferior shoulder dislocation, (*luxatio erecta*) is extremely rare but is easiest to diagnose clinically, as the patient's arm tends to be permanently held upward, in fixed abduction, as if the patient were raising their hand.

d. Case #4: A different young patient is complaining of nonspecific shoulder pain and swelling after trauma. A radiograph is obtained. What injury is demonstrated?

See Fig. 61.9.

Answer: There is widening of the acromioclavicular and coracoclavicular joint spaces with elevation of the clavicle with respect to the acromion, consistent with an acromioclavicular joint separation. These injuries are characterized under the "Rockwood" classification system, with lower grades demonstrating less separation and being treated conservatively, and with higher grades (greater separation) often requiring orthopedic surgery. Imaging of the patient's other clavicle for comparison and stress views are sometimes added if there is a questionable finding.

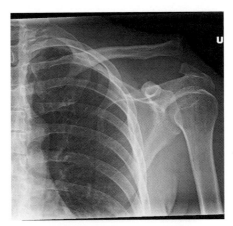

Fig. 61.9 Acromioclavicular joint separation.

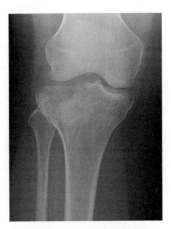

Fig. 61.10 Tibial plateau fracture.

e. Case #5: A patient presents with knee pain following a fall from a ladder. A knee radiograph was obtained. What injury is demonstrated?

Answer: A tibial plateau fracture is demonstrated (Fig. 61.10). In this case, fracture lines are seen extending from the lateral proximal aspect of the tibial metaphasis to the lateral tibial plateau. Fractures of the lateral plateau are more common than medial, and the fracture pattern tends to change with different mechanisms of injury. Tibial plateau fractures are classified based on the "Schatzker" classification, with more severe injuries involving both lateral and medial plateaus.

f. Case #6: An elderly patient presents following a fall on the hip. Radiograph was obtained. What injury is demonstrated?

See Fig. 61.11.

Answer: Left femoral neck fracture. Femoral neck fractures are unfortunately common in elderly patients following falls, due to unsteadiness and bone fragility associated with aging. There are several common types of femoral neck fractures based on the location of fracture: "subcapital" fractures at the head-neck junction, "transcervical" fractures at the midportion of the femoral neck, "basicervical" fractures at the base of the femoral neck, "intertrochanteric" fractures crossing the greater and lesser trochanters (suggested in Fig. 61.11), and "subtrochanteric" fractures. Depending on the condition of the patient and the location and severity of the fracture, treatment may include nonoperative management or surgery such as internal fixation or hip replacement.

g. Case #7: A pediatric patient falls off a swing set onto an outstretched arm and complains of elbow pain. What injury is demonstrated?

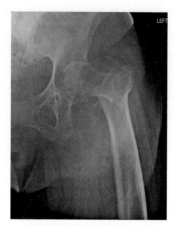

Fig. 61.11 Femoral neck fracture.

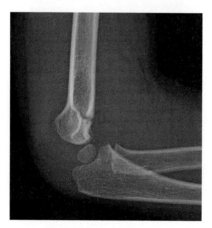

Fig. 61.12 Supracondylar fracture.

Answer: One of the more common elbow injuries in children is the supracondylar fracture. These can be challenging on radiograph, as many are incomplete or nondisplaced. You will often see a subtle transparent line or cortical step-off of the supracondylar portion of the distal humerus, often most visible along the anterior cortex in the lateral view. But even if the fracture itself is invisible, an associated elbow joint effusion may suggest an underlying injury. Elevation of the anterior fat pad ("sail sign") and elevation of the posterior fat pad (See Fig. 61.12) in the lateral view should make you suspicious for an osseous injury, even when a fracture line is not definitively seen.

h. Case #8: Neck pain following a dive into a shallow pool. What does the radiograph show?

Answer: Sometimes known as the "Jefferson" fracture, this is a multipart "burst" fracture of the atlas, involving a two-to-four-part fracture of the anterior and posterior arches of C1. It is due to axial loading on the cervical spine, resulting in the occipital condyles of the skull being driven into the lateral masses of C1. On radiograph, you will generally only see asymmetry of the spaces between the lateral masses and the odontoid process (see Fig. 61.13). More significant displacement suggests ligamentous injury. It is therefore important that you have a true frontal projection, as rotation may augment the degree of asymmetry. Simple burst fractures themselves are often treated conservatively but tend to be associated with other cervical spine fractures, so cross-sectional imaging (CT) follow-up is generally warranted.

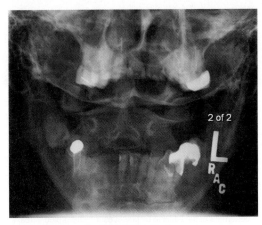

Fig. 61.13 C1 burst fracture.

KEY POINTS

1. When reviewing imaging, search patterns are important. For example, when reviewing a chest x-ray, using a systemic approach (e.g., ABCD) is helpful to avoid overlooking subtle findings. Find one you're comfortable with and use it consistently.
2. Be on alert for common patterns of fracture. While every injury is slightly different, there are some patterns that are seen so often that they have their own names.
3. Use natural symmetry. If something looks wrong in a bone or joint, consider imaging the other side for comparison. This goes doubly in the pediatric population, since growing bones can have a wide variety of normal appearances.
4. Be aware that rings like to fracture/dislocate in more than one place. When a patient has an unstable ankle fracture, obtain imaging of the proximal tibia/fibula; forces may have translated up the fibular shaft. Similarly, in cases of a wrist/forearm fracture or dislocation, imaging at the elbow is warranted.
5. If a patient has an elbow joint effusion, manifested by elevation of the anterior ("sail sign") and posterior fat pads, this may suggest an occult fracture. Consider additional imaging or treat it as a fracture and follow up to look for interval displacement or healing.

BIBLIOGRAPHY

Donnelly LF. *Pediatric Imaging: The Fundamentals*. Saunders Elsevier; 2009.
Jones J. Chest X-ray review: ABCDE, Radiopaedia, www.radiopaedia.org (2021). Accessed September 5, 2022.
Lee P, Hunter TB, Taljanovic M. Musculoskeletal colloquialisms: how did we come up with these names? *Radiographics*. 2004;24(4):1009–1027.
Smithuis R. Elbow fractures in children. Radiology Assistant, www.radiologyassistant.nl. Accessed September 5, 2022.
Truszkiewicz K, Poreba R, Gac P. Radiological cardiothoracic ratio in evidence-based medicine. *J Clin Med*. 2021;10(9):2016.

CHAPTER 62

DIAGNOSTIC ULTRASOUND

Munaza Batool Rizvi, MD, Joni E. Rabiner, MD

TOP SECRETS

1. Point-of-care ultrasound (POCUS) is a dynamic test that is performed by the clinician at the bedside for diagnosis, procedures, and to facilitate management.
2. Familiarity with normal sonographic landmarks and findings is essential for identification of pathology.

INTRODUCTION TO ULTRASOUND

1. **What is point-of-care ultrasound (POCUS)?**
   POCUS is an ultrasound performed at the bedside by practitioners, interpreted in real time, and used to answer specific clinical questions to improve patient care or procedural performance. Most US applications have a higher specificity than sensitivity, making it a better "rule-in" tool for pathology.

2. **What are the advantages of POCUS in the urgent care setting?**
   When available to the trained provider, POCUS is noninvasive, dynamic, portable, and easy to repeat at the bedside. It can be used in both resource-rich and resource-poor settings.

3. **What common terminology is used to describe ultrasound (US) images?**
   - Anechoic: a complete absence of returning sound waves, appears black
   - Hypoechoic: structure appears darker than the surrounding tissue
   - Isoechoic: structure has a similar appearance to the surrounding tissue
   - Hyperechoic: structure appears brighter than the surrounding tissue, appears white
     Fluids, including water and blood, are anechoic or hypoechoic (black or dark gray), and bone and air are hyperechoic (white) in US images. Soft tissue and muscle have echotextures with varying shades of gray.

4. **What are the four main types of US probes and for what applications are they typically used?**
   - Phased Array: FAST, cardiac, abdominal imaging
   - Curvilinear: abdominal imaging, transabdominal obstetrical and gynecological imaging
   - Linear: thoracic, musculoskeletal, ocular, procedural guidance
   - Intracavitary probe: transvaginal obstetrical and gynecological imaging, peritonsillar abscess evaluation

FAST

5. **What is the Focused Assessment with Sonography for Trauma (FAST) examination?**
   The FAST exam can provide quick and reliable information on potential bleeding into the peritoneal, pericardial, or pleural spaces in patients with trauma. The Extended FAST, or EFAST, adds views of the lungs to assess for pneumothorax.

6. **How is an EFAST exam performed?**
   The EFAST consists of four abdominal views and two hemithorax views and is a highly specific test (specificity 94–95%). The phased array or curvilinear probes are used to obtain abdominal images for the FAST exam. Free fluid, which is likely blood in the setting of trauma, appears anechoic on ultrasound. There are four abdominal FAST views:
   1. Right upper quadrant (RUQ): the probe is placed in the right midaxillary line in the seventh to ninth intercostal spaces (ICS), indicator toward the patient's head. This view assesses for free fluid in Morison's pouch and in the paracolic gutter. A complete scan should include views of the subphrenic space, superior and inferior poles of the kidney, and the liver tip. The RUQ view is the most sensitive for free fluid assessment in adult patients (Fig. 62.1).
   2. Left upper quadrant (LUQ): the probe is placed in the left posterior axillary line in the fifth to seventh ICS, indicator toward the patient's head. Free fluid is assessed in the splenorenal recess and in the subphrenic space. A complete scan includes the superior and inferior poles of the kidney and the splenic tip.
   3. Suprapubic: the probe is placed superior to the pubis symphysis and angled toward the patient's feet. Both sagittal and transverse views are obtained. This view assesses for free fluid in the rectovesical pouch in males and in the pouch of Douglas in females.
   4. Subxiphoid: the probe is placed flat on the patient's abdomen just inferior to the xiphoid process, with the indicator toward the patient's right and the probe directed toward the patient's left shoulder. This view assesses for free fluid in the pericardium.

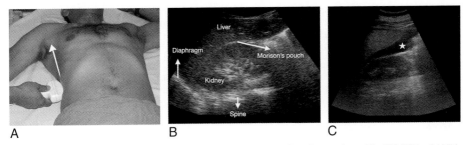

Fig. 62.1 (A) Probe position for the FAST exam right upper quadrant (RUQ) view. (B) Normal sonoanatomy of the RUQ. (C) Free fluid (*) in Morison's pouch and at the liver tip.

7. **What are the lung EFAST views?**
   - Hemothorax: in the RUQ and LUQ views, the probe may be moved superiorly above the diaphragm to assess for free fluid in the pleural space.
   - Pneumothorax: the linear or phased array probe is placed over the anterior chest in the second to fourth ICS bilaterally to evaluate the hyperechoic pleural line between two ribs. The normal aerated lung will have lung sliding which appears as a shimmering white pleural line. In a pneumothorax, there will be a static pleural line. Motion mode, or M-mode, demonstrates a sandy beach sign in normal lungs and a barcode sign in pneumothorax.

8. **What are the limitations of the EFAST exam?**
   The EFAST exam is not reliable for solid organ, retroperitoneal, or hollow viscous injuries. Additionally, small fluid collections may be challenging to visualize initially. Serial FAST exams will increase the sensitivity of the exam.

PULMONARY

9. **What is the utility of lung POCUS?**
   POCUS of the lung can be used to evaluate patients with acute dyspnea or other respiratory complaints to look for pathology including pneumothorax, pulmonary edema, pneumonia, and pleural effusions.

10. **How is lung POCUS performed?**
    The linear, curvilinear, or phased array probes may be used for lung POCUS. Longitudinal and transverse images in anterior, lateral, and posterior lung fields bilaterally are needed for a complete lung POCUS scan.

11. **What are the findings on lung POCUS?**
    In longitudinal views, ribs are visualized as curvilinear, hyperechoic lines with posterior shadowing, and the bright white pleural line is visualized shimmering between the ribs (Fig. 62.2).
    1. A-lines: horizontal hyperechoic reflection artifacts arising from the reverberations produced between the pleural line and the probe in a normal lung
    2. B-lines (comet tail artifacts): discrete, hyperechoic, vertical artifacts arising from the pleural surface and extending to the bottom of the screen, obliterating A-lines at their intersection

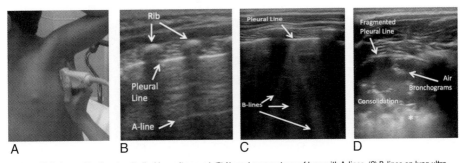

Fig. 62.2 (A) Probe position for a longitudinal lung ultrasound. (B) Normal sonoanatomy of lung with A-lines. (C) B-lines on lung ultrasound. Hepatization of lung in pneumonia with air bronchograms and shred sign (*).

3. Consolidations: soft tissue appearance (lung hepatization) with irregular borders (shred sign) and pleural line abnormalities; they often have air bronchograms, which are hyperechoic dots or lines representing the air-filled bronchi surrounded by fluid-filled lungs
4. Pleural effusion: anechoic fluid collections above the diaphragm

12. **How are B-lines interpreted on lung POCUS?**
The presence of >3 B-lines per intercostal space is considered pathological. B-lines in a focal pattern can be seen in pneumonia, atelectasis, pulmonary embolism, or neoplasm. A more diffuse pattern of B-lines can be seen in cardiogenic pulmonary edema, ARDS, and pulmonary fibrosis.

AORTA

13. **What is the utility of POCUS of the aorta?**
POCUS is a highly sensitive and specific test to diagnose abdominal aortic aneurysm (AAA). Early diagnosis is paramount to reduce its exceptionally high mortality rate.

14. **What are the landmarks of the aorta on POCUS?**
Start with the phased array/curvilinear probe below the xiphoid process, to the left of the midline. Scan inferiorly to visualize the following landmarks:
1. Proximal aorta: a thick-walled, hypoechoic, pulsatile circle just above the vertebral body in the transverse view. The celiac trunk is seen branching into the common hepatic artery and splenic artery (seagull sign) anteriorly. Slightly inferiorly, the superior mesenteric artery will appear as a smaller, circular, hypoechoic structure anterior to the abdominal aorta.
2. Mid-aorta: near the level of the renal arteries
3. Distal aorta: most superficial segment, near the umbilicus
4. Aortic bifurcation: aorta divides into two iliac vessels
    It is important to distinguish the aorta from the IVC, which is thin walled, usually not as circular as the aorta, lies to the patient's right, and is usually collapsible with respirations.

15. **What are the measurements concerning aortic aneurysm?**
An aortic diameter measured from outer wall to outer wall in the anteroposterior plane ≥3 cm for the abdominal aorta and ≥1.5 cm diameter for the iliac arteries is concerning for aortic aneurysm.

BILIARY

16. **What is the utility of POCUS in patients with right upper quadrant pain?**
POCUS can evaluate for gallstones and cholecystitis. Acute cholecystitis is one of the most common reasons for hospital admission with acute abdominal pain.

17. **How is POCUS of the gallbladder performed and what are the landmarks?**
The phased array or curvilinear probe is placed in the RUQ/epigastric area with the indicator toward the patient's head. The gallbladder appears as a thin-walled, anechoic, pear-shaped structure. The portal triad appears as the Mickey Mouse Sign in short axis, where the CBD and hepatic artery are the "ears," and the portal vein is the "head." The CBD has an absence of flow on color Doppler imaging (Fig. 62.3).

18. **What are the POCUS findings for gallstones?**
Gallstones appear as mobile, echogenic foci casting posterior acoustic shadows. A wall-echo-shadow (WES) sign may be observed when the gallbladder has multiple gallstones. Obstructive cholelithiasis leads to CBD dilation with a measurement >0.6 cm, measured from inner-to-inner wall. However, with every decade of life after 60, the expected diameter increases by 1 millimeter (e.g., CBD dilation for a 70-year-old patient would be >0.7 cm).

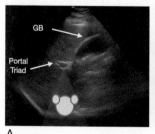 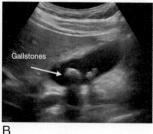 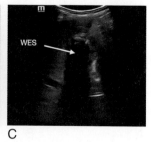

A   B   C

Fig. 62.3 (A) Gallbladder (GB) in long axis with portal triad Mickey Mouse sign. (B) Gallstones casting posterior acoustic shadow. (C) Wall-echo-shadow (WES) sign.

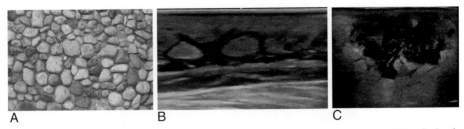

Fig. 62.4 (A) Cobblestoning. (B) Cobblestoning of soft tissue on ultrasound consistent with cellulitis. (C) An abscess with a collection of hypoechoic fluid that has purulent debris.

19. **What are the POCUS findings for acute cholecystitis?**
    1. Gallbladder edema with an anterior gallbladder wall >0.3 cm
    2. Presence of pericholecystic or perihepatic fluid
    3. Sonographic Murphy's sign: abdominal tenderness from pressure of the probe over the gallbladder
    4. Gallbladder distention measuring >4 cm on the short axis or >8 cm on the long axis

SKIN AND SOFT TISSUE

20. **What is the utility of POCUS for soft tissue infections?**
    POCUS improves the ability to detect the presence of drainable abscesses in the setting of soft tissue infections and is very useful as an adjunct to the history and physical examination.

21. **How is POCUS for soft tissue performed?**
    The linear probe is used to scan the area of interest. Comparison with the contralateral normal side or a normal area adjacent to the area of interest may be helpful for identifying pathology.

22. **How do cellulitis and abscesses appear on POCUS?**
    Cellulitis appears as soft tissue swelling and cobblestoning, representing hypoechoic edema in the interstitial space separating the hyperechoic fat lobules. An abscess appears as a collection of hypoechoic fluid that has an absence of internal vascular flow on Color Doppler. POCUS allows measurement of abscess size and aids in identifying important surrounding structures for procedure planning and execution. Abscess contents such as purulent matter with swirling debris and loculation can be seen on POCUS (Fig. 62.4).

INTRAUTERINE PREGNANCY

23. **What is the utility of first-trimester POCUS?**
    POCUS may establish an IUP, thereby helping rule out an ectopic pregnancy, with 99% sensitivity.

24. **How is first-trimester obstetric ultrasound performed?**
    The phased array or curvilinear probe is used for the transabdominal approach (TA). The endocavitary probe is used for the transvaginal approach (TV). A full bladder for TA and an empty bladder for TV is advised. Obtain longitudinal and transverse views, scanning the entire pelvis to evaluate the uterus, bilateral ovaries, and pouch of Douglas for free fluid.

25. **What are the criteria for diagnosis of an intrauterine pregnancy (IUP) on POCUS?**
    The presence of a gestational sac and a yolk sac, fetal pole, or fetal heart rate is necessary to confirm an IUP. A gestational sac is a fluid collection in the uterus surrounded by two concentric echogenic rims called the double decidual reaction. A yolk sac is a circular thick-walled echogenic structure with an anechoic center within the gestational sac. The fetal pole initially appears as thickening at the margin of the yolk sac. When the fetal pole is ≥7 mm, a fetal heartbeat should be detected (Fig. 62.5).

26. **When is an ectopic pregnancy suspected on POCUS?**
    The estimated rate of ectopic pregnancy is 1–2% in the general population and 2–5% among patients utilizing assisted reproductive technology. The absence of an IUP on POCUS in a female with a positive pregnancy test is highly suspicious for ectopic pregnancy. The presence of free fluid in the pelvis and/or RUQ with hemodynamic instability is considered a ruptured ectopic pregnancy until proven otherwise.

RENAL

27. **What is the utility of POCUS of the kidneys?**
    POCUS of the kidneys can diagnose hydronephrosis, which may be caused by a renal stone.

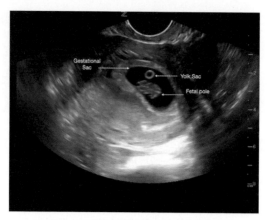

Fig. 62.5 A transvaginal ultrasound demonstrating an IUP.

28. How is POCUS of the kidneys performed?

Place the curvilinear or phased array probe at the right **midaxillary line** around the tenth to eleventh ICS and at the left posterior axillary line around the eighth to tenth ICS. Obtain sagittal and transverse views.

29. What are the grades of hydronephrosis on POCUS?

Hydronephrosis on POCUS appears as dilation of the urinary spaces. Grade 1 (mild) hydronephrosis has dilation of the renal pelvis only. Grade 2 (mild to moderate) hydronephrosis has dilation of the renal pelvis and major calyces. Grade 3 (severe) hydronephrosis has dilation of the renal pelvis and major and minor calyces.

KEY POINTS

1. Fluid appears hypoechoic or anechoic (black), soft tissues and muscles are gray, and bones and air appear hyperechoic (white) on ultrasound.
2. POCUS can be used to rule in pathology due to its high specificity for most applications.
3. POCUS can be lifesaving when used in a high-risk patient population.

BIBLIOGRAPHY

Fleming C, Whitlock E, Beil T, Lederle F. Screening for abdominal aortic aneurysm: a best-evidence systematic review for the U.S. Preventive Services Task Force. *Ann Intern Med*. 2005;142(3):203. https://dx.doi.org/10.7326/0003-4819-142-3-200502010-00012.

Lobo V, Hunter-Behrend M, Cullnan E, et al. Caudal edge of the liver in the right upper quadrant (RUQ) view is the most sensitive area for free fluid on the FAST exam. *West J Emerg Med*. 2017;18(2):270–280. doi:10.5811/westjem.2016.11.30435.

Netherton S, Milenkovic V, Taylor M, Davis PJ. Diagnostic accuracy of eFAST in the trauma patient: a systematic review and meta-analysis. *CJEM*. 2019;21(6):727–738. doi:10.1017/cem.2019.381.

Rizvi MB, Rabiner JE. Pediatric point-of-care lung ultrasonography: a narrative review. *West J Emerg Med*. 2022;23(4):497–504. doi:10.5811/westjem.2022.3.54663. Published 2022 Jun 5.

Stein JC, Wang R, Adler N, et al. Emergency physician ultrasonography for evaluating patients at risk for ectopic pregnancy: a meta-analysis. *Ann Emerg Med*. 2010;56(6):674–683. doi:10.1016/j.annemergmed.2010.06.563.

OBSTETRICAL COMPLAINTS

Andrew Lutzkanin, MD, FAAFP, Justine Bensur, DO, MSMedEd

CHAPTER 63

1. **What patients need to be urgently evaluated by an OB/GYN?**
   If encountered, the following pregnancy-related complications should be immediately assessed by an OB/GYN:
   - Patients presenting with early miscarriage featuring heavy vaginal bleeding and/or hemodynamic instability
   - Patients presenting with symptoms concerning for ectopic pregnancy (vaginal bleeding and/or abdominal or pelvic pain with no intrauterine pregnancy established)
   - Patients >20 weeks of gestation with blood pressure >140/90 with new-onset headache, blurred vision, chest pain, shortness of breath, right upper quadrant abdominal pain, decreased urination, or blood pressure >160/110 alone
   - Patients in the third trimester (>28 weeks) with vaginal bleeding
   - Patients with vaginal discharge or leaking fluid concerning for rupture of membranes, particularly prior to 34 weeks of gestation

2. **What causes of vaginal bleeding in the first trimester should be considered?**
   Ectopic pregnancy, early pregnancy loss, threatened abortion, or physiologic/implantation bleeding can occur. Additional sources not caused by the pregnancy include inflammation or infection (vaginitis, cervicitis), trauma (including intercourse), ectropion, cervical polyps, tumors, warts, or fibroids. Vaginal bleeding is common in the first trimester, occurring in 20–40% of pregnancies.

3. **How should first-trimester vaginal bleeding be evaluated in the hemodynamically stable patient?**
   - Abdominal exam to rule out peritoneal signs
   - Obtain ultrasound (transvaginal preferred) to confirm pregnancy location.
   - Obtain bHCG, hemoglobin level, and Rh factor evaluation.
     - Gestational sac expected on transvaginal ultrasonography when β-hCG levels reach 1500–3000 mIU per mL
     - Administer Rhogam to Rh-negative women experiencing early pregnancy loss or ectopic pregnancy
   - Pelvic examination with speculum examination
   - Rule out nonobstetric causes and treat accordingly: vaginitis, cervicitis, ectropion, trauma, tumor, warts, polyps, and fibroids.
   - Look for cervical os dilation and products of conception.
   - If products of conception are present in the vagina, patient has experienced an incomplete or complete abortion.
   - If no other causes of bleeding are identified and the cervical os is closed, ultrasound findings are helpful in determining if the patient is experiencing the following:
     - Pregnancy of unknown location – pregnancy not yet visualized; follow-up with maternity clinician, serial bHCG, and ultrasound
     - Intrauterine pregnancy with viability uncertain: repeat TVUS in 7–14 days
     - Viable intrauterine pregnancy: threatened abortion, repeat TVUS if bleeding continues
     - Nonviable intrauterine pregnancy: patient is experiencing early pregnancy loss; expectant management, medical management, and uterine aspiration are safe and effective treatments for early pregnancy loss in hemodynamically stable patients.

4. **What are common causes of second-trimester bleeding before 20 weeks of gestation?**
   Early pregnancy loss, cervical insufficiency, placental abruption, ectopic pregnancy (rare; often locations other than tubal).

5. **How should a pregnant patient with vaginal bleeding before 20 weeks of gestation be evaluated?**
   - Similar to first-trimester evaluation
   - Quantify bleeding.
     - Light, painless, intermittent: cervical insufficiency, small marginal placental separation, cervical/vaginal lesions
   - Heavy, painful: impending pregnancy loss, placental abruption
   - Auscultate fetal heart tones by Doppler
   - Abdominal examination: palpate for pain, uterine fundus

- Speculum examination: visualize cervix/cervical os, assess for dilation, prolapse of membranes, nonpregnancy sources of bleeding
  - Dilated cervical os or fetal membranes visualized: impending pregnancy loss (contractions often present) or cervical insufficiency (contractions often absent)
- Obtain transvaginal ultrasound.
  - Look for placenta previa, placental abruption, cervical insufficiency.

6. **What are common causes of second- and third-trimester bleeding after 20 weeks of gestation?**
Bloody show associated with labor onset or cervical insufficiency, placenta previa, vasa previa, and placental abruption should all be considered. Vaginitis, trauma, tumor, warts, polyps, fibroids, and ectropion can continue to cause vaginal bleeding throughout pregnancy as above. Rarer but also of consideration are gestational trophoblastic disease and choriocarcinoma.

7. **How should a pregnant patient with vaginal bleeding after 20 weeks of gestation be evaluated?**
- Evaluate for labor.
- Perform abdominal exam and sterile speculum exam. Exclude placenta previa via ultrasound before performing digital examination.
- Obtain hemoglobin and hematocrit. If not in early labor or bleeding from a nonobstetric cause, obtain Rh testing, consider blood type and crossmatch.
  - Rho(D) immune globulin (Rhogam) for Rh-negative patients and obtain Kleihauer-Betke test to determine appropriate dose
- Management of pregnant patients with vaginal bleeding in the second and third trimesters is highly dependent on the cause of the bleeding.
- Immediate transfer to a facility with obstetric care capacity if in labor or if placenta previa, vasa previa, placental abruption, or uterine rupture are suspected
  - Placenta previa: often painless vaginal bleeding, sometimes after sexual intercourse
  - Vasa previa: hemorrhage following suspected rupture of membranes
  - Placental abruption: vaginal bleeding, abdominal or back pain, or uterine tenderness
  - Uterine rupture: vaginal bleeding, abdominal pain, in labor or recent abdominal trauma, may have history of previous cesarean birth or transmyometrial surgery

8. **How do you manage nausea and vomiting (including hyperemesis) in pregnancy?**
- Benign nausea and vomiting of pregnancy: begins around 4 weeks of estimated gestational age, typically resolves around 12 weeks of gestational age
- If outside of the 4–12 weeks gestational age window or is severe/refractory, consider less common causes: molar pregnancy, multiple gestation, thyroid disease, gallbladder disease.
  - Obtain beta human chorionic gonadotropin levels, comprehensive metabolic panel, thyroid-stimulating hormone, and transabdominal ultrasonography.
- If n/v is accompanied by abdominal pain or tenderness: obtain CBC, confirm intrauterine pregnancy, consider ultrasonography of gallbladder or appendix.

9. **What distinguishes hyperemesis gravidarum from nausea and vomiting of pregnancy?**
When vomiting unrelated to other causes continues, the patient demonstrates signs of acute starvation (such as ketonuria), and weight loss of at least 5% from prepregnancy weight occurs, the clinical diagnosis of hyperemesis gravidarum is considered.

10. **What are the treatment options for nausea and vomiting of pregnancy/hyperemesis gravidarum?**
- First-line treatment: nonpharmacologic options include frequent small meals, converting prenatal vitamin to folic acid only, and trial of ginger capsules (not to exceed 1500 mg/day); consider P6 acupressure wristbands
- If symptoms persist: trial of vitamin B6 (pyridoxine) +/− doxylamine; if unresolved, consider diphenhydramine, prochlorperazine, or promethazine. If still unresolved, consider adding metoclopramide, ondansetron, or trimethobenzamide.
- Consider PR medications when PO medications are not tolerated.
- Consider hospitalization for IV fluid and electrolyte replacement when there is no response to outpatient management and the patient is dehydrated/unable to tolerate liquids without vomiting. These cases may also require chlorpromazine or methylprednisolone.

11. **How common are urinary tract infections in pregnancy?**
Infections of the urinary tract are more common during pregnancy, with asymptomatic bacteriuria occurring in 2–7% of patients. Left untreated, 30–40% will develop symptomatic infection. Relaxation of ureteral smooth muscle increases the risk of pyelonephritis, particularly in the second and third trimesters.

12. **Should asymptomatic bacteriuria be treated during pregnancy?**
Yes; per the Infectious Diseases Society of America (IDSA), asymptomatic bacteriuria should be treated during pregnancy. Asymptomatic bacteriuria is associated with an increased risk of preterm birth and low birth weight. The IDSA recommends universal screening of all pregnant women with a urine culture at the first visit.

13. **How do you treat urinary tract infections in pregnancy?**
Safe antibiotics during pregnancy include penicillins, cephalosporins, and aztreonam. Nitrofurantoin should not be used in the first trimester or at term (>37 weeks). Fluoroquinolones, tetracyclines, trimethoprim-sulfamethoxazole, and aminoglycosides should all be avoided during pregnancy.

14. **How do you treat heartburn in pregnancy?**
- Gastroesophageal reflux symptoms can occur at any time throughout pregnancy but are most common during the third trimester.
- First-line treatment consists of lifestyle modifications including eating smaller, more frequent meals and dietary changes to avoid triggering foods.
- Medication options include antacids (calcium carbonate, aluminum hydroxide), H2-receptor blockers (famotidine, cimetidine), and sucralfate.
- Proton pump inhibitors should be considered only if the above treatments are not effective. Omeprazole is a Category C medication; all other PPIs are Category B.

15. **What are common musculoskeletal complaints during pregnancy?**
Pregnant patients commonly develop pain in the lower back and pelvic girdle. Weight gain, uterine enlargement, and hormonal changes alter the biomechanics of the axial skeleton and pelvis. Pregnant persons also experience exaggerated lumbar lordosis and forward neck flexion, ligamentous laxity, joint laxity, and fluid retention.

16. **What are musculoskeletal causes of back pain in pregnancy?**
- Lumbar musculoskeletal strain, SI joint pain, joint laxity, sciatic nerve/lumbar plexus pressure
- Rule out neurologic red flags (saddle anesthesia, incontinence or retention of bowel or bladder, neurologic exam deficits) and urologic red flags (fever, costovertebral angle tenderness).
- Presence of vaginal bleeding or contractions may suggest obstetric causes of lower back pain, such as labor or placental abruption. Patients with a history of falls/trauma should undergo obstetric monitoring for signs of placental abruption.

17. **Safe treatments for lower back pain in pregnancy.**
Acetaminophen, physical therapy, lower back stretching exercises, water exercises, job and activity modification, heat, supportive devices (pregnancy belly bands, sacroiliac joint belts)

18. **Pubic symphysis pain.**
Pain and tenderness of the suprapubic region with radiation to the hips. Pelvic girdle syndrome can also develop, which is when pubic symphysis pain and bilateral SI joint pain occur. Again, signs of labor should be ruled out in the patient history. Treatment for musculoskeletal pelvic pain in pregnancy is similar to that of lower back pain.

19. **What should be considered in headache evaluation of the pregnant patient?**
Pregnant patients are susceptible to the same headache etiologies of nonpregnant adults requiring a full history, physical examination, and consideration of secondary causes or alarm features. **However, additional consideration should be made for headaches as a sign of preeclampsia with severe features in patients >20 weeks pregnant or patients who are recently postpartum.** If a headache without other clear etiology is not relieved with analgesics and rest, or there is scotoma, photopsia, or elevated blood pressure, obtain CBC, LFTs, renal function, and urine protein/creatinine ratio, and consult with a maternity care clinician if needed.

20. **What are safe headache treatments in pregnancy?**
- Acetaminophen is a safe option for all headaches in pregnancy.
- For migraine headaches, acetaminophen with antiemetic (such as metoclopramide or prochlorperazine plus diphenhydramine) with rest in a dark, quiet environment is preferred. Acetaminophen with caffeine may also be used.
- Second trimester prior to 20 weeks: NSAIDs may be considered.
- For severe or refractory migraines, sumatriptan (Imitrex), magnesium sulfate, or glucocorticoids may be considered.
- ACOG recommends against the use of butalbital-acetaminophen-caffeine or opioids for headaches. Ergot, alkaloid-containing products are contraindicated in pregnancy.

21. **How do you manage acute upper respiratory infections during pregnancy?**
Pregnant women are more susceptible to upper respiratory infections (URIs), both viral and bacterial. Common colds can be managed symptomatically (see table below) with appropriate antibiotic avoidance.

22. **What over-the-counter medications are safe during pregnancy?**
See Table 63.1.

Table 63.1 Over-the-Counter Medications Safe for Use in Pregnancy

SYMPTOM	MEDICATIONS
Fever/pain	Acetaminophen
Decongestants	Chlorpheniramine Pseudoephedrine* Phenylephrine*
Cough suppressants	Dextromethorphan Benzonatate†
Antihistamines	Diphenhydramine Fexofenadine Loratadine Cetirizine
Nasal sprays	Azelastine Ipratropium bromide Corticosteroids Oxymetazoline
Other	Humidifier Nasal saline

*Use with caution; may increase blood pressure.
†Use with caution; do not use if breastfeeding.

Table 63.2 Antibiotics Safe and Unsafe for Use in Pregnancy

SAFE	UNSAFE
Penicillins	Fluoroquinolones
Cephalosporins	Tetracyclines
Clindamycin	Aminoglycosides
Vancomycin	Trimethoprim-sulfamethoxazole
Macrolides (>13 weeks)	
Nitrofurantoin (13–37 weeks)	

23. **What seasonal vaccines are safe during pregnancy?**
    The seasonal influenza vaccine and the COVID-19 vaccines are both safe to administer during pregnancy. Due to the higher risk of severe infection, all pregnant women should be vaccinated against influenza and COVID-19.

24. **How do you treat influenza during pregnancy?**
    Oseltamivir is safe and effective to use and is recommended for the treatment of influenza during pregnancy. The authors recommend treatment at any time during illness to reduce the risk of complications from an infection.

25. **How do you treat bronchitis during pregnancy?**
    Albuterol is a safe and effective choice for the treatment of bronchitis in pregnancy.

26. **What antibiotics are safe during pregnancy?**
    See Table 63.2.

27. **What are common rashes seen during pregnancy?**
    - Polymorphic eruption of pregnancy/pruritic urticarial papules and plaques of pregnancy [PUPPP]
        - Pruritic, erythematous papules, often within striae
        - May start on the abdomen and spread to the extremities, chest, and back; usually spares the umbilicus, face palms, and soles
        - Typically primiparous women in late third trimester or postpartum
        - No increased risk to the fetus
        - Treat with mid- to high-potency topical corticosteroids until improvement occurs; a short course of systemic corticosteroids for severe cases. Oral antihistamines may also help.

- Atopic eruption of pregnancy:
  - Eczematous or papular lesions, flexural distribution
  - Patients typically have a history of atopy.
  - No adverse effects to the fetus
  - Manage with emollients, low- to mid-potency topical corticosteroids, and oral antihistamines.
- Pemphigoid gestationis:
  - Autoimmune bullous disease presenting in the second or third trimester of pregnancy or postpartum period
  - Intense pruritus, usually beginning on the trunk, often has early urticarial plaques similar to polymorphic eruption of pregnancy; distinguished by rapid spread and formation of tense blisters
  - May be associated with increased fetal risk
  - Requires immediate referral to dermatologist for diagnosis and treatment with high-potency topical corticosteroids, systemic corticosteroids, or other systemic immunosuppressive agents
- Pustular psoriasis of pregnancy:
  - Erythematous plaques, sterile pustules situated at the edges of plaques; eruption begins on flexural surfaces and spreads to the trunk. Pruritus is usually absent.
  - Associated with fetal risk
  - Requires immediate referral to a dermatologist for diagnosis and treatment with systemic corticosteroids, cyclosporine, or other suppressive therapies
- Herpes simplex, herpes zoster, and varicella infections require antiviral therapy.
- Generalized pruritus with no rash, especially on the palms and soles, is suggestive of intrahepatic cholestasis of pregnancy, requiring laboratory workup (bile acid level, LFTs) and treatment with ursodiol. Obstetric consultation is needed, as delivery timing is often affected by this condition.

KEY POINTS

1. Vaginal bleeding is common in the first trimester, occurring in 20–40% of pregnancies.
2. Administer Rhogam to Rh-negative women experiencing early pregnancy loss or ectopic pregnancy.
3. Benign nausea and vomiting of pregnancy begin around the estimated 4 weeks of gestational age and typically resolve around 12 weeks of gestational age.
4. First-line treatment for hyperemesis gravidarum includes nonpharmacologic options: frequent small meals, convert prenatal vitamin to folic acid only, and trial ginger capsules (not to exceed 1500 mg/day); consider P6 acupressure wrist bands.
5. Infections of the urinary tract are more common during pregnancy, with asymptomatic bacteriuria occurring in 2–7% of patients. Left untreated, 30–40% will develop symptomatic infection.

BIBLIOGRAPHY

ACOG Committee on Clinical Practice Guidelines—Obstetrics. Headaches in pregnancy and postpartum. *Obstet Gynecol.* 2022;139(5):944–972.
ACOG Committee on Obstetric Practice. Nausea and vomiting of pregnancy. *Obstet Gynecol.* 2018;131(1):e15–e30.
ACOG Committee on Practice Bulletins—Gynecology. Early pregnancy loss. *Obstet Gynecol.* 2018;132(5):e197–e207.
Bermas, B. Maternal adaptations to pregnancy: musculoskeletal changes and pain. UpToDate. Updated June 22, 2022. https://www.uptodate.com. Accessed September 20, 2022.
Gregory DS, Wu V, Tuladhar P. The pregnant patient: managing common acute medical problems. *Am Fam Physician.* 2018;98(9):595A–602A.
Hendriks E, MacNaughton H, MacKenzie MC. First trimester bleeding: evaluation and management. *Am Fam Physician.* 2019;99(3):166–174.
Hendriks E, Rosenberg R, Prine L. Ectopic pregnancy: diagnosis and management. *Am Fam Physician.* 2020;101(10):599–606.
Infectious Diseases Society of America. www.idsociety.org.
Medina TM, Hill DA. Preterm premature rupture of membranes: diagnosis and management. *Am Fam Physician.* 2006;73(4):659–664.
Norwitz ER, Park JS. Overview of the etiology and evaluation of vaginal bleeding in pregnancy. UpToDate. Updated March 18, 2022. https://www.uptodate.com. Accessed September 20, 2022.
Pomeranz MK. Dermatoses of pregnancy. UpToDate. Updated August 29, 2022. https://www.uptodate.com. Accessed September 20, 2022.
Sakornbut E, Leeman L, Fontaine P. Late pregnancy bleeding. *Am Fam Physician.* 2007;75(8):1199–1206.

INDEX

Note: Pages followed by *b*, *t*, or *f* refer to boxes, tables, or figures, respectively.